Advances in Sleep Disorders

Advances in Sleep Disorders

Edited by **Slaton Channing**

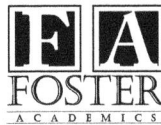

FOSTER
ACADEMICS

New Jersey

Published by Foster Academics,
61 Van Reypen Street,
Jersey City, NJ 07306, USA
www.fosteracademics.com

Advances in Sleep Disorders
Edited by Slaton Channing

© 2016 Foster Academics

International Standard Book Number: 978-1-63242-442-6 (Hardback)

Printed in the United States of America.

Contents

Preface

The purpose of the book is to provide a glimpse into the dynamics and to present opinions and studies of some of the scientists engaged in the development of new ideas in the field from very different standpoints. This book will prove useful to students and researchers owing to its high content quality.

Sound sleep is the reason behind a perfectly balanced mental, physical and social well-being of people. Excess or lack of sleep could cause severe behavioral problems in human beings. Sleep disorders could be caused by stress, traumatic childhood experiences and hereditary factors. There are a number of problems and diagnostic methods related to sleep disorders. This book explains a wide variety of them such as obstructive sleep apnea, insomnia, etc. This book is compiled in such a manner, that it will provide an in-depth understanding of the concepts, diagnostic methods and emerging treatments related to sleep disorders. It provides comprehensive insights into the field of sleep related disorders. A number of latest researches have been included to keep the readers up-to-date with the global concepts in this area of study.

At the end, I would like to appreciate all the efforts made by the authors in completing their chapters professionally. I express my deepest gratitude to all of them for contributing to this book by sharing their valuable works. A special thanks to my family and friends for their constant support in this journey.

Editor

Depictions of Insomniacs' Behaviors and Thoughts in Music Lyrics

Constance H. Fung,[1,2] Stella Jouldjian,[1] and Lara Kierlin[3]

[1] *Geriatric Research Education and Clinical Center (GRECC), Veterans Administration Greater Los Angeles Healthcare System, North Hills, CA 91343, USA*
[2] *David Geffen School of Medicine, University of California, Los Angeles, CA 90095, USA*
[3] *Oregon Sleep Associates, Portland, OR 97210, USA*

Correspondence should be addressed to Constance H. Fung; constance.h.fung@gmail.com

Academic Editor: Marco Zucconi

Study Objectives. Studies have found that depictions of unhealthy behaviors (e.g., illicit substance use, violence) are common in popular music lyrics; however, we are unaware of any studies that have specifically analyzed the content of music lyrics for unhealthy sleep-related behaviors. We sought to determine whether behaviors known to perpetuate insomnia symptoms are commonly depicted in the lyrics of popular music. *Methods.* We searched three online lyrics sites for lyrics with the word "insomnia" in the title and performed content analysis of each of the lyrics. Lyrics were analyzed for the presence/absence of the following perpetuating factors: extending sleep opportunity, using counter fatigue measures, self-medicating, and engaging in rituals or anti-stimulus control behaviors. *Results.* We analyzed 83 music lyrics. 47% described one or more perpetuating factor. 30% described individual(s) engaging in rituals or antistimulus control strategies, 24% described self-medicating, 7% described engaging in counter fatigue measures, and 2% described extending sleep opportunity (e.g., napping during daytime). *Conclusion.* Maladaptive strategies known to perpetuate insomnia symptoms are common in popular music. Our results suggest that listeners of these sleep-related songs are frequently exposed to lyrics that depict maladaptive coping mechanisms. Additional studies are needed to examine the direct effects of exposing individuals to music lyrics with this content.

1. Introduction

Insomnia is a prevalent condition among adolescents and adults, with an estimated prevalence of 22.1% when using DSM-IV-TR criteria [1]. Insomnia frequently presents in the context of comorbid conditions, ranging from substance use disorders to medical or psychiatric disorders, or even other sleep disorders such as obstructive sleep apnea. Less commonly, insomnia may be seen as a primary disorder, with the sleep complaint existing outside of other discernible medical or psychiatric cause [2]. In Spielman's 3-P model of insomnia, predisposing (biological and psychological inputs), precipitating (acute stressors), and perpetuating factors (behaviors such as napping that maintain or exacerbate sleep difficulties) contribute to individual sleep disturbance to varying degrees [3]. In particular, perpetuating factors can

be seen as modifiable behaviors that may serve as intervention points in insomnia treatment and public health awareness campaigns [4–6].

As described by Perlis et al., the four major types of perpetuating factors include (1) extending sleep opportunity (e.g., napping), (2) using counter fatigue measures (e.g., increasing coffee consumption), (3) self-medicating (e.g., drinking alcohol to promote sleep), and (4) using strategies that reduce stimulus control (e.g., reading in bed) or result in anticipatory anxiety if the strategy becomes unavailable (e.g., drinking special teas) [7]. These perpetuating factors contrast with recommended strategies for coping with insomnia, such as keeping a consistent wake up time and getting out of bed when unable to fall asleep. Cognitive behavioral therapy for insomnia, which is the most effective treatment for chronic insomnia, addresses these perpetuating factors through sleep restriction, stimulus control, sleep hygiene, and cognitive restructuring [4]. From a public health perspective, chronic insomnia could potentially be prevented if individuals avoided maladaptive compensatory behaviors when faced with factors that precipitate insomnia.

Studies of other health conditions suggest that the content of popular media may be of interest to clinicians, researchers, and public health programs, because popular media can influence the behaviors of individuals [8, 9]. For example, a systematic review found that exposure to alcohol advertising or alcohol promotional activity in print or broadcast media was associated with subsequent alcohol consumption in young people [8], and a recent study found an association between exposure to cannabis in popular music and early cannabis use among urban American adolescents [9]. Popular media could also affect the way individuals approach their own insomnia symptoms [10]. A study of British print media found that insomnia is couched in terms of stress and anxiety, and that treatments discussed in the media ranged from sleep hygiene to cognitive behavioral therapy to self-help remedies [10]. We are not aware of any published studies of popular music that have assessed the frequency with which perpetuating factors are conveyed.

The goal of this study was to assess the prevalence of the four types of perpetuating factors (extending sleep opportunity, using counter fatigue measures, self-medicating, and engaging in rituals or antistimulus control behaviors) found in the lyrics of popular music.

2. Materials and Methods

We searched three online music lyrics sites (http://www.lyrics.com/, http://www.metrolyrics.com/, and http://www.lyricsmode.com/) for lyrics with the word "insomnia" in the title (search completed in August 2012). We selected these licensed and authorized sites, because they pay royalty fees to songwriters and publishers based upon legal agreements between parties involved, unlike other sites that do not have the endorsement of those owning the music being referenced. We downloaded the music lyrics of all songs that appeared in the search results (N = 119). These three online sites did provide some lyrics in languages other than English. These were included in the sample, and were translated into English using Google translator. Non-English language lyrics that could not be translated using Google Translate (http://www.translate.google.com/) were attempted to be translated using Microsoft Translator (http://www.bing.com/translator/).

Two trained coders (CHF and LK) reviewed the content of all of the music lyrics downloaded. The ratings of the two coders were compared for each set of music lyrics, and differences were discussed. Residual differences in ratings were resolved completely with the input of a third coder (SJ), who independently reviewed the music lyrics blinded to the initial ratings of the first two coders. During their initial assessment, the coders independently assessed whether the lyrics were interpretable (e.g., sufficient amount of translation

from non-English language; N = 101) and contained unique lyrics (some lyrics were the same for two different artists; N = 112). Music lyrics that were deemed interpretable and that contained unique lyrics were further assessed to determine if the music lyrics provided content pertaining to insomnia. A total of 83 music lyrics were rated as having insomnia content and underwent further evaluation for the presence of maladaptive strategies for coping with insomnia [7] as described below.

Our research project was approved by VA Greater Los Angeles Healthcare Institution Research and Development.

2.1. Measures

(1) Extending sleep opportunity (e.g., going to bed early, waking up later, or napping). These strategies may deprime the sleep homeostat (reduce the propensity for sleep) and may result in circadian dysregulation.

(2) Engaging in counter fatigue measures (e.g., using stimulants or decreasing physical activity). Ingesting stimulants may increase arousal at inappropriate times, and decreasing physical activity may deprime the sleep homeostat, which could lead to conditioned arousal over time if the individual also spends more time resting in bed.

(3) Engaging in rituals or antistimulus control strategies (e.g., engaging in behaviors in the bedroom, sleeping outside the bedroom, using special herbs, teas, etc., to promote sleep and avoiding behaviors thought to inhibit sleep). These strategies may lead to a lack of stimulus control or may lead to anticipatory anxiety if the ritual becomes unavailable.

(4) Self-medicating: sedation with nonprescription substances (e.g., increase alcohol intake before bedtime, use of marijuana, use of over-the-counter antihistamines, use of melatonin as a hypnotic, or use of prescription medications not approved for hypnotic use such as opioids or certain benzodiazepines). These substances may disrupt the sleep stages, lead to psychological dependence, decrease sleep-related self-efficacy, cause rebound insomnia, or have the potential to shift circadian phase in the case of melatonin.

Frequency counts (presence/absence of each strategy type) were summarized using Microsoft Office Excel 2007.

3. Results

Table 1 provides a list of the music lyrics included in the analysis. Table 2 provides the frequency of perpetuating factors identified through content analysis. Overall, analysis of the lyrics containing insomnia content revealed that 47% described one or more perpetuating factor, and 14% described two or more perpetuating factors. The most frequent type of perpetuating factor described an individual

TABLE 1: Song titles and artist names of music lyrics analyzed (*N* = 83).

Artist Name	Song Title
Abgott	Shining Insomniac
Abysmalia	Whispering Insomnia
A C T	Insomniac
Annihilator	Insomniac
Anssi Kela	Insomnia
Anxiety of Influence	Insomniac
Bif Naked	Insomnia
Big K R I T	Insomnia
Billy Pilgrim	Insomniac
Bleeding Through	Insomniac
Boiler Room	Insomnia
Carpathian	Insomnia
Charlie	Insomnia's Lullaby
Counting Crows	Up All Night (Frankie Miller Goes To Hollywood)— The Song Formely Known As Insomnia
Craig David	Insomnia
Crüxshadows	Insomnia (A Ghost Story)
Dark Age	Insomnia
Deinonychus	Nightfall Guides Insomnia to be an everlasting mental torture, With This Being The Concequence
Dirty Heads	Insomnia
Dr. Sin	Insomnia
Duna Hill	Jack Insomniac
Echobelly	Insomniac
Electric President	Insomnia
Empyrios	Insomnia
Enter Shikari	Insomnia
Entwine	Insomniac
Faithless	Insomnia
Feeder	Insomnia
Finch	Insomniatic Meat
Government Issue	Insomniac
Grave Flowers	Insomnia
Gutter Demons	Insomnia
Haken	Insomnia
Her Six Daughters	Insomnia
Imago Mortis	Insomnia
Isole	Insomnia
Jester's Funeral	Insomnia l
Jill Scott	Insomnia
Katatonia	Tomb of Insomnia
Kylesa	Insomnia for Months
Ligion	Insomniacs Dreams
Live	Insomnia and the hole in the universe
Luka Belani	Love Insomnia
Lumine Criptica	Insomnia
Lunachicks	Insomnia

TABLE 1: Continued.

Artist Name	Song Title
Make Do And Mend	Insomniac Jams
Marillion	Insomnia
Megadeth	Insomnia
Minus	Insomniac
Music Emporium	Insomnia
Mustard Plug	Insomnia
Nephenzy Chaos Order	Insomnia
No More Heroes	Insomnia
Noe Venable	My insomnia
Pensive	Insomnia
Periphery	Insomnia
Raventhrone	Malicia The 3rd (Empress Of Insomnia)
Rentals	Insomnia
RZA	Insomnia
Salad	Insomnia
Sea Of Desperation	Insomnia
Shawn Desman	Insomniac
Shining Star	Insomnia
Silverchair	Insomnia
Slaine	Insomnia
Slowmotion Apocalypse	The Insomniac
Sum 41	Hyper-Insomnia
The Glass Child	Insomnia
The Veronicas	Insomnia
Tyler Hilton	Insomnia
Vader	Insomnia
Various Artist	Insomnia
Vivacity	Insomnia
War From A Harlots Mouth	Insomnia
Wheesung and Craig David	Insomnia
White Willow	Insomnia
Wintersleep	Insomnia
Wishbone Ash	Insomnia
Wynter Gordon	Insomnia
Wyrd	Ominous Insomnia
Yellow 5	Heart Break Insomnia

engaging in rituals or other maladaptive strategies. The following examples depict antistimulus control behaviors:

> *"I lie there staring at the dark ceiling and wait… My neurotic brain races for hours about everything possible."*

> *"Hypnotized by the strips on my TV."*

> *"I sit alone and I watch the clock. I breathe in on the tick and out on the tock."*

The second most frequent perpetuating factor described the use of substances for promoting sleep. The following three examples depict the use of substances for promoting sleep:

"Poured a bottle off NyQuil in my veins."

"Insomnia's lullaby, drinking wine and counting down the time."

"I only smoke weed when I need to."

A few music lyrics described an individual engaging in counter fatigue measures. The following is an example: "But now I keep myself pepped." Descriptions of an individual's attempt to extend sleep opportunity such as napping during the daytime were the least frequent type of perpetuating factor. The following are two examples of extending sleep opportunity: "I might sleep all day" and "Gotta try sleep through to Saturday."

4. Discussion

To our knowledge, this is the first study to evaluate the content of popular music for insomnia coping strategies. Our study found that maladaptive strategies for coping with insomnia symptoms are common in popular music, with close to half of the music lyrics referencing at least one perpetuating factor. Behaviors that adversely affect stimulus control (e.g., tossing and turning in bed) and the use of substances such as alcohol, marijuana, or opioids were the most commonly described behaviors. Our results suggest that listeners of these sleep-related songs are frequently exposed to unhealthy coping mechanisms for addressing insomnia symptoms.

The high prevalence of maladaptive strategies contained in popular music lyrics is colored by the dramatic nature of the medium, but it is also a reflection of the ways in which the public, in general, copes with sleep disturbances. A 2005 National Sleep Foundation survey found that 14% of Americans surveyed used sleep aids at least a few nights per week, 13% used alcohol within one hour of going to bed at least a few nights per week, and 35% took naps at least two times per week [11]. One market research study estimated that the worldwide market for sleeping pills may expand to $9.0 billion by 2015 [12]. Research has demonstrated that insomniacs tend to have increased belief in the negative sequelae of their sleep difficulty, which may itself be a perpetuating factor, and presentation of insomnia as highly dramatic and worthy of distress (e.g., "I'm hangin on by a thread to my sanity") may itself increase anxiety relating to sleep and worsen insomnia [13].

Our findings are important because popular music reaches a wide audience and can impact the sleep of listeners. American adolescents and younger children listen to 1.5–2.5 hours per day to music [14]. Many songs have been written to influence sleep (e.g., Johannes Brahms's *Guten Abend, gute Nacht*). A positive relationship between music and initiating sleep has been recognized for many years. In 1928, Frederico Garcia Lorca delivered his lecture, "On Lullabies," which describes the soothing effects of lullaby lyrics on children's

TABLE 2: Characteristics of perpetuating factors identified in music lyrics ($N = 83$).

Number of perpetuating factor(s) per music lyric	N (%)
None	44 (53)
One	27 (32)
Two	8 (10)
Three	4 (5)
Four	0 (0)
Type of perpetuating factor	N (%)
Engaging in rituals or anti-stimulus control strategies	25 (30)
Self-medicating	20 (24)
Engaging in counter fatigue measures	6 (7)
Extending sleep opportunity	4 (2)

sleep [15]. More recently, two randomized controlled studies that assessed the effects of listening to music at bedtime found that music improves self-reported sleep duration and sleep efficiency [16, 17]. Another study of young adults found that listening to classical music at bedtime improves sleep quality and reduces depressive symptoms as compared with an audiobook or control [18]. Although studies examining the effect of negative lyric content on sleep behaviors are not available, studies of other types of behaviors show an association between music lyrics and behavior. For instance, a strong relationship has been found between violent music lyrics and aggressive behavior [19, 20]. Other studies suggest that exposure to sexual messages and use of substances in music videos might change adolescents' behaviors and attitudes [21].

The 2006 Institute of Medicine report, "Sleep Disorders and Sleep Deprivation: An Unmet Public Health Problem" [22], described a need for a multimedia public education and awareness campaign to promote healthy sleep practices. Popular music remains untapped as a vehicle for raising awareness about sleep deprivation from insomnia and the behaviors that perpetuate insomnia symptoms. We already know that music lyrics can also have a positive impact on behavior. A study by Greitemeyer found that listening to songs with prosocial, relative to neutral, lyrics increased helping behavior. In theory, music lyrics could promote healthy sleep habits and encourage use of recommended strategies for dealing with events that trigger insomnia. Highlighting healthy sleep habits in songs that have been released and/or offering incentives for artists to write prosleep lyrics are two ways public health campaigns could use popular music to promote healthy sleep. Lyrics by Milk Inc, for example, describe an individual who has gotten out of bed due to insomnia symptoms, which is a behavior that promotes stimulus control: "At the count of three I pull back the duvet. Make my way to the refrigerator…But there's no relief. I'm wide awake in my kitchen." The following lyrics by Vivacity provide an example of an individual who challenges his/her beliefs about poor sleep, which may reduce the anxiety and arousal that can perpetuate insomnia (cognitive restructuring): "Go on just leave me here, cause this night is going to hell. Well it's just one more night, We'll make this time turn out well." Other forms of media such as television have successfully incorporated positive health messages into programming. For example, The Henry J. Kaiser Family Foundation has partnered with MTV, Univision, and Fox Networks Group to reduce sexually transmitted diseases, substance abuse, and obesity [23].

Our study has several limitations. First, because we only searched for music lyrics with the word "insomnia" in the title, we did not capture the lyrics focusing on insomnia whose song titles did not include "insomnia." Our search strategy, however, identified music lyrics that would have a high likelihood of containing content about insomnia. Second, although we captured some non-English lyrics, which we attempted to translate using publically available translation tools, we found that we were not able to translate all of the non-English lyrics and had limited access to other means of translation. Similarly, we were not able to use other languages for our search term because our research team did not have the capability to translate other languages. It should also be noted that since the sample included few non-English language lyrics, generalizing the findings to all music and/or English language media should be done with caution.

5. Conclusion

Many popular music lyrics that focus on insomnia depict unhealthy coping strategies for addressing sleep disturbance. Future studies should examine the direct effect of exposing individuals to music lyrics with a range of content (perpetuating factors versus recommended strategies for coping with insomnia). Additional studies of other forms of popular media, such as music videos, television, and social media exchanges, are needed to obtain better understanding of the types of messages that are conveyed in other forms of media and their influence on health behavior. Public health campaigns could consider using popular music to promote healthy sleep habits. Studying media's depictions of insomnia symptoms not only may inform our understanding of its impact on individual behavior and perceptions, but also could result in more targeted public health campaigns.

Conflict of Interests

The authors declared no conflict of interests. This study did not involve any off-label or investigational use.

Acknowledgments

This work funded by the Department of Veterans Affairs Advanced Geriatrics Fellowship Program and the Veterans Administration Greater Los Angeles Geriatric Research Education and Clinical Center. All work was completed at VA Greater Los Angeles Healthcare System and Oregon Sleep Associates.

References

[1] T. Roth, C. Coulouvrat, G. Hajak et al., "Prevalence and perceived health associated with insomnia based on DSM-IV-TR; international statistical classification of diseases and related health problems, tenth revision; and research diagnostic criteria/international classification of sleep disorders, second edition criteria: results from the America insomnia survey," *Biological Psychiatry*, vol. 69, no. 6, pp. 592–600, 2011.

[2] J. D. Edinger, M. H. Bonnet, R. R. Bootzin et al., "Derivation of research diagnostic criteria for insomnia: report of an American Academy of Sleep Medicine work group," *Sleep*, vol. 27, no. 8, pp. 1567–1596, 2004.

[3] A. J. Spielman, L. S. Caruso, and P. B. Glovinsky, "A behavioral perpective on insomnia treatment," *Psychiatric Clinics of North America*, vol. 10, no. 4, pp. 541–553, 1987.

[4] "NIH State-of-the-Science Conference Statement on Manifestations and Management of Chronic Insomnia in Adults," National Institutes of Health, vol. 22, no. 2, 2005, http://consensus.nih.gov/2005/insomniastatement.pdf.

[5] S. S. Kraus and L. A. Rabin, "Sleep America: managing the crisis of adult chronic insomnia and associated conditions," *Journal of Affective Disorders*, vol. 138, no. 3, pp. 192–212, 2012.

[6] American Sleep Association, "Sleep Hygiene Tips," 2007, http://www.sleepassociation.org/index.php?p=sleephygiene-tips.

[7] M. Perlis, C. Jungquist, M. Smith, and D. Posner, *Cognitive Behavioral Treatment of Insomnia*, Springer Science+Business Media, New York, NY, USA, 2005.

[8] L. A. Smith and D. R. Foxcroft, "The effect of alcohol advertising, marketing and portrayal on drinking behaviour in young people: systematic review of prospective cohort studies," *BMC Public Health*, vol. 9, article no. 51, 2009.

[9] B. A. Primack, E. L. Douglas, and K. L. Kraemer, "Exposure to cannabis in popular music and cannabis use among adolescents," *Addiction*, vol. 105, no. 3, pp. 515–523, 2010.

[10] S. J. Williams, C. Seale, S. Boden, P. Lowe, and D. L. Steinberg, "Medicalization and beyond: the social construction of insomnia and snoring in the news," *Health*, vol. 12, no. 2, pp. 251–268, 2008.

[11] National Sleep Foundation, "Sleep in America poll: summary of findings," National Sleep Foundation, 2005, http://www.sleepfoundation.org/sites/default/files/2005_summary_of_findings.pdf.

[12] Global Industry Analysts I., "Global Sleeping Pills Market to Reach US$9.0 billion by 2015, According to New Report by Global Industry Analysts, Inc.," Global Industry Analysts, Inc., 2010, http://www.prweb.com/releases/sleeping_pills/sleeping_tablets/prweb4318034.htm.

[13] C. M. Morin, J. Stone, D. Trinkle, J. Mercer, and S. Remsberg, "Dysfunctional beliefs and attitudes about sleep among older adults with and without insomnia complaints," *Psychology and Aging*, vol. 8, no. 3, pp. 463–467, 1993.

[14] American Academy of Pediatrics, "Policy statement—impact of music, music lyrics, and music videos on children and youth," *Pediatrics*, vol. 124, no. 5, pp. 1488–1494, 2009.

[15] A. S. Kline, "Federico García Lorca," 2008, http://www.poetry-intranslation.com/PITBR/Spanish/Lullabies.htm.

[16] H. L. Lai and M. Good, "Music improves sleep quality in older adults," *Journal of Advanced Nursing*, vol. 49, no. 3, pp. 234–244, 2005.

[17] L. P. Tan, "The effects of background music on quality of sleep in elementary school children," *Journal of Music Therapy*, vol. 41, no. 2, pp. 128–150, 2004.

[18] L. Harmat, J. Takács, and R. Bódizs, "Music improves sleep quality in students," *Journal of Advanced Nursing*, vol. 62, no. 3, pp. 327–335, 2008.

[19] S. Villani, "Impact of media on children and adolescents: a 10-year review of the research," *Journal of the American Academy of Child and Adolescent Psychiatry*, vol. 40, no. 4, pp. 392–401, 2001.

[20] P. Fischer, T. Greitemeyer, A. Kastenmüller, C. Vogrincic, and A. Sauer, "The effects of risk-glorifying media exposure on risk-positive cognitions, emotions, and behaviors: a meta-analytic review," *Psychological Bulletin*, vol. 137, no. 3, pp. 367–390, 2011.

[21] B. A. Primack, E. L. Douglas, M. J. Fine, and M. A. Dalton, "Exposure to sexual lyrics and sexual experience among urban adolescents," *American Journal of Preventive Medicine*, vol. 36, no. 4, pp. 317–323, 2009.

[22] "Sleep disorders and sleep deprivation: an unmet public health problem," National Academies Press, Washington, DC, USA, March 2006, http://www.iom.edu/~/media/Files/Report%20Files/2006/Sleep-Disorders-and-Sleep-Deprivation-An-Unmet-Public-Health-Problem/Sleepforweb.pdf.

[23] Health Communication and Media Partnerships, "The Henry J. Kaiser Family Foundation," 2012, http://www.kff.org/entpartnerships/.

2

The Relationship between Diabetic Neuropathy and Sleep Apnea Syndrome: A Meta-Analysis

Kazuya Fujihara,[1,2] **Satoru Kodama,**[1,2] **Chika Horikawa,**[1,2]
Sakiko Yoshizawa,[1,2] **Ayumi Sugawara,**[1,2] **Reiko Hirasawa,**[1,2] **Hitoshi Shimano,**[1]
Yoko Yachi,[2] **Akiko Suzuki,**[2] **Osamu Hanyu,**[2] **and Hirohito Sone**[2]

[1] *Department of Internal Medicine, Faculty of Medicine, Tsukuba University, Japan*
[2] *Department of Internal Medicine, Faculty of Medicine, Niigata University, 1-754 Asahimachi, Niigata, Niigata 951-8510, Japan*

Correspondence should be addressed to Hirohito Sone; sone@med.niigata-u.ac.jp

Academic Editor: Mehdi Tafti

Aims. High prevalence of sleep apnea syndrome (SAS) has been reported in patients with diabetes. However, whether diabetic neuropathy (DN) contributes to this high prevalence is controversial. Our aim of this study is to compare the prevalence of SAS between patients with and without DN. *Methods.* Systematic literature searches were conducted for cross-sectional studies that reported the number of patients with DN and SAS using MEDLINE (from 1966 to Nov 5, 2012) and EMBASE (from 1974 to Nov 5, 2012). Odds ratios (ORs) of SAS related to DN were pooled with the Mantel-Haenszel method. *Results.* Data were obtained from 5 eligible studies (including 6 data sets, 880 participants, and 429 cases). Overall, the pooled OR of SAS in patients with DN compared with that in non-DN patients was significant (OR (95% CI), −1.95 (1.03–3.70)). The pooled OR of SAS was 1.90 (0.97–3.71) in patients with type 2 diabetes. Excluding data on patients with type 1 diabetes, a higher OR was observed in younger patients (mean age <60 years) than in those ≥60 years among whom the OR remained significant (3.82; 95% CI, 2.24–6.51 and 1.17; 95% CI, 0.81–1.68). *Conclusions.* Current meta-analysis suggested the association of some elements of neuropathy with SAS in type 2 diabetes. Further investigations are needed to clarify whether the association is also true for patients with type 1 diabetes.

1. Introduction

Sleep apnea syndrome (SAS) is characterized by nocturnal sleep restriction, sleep fragmentation, and intermittent hypoxia, resulting in poor sleep quality and daytime sleepiness [1, 2]. The prevalence of SAS, in particular obstructive sleep apnea, is dramatically increasing with the increased prevalence of obesity, which is the main cause of the upper airway obstruction typically observed as snoring while sleeping [3]. SAS not only causes a lower quality of life due to sleepiness but also has clinical consequences that include hypertension, diabetes, cardiovascular disease, and sudden death [1, 2, 4].

A recent meta-analysis indicated that obstructive sleep apnea is associated with an increased risk of future type 2 diabetes, [5] clearly suggesting that individuals with diabetes had a higher prevalence of SAS compared to those without diabetes. The higher prevalence of SAS is partially explained by the higher prevalence of obesity among individuals with diabetes compared with those without diabetes [6, 7]. Diabetic neuropathy (DN) [8, 9] has been suggested as another explanation for the presence of SAS because it is diabetes-specific [10]. However, epidemiological findings regarding the association between DN with SAS are inconsistent [11]. Therefore, our aim of this meta-analysis is to compare the prevalence of SAS between patients with and without DN.

2. Materials and Methods

2.1. Search Strategy. Electronic literature searches (MEDLINE, from January 1966 to November 2012 and EMBASE, from January 1974 to November 2012) were conducted for studies investigating the relationships between DN and SAS. Study keywords were related to diabetes, neuropathy, and sleep apnea, which were combined using the Boolean logical operator "AND" (see Supplementary Material available online at http://dx.doi.org/10.1155/2013/150371). We added a manual search using reference lists of the relevant articles. This process was repeated until no additional articles could be identified. No language restriction was imposed.

For inclusion in the meta-analysis, a study had to fulfill the following criteria: (1) all patients had diabetes; (2) cross-sectional design was used; and (3) data on the number of cases and noncases of SAS according to the prevalence of DN were provided. However, we limited the meta-analysis to studies in which the presence of SAS was determined by instruments such as the apnea hypoxia index (AHI) or respiratory disturbance index (RDI) or pulse oximetry that calculated the oxygen desaturation index (ODI: number of desaturation events ≥4%/h). Therefore, we excluded one study [12] because the presence of SAS was judged by the existence of breathing pauses while sleeping and another study [13] because the criteria of SAS were not clarified. We also excluded studies that did not specify the type of diabetes [12, 14–17] because the characteristics of neuropathy, such as severity, resulting from type 1 diabetes and type 2 diabetes are different [18].

2.2. Data Extraction.
Two of the investigators (Kazuya Fujihara and Satoru Kodama) independently identified eligible studies and reviewed all relevant articles, including extraction of all relevant data and assessment of study quality. Discrepancies were resolved by the third investigator (Hirohito Sone). We extracted the following data from each publication: the first author's name, year of publication, geographic region, type of diabetes, participants' characteristics (i.e., age (mean), body mass index (mean), and duration of diabetes (mean)), proportion of men, definitions of SAS, number of SAS categories, type of DN (autonomic or peripheral), definitions of DN, number of participants and cases, and adjustment for age and sex or for obesity-related variables. Quality assessment was conducted by modifying the Newcastle-Ottawa Scale (NOS) for case-control studies so that it would be applicable to this meta-analysis [19]. Supplementary Material 2 shows the questions used in this assessment. Each "Yes" answer was awarded one point, with 8 as the highest possible score. Study quality was judged by the total of awarded points as follows: low (<4 points) and high (≥4 points).

2.3. Data Synthesis.
Odds ratios (ORs) for DN related to SAS were pooled with the Mantel-Haenszel method using DerSimonian and Laird's random-effects model [20]. This model considers between-study heterogeneity assessed by I-squared [21]. Primarily, in pooling the relationship between DN and SAS, we gave priority to SAS diagnosed using AHI if data on both the prevalence of abnormal AHI and ODI were given [22]. In addition, priority was given to data on mild SAS cases if multiple data were provided according to the severity of SAS using AHI or ODI [22–24].

Analyses were stratified by the following prespecified confounders that potentially influenced the study results: mean age (≥60 or <60 years); mean BMI (≥30 kg/m² or <30 kg/m²); country (Asian or non-Asian); type of DN (autonomic, peripheral, or unknown); and study quality (high or low). To explore the effect of study characteristics on the risk of SAS, meta-regression analysis was conducted where each confounder that we described above was entered as an explanatory variable and log OR as a dependent variable. Publication bias was statistically assessed using Egger's regression test [25]. A two-sided P value less than 0.05 was statistically significant. All analyses were conducted with STATA software version 11 (STATA Corporation, College Station, TX, USA).

3. Results

3.1. Literature Research.
Supplementary Material 3 shows details of the literature searches. First, 270 citations were identified. Of these, 237 articles were excluded according to their titles and abstracts. Forty articles, including 7 articles obtained from the manual search, were included for a more detailed review. After this review, 35 were excluded for the reasons shown in Supplementary Material 3. Finally, 5 eligible studies were included in this meta-analysis.

3.2. Study Characteristics.
Characteristics of the 5 selected studies comprising 6 data sets, 880 participants, 442 cases of DN, and 429 cases of SAS are shown in Table 1. All 5 studies included both males and females [22–24, 26, 27]. Mean age of participants was under 60 years in 3 studies [22, 24, 26] and was 60 years or over in 2 studies [23, 27]. Two studies [24, 27] were of the Asian region and 3 of non-Asian regions [22, 23, 26]. Mean duration was over 10 years in all 5 studies [22–24, 26, 27]. Three studies [22, 24, 26] used the AHI to diagnose SAS, whereas 1 study [27] used the ODI. One study [23] used the RDI. Among the 5 included studies, 1 [22] and 3 [23, 26, 27] investigated participants with autonomic neuropathy and peripheral neuropathy, respectively. According to the NOS scale, 3 studies were judged to be of high quality [22, 26, 27] and the other 2 were judged to be of low quality [23, 24] (Supplementary Material 2). One study [22] separately allowed estimation of the OR for SAS based on type 1 and type 2 diabetes. These ORs were separately pooled after the overall analysis. We first calculated the OR for both type 1 diabetes and type 2 diabetes, then calculated the OR for only type 2 diabetes since we only obtained data from one study for type 1 diabetes.

3.3. Overall Estimate of Prevalence of Sleep Apnea Syndrome Associated with Diabetic Neuropathy.
Figure 1 shows the pooled estimates for SAS in persons with DN. The overall pooled OR of SAS for DN participants compared with that for the non-DN participants was 1.95 (95% CI, 1.03–3.69; $P < 0.041$). However, between-study heterogeneity in the strength of the association was highly significant ($I^2 = 64.8\%$; $P = 0.014$). After excluding one data set on patients with type 1 diabetes expressing 4.76 of OR for SAS, the overall pooled OR of SAS for DN participants compared with that for the non-DN participants was 1.90 (95% CI, 0.97–3.71 $P = 0.060$) in those with type 2 diabetes (Figure 2).

TABLE 1: Characteristics of studies included in the meta-analysis.

(a)

Author	Country	Type of diabetes	Age (yrs), mean	BMI (kg/m²), mean	Duration of diabetes (yrs)	% Men	No. of subject					SA definition	Risk group	Referent group
							Total	DN (+) SA (+)	DN (+) SA (−)	DN (−) SA (+)	DN (−) SA (−)			
Nomura et al. (2013) [27]	Japan	T2DM	62.8	24.9	11.6	62	261	36	107	28	90	ODI 4% ≥ 5	ODI 4% ≥ 5	ODI 4% < 5
Tahrani et al. (2012) [26]	UK	T2DM	58.0	32.9	10.3	58	234	90	23	61	60	AHI ≥ 5	AHI ≥ 5	AHI < 5
Laaban et al. (2009) [23]	France	T2DM	61.0	31.1	14.4	53	303	90	47	101	65	RDI ≥ 5	RDI ≥ 5	RDI < 5
Takahashi et al. (2003) [24]	Japan	T2DM	58.0	24.4	ND	59	34	14	12	3	5	AHI ≥ 5	AHI ≥ 5	AHI < 5
Ficker et al. (1998) [22]	Germany	T1DM 22 / T2DM 26	51.3	25.1	17.5	48	22 / 26	1 / 5	8 / 9	0 / 0	13 / 12	AHI ≥ 10	AHI ≥ 10	AHI < 10

(b)

Author	Neuropathy definition			Matched age and sex	Matched obesity
	Peripheral	Autonomic	Evaluation of diabetic neuropathy		
Nomura et al. (2013) [27]	Yes	No	DTR, vibration, dysesthesia	Yes	Yes
Tahrani et al. (2012) [26]	Yes	No	MNSI examinations scores, MNSI questionnaire scores	Yes	Yes
Laaban et al. (2009) [23]	Yes	No	Patient's records	No	No
Takahashi et al. (2003) [24]	No	No	Not described	No	No
Ficker et al. (1998) [22]	No	Yes	CV, RMSSD, E-I difference, E/I ratio, maximum/minimum 30 : 15 ratio	No	No

Abbreviations: AHI: apnea hypoxia index; BMI: body mass index; CV: coefficient of variation; DM: diabetes mellitus; DN: diabetic neuropathy; DTR: deep tendon reflexes; MNSI: Michigan neuropathy screening instrument; ODI: oxygen desaturation index; RMSSD: root mean square of successive difference; RDI: respiratory disturbance index; SA: sleep apnea; T1DM: type 1 diabetes mellitus; T2DM: type 2 diabetes mellitus.

First author (year)	OR (95% CI)	DN + SAS cases/N	DN − SAS cases/N
Nomura et al. (2013)	1.08 (0.61, 1.91)	36/143	28/118
Tahrani et al. (2012)	3.85 (2.15, 6.88)	90/113	61/121
Laaban et al. (2009)	1.23 (0.77, 1.97)	90/137	101/166
Takahashi et al. (2003)	1.94 (0.38, 9.88)	14/26	3/8
Ficker et al. (1998) Type 1 DM	4.76 (0.17, 130.96)	1/9	0/13
Ficker et al. (1998) Type 2 DM	14.47 (0.71, 295.24)	5/14	0/12
Overall ($I^2 = 64.8\%$, $P = 0.014$)	1.95 (1.03, 3.69)	236/442	193/438

Note: weights are from random effects analysis

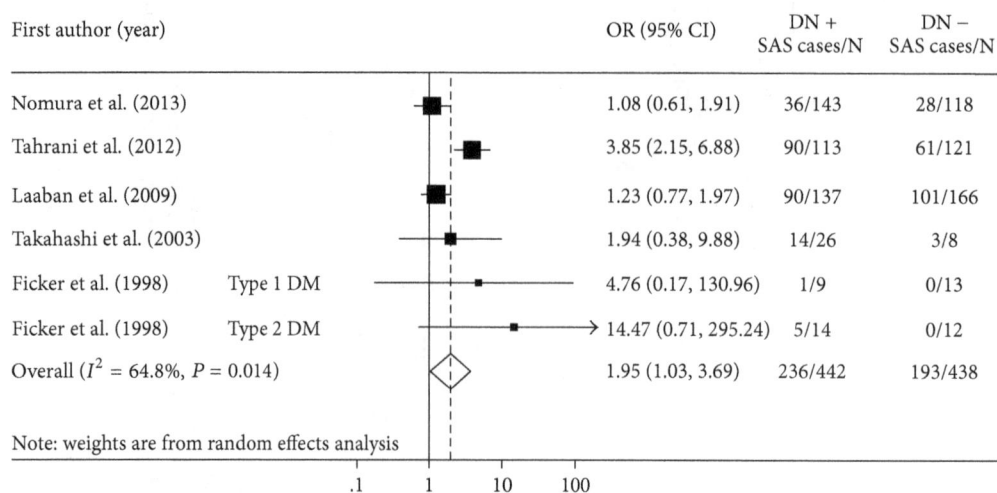

FIGURE 1: Forest plot showing the odds ratios (ORs) with 95% confidence interval (95% CI) of sleep apnea syndrome (SAS) for participants with diabetic neuropathy (DN) compared to participants without DN. Pooled OR is indicated by a diamond. The 95% CI of each OR is indicated by a vertical line. Size of squares reflects the statistical weight of each study.

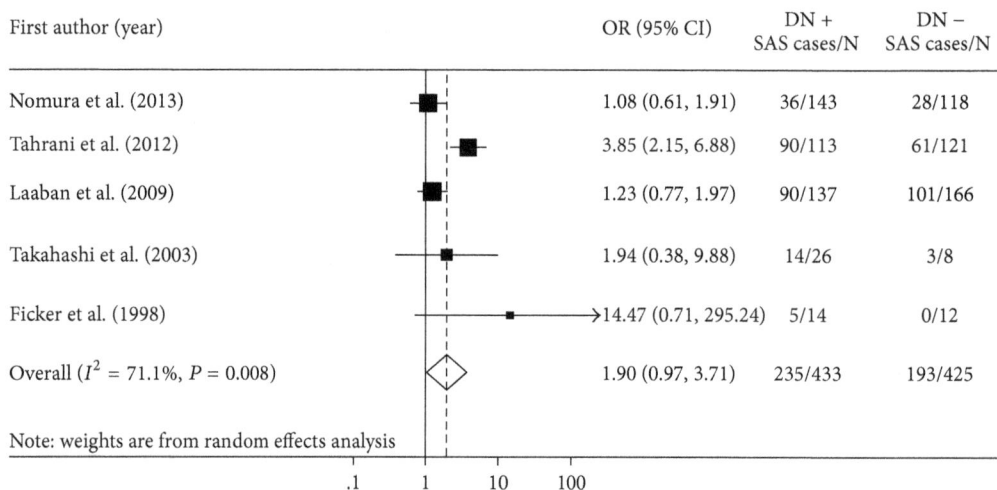

First author (year)	OR (95% CI)	DN + SAS cases/N	DN − SAS cases/N
Nomura et al. (2013)	1.08 (0.61, 1.91)	36/143	28/118
Tahrani et al. (2012)	3.85 (2.15, 6.88)	90/113	61/121
Laaban et al. (2009)	1.23 (0.77, 1.97)	90/137	101/166
Takahashi et al. (2003)	1.94 (0.38, 9.88)	14/26	3/8
Ficker et al. (1998)	14.47 (0.71, 295.24)	5/14	0/12
Overall ($I^2 = 71.1\%$, $P = 0.008$)	1.90 (0.97, 3.71)	235/433	193/425

Note: weights are from random effects analysis

FIGURE 2: Forest plot showing the odds ratios (ORs) with 95% confidence interval (95% CI) of sleep apnea syndrome (SAS) for participants with diabetic neuropathy (DN) compared to participants without DN. Pooled OR is indicated by a diamond. The 95% CI of each OR is indicated by a vertical line. Size of squares reflects the statistical weight of each study.

3.4. Sensitivity Analysis. Table 2 and Supplementary Material 4 show the results of stratified and meta-regression analyses across a number of key study characteristics to explore the origin of the heterogeneity and the influence of those characteristics on study results. A statistically stronger association between DN and SAS prevalence was remarkable in the younger participants (mean age < 60 years) in comparison with those ≥60 years. The difference was statistically significant (3.82; 95% CI, 2.24–6.51 and 1.17; 95% CI, 0.81–1.68; $P = 0.04$) (Supplementary Material 4 and Table 2).

3.5. Publication Bias. Egger's test revealed that there was no publication bias in both overall analysis and studies of only type 2 diabetes ($P = 0.42$ and $P = 0.50$, resp.).

4. Discussion

The current meta-analysis indicated that DN patients had approximately 2-fold higher prevalence of SAS than diabetic patients without neuropathy. Every 10 years of aging has been associated with a 1.24-fold increased risk of SAS in the general population [28]. If these data were applied to the current results, DN individuals would be estimated to develop SAS more than 30 years earlier than diabetic patients without neuropathy. Another main finding of the stratified analysis was that the effect of DN on the prevalence of SAS was remarkable in studies targeting relatively young diabetic patients (OR = 3.8) compared with those targeting relatively elderly patients (OR = 1.2). This result could be interpreted to mean that the association between DN and SAS is prominent

TABLE 2: Univariate meta-regression analysis of risk of SAS related to study characteristics*.

Variable	Coefficient	SE	P value
Mean age $\geq$ 60 years	−1.16	0.33	0.04
BMI $\geq$ 30 kg/m^2	0.21	0.80	0.81
Asian population	−0.65	0.74	0.44
DN diagnosis**			
Autonomic and peripheral	0.13	1.12	0.92
Autonomic only	2.14	1.72	0.34
High study quality***	0.53	0.77	0.54

*Logarithm of odds ratio for SAS was a dependent variable, and each variable was entered as an explanatory variable.
**Peripheral only was referent.
***Quality score $\geq$ 4 was regarded as high study quality.
Abbreviation: SE: standard error.

in a young diabetic population among which the effect of aging is relatively weak, whereas an association between DN and SAS might be masked by the effect of aging in the more elderly patients. Consequently, it is suggested that DN was significantly associated with high prevalence of SAS without regard to the effect of aging.

A meta-analysis of observational studies in principle can never prove causality. However, there are possible mechanisms as to why both autonomic and peripheral DN could lead to progression of SAS. An association between impairment of autonomic dysfunction and SAS was reported. The impairment in the central generation of respiratory movements that have been seen in autonomic disorders, such as Shy-Drager syndrome, may lead to collapse of the upper airway [29]. Another mechanism is that the reduction in sympathetic afferent nerves from the lung or CO_2-induced sympathetic activity controlling the ventilatory output may lead to an enhanced response to hypercapnia [30]. This abnormal respiratory control may account for central sleep apnea [12]. On the other hand, the association between impairment of peripheral nerve dysfunction and SAS also has been reported. The impairment of the pharyngeal sensory nerve, which fails to compensate for the compromised upper airway through protective reflexes, thereby increasing upper airway dilating muscle activity, finally leads to pharyngeal collapse and obstructive sleep apnea [31]. This impairment is known to be observed in a generalized neuropathy such as Charcot-Marie-Tooth [32]. Interestingly, deterioration of the reflexes protecting the upper airway is known to correlate with aging [33]. Another possible mechanism is that painful peripheral neuropathy might disturb sleep. However, it is obvious that the detailed mechanism elucidating the relationship between DN and SAS should be studied in the future.

Study Limitations. Several limitations need be addressed regarding this meta-analysis. First, this meta-analysis could not access individual data in each included study because it was study-based but not individual-based. Therefore, it is impossible to perfectly control for confounders linking DN and SAS. In addition, unfortunately, adjustment for possible residual confounders (e.g., cognitive heart failure,

smoking, glycemic control, and dyslipidemia) [1, 34–36] in each included study was generally poor. For example, higher prevalence of chronic heart failure or poor glycemic control was observed in patients with DN than that in patients without DN [1, 34–36]. The failure of adjustment for these confounders might have been responsible for the apparent association between DN and SAS. Second, meta-analyses of cross-sectional studies do not have the ability to distinguish an exposure from an outcome. We discussed the possibility that DN was associated with incident SAS. However, a reverse association could not be ruled out. A recent meta-analysis indicated that obstructive sleep apnea is associated with an increased risk of type 2 diabetes [5]. Therefore, it is possible that patients having SAS had developed diabetes and, at a later time, developed DN due to poor diabetes care. Third, few of the studies randomly selected their participants. It might not be sufficient to ascertain external validity since subjects in these studies might not be representative of average populations of diabetic patients.

In conclusion, the results of the current meta-analysis suggested an association of elements of neuropathy with SAS in type 2 diabetes. Further investigations are needed to clarify whether the association is true in patients with type 1 diabetes.

Conflict of Interests

The authors declare that there is no conflict of interests associated with this paper.

Authors' Contribution

Hirohito Sone has full access to all of the data in the study and takes responsibility for the integrity of the data and the accuracy of the data analysis. Study members that contributed significantly to this work are as follows. Study concept and design were done by Kazuya Fujihara, Satoru Kodama, and Hirohito Sone. Acquisition of data was done by Kazuya Fujihara, Sakiko Yoshizawa, and Chika Horikawa. Analysis and interpretation of data were done by Kazuya Fujihara, Satoru Kodama, and Osamu Hanyu. Drafting of the manuscript was done by Kazuya Fujihara, Satoru Kodama, Ayumi Sugawara, Sakiko Yoshizawa, Chika Horikawa, Ayumi Sugawara, Reiko Hirasawa, and Osamu Hanyu. Critical revision of the manuscript for important intellectual content was done by Kazuya Fujihara, Satoru Kodama, Hitoshi Shimano, Osamu Hanyu, and Hirohito Sone. Statistical analysis was done by Kazuya Fujihara and Satoru Kodama. Administrative, technical, or material support was done by Kazuya Fujihara and Satoru Kodama. Study supervision was done by Osamu Hanyu and Hirohito Sone.

Acknowledgments

This work is supported in part by the Ministry of Health, Labour, and Welfare, Japan. Dr. Sone and Dr. Kodama are recipients of a Grant-in-Aid for Scientific Research and Postdoctoral Research Fellowship, respectively, both from the Japan Society for the Promotion of Science (JSPS). This work is also financially supported by the Japan Cardiovascular Research Foundation and Ministry of Health, Labour, and Welfare, Japan. However, these sponsors had no role in the study design, collection, analysis, and interpretation of data, writing the report, and the decision to submit the report for publication. Thanks are also extended to Ms. Satomi Fukuya for her excellent secretarial assistance.

References

[1] V. K. Somers, D. P. White, R. Amin et al., "Sleep apnea and cardiovascular disease. An American heart association/American college of cardiology foundation scientific statement from the American heart association council for high blood pressure research professional education committee, council on clinical cardiology, stroke council, and council on cardiovascular nursing in collaboration with the national heart, lung," *Journal of the American College of Cardiology*, vol. 52, no. 8, pp. 686–717, 2008.

[2] J. E. Shaw, N. M. Punjabi, J. P. Wilding, K. G. M. M. Alberti, and P. Z. Zimmet, "Sleep-disordered breathing and type 2 diabetes. A report from the International diabetes federation taskforce on epidemiology and prevention," *Diabetes Research and Clinical Practice*, vol. 81, no. 1, pp. 2–12, 2008.

[3] A. R. Schwartz, S. P. Patil, A. M. Laffan, V. Polotsky, H. Schneider, and P. L. Smith, "Obesity and obstructive sleep apnea: pathogenic mechanisms and therapeutic approaches," *Proceedings of the American Thoracic Society*, vol. 5, no. 2, pp. 185–192, 2008.

[4] O. Ludka, T. Konecny, and V. Somers, "Sleep apnea, cardiac arrhythmias, and sudden death," *Texas Heart Institute Journal*, vol. 38, no. 4, pp. 340–343, 2011.

[5] X. Wang, Y. Bi, Q. Zhang, and F. Pan, "Obstructive sleep apnoea and the risk of type 2 diabetes: a meta-analysis of prospective cohort studies," *Respirology*, vol. 18, no. 1, pp. 140–146, 2013.

[6] H. E. Resnick, S. Redline, E. Shahar et al., "Diabetes and sleep disturbances: findings from the sleep heart health study," *Diabetes Care*, vol. 26, no. 3, pp. 702–709, 2003.

[7] B. Balkau, S. Vol, S. Loko et al., "High baseline insulin levels associated with 6-year incident observed sleep apnea," *Diabetes Care*, vol. 33, no. 5, pp. 1044–1049, 2010.

[8] A. I. Vinik, M. T. Holland, J. M. Le Beau, F. J. Liuzzi, K. B. Stansberry, and L. B. Colen, "Diabetic neuropathies," *Diabetes Care*, vol. 15, no. 12, pp. 1926–1975, 1992.

[9] A. I. Vinik, T. S. Park, K. B. Stansberry, and G. L. Pittenger, "Diabetic neuropathies," *Diabetologia*, vol. 43, no. 8, pp. 957–973, 2000.

[10] K. O. Lee, J. S. Nam, C. W. Ahn et al., "Insulin resistance is independently associated with peripheral and autonomic neuropathy in Korean type 2 diabetic patients," *Acta Diabetologica*, vol. 49, no. 2, pp. 97–103, 2012.

[11] P. Bottini, L. Scionti, F. Santeusanio, G. Casucci, and C. Tantucci, "Impairment of the respiratory system in diabetic autonomic neuropathy," *Diabetes, Nutrition and Metabolism*, vol. 13, no. 3, pp. 165–172, 2000.

[12] P. J. Rees, J. G. Prior, G. M. Cochrane, and T. J. H. Clark, "Sleep apnea in diabetic patients with autonomic neuropathy," *Journal of the Royal Society of Medicine*, vol. 74, no. 3, pp. 192–195, 1981.

[13] S. Mondini and C. Guilleminault, "Abnormal breathing patterns during sleep in diabetes," *Annals of Neurology*, vol. 17, no. 4, pp. 391–395, 1985.

[14] A. Schober, M. F. Neurath, and I. A. Harsch, "Prevalence of sleep apnoea in diabetic patients," *Clinical Respiratory Journal*, vol. 5, no. 3, pp. 165–172, 2011.

[15] P. Bottini, S. Redolfi, M. L. Dottorini, and C. Tantucci, "Autonomic neuropathy increases the risk of obstructive sleep apnea in obese diabetics," *Respiration*, vol. 75, no. 3, pp. 265–271, 2008.

[16] T. Keller, C. Hader, J. de Zeeuw, and K. Rasche, "Obstructive sleep apnea syndrome: the effect of diabetes and autonomic neuropathy," *Journal of Physiology and Pharmacology*, vol. 58, no. 5, pp. 313–318, 2007.

[17] P. Bottini, M. L. Dottorini, M. C. Cordoni, G. Casucci, and C. Tantucci, "Sleep-disordered breathing in nonobese diabetic subjects with autonomic neuropathy," *European Respiratory Journal*, vol. 22, no. 4, pp. 654–660, 2003.

[18] A. A. F. Sima and H. Kamiya, "Diabetic neuropathy differs in type 1 and type 2 diabetes," *Annals of the New York Academy of Sciences*, vol. 1084, pp. 235–249, 2006.

[19] G. A. Wells, B. O. C. D. Shea, J. Peterson, V. Welch, and M. Losos, "The Newcastle-Ottawa scale (NOS) for assessing the quality if nonrandomized studies in meta-analyses," http://www.ohri.ca/programs/clinical_epidemiology/.

[20] N. Mantel and W. Haenszel, "Statistical aspects of the analysis of data from retrospective studies of disease," *Journal of the National Cancer Institute*, vol. 22, pp. 719–748, 1959.

[21] R. DerSimonian and N. Laird, "Meta-analysis in clinical trials," *Controlled Clinical Trials*, vol. 7, no. 3, pp. 177–188, 1986.

[22] J. H. Ficker, S. H. Dertinger, W. Siegfried et al., "Obstructive sleep apnoea and diabetes mellitus: the role of cardiovascular autonomic neuropathy," *European Respiratory Journal*, vol. 11, no. 1, pp. 14–19, 1998.

[23] J. P. Laaban, S. Daenen, D. Léger et al., "Prevalence and predictive factors of sleep apnoea syndrome in type 2 diabetic patients," *Diabetes and Metabolism*, vol. 35, no. 5, pp. 372–377, 2009.

[24] S. Takahashi, S. Sakurai, T. Nishijima et al., "The prevalence of obstructive sleep apnea syndrome in the diabetes mellitus patients who require educational hospitalization," *Respiration and Circulation*, vol. 51, no. 6, pp. 617–621, 2003.

[25] M. Egger, G. D. Smith, M. Schneider, and C. Minder, "Bias in meta-analysis detected by a simple, graphical test," *The British Medical Journal*, vol. 315, no. 7109, pp. 629–634, 1997.

[26] A. A. Tahrani, A. Ali, N. T. Raymond et al., "Obstructive sleep apnea and diabetic neuropathy: a novel association in patients with type 2 diabetes," *The American Journal of Respiratory and Critical Care Medicine*, vol. 186, no. 5, pp. 434–441, 2012.

[27] K. Nomura, H. Ikeda, K. Mori et al., "Less variation of R-R interval of electrocardiogram in nonobese type 2 diabetes with nocturnal intermittent hypoxia," *Endocrine Journal*, vol. 60, no. 2, pp. 225–230, 2013.

[28] T. Young, E. Shahar, F. J. Nieto et al., "Predictors of sleep-disordered breathing in community-dwelling adults: the sleep heart health study," *Archives of Internal Medicine*, vol. 162, no. 8, pp. 893–900, 2002.

[29] F. E. Munschauer, L. Loh, R. Bannister, and J. Newsom-Davis, "Abnormal respiration and sudden death during sleep in multiple system atrophy with autonomic failure," *Neurology*, vol. 40, no. 4, pp. 677–679, 1990.

[30] C. Tantucci, L. Scionti, P. Bottini et al., "Influence of autonomic neuropathy of different severities on the hypercapnic drive to breathing in diabetic patients," *Chest*, vol. 112, no. 1, pp. 145–153, 1997.

[31] P. Lévy, J. Pépin, and M. Dematteis, "Pharyngeal neuropathy in obstructive sleep apnea: where are we going?" *The American Journal of Respiratory and Critical Care Medicine*, vol. 185, no. 3, pp. 241–243, 2012.

[32] M. Dematteis, J. L. Pépin, M. Jeanmart, C. Deschaux, A. Labarre-Vila, and P. Lévy, "Charcot-Marie-Tooth disease and sleep apnoea syndrome: a family study," *The Lancet*, vol. 357, no. 9252, pp. 267–272, 2001.

[33] C. L. Marcus, L. B. F. Do Prado, J. Lutz et al., "Developmental changes in upper airway dynamics," *Journal of Applied Physiology*, vol. 97, no. 1, pp. 98–108, 2004.

[34] R. E. Maser, A. R. Steenkiste, J. S. Dorman et al., "Epidemiological correlates of diabetic neuropathy. Report from Pittsburgh epidemiology of diabetes complications study," *Diabetes*, vol. 38, no. 11, pp. 1456–1461, 1989.

[35] J. Partanen, L. Niskanen, J. Lehtinen, E. Mervaala, O. Siitonen, and M. Uusitupa, "Natural history of peripheral neuropathy in patients with non-insulin-dependent diabetes mellitus," *The New England Journal of Medicine*, vol. 333, no. 2, pp. 89–94, 1995.

[36] S. Tesfaye, N. Chaturvedi, S. E. M. Eaton et al., "Vascular risk factors and diabetic neuropathy," *The New England Journal of Medicine*, vol. 352, no. 4, pp. 341–350, 2005.

3

Healthcare Providers' Knowledge of Disordered Sleep, Sleep Assessment Tools, and Nonpharmacological Sleep Interventions for Persons Living with Dementia: A National Survey

Cary A. Brown,[1] Patricia Wielandt,[2] Donna Wilson,[3] Allyson Jones,[4] and Katelyn Crick[4]

[1] *Department of Occupational Therapy, University of Alberta, 2-64 Corbett Hall, Edmonton, AB, Canada T6G 2G4*
[2] *Occupational Therapy, Central Queensland University, Building 6, Bruce Highway, Rockhampton, QLD 4702, Australia*
[3] *Faculty of Nursing, Edmonton Clinic Health Academy, University of Alberta, 87 Avenue, Edmonton, AB, Canada T6G 1C9*
[4] *Department of Physical Therapy, University of Alberta, 3-44C Corbett Hall, Edmonton, AB, Canada T6G 2G4*

Correspondence should be addressed to Cary A. Brown; cary.brown@ualberta.ca

Academic Editor: Luigi J. Ferini-Strambi

A large proportion of persons with dementia will also experience disordered sleep. Disordered sleep in dementia is a common reason for institutionalization and affects cognition, fall risk, agitation, self-care ability, and overall health and quality of life. This report presents findings of a survey of healthcare providers' awareness of sleep issues, assessment practices, and nonpharmacological sleep interventions for persons with dementia. There were 1846 participants, with the majority being from nursing and rehabilitation. One-third worked in long-term care settings and one-third in acute care. Few reported working in the community. Findings revealed that participants understated the incidence of sleep deficiencies in persons with dementia and generally lacked awareness of the relationship between disordered sleep and dementia. Their knowledge of sleep assessment tools was limited to caregiver reports, self-reports, and sleep diaries, with few using standardized tools or other assessment methods. The relationship between disordered sleep and comorbid conditions was not well understood. The three most common nonpharmacological sleep interventions participants identified using were a regular bedtime routine, increased daytime activity, and restricted caffeine. Awareness of other evidence-based interventions was low. These findings will guide evidence-informed research to develop and test more targeted and contextualized sleep and dementia knowledge translation strategies.

1. Introduction

Disordered sleep (DS) is defined as a range of sleep problems including hypersomnia conditions (such as sleep apnea and narcolepsy), parasomnia conditions (such as confusional arousal, restless leg syndrome, and sleep walking), insomnia, and sleep-wake cycle disturbances [1]. All of these DS conditions share the outcome of nonrestorative sleep. Disordered sleep in older persons is a largely overlooked contributing factor for psychosocial dysfunction, decreased cognitive function, depression, agitation, numerous health problems [2], and a major reason for institutionalization in later life. The relationships between DS and decreased cognitive, emotional, and physical functioning, substance misuse, and

various mental health problems are well documented [3]. Research suggests that this is a bidirectional relationship such that poor sleep influences health and dementia, and vice versa. This presents an exciting proposition because interventions for DS may reduce the risk for, or lessen the severity of, mental and physical health problems. Promoting better sleep can therefore contribute to health, wellbeing, and continued independent community living for persons with dementia (PWD).

Older adults, and particularly PWD, are at significant risk for altered sleep patterns and DS [4]. Disordered sleep is both a consequence of poor health and a risk factor for the onset of various mental and physical health conditions. For example, animal studies have demonstrated a relationship between sleep deprivation of only three weeks and accelerated development of the amyloid plaques associated with Alzheimer's disease [5]. Other researchers have revealed clear links between insomnia and cognitive tasks such as vigilance [6], concentration, memory, and executive function [7, 8].

The relationship between DS and a range of health conditions common in older persons has been demonstrated. Traumatic brain injury [9], Parkinson's disease [10], and stroke/CVA [11], for example, carry an increased risk of reduced or altered cognitive functioning. Adding DS contributes an additional risk to cognitive decline and the increased likelihood of reduced independence, deteriorated quality of life, and increased caregiver/family burden. DS is a significant predictor of depression among well community-dwelling older adults [12] and, cyclically, depression is a risk factor for dementia [12]. Disordered sleep is also an issue for family caregivers. Providing home-based care to PWD can significantly affect the sleep of family members, and therefore their health and ability to cope with the emotional and physical demands of caregiving [4], all to the detriment of their continued ability to maintain the PWD at home. Support for caregivers is now understood as key for preventing institutionalization [13].

Healthcare providers, service organizations, and care providers lack awareness regarding DS and sleep interventions for both PWD and for their sleep-deprived caregivers [14]. Although nonpharmacological sleep interventions (NPSIs) are effective for improving restorative sleep among older persons [15, 16], the inaccurate belief that reduced hours of sleep and decreased ability to sleep well in old age are "normal" aspects of aging is pervasive [17]. This mistaken belief on the part of both healthcare providers and the general public, coupled with both PWD and their family members reluctance to seek help for sleep issues, contributes to the underdiagnosis and undertreatment of DS in this high need and growing population.

The survey goal was to identify HCP's sleep and dementia evidence-to-practice gaps so as to guide development of knowledge translation (KT) strategies and, ultimately, facilitate better management of DS in PWD. Specifically we surveyed healthcare providers across Canada working in the area of older adult care to identify (1) their level of knowledge related to risk factors for DS in PWD, (2) screening practices and knowledge of sleep assessment tools relevant to DS in PWD, and (3) participants' use of, and perceptions about, the practicality of NPSI for PWD.

2. Materials and Methods

2.1. Sample. An Internet search, followed by a snowball technique, identified 318 national and provincial Canadian healthcare provider professional organizations and associations. Each was contacted, requesting them to disseminate an online survey to their members. A small number did not respond to repeated emails and presumably did not forward the invitation to their members. Some allowed us access to membership email lists, others disseminated the survey invitation through their internal communication networks, and

others forwarded the request to different groups we were unaware of at that time. We estimate that 65–80 organizations participated in distributing the survey invitation. This range of strategies was highly effective for achieving a large and diverse participant group across Canada, but this meant ultimately that we were unable to tally exactly how many healthcare providers were invited to participate. Although we originally intended to have the survey in both the English and French languages, circumstances precluded having a French language survey tool and this report deals only with the English language responses.

2.2. Survey. The extant evidence for NPSIs for PWD [1] formed the evidence base for the survey questions. We asked what healthcare providers knew about risk factors for DS in PWD, the consequences of DS, sleep assessment methods, and NPSIs for PWD. We also gathered background demographics. The draft survey was piloted and revised before its distribution. The online survey, approved by the Health Research Ethics Board of the University of Alberta, Edmonton, Canada, and built on the open access software platform "FluidSurvey," ran between October 2011 and March 2012. The Northwest Territories was not included as regulatory issues precluded surveying in this jurisdiction.

2.3. Analysis. The quantitative data received had descriptive statistical analyses done using SPSS (version 19.0). We performed 2-tailed statistical testing, with Bonferroni correction, at the .01 level of significance.

3. Results

3.1. Demographics and Practice Profile. There were 1,846 survey participants who completed the survey in whole or in part. Participants were not required to answer all of the questions and could make more than one selection for many of the questions. Consequently the total number of participants and responses for each question varied. Participants were able to select multiple practice settings so as to best reflect their actual working patterns. For example, a number of participants indicated they worked both in long-term care (LTC) and in acute care settings. Long-term care (LTC) (33.6%, $n = 680$), followed by acute care (32.2%, $n = 652$), accounted for the majority of work settings. Healthcare providers working in the community appeared to be underrepresented (17.4%, $n = 351$) (Table 1 provides the full breakdown by work setting).

Postal codes were provided by 1052 (57.0%) participants and revealed a cross-Canada distribution with the exception of the Northwest Territories. Alberta (38.7%), Ontario (18.9%), and New Brunswick (14.6%) had the highest rates of participation. Respondents worked primarily in nursing (61.1%), physiotherapy (PT) (10.8%), or occupational therapy (OT) (6.2%). Thirty-nine percent (38.8%) of the participants reported that "50% or greater of their patients with dementia resided in the community." Similarly, 37.9% reported that "50% or greater of their patients with dementia resided in institutional settings."

TABLE 1: Practice setting.

Long-term care facility	33.9% (616)
Acute care facility	33.1% (602)
Community/homecare service	16.3% (295)
Family practice/primary care	8.8% (159)
Rehabilitation service	8.5% (154)
Supported living facility	7.3% (133)
Geriatric clinic	6.9% (125)
Private practice	5.6% (101)
Research centre	2.4% (44)
Other	14.4% (261)

Note. Participants could select >1 category; therefore, the total exceeds 100%.

3.2. Awareness of Sleep Issues for Persons with Dementia. Of 1526 participants responding to the question *"what percentage of patients with dementia are likely to have sleep problems?,"* 10.7% ($n = 164$) indicated they believe that this was the case for "less than 25%" of their patients, and 42.9% ($n = 655$) indicated "25–50%." Of the other participants, 30.5% ($n = 534$) indicated they believe "51–75%" of their patients with dementia have sleep problems and 11.3% ($n = 173$) indicated "76–100%".

Participants reported they most often became aware of sleep problems during their usual assessment practices (32.3%, $n = 837$) or from another member of the team (26.9%, $n = 699$). Few reported they became aware through family or patient reports (18.6% and 15.8%%, resp.). Many selected more than one option for this question indicating that sources of information may be quite individual depending on the patient.

3.3. Awareness of Sociocultural and Behavioral Factors Associated with Sleep Problems in Persons with Dementia. Participants were asked to select factors from a total of 16 behavioral and sociocultural factors they believe to be associated with the likelihood of sleep problems in PWD (Table 2). All 16 factors were evidence based with no distractors. The most frequently selected factor was "daytime sleepiness" (88.9%) and least selected factor was "smoking" (1.5%). Awareness of sleep-related factors varied across professional groups but participant knowledge was generally low. Table 2 illustrates for each of the 16 factors which profession had the highest and lowest selection rate, and the percentage of the participants within these two groups making the selection. For example, physicians had the highest selection of the factor "alcohol use" (38.3%), while the lowest selection of this factor was by recreation therapists (5.1%). Table 2 also displays where statistically significant differences were found between the two professions with the highest and the lowest selection rate for each factor. For example, the difference between the percentage of physicians who identified "falls" as related to DS in PWD compared to pharmacists (51.2% and 26.9%, resp.) was statistically significant ($P = .006$).

3.4. Awareness of Comorbidities Associated with Sleep Problems in Persons with Dementia. Participants selected from 15 physical comorbidities and one category labeled "mental health" those comorbidities they believed were associated with the likelihood of sleep problems in PWD (Table 3). There were no distractors. Table 3 details which profession had the highest or the lowest selection rate, and what percentage of the participants within these two professional groups made the selection. The most frequently selected comorbid condition was "mental health" identified by 92.9% of psychiatrists and the least frequently selected "allergies" (1.7%) made by recreation therapists. There was high between-group variation in selection. For example, 32.1% of nursing participants selected "gastrointestinal (GI) disorders" as related to poor sleep but only 19.0% of psychiatrists selected this factor. Overall, psychiatrists most often had the highest selection rate for the sixteen factors. Only two of the 16 factors, "mental health" and "pain" (selected by 92.9% and 85.7%, resp., of psychiatrists), were also selected frequently by other participants. However, aside from "urological conditions" (selected by 74.1% of physicians), all other physical comorbidities were selected by less than 65% of any of the members of each profession. Table 3 also displays any statistically significant differences between the two professions with the highest and the lowest selection rate for each factor. The difference between the highest and lowest selection rate was statistically significant for all comorbidities except "allergies," "gastrointestinal disorders," and "rheumatic disease." These three were infrequently selected by all participants.

3.5. Experience and Awareness of Standardized Sleep Assessment Tools. Participants were asked to identify sleep assessment tools they had used, ones they were aware of but had not used, and ones they felt were not practical in their practice setting. All of the assessment tools were derived from the evidence base. Three nonstandardized tools, "caregiver report" (selected by 97.2% of social workers), "patient self-report" (92.5% of physicians), and "sleep diaries" (78.9% of psychiatrists), were found as having been used by higher numbers of the participants in each professional group. Of the standardized tools, "polysomnography assessment in a sleep lab" had been most often used, but by only 31.2% of psychiatrists and 24.7% of physicians. Of the other standardized tools, less than 30% of any of respondents in any of the professional groups had used the "Epworth" (28.6% of physicians), the "SDI (Sleep Disturbances Index)" (14.3% of social workers), the "SSS (Stanford Sleepiness Scale)" (6.6% of physicians), the "PSQI (Pittsburg Sleep Quality Index)" (6.2% of psychiatrists), the "MOS-SS (Medical Outcomes of Sleep Study Scale)" (3.7% of recreation therapists), and the "Verran Snyder-Halpern Sleep scale" (2.6% of physicians).

We found minimal experience with sleep scales designed specifically for populations where high rates of dementia would be expected; the "PDSS (Parkinson's Disease Sleep Scale)" had been used by 3.9% of physicians, followed by the "SCOPA (Scales for Outcomes in Parkinson's Disease-Sleep Scale)" which had been used by 1.9% of recreation therapists. "Actigraphy," although considered in the literature as a reasonably affordable objective measure of a number of sleep parameters [18], was very seldom used (5.0% of the

TABLE 2: Awareness of relationship between risk factors and disordered sleep (%).

Related factor	Psychiatrist	Physician	Social worker	OT	PT	Nursing	Pharmacist	RT	Stat Sig.
Appetite	11.9*					33.0^			$P < 0.001$
Falls		51.2^					26.9*		0.006
Social withdrawal			37.8*					57.6^	
Problem solving				39.8*				54.2^	
Aggression					29.3*			61.0^	$P < 0.001$
Depression	81.0^		23.3*						0.003
Daytime sleepiness		88.9^	70.3*						
Night wakefulness	82.1^						62.7*		
Napping	76.2^				58.8*				0.008
Medication		69.1^			42.7*				$P < 0.001$
Cognitive decline	79.0^							40.6*	$P < 0.001$
Comorbidity	67.9^					33.4		25.4*	$P < 0.001$
Decreased mobility			51.4*		69.8^				
Alcohol use		38.3^						5.1*	$P < 0.001$
Smoking	14.3^						1.5*		
Caregiver beliefs		21.0^	3.4*						0.011

Key. ^highest endorsement, *lowest endorsement, OT: occupational therapist, PT: physical therapist, RT: recreation therapist. Note. Insufficient sample of psychologists, respiratory technicians, and assistants for analysis.

TABLE 3: Awareness of relationship between comorbidity and disordered sleep (%).

Condition	Psychiatrist	Physician	Social worker	OT	PT	Nursing	Pharmacist	RT	Stat sig.
Allergies			8.1^					1.7*	
Cardiovascular	61.9^							30.5*	$P < 0.001$
Substance abuse	55.4^							11.9*	$P < 0.001$
Endocrine disorder		16.0^						1.7*	$P < 0.001$
Obesity	50.0^			19.6*					$P < 0.001$
GI disorders	19.0*				32.1^				
Infection							9.0*	35.6^	$P < 0.001$
Pain	85.7^		64.9*						$P < 0.011$
Neurological		60.5^						35.6*	
Skin condition		25.9^			4.0*				$P < 0.001$
Mental health	92.9^				63.8*				$P < 0.001$
Pulmonary	50.0^						28.4*		$P = 0.006$
Renal disorder	2.4*		16.2^						$P = 0.003$
Rheumatic disease		24.7^						10.2*	
Sensory deficit					7.5*			23.7^	$P < 0.001$
Urological cond.		74.1^						47.5*	$P < 0.001$

Key. ^highest endorsement, *lowest endorsement, OT: occupational therapist, PT: physical therapist, RT: recreation therapist. Note. insufficient sample of psychologists, respiratory technicians, and assistants for analysis.

physicians). Full details by profession are available from the author on request.

3.6. Use and Perceived Practicality of Nonpharmacological Sleep Interventions.

The respondents were also presented with a list of NPSIs derived from the evidence base specific to persons with dementia. Participants were asked to select responses for each in four categories so as to capture the breadth of experience with, and perceptions about, each NPSI. The categories were (1) "*recommended in the past and practical for patients to use*," (2) "*recommended in the past BUT not practical for patients to use*," (3) "*not previously recommended but may be practical for patients*," and (4) "*not recommended and not practical*." Overall, participants indicated they had minimal experience with most NPSIs listed, with the exception of "increased daytime activity" and "decreased daytime napping." They were positively disposed to many of the interventions as indicated by participants' rating a number of NPSIs as potentially useful despite having no experience with them. There were four NIPSs that participants selected as having previously used but now believed to be impractical: "increased time outside" (24.0%), "warm bath before bed" (19.6%), "sleep restriction regime" (16.2%), "PWD sets own bedtime" (16.8%), and "adjust caregiver bedtime to that of PWD" (15.2%). Full details by profession are available from the authors on request.

4. Discussion

The representativeness of the participants, the implications of findings, and emergent points for action are discussed below.

4.1. Representativeness of Survey Participants. Nurses comprised 61.1% of the participants, followed by PT (10.8%) and OT (6.2%). This is considered a fairly representative healthcare professional sample, and particularly for PT and OT, because only 11.7% (686/5841) of OT members of the Canadian Association of Occupational Therapists (CAOT) report working in the area of older adult rehabilitation (CAOT, 2012). The 113 OTs participants in this survey potentially represent 1 in 6 of these therapists. For PT, their national organization reports that 5.6% (574/10,253) of their members are identified as working in the area of older adult rehabilitation. The 199 PTs participants in this survey potentially represent 35%, or 1 in 3, of these therapists (personal correspondence 25/10/2012).

This representation from nurses, PT, and OT is a research strength because these healthcare providers typically have frequent, in some cases weekly or even daily, contact with PWD and their families. As such, they may be best suited to assume a triage and advocacy role to alert other team members to possible DS. The low proportion of participants who were physicians (4.0%), psychiatrists (4.2%), or psychologists (<1%) is unsurprisingly given the scarcity of geriatricians and psychogeriatricians in Canada. The Canadian Academy of Geriatric Psychiatry reported in 2012 that only 217 psychiatrists worked predominantly in geriatrics (personal correspondence 29/10/2012). While membership in this national organization is voluntary, it is presumably indicative of the low number of psychiatrists in Canada who work with persons who have dementia. However, a total of 86 psychiatrists completed a survey, and we cautiously propose this is a sufficiently representative sample from which we can draw some conclusions.

4.2. Knowledge of the Prevalence of DS and Risk Factors for DS in PWD. The prevalence of sleep problems in community-dwelling persons with dementia is conservatively estimated at 40% [3, 19]. The prevalence in LTC settings, because of the residents' poorer health, decreased activity levels, noise, light, and temperature that is nonsleep conducive at night, and staffing practices and routines, requiring activity at night, would be higher. It has been proposed that some LTC residents do not get a full hour of sleep in any 24-hour period [20]. Close to one-half of the survey participants estimated that 50% or more of their patients had sleep problems. Given that over 60% of our participants are identified as working in long-term care or other institutional care settings, it appears that they underestimate the prevalence of the problem as presented in the literature.

Knowledge about indicators of risk related to DS, aside from "daytime sleepiness," was generally low. None of the risk factors were identified by 85% or greater of the respondents within any professional group. Notable deficits in awareness were evident about the relationship between sleep and "appetite," "falls," "problem solving," "alcohol," "smoking," and "caregiver beliefs." In these categories, none of the professional groups had greater than 55% awareness of the relationship between the factor and DS (Table 2) and in some awareness fell to less than 5%. "Smoking" and "caregiver beliefs" were the least frequently selected although the evidence is clear that smoking, which contributes to apnea, is related to poor sleep [21]. Similarly, the influence of caregiver beliefs as influencing DS was underrecognized [22]. It is possible that participants, over half who are working in institutional settings, did not select "smoking" because it is largely controlled by staff in LTC settings. However, previous smoking habits can influence respiratory function and apnea. Caregiver beliefs are very important as they assume increasing responsibility and decision making for their family member with dementia. Healthcare providers who understand caregiver beliefs about sleep can address misunderstandings or values that pose challenges to effective sleep management. It is also notable that awareness of different factors varied across professions such that not one profession appeared to be consistently most aware of the evidence-based link between specific risk factors and DS. This is important because it reinforces current guidelines emerging from knowledge translation (KT) research recommending that targeted educational and KT strategies, building on existing awareness and addressing specific knowledge gaps within individual groups, are likely to be more effective compared to "one-size-fits-all" generic education strategies [23].

4.3. Knowledge of the Relationship between Sleep and Other Comorbidities. Overall knowledge about relationships between sleep and evidence-based comorbid health conditions was low. Of particular concern were the low (less than 25% in any professional group) endorsement rates for a relationship between DS in PWD and the comorbid conditions of "allergies," "endocrine disorders," "renal disorders," "rheumatic diseases," and "sensory deficits." This lack of knowledge matters because of the growing evidence base supporting a bidirectional, reciprocal relationship between these health conditions and DS in PWD [20, 24]. Sleep problems tend to be underrecognized in PWD as the complexity of comorbidities increases and managing the other aspects of dementia becomes an increasing challenge [4]. It is possible that among the survey respondents comorbid conditions, such as these, which routinely alert HCPs to the possibility of DS in noncognitively impaired populations, tend to be overlooked in PWD.

4.4. Awareness of Sleep Problems. Participants became aware of sleep problems either through their usual assessment practices (32.3%) or when reported by another team member (26.9%). Family member reporting was identified less than 20% of the time, so it appears that responsibility for recognizing a potential sleep problem rests with the HCP directly or through a referral from another member of the formal healthcare team. However, it is possible that families do not routinely bring concerns about DS to the attention of any HCP, who then must rely more on their own practice and colleagues. Given these findings and the complexities of detecting DS in PWD, it would be of benefit to identify opportunities to include basic sleep-related screening questions in existing, routinely administered, geriatric assessments. For example, DS is a risk factor for falls [25], and significant resources have been dedicated to falls reduction and prevention programs in many countries. However, the Morse Falls Scale (available at http://www.patientsafety.gov/SafetyTopics/fallstoolkit/media/morse_falls_pocket_card.pdf) and the St. Thomas's Risk Assessment Tool in Falling Elderly Inpatients—STRATIFY [26], two of the most widely used, psychometrically sound falls assessment tools, do not contain any sleep-related questions. A literature search for falls risk assessment tools revealed one in-house tool, the FARAM, developed by Bayside Health in Victoria, Australia (available at http://www.health.vic.gov.au/qualitycouncil/downloads/falls/tools.pdf) that incorporated sleep-related questions. Although not yet validated, the sleep-related questions in the FARAM tool could serve as model. Given the clear evidence-based relationship between falls and sleep disorders [25] embedding basic sleep screening in falls assessment tools seems to be a practical step forward to facilitate busy HCPs' routine sleep screening.

4.5. Knowledge and Use of Sleep Assessment Tools. Assessment tool knowledge was limited for any assessments beyond nonstandardized self-report measures such as sleep diaries and caregiver reports. These types of self-report tools, while important, are often insufficient to capture a full picture of the extent and characteristics of DS. Current guidelines recommend a combination of self-report, observational, and standardized tools so as to best understand the complexity of DS in PWD [2]. Encouragingly, none of the tools were perceived as highly impractical by the respondents, with the exception of polysomnography. This is not surprising, given the challenges to ensure a sufficient degree of reliability when using polysomnography with PWD. These findings may indicate that, although awareness and experience with standardized tools were low, HCP saw the relevance of sleep assessment and did not regard these tools as impractical. This is a promising finding and interdisciplinary strategies to deliver education about available sleep assessment are indicated. Sleep assessment tools of particular relevance to PWD include actigraphy [18], the Sleep Disturbance Index (SDI) [4], the Pittsburg Sleep Quality Index (PSQI), and the Epworth Sleepiness Scale (ESS) [27]. There is a scarcity of assessment and screening tools specific to SD in PWD, with scope then for further research and development.

4.6. Awareness of, and Experience with, Nonpharmacological Sleep Interventions. Only three of the 22 evidence-based nonpharmacological sleep intervention strategies listed in the survey (i.e., "regular bedtime routine," "increased daytime activity," and "restricted caffeine") were reported as having been recommended and perceived as practical by greater than 80% of the entire sample (86.2, 84.2, and 83.2%, resp.). Four of the remaining interventions were endorsed as practical by between 70 and 79% of participants: "regular exercise routine" (76.0%), "restricted daytime naps" (75.7%), "decreased evening noise levels" (73.9%), and "restricted evening fluids" (70.4%). As such, there was reasonable knowledge of these interventions.

The remaining 15 interventions were selected with much less frequency and with greater between-group variation. "Education about sleep surfaces" was more likely to be recommended by OT and PT than other participants, while "evening warm bath" was endorsed most often by psychiatrists and social workers. "Use of a white noise machine" was most likely to be endorsed by social workers and "reduced ambient lighting at night" was more likely to be endorsed by psychiatrists and physicians. "Sleep restriction regime" was most likely to be endorsed by psychiatrists and physicians were more likely to endorse "increased daytime ambient lighting." Physiotherapists were less likely to endorse "adjustment of caregiver sleep schedule" and "allowing PWD to self-determine sleep schedule." While social workers were most likely to endorse "caregiver respite care," physicians and psychiatrists were more likely to endorse "respite care for PWD." While we can only speculate as to the reason for these professional-specific differences, it may reflect professional training and differing priorities for healthcare or rehabilitation that would promote experience with, and a preference for, certain interventions over others.

Interestingly, interventions targeting modification to the nighttime sleep environment showed weak endorsement overall. It may be that the significant role that the environment plays in sleep is not well understood. While reduced nighttime light may not have been strongly endorsed by HCP working in LTC settings because of potential safety concerns, white noise machines and modification of sleep surfaces/bedding are relatively pragmatic considerations with no evident safety barriers that would preclude selection of these interventions by LTC workers.

It is noteworthy that only 44.6% of participants overall had knowledge of and endorsed "increased time outdoor" while other interventions such as "increased exercise" (76.0%) and "relaxation techniques" (67.5%) were identified much more frequently as having been tried and as also being practical. This apparent preference for active interventions may reflect the current social trend to view exercise as a form of medication for many conditions (e.g., http://exerciseismedicine.org/). Additionally, a lack of awareness among the respondents overall was noted about the significant role exposure to daylight plays in sleep regulation. It is possible that the high number of participants who report working in LTC and other institutional settings may have skewed the findings since daylight exposure is a much less realistic option in these settings compared to PWD living with family caregivers in the community.

(1) Build capacity for screening and advocacy related to sleep and dementia in professions (nursing, physiotherapy, occupational therapy) whose practices have the highest frequency and duration of patient/family interaction.

(2) Prioritize sleep and dementia education by profession so as to build on existing awareness when introducing information. For example, as physicians already report awareness of the relationship between DS and depression and nighttime wakefulness, KT efforts should not focus on these elements. Rather, clear knowledge gaps should be targeted.

(3) Education about the relationship between caregiver beliefs and DS in PWD should be a priority for all HCPs.

(4) Education about comorbid conditions with known association with DS is required across professional groups with particular emphasis on allergies, endocrine conditions, and sensory deficits.

(5) Embedding sleep-related questions in widely used screening tools for other conditions would be congruent with HCPs current practice and promote more routine screening in a practical format.

(6) Healthcare providers need information about, and access to, appropriate assessment tools for PWD. Particular emphasis should be on actigraphy, PSQI, ESS, and SDI.

(7) Healthcare providers need education about NPSI that is tailored to knowledge gaps within their own profession.

(8) All healthcare providers need education about NPSI focused on modifications to the sleep environment and the critical role of passive exposure to daylight.

(9) Develop KT strategies that incorporate awareness of organizational context and that focus on the level of those stakeholders who are able to influence organizational culture.

(10) Deliver KT with as much local context as possible, in a range of formats that accommodate learners' preferences and that reduce the amount of time spent in learning new technology to access the material as opposed to time spent in learning the new material specifically.

Box 1: Action points for NPSI KT strategies.

4.7. Emerging Needs and Recommendations. Box 1 outlines ten recommendations to increase healthcare providers' awareness of sleep and dementia that emerge from our discussion of the survey findings. Recommendations include the need for capacity building across HCP groups to help them better understand the factors that influence sleep, the range of evidence-based risk factors, and the relationship between insufficient sleep and comorbidities. Additional recommendations address HCPs' need for more information about assessment tools and NPSI strategies—particularly pragmatic, evidence-based, environmental modifications. Because home-care nurses, OTs, and PTs have the most extended and frequent contact with PWD and their families, they may be best suited to a sleep triage role. We recommend that these HCPs should be a priority for more in-depth education. Other recommendations, informed by KT best-practice guidelines, highlight that KT strategies should be strength based, target clear knowledge gaps, include family members and other stakeholders when possible, and address the importance of family caregiver beliefs and values about sleep. Final recommendations focus on the cross-disciplinary need for understanding the foundational physiological role that light exerts on sleep, the need to educate both individual HCPs and organizational decision-makers so that sleep-friendly sustainable environments and routines are created, and the importance of contextualized information delivered with attention to the audiences' preferred learning styles.

An evidence-informed approach to HCPs' unmet need for sleep and dementia knowledge is important. Lessons from the examples of KT initiatives in diabetes, cardiovascular care, medication adherence, and guideline implication [23, 28, 29] will help us move forward more effectively in addressing this challenge. Knowledge translation evidence, applied to the survey findings, reinforces the need to plan dissemination strategies addressing demonstrated knowledge gaps and building on existing awareness within individual professional groups. This KT approach, as opposed to delivering less targeted, generic sleep education, can help address HCPs' need for learning that accommodates time constraints. Targeting identified knowledge gaps increases the relevance of information to the recipient. Building on existing knowledge that is already familiar and comfortable for the learner helps achieve knowledge user engagement and perceived self-efficacy with new information [28]. Elwyn et al. [28] propose that KT research neglects the important elements of communication theory and the evidence generated in the field of business and marketing. Drawing from these fields they developed the "sticky knowledge" conceptual model which suggests that the existence of ambiguity and uncertainty, the degree of credibility of both the source of information and the information itself, the learners' absorptive and retentive capacity for new information, the contextual elements influencing the organization's receptivity, and the existence of challenging arduous relationships will all influence the flow of information between sender and receiver. Importantly, these factors also influence how well the information "sticks" to the receiver and then, in turn, flows to the next recipient. As in other KT models, the importance of contextualized information so that the relevance is clearly evident to the recipient is highlighted. These concepts can be applied to help refine KT strategies addressing HCPs' gaps in sleep and dementia knowledge and practice.

Summary. These findings indicate that awareness is generally low and knowledge varies between professional groups. This again highlights that, consistent with examples of KT in other areas with evidence-to-practice [23], sleep and dementia awareness and intervention strategies may benefit from targeting specific professions and their identified knowledge gaps instead of focusing efforts into more generic sleep educational approaches intended for all service providers.

Limitations. The survey had several limitations. The sample was one of convenience and we have no certainty that it was representative. Additionally, because participants were able to select more than one response for some questions, we cannot conclude that responses were rank ordered. Losing our ability to complete all aspects of the survey in French as well as English language leaves Francophone HCPs working with PWD underrepresented. Finally, and most importantly, healthcare providers working with PWD living in the community were also underrepresented. This is a critical setting for attention as effective and early sleep intervention in the community can act as a preventative measure to support caregivers' wellbeing, optimize PWD's functional capacity, and possibly reduce the risk of institutionalization.

5. Conclusions

At the start of the study we knew from clinical experience and from the research literature that sleep problems for PWD were largely unrecognized and often undertreated. As a consequence of this survey, we now know that HCP groups have different knowledge strengths and knowledge gaps. These findings will guide future, evidence-informed, research to develop and test the outcomes of more targeted and contextualized sleep and dementia KT strategies.

Conflict of Interests

The authors declare that there is no conflict of interests regarding the publication of this paper.

Author's Contributions

Cary A. Brown was the principal investigator on the research project and drafted the paper, Patricia Wielandt, Donna Wilson, and Allyson Jones assisted with the writing, and Allyson Jones and Katelyn Crick assisted with the statistical analysis and writing of those sections.

Acknowledgment

The authors would like to acknowledge the support of the Addiction & Mental Health Research Partnership Program: Alberta Health Services (AHS) (http://www.albertahealthservices.ca/2770.asp), which provided funding for this project.

References

[1] C. A. Brown, R. Berry, M. C. Tan, A. Khoshia, L. Turlapati, and F. Swedlove, "A critique of the evidence-base for non-pharmacological sleep interventions for persons with dementia," *Dementia*, vol. 12, no. 2, pp. 174–201, 2011.

[2] H. G. Bloom, I. Ahmed, C. A. Alessi et al., "Evidence-based recommendations for the assessment and management of sleep disorders in older persons," *Journal of the American Geriatrics Society*, vol. 57, no. 5, pp. 761–789, 2009.

[3] S. Ancoli-Israel, "Sleep and its disorders in aging populations," *Sleep Medicine*, vol. 10, supplement 1, pp. S7–S11, 2009.

[4] R. E. Tractenberg, C. M. Singer, J. L. Cummings, and L. J. Thal, "The Sleep Disorders Inventory: an instrument for studies of sleep disturbance in persons with Alzheimer's disease," *Journal of Sleep Research*, vol. 12, no. 4, pp. 331–337, 2003.

[5] J.-E. Kang, M. M. Lim, R. J. Bateman et al., "Amyloid-β dynamics are regulated by orexin and the sleep-wake cycle," *Science*, vol. 326, no. 5955, pp. 1005–1007, 2009.

[6] E. Altena, Y. D. Van Der Werf, R. L. M. Strijers, and E. J. W. Van Someren, "Sleep loss affects vigilance: effects of chronic insomnia and sleep therapy," *Journal of Sleep Research*, vol. 17, no. 3, pp. 335–343, 2008.

[7] C. H. Bastien, E. Fortier-Brochu, I. Rioux, M. LeBlanc, M. Daley, and C. M. Morin, "Cognitive performance and sleep quality in the elderly suffering from chronic insomnia: relationship between objective and subjective measures," *Journal of Psychosomatic Research*, vol. 54, no. 1, pp. 39–49, 2003.

[8] M. Cricco, E. M. Simonsick, and D. J. Foley, "The impact of insomnia on cognitive functioning in older adults," *Journal of the American Geriatrics Society*, vol. 49, no. 9, pp. 1185–1189, 2001.

[9] R. J. Castriotta and J. M. Lai, "Sleep disorders associated with traumatic brain injury," *Archives of Physical Medicine and Rehabilitation*, vol. 82, no. 10, pp. 1403–1406, 2001.

[10] W. G. Ondo, K. Dat Vuong, H. Khan, F. Atassi, C. Kwak, and J. Jankovic, "Daytime sleepiness and other sleep disorders in Parkinson's disease," *Neurology*, vol. 57, no. 8, pp. 1392–1396, 2001.

[11] M. Arzt, T. Young, L. Finn, J. B. Skatrud, and T. D. Bradley, "Association of sleep-disordered breathing and the occurrence of stroke," *American Journal of Respiratory and Critical Care Medicine*, vol. 172, no. 11, pp. 1447–1451, 2005.

[12] G. Livingston, B. Blizard, and A. Mann, "Does sleep disturbance predict depression in elderly people? A study in inner London," *British Journal of General Practice*, vol. 43, no. 376, pp. 445–448, 1993.

[13] J. Kochar, L. Fredman, K. L. Stone, and J. A. Cauley, "Sleep problems in elderly women caregivers depend on the level of depressive symptoms: results of the caregiver-study of osteoporotic fractures," *Journal of the American Geriatrics Society*, vol. 55, no. 12, pp. 2003–2009, 2007.

[14] S. A. Beaudreau, A. P. Spira, H. L. Gray, J. Long, M. Rothkopf, and D. Gallagher-Thompson, "The relationship between objectively measured sleep disturbance and dementia family caregiver distress and burden," *Journal of Geriatric Psychiatry and Neurology*, vol. 21, no. 3, pp. 159–165, 2008.

[15] E. J. Stepanski and J. K. Wyatt, "Use of sleep hygiene in the treatment of insomnia," *Sleep Medicine Reviews*, vol. 7, no. 3, pp. 215–225, 2003.

[16] S. Koch, E. Haesler, A. Tiziani, and J. Wilson, "Effectiveness of sleep management strategies for residents of aged care facilities:

findings of a systematic review," *Journal of Clinical Nursing*, vol. 15, no. 10, pp. 1267–1275, 2006.

[17] J. Ellis, S. E. Hampson, and M. Cropley, "The role of dysfunctional beliefs and attitudes in late-life insomnia," *Journal of Psychosomatic Research*, vol. 62, no. 1, pp. 81–84, 2007.

[18] S. Ancoli-Israel, R. Cole, C. Alessi, M. Chambers, W. Moorcroft, and C. P. Pollak, "The role of actigraphy in the study of sleep and circadian rhythms," *Sleep*, vol. 26, no. 3, pp. 342–392, 2003.

[19] Y. Song, G. A. Dowling, M. I. Wallhagen, K. A. Lee, and W. J. Strawbridge, "Sleep in older adults with Alzheimer's disease," *Journal of Neuroscience Nursing*, vol. 42, no. 4, pp. 190–198, 2010.

[20] J. L. Martin and S. Ancoli-Israel, "Sleep disturbances in long-term care," *Clinics in Geriatric Medicine*, vol. 24, no. 1, pp. 39–50, 2008.

[21] B. Phillips and S. Ancoli-Israel, "Sleep disorders in the elderly," *Sleep Medicine*, vol. 2, no. 2, pp. 99–114, 2001.

[22] C. M. Morin, J. Stone, D. Trinkle, J. Mercer, and S. Remsberg, "Dysfunctional beliefs and attitudes about sleep among older adults with and without insomnia complaints," *Psychology and Aging*, vol. 8, no. 3, pp. 463–467, 1993.

[23] S. Straus, J. Tetroe, and I. D. Graham, Eds., *Knowledge translation in health care: moving from evidence to practice*, Blackwell, Oxford, UK, 2009.

[24] P. Voyer, R. Verreault, P. N. Mengue, and C. M. Morin, "Prevalence of insomnia and its associated factors in elderly long-term care residents," *Archives of Gerontology and Geriatrics*, vol. 42, no. 1, pp. 1–20, 2006.

[25] R. J. St George, K. Delbaere, P. Williams, and S. R. Lord, "Sleep quality and falls in older people living in self- and assisted-care villages," *Gerontology*, vol. 55, no. 2, pp. 162–168, 2009.

[26] D. Oliver, M. Britton, P. Seed, F. C. Martin, and A. H. Hopper, "Development and evaluation of evidence based risk assessment tool (STRATIFY) to predict which elderly inpatients will fall: case-control and cohort studies," *British Medical Journal*, vol. 315, no. 7115, pp. 1049–1053, 1997.

[27] D. R. Lee and A. J. Thomas, "Sleep in dementia and caregiving–assessment and treatment implications: a review," *International Psychogeriatrics*, vol. 23, no. 2, pp. 190–201, 2011.

[28] G. Elwyn, M. Taubert, and J. Kowalczuk, "Sticky knowledge: a possible model for investigating implementation in healthcare contexts," *Implementation Science*, vol. 2, no. 44, 2007.

[29] G. M. Grimshaw, M. P. Eccles, J. N. Lavis, S. J. Hill, and J. E. Squires, "Knowledge translation of research findings," *Implementation Science*, vol. 7, article 50.

4

The Role of Daytime Sleepiness in Psychosocial Outcomes after Treatment for Obstructive Sleep Apnea

Esther Yuet Ying Lau,[1] Gail A. Eskes,[2,3,4] Debra L. Morrison,[4,5] Malgorzata Rajda,[2,5] and Kathleen F. Spurr[6]

[1] *Sleep Laboratory, Department of Psychology, 6/F Jockey Club Tower, The University of Hong Kong, Pokfulam Road, Hong Kong*
[2] *Department of Psychiatry, Dalhousie University, Halifax, NS, Canada*
[3] *Department of Psychology, Dalhousie University, Halifax, NS, Canada*
[4] *Department of Medicine, Dalhousie University, Halifax, NS, Canada*
[5] *Sleep Clinic and Laboratory, Queen Elizabeth II Health Sciences Centre, Halifax, NS, Canada*
[6] *School of Health Sciences, Dalhousie University, Halifax, NS, Canada*

Correspondence should be addressed to Esther Yuet Ying Lau; eyylau@hku.hk

Academic Editor: Marco Zucconi

We investigated the role of daytime sleepiness and sleep quality in psychosocial outcomes of patients with obstructive sleep apnea (OSA) treated with continuous positive airway pressure (CPAP). Thirty-seven individuals with moderate to severe OSA and compliant with CPAP treatment for at least 3 months were compared to 27 age- and education-matched healthy controls. The OSA group and the control group were studied with overnight polysomnography (PSG) and compared on measures of daytime sleepiness (Epworth Sleepiness Scale), sleep quality (Pittsburg Sleep Quality Index), mood (Beck Depression Inventory, Profile of Mood States), and functional outcomes (Functional Outcomes of Sleep Questionnaire). After CPAP treatment, the OSA group improved on sleep quality and sleepiness. As a group, they did not differ from controls on sleep architecture after CPAP. The OSA group also showed significant improvements in functional outcomes and was comparable to controls on mood and functional outcomes. Persistent difficulties included lowered activity level and residual sleepiness in some individuals. Sleepiness was found to be a significant predictor of mood and affective states, while both sleepiness and sleep quality predicted functional outcomes. These results highlight the importance of assessment and intervention targeting psychosocial functioning and sleepiness in individuals with OSA after treatment.

1. Introduction

Individuals with obstructive sleep apnea-hypopnea syndrome (OSA) experience excessive daytime sleepiness and fatigue, decreased cognitive function and mood changes, resulting in significant, negative consequences in work and driving performance, and lowered quality of life (see review by [1]). Therefore, the evaluation of OSA treatment on both nighttime and daytime consequences of OSA is critical.

The most obvious consequence and manifestation of untreated OSA are probably subjective sleepiness and high propensity to fall asleep during the daytime. Engleman and Douglas [2] reviewed 29 studies that measured sleepiness and concluded that at least moderate impairments in terms of excessive daytime sleepiness are indicated in patients with OSA. Accumulating evidence suggests that the main causes of daytime sleepiness in patients with OSA are sleep fragmentation and sleep architecture disruptions [3]. Some propose that sleepiness of patients with more severe OSA may be more related to the breathing disruptions and the associated nocturnal hypoxemia (e.g., [4]).

An association between OSA and mood disorders is revealed by studies reporting their comorbidity (e.g., [5]). Previous studies also showed that individuals with OSA showed elevated scores on measures of depression, and 58% met the DSM criteria for depression [6]. In the Wisconsin

Sleep Cohort Study, longitudinal data demonstrated a dose-response association between OSA and depression in a community sample of 1408 participants [7]. On the contrary, other studies do not find an association between OSA and psychological problems (e.g., [8]). Authors like Cassel contend that the so-called personality change or psychological consequence of OSA is due to a misinterpretation of sleepiness by medical staff and the overlap of symptoms like fatigue between OSA and depression. The implication is that symptoms of fatigue and depression have to be distinguished in studies investigating mood in patients with OSA. Bardwell et al. [9] concluded from their study that many of the previously reported links between mood and OSA dissipate after controlling for covariates such as age, BMI, and hypertension. But it should be noted that a strong relationship between OSA and mood was demonstrated even after potential confounds were controlled in a later study (see above) [5].

The relationship between OSA and psychological problems is still uncertain, and the mechanisms of OSA-related mood symptoms are unknown. Depressive symptoms in patients with OSA have been proposed to be related to oxygen desaturation and nocturnal hypoxemia (e.g., [10]) or to sleep fragmentation and excessive daytime sleepiness [11]. It has also been shown that experimental sleep fragmentation produces significant mood symptoms [12], supporting the potential effects of sleep disruption and daytime sleepiness on mood. However, it is difficult, if not impossible, for previous studies to distinguish the more direct effects of the illness itself (i.e., the hypoxic insults) and the indirect effects of daytime sleepiness on mood in patients with untreated OSA. Investigating stably treated individuals in which hypoxemia is eliminated or minimized would help elucidate the remaining effects of any persistent daytime sleepiness.

Continuous Positive Airway Pressure (CPAP) has been reported to be effective in improving subjective and objective measures of sleepiness in patients with OSA [13], with therapeutic effects ranging from moderate to large [2, 14]. The average improvement for patients with severe OSA was 4.75 points on the Epworth Sleepiness Scale (ESS, [13]). However, it is not uncommon for individual patients to continue to experience excessive daytime sleepiness with CPAP treatment (e.g., [4]). A number of authors have reported improvements of psychological functioning after CPAP treatment (e.g., [15]). Several placebo-controlled studies on the reversibility of psychopathology (mainly depression) have been conducted with mixed results [16, 17]. Sateia [18] concluded that while the clinical impression suggests that OSA may be directly related to psychopathology and that treatments can reverse the impairments, the literature does not provide unequivocal support for these associations. In addition, another question that is left unanswered is whether the psychosocial functioning of stably treated patients is comparable to their peers without OSA.

The purpose of the current study was to investigate the relationship between any residual sleepiness or sleep issues and psychosocial functioning in individuals with stably treated OSA to understand their long-term outcomes. In order to ensure that the patients were indeed properly treated

with CPAP, data on their pre-treatment status (i.e., PSG data, sleepiness scores, subjective sleep quality) were collected and compared with posttreatment data. Improvements on hypoxemia indices, sleepiness, and sleep quality were previously reported in an earlier paper focusing on cognitive functions [19] and will be summarized in the results section. Here, we report in detail on how changes in sleepiness and sleep quality relate to psychosocial functioning posttreatment. The OSA group was also asked to rate their pre-treatment functional outcomes retrospectively to understand if and to what extent they perceived CPAP helped in terms of subjective daytime functions. We then investigated the predictors of the psychosocial functioning of individuals with treated OSA. Outcome variables included the mood measures and functional outcomes. Predictors examined were demographics, pretreatment disease severity, and posttreatment sleep-related variables.

Based on the findings of previous studies, we hypothesized that (1) the OSA group will show improvements in their daytime sleepiness, sleep quality, and functional outcomes after CPAP treatment as compared to their pre-CPAP status; (2) current sleep variables would be more important in predicting psychosocial outcomes in individuals with stably treated OSA compared to pre-treatment diagnostic variables; (3) the associations between sleepiness, sleep quality, and psychosocial functioning would also apply to healthy age-matched controls.

2. Methods

2.1. Participants and Procedures. Thirty-seven individuals with OSA treated with CPAP and 27 healthy control participants were studied. Details of the inclusion and exclusion criteria were reported in Lau et al. [19]. Briefly, patients had moderate to severe OSA and had been on CPAP treatment for at least three months with compliance of at least 4 hours per night for 80% of the week; exclusion criteria were other sleep pathologies as verified by overnight PSG and clinical interview by attending physicians, diagnosed psychiatric disorders (e.g., psychotic disorders, major depression with suicidal ideation), or neurological conditions (e.g., stroke, epilepsy), current alcohol or drug abuse, current use of medication that could affect cognitive function (e.g., benzodiazepine), and undertreatment of OSA other than CPAP. The protocol was approved by the Research Ethics Board of the Queen Elizabeth II Health Sciences Centre and was prepared in accordance with the Helsinki Declaration. After the initial screening and consenting procedure, all participants filled out questionnaires of subjective sleep quality, sleepiness, and psychosocial measures (see below). Then, participants completed experimental tasks of working memory and a comprehensive neuropsychological battery (findings reported in Lau et al. [19]). All participants also received an overnight PSG using standardized procedures and scoring within eight weeks of psychological testing [20]. Relevant information was extracted from patients' medical charts at the Sleep Clinic and Laboratory, including pretreatment data on PSG, daytime sleepiness, sleep quality, and other relevant medical history and medications.

2.2. Measures

2.2.1. Epworth Sleepiness Scale (ESS) [21, 22].

All participants completed the ESS, a self-administered eight-item questionnaire for measuring daytime sleepiness by rating the chances of dozing off or falling asleep in eight different situations commonly encountered in daily life, on a scale from 0 (would never doze) to 3 (high chance of dozing). An ESS score > 10 (out of 24) is conventionally considered as clinically significant [23]. ESS is a validated clinical and research tool in assessing daytime sleepiness with high test-retest reliability ($r = 0.82$) and internal consistency (Cronbach's alpha = 0.88) [21, 24, 25]. The reliable change index of 5.89 on the ESS as calculated by a formula with the mean change score, the standard deviation, and the reliability coefficient are used in the current study to evaluate the extent of change in our OSA group [26].

2.2.2. Pittsburgh Sleep Quality Index (PSQI).

The PSQI is a self-rated questionnaire which assesses sleep quality and disturbances over a one-month time interval. Nineteen individual items generate seven "component" scores including subjective sleep quality, sleep latency, sleep duration, habitual sleep efficiency, sleep disturbances, use of sleeping medication, and daytime dysfunction. Component scores ranging from 0 to 3 are then summed to yield one global score (0–21) with higher scores indicating worse sleep quality. The global score is used to distinguish good and poor sleepers (>5 as poor sleepers) with a diagnostic sensitivity of 89.6% and specificity of 86.5%. Evidence of internal homogeneity (Cronbach's $\alpha = 0.83$) and consistency (test-retest reliability coefficient = 0.85) was reported by Buysse et al. [27].

2.2.3. Beck Depression Inventory (BDI) [28].

On the well-validated BDI, mild, moderate, and severe levels of depressive symptomatology are indicated by a raw score of 14 to 19, 20 to 28, and 29 to 63, respectively.

2.2.4. Profile of Mood States (POMS) [29].

Affective states were measured by the POMS. Participants rate their feelings during the past week on 65 adjective scales using a 5-point rating system from 0 (not at all) to 4 (extremely). The profile includes a total score and scores of six affective states: tension anxiety, depression dejection, anger hostility, vigor activity, fatigue inertia, and confusion bewilderment. These subscales separate out somatic symptoms (sleepiness, fatigue) from affective symptoms (anxiety, depression), providing useful evidence to validate the potential effectiveness of CPAP in improving mood, without the confound of physical symptoms. The reliability and validity of the POMS have been demonstrated in numerous studies in a variety of normal as well as chronically ill populations [29–31].

2.2.5. Functional Outcomes of Sleep Questionnaire (FOSQ) [32].

The FOSQ was used to evaluate the specific impact of excessive sleepiness or tiredness on multiple activities of everyday living. A total score can be generated from five factors including activity level, vigilance, intimacy, sexual relationships, general productivity, and social outcome. The FOSQ has been found to be capable of discriminating between normal participants and untreated sleep apnea patients [32]. It has very high content validity, test-retest reliability ($r = 0.91$), and internal consistency (Cronbach's alpha = 0.96). A total score of less than 18 is considered as clinically significant [23]. Participants were asked to fill out the questionnaires according to their current condition and then their condition before using CPAP. This is the "Then-Test" approach designed to eliminate treatment-induced response-shift effects and used to provide an unconfounded indication of treatment effects [33].

2.3. Data Analytical Strategies.

Significant improvements in PSG variables, daytime sleepiness, and subjective sleep quality were reported in Lau et al. [19]. In the current study, we first assessed the posttreatment changes in functional outcomes in the OSA group using paired sample t-test. To understand the clinical significance of the changes, the percentages of patients and healthy controls whose scores were in the clinical range also were compared using chi-square analyses. Between-group independent t-tests were used to compare the scores of the OSA group and healthy controls on sleepiness (ESS), sleep quality (PSQI), and on psychosocial outcomes, namely, mood (BDI, POMS) and daytime functioning (FOSQ).

To explore the predictors of patients' psychosocial outcomes, mood measures (BDI, POMS), and subjective daytime functioning (FOSQ) were regressed on predictors, including age, BMI, diagnostic RDI, diagnostic minimum SpO$_2$, posttreatment sleep efficiency, current sleepiness (ESS), and subjective sleep quality (PSQI) using stepwise regression procedures.

Due to the number of analyses, a significance level of .01 was used for all between-group comparisons to control for Type I error. Significance level for regression analyses was set at .05 due to their exploratory nature.

3. Results

3.1. Participants' Characteristics.

Participants' characteristics and the OSA group's clinical information were reported by Lau et al. [19] and summarized in Table 1. Briefly, the two groups were of comparable age and education level but as expected, the mean BMI of the OSA group was significantly higher than that of the control group, and the gender ratio differed between the two groups with more males in the OSA group and more females in the control group.

3.2. Effects of CPAP Treatment on Nighttime Sleep, Daytime Sleepiness, and Functional Outcomes.

Significant improvements on respiratory and oxygen saturation indices (RDI, minimum SpO$_2$, and mean SpO$_2$), sleepiness (ESS), and sleep quality (PSQI) were reported by Lau et al. [19] and briefly reported in Table 1. There were also significant posttreatment improvements in functional outcomes (FOSQ), $t = 7.64$ (32), $P < .000$, and $d = 0.91$. For measures that have established clinical cut-offs, the percentage of individuals of the OSA

TABLE 1: Participants' characteristics and OSA group CPAP treatment information.

	OSA before CPAP (A) (n = 37)	OSA after CPAP (B) (n = 37)	Controls (C) (n = 27)	A versus B t (df)	B versus C t (df)
Age (years)		57.9 (9.5)[a]	56.7 (10.5)		0.48 (62)
Sex (F : M)		15 : 22	19 : 8		
Education (years)		15.1 (3.6)	15.7 (3.2)		0.61 (62)
Body mass index (BMI)		33.5 (7.4)	25.5 (5.0)		4.83 (62)***
Time since diagnosis of OSA (months)		25.6 (21.1)			
Duration of CPAP treatment (months)		17.8 (11.4)			
Usage of CPAP per week (hours)		51.4 (6.7)			
CPAP compliance[b]		96.1 (5.6)			
Respiratory disturbance index (RDI)	42.2 (24.9)	1.7 (1.5)	4.0 (3.4)	9.52 (32)***	3.25 (62)**
Minimum oxygen saturation (min SpO2)	80.2 (9.8)	90.3 (3.6)	88.6 (3.3)	5.61 (27)***	1.90 (60)
Mean oxygen saturation (mean SpO2)	93.7 (3.5)	95.7 (1.6)	95.7 (0.9)	3.17 (29)**	0.10 (62)
Epworth Sleepiness Scale (ESS)	14.4 (5.2)	8.3 (4.5)	6.6 (4.7)	7.52 (36)***	1.48 (62)
Pittsburg Sleep Quality Index—global score	8.5 (3.3)	4.4 (2.4)	4.6 (2.8)	5.85 (27)***	0.20 (62)

CPAP: continuous positive airway pressure.
[a] Mean (SD).
[b] CPAP compliance is defined as percentage of days with usage >4 hours in the last 3 months. Compliance was determined objectively by downloading data from the built-in smart card of the CPAP machines for 73% of the participants. Self-report of usage was used for the rest of the participants whose machines were not equipped with a smart card.
** $P < .01$, *** $P < .001$.

group and that of the control group passing the thresholds for the clinically problematic range are shown in Figure 1. Overall, there were large reductions in the percentages of individuals with OSA in the clinically significant range on ESS, PSQI, and FOSQ after CPAP treatment. However, 30% of the posttreatment OSA group still reported excessive daytime sleepiness, twice the percentage in the healthy control group. Also, 43% of OSA group (posttreatment) had significant problems in functional outcomes, as compared to 33% of the controls. These differences in the percentages of clinically significant scores between the two groups were not statistically significant using chi-square analyses, however.

3.3. Comparisons between Treated OSA Group and Healthy Controls on Sleep and Psychosocial Outcomes.

Results of the between-group comparisons are summarized in Table 2. There was a trend for a difference between the two groups in the component score of daytime dysfunction on the PSQI, $t(62) = 2.14$, $P = .036$, with the OSA group reporting more sleep-related daytime dysfunction than the controls did.

No significant differences between the two groups were detected on the two mood measures, BDI and POMS. On the BDI, 5% of patients (versus none in the control group) showed an elevated score in the mild range (14–19). In the FOSQ, the only difference found was on the FOSQ subscale of "activity level," with the OSA group having a lower activity level than controls, $t(62) = 3.00$, $P < .01$.

3.4. Predictors of Psychosocial Outcomes in Treated OSA Group

3.4.1. Emotional Functioning.

BDI was predicted by posttreatment ESS score, with sleepier patients having a higher level of depressive symptoms (Table 3). Posttreatment ESS also predicted POMS-total score, with worse affective states associated with sleepiness. To delineate the affective versus the physical components underlying mood states, individual subscales of POMS were regressed on the same set of variables (Table 4). Posttreatment ESS predicted all subscales except for vigor activity, which was predicted by PSQI, with poorer sleep quality associated with lower vigor activity. In addition to ESS, BMI also predicted fatigue inertia, with higher BMI associated with worse fatigue inertia. To investigate whether these associations apply also to the control group, post hoc analyses on the correlations between ESS scores with BDI and POMS were conducted. Significant correlation between ESS and POMS was found in the control group (total score— $r = .57$, $P < .01$, tension anxiety— $r = .40$, $P < .05$, depression dejection— $r = .53$, $P < .01$, fatigue inertia— $r = .69$, $P < .001$).

3.4.2. Functional Outcomes.

Posttreatment FOSQ—total score was predicted by posttreatment ESS score and posttreatment PSQI—global score. Better functional outcomes were associated with less sleepiness and better sleep quality (Table 5). FOSQ—activity level was associated with lower scores on the ESS, lower scores on the PSQI, and older age. FOSQ—vigilance was associated with lower ESS scores.

TABLE 2: Comparison between the OSA group treated with CPAP and the control group in sleep and mood questionnaires.

	OSA ($n = 37$)	Controls ($n = 27$)	t (df = 62)	P	d
Epworth sleepiness scale (ESS)	8.3 (4.5)[a]	6.6 (4.7)	1.48	.144	0.38
Pittsburg sleep quality index (PSQI)					
Global score	4.4 (2.4)	4.6 (2.8)	0.29	.776	0.08
Subjective sleep quality	0.7 (0.6)	0.8 (0.7)	0.64	.526	0.17
Sleep latency	0.4 (0.6)	0.7 (0.6)	1.87	.066	0.50
Sleep duration	0.6 (0.8)	0.6 (0.7)	0.15	.880	0
Habitual sleep efficiency	0.3 (0.7)	0.6 (0.9)	1.38	.173	0.43
Sleep disturbances	1.2 (0.5)	1.2 (0.5)	0.47	.641	0
Use of sleep medication	0.2 (0.6)	0.1 (0.5)	0.29	.771	0.17
Daytime dysfunction	0.9 (0.7)	0.6 (0.6)	2.14	.036*	0.43
Beck Depression Inventory (BDI)	2.8 (4.7)[a]	2.9 (2.4)	0.01	.989	0.02
Profile of Mood States (POMS)					
Global score	67.4 (24.0)	60.3 (18.2)	1.29	.204	0.30
Tension anxiety	6.1 (5.0)	5.0 (4.7)	0.89	.375	0.22
Depression dejection	5.0 (7.1)	5.2 (6.1)	0.11	.913	0.03
Anger hostility	4.7 (6.2)	3.7 (4.0)	0.74	.465	0.16
Vigor activity	17.5 (6.7)	19.0 (5.2)	0.96	.342	0.22
Fatigue inertia	7.4 (6.2)	4.7 (4.9)	1.89	.064	0.44
Confusion bewilderment	6.2 (4.6)	5.3 (4.5)	0.78	.436	0.20
Functional Outcomes of Sleep Questionnaire (FOSQ)					
Total score	17.6 (2.2)	18.4 (1.5)	1.61	.113	0.36
Activity level	3.3 (0.6)	3.7 (0.3)	2.99	.004**	0.67
Vigilance	3.4 (0.5)	3.5 (0.5)	0.96	.341	0.20
Intimacy	3.6 (0.6)	3.8 (0.5)	1.04	.304	0.33
General productivity	3.6 (0.5)	3.8 (0.3)	1.48	.143	0.40
Social outcome	3.7 (0.5)	3.7 (0.5)	0.06	.953	0

Higher scores indicate more difficulties in all questionnaires, except for FOSQ.
[a]Mean (SD); *$P < .05$; **$P < .01$.

FOSQ—intimate relationships and sexual activity, general productivity, and social outcomes were all associated with lower PSQI scores. These associations were not found in the control group.

4. Discussion

This study aimed at elucidating the role of daytime sleepiness in psychosocial outcomes of individuals with OSA treated with CPAP. Pre- and posttreatment comparisons on subjective sleep quality (PSQI), daytime sleepiness (ESS), and functional outcomes (FOSQ) revealed significant improvements, consistent with findings of some previous studies [13, 15, 34].

4.1. Is Daytime Sleepiness an Issue in Stably Treated Individuals with OSA? The percentage of individuals in the OSA group with self-reports of pathological sleepiness dropped from 76% to 30% after treatment, with a significant mean change of 6.1 (c.f. the reliable change index score of 5.9 [26] and consistent with the mean reduction of 4.75 points as reported by a comprehensive review [35]). It could be concluded that sleepiness was significantly reduced in the OSA group after CPAP treatment, although one-third of individuals continued to show excessive sleepiness during

the day (compared to 15% of controls). Given that sleepiness was found to consistently predict psychosocial outcomes in this study, the question of what predicts residual sleepiness in treated individuals with OSA is relevant. No significant predictors of posttreatment ESS scores were identified in post hoc analyses. We also investigated the potential causes as suggested by Santamaria et al. [35], including inadequate CPAP treatment or titration, insufficient sleep, depression, or other sleep disorders. Issues with compliance or titration were unlikely to be the culprit as our study participants had good compliance and titration level was deemed suitable as validated by PSG. In addition, mean hours of CPAP usage were not correlated with ESS scores ($r = -.259$, $P = .122$). With regards to sleep restriction, ESS scores were also not correlated with sleep duration in either the OSA group or the control group. Other sleep pathologies were ruled out by PSG as well. There was an association between ESS scores and BDI scores, but it could not be concluded that the residual sleepiness was related to depression as the mean BDI score was well within the normal range (details discussed below). With the lack of statistical difference in self-reported sleepiness between the two groups, one could argue that the sleepiness in the OSA group could just be a normal age-related phenomenon. To investigate the potential aging

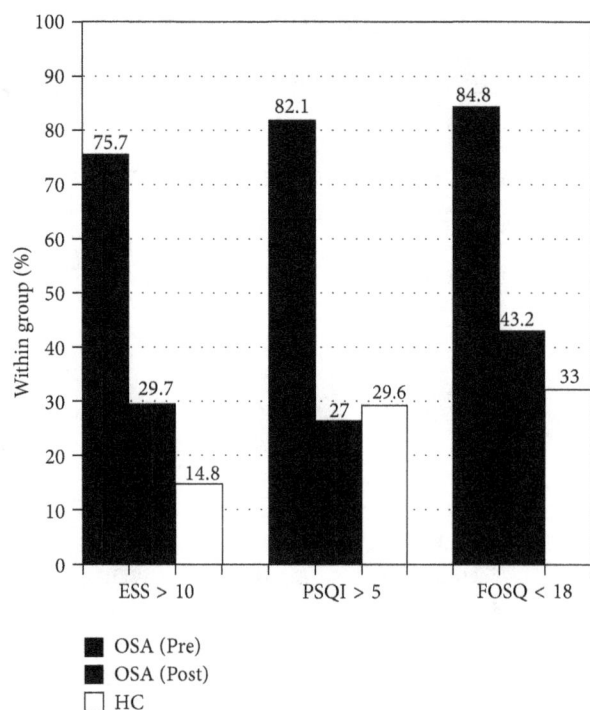

FIGURE 1: Percentages of participants with OSA pre- and post-treatment and of controls scoring in the clinically significant range on the Epworth Sleepiness Scale (ESS), Pittsburg Sleep Quality Index (PSQI—global score), and Functional Outcomes of Sleep Questionnaire (FOSQ—total score).

TABLE 3: Prediction of psychosocial outcomes in participants with OSA treated with CPAP using stepwise regression.

Predictors	BDI	POMS	FOSQ
ESS (post)			
β	0.45	0.54	−0.42
ΔR^2	.20	.29	.29
t (df)	2.59 (27)	3.33 (27)	−2.67 (26)
P	.015	.002	0.013
PSQI (post)			
β			−.37
ΔR^2			0.13
t (df)			−2.36 (26)
P			.026
Model R^2	.20	.29	.42
Adjusted R^2	.17	.27	.37
F (df)	6.71 (1, 27)	11.12 (1, 27)	9.31 (2, 26)
P	.015	.002	.001

Nonsignificant predictor variables including age, education, diagnostic respiratory disturbance index (RDI), diagnostic peripheral oxygen saturation (SpO$_2$), and post-treatment sleep efficiency are not shown in the table.
ESS: Epworth Sleepiness Scale; PSQI: Pittsburg Sleep Quality Index; BDI: Beck Depression Inventory; POMS: Profile of Mood States; FOSQ: Functional Outcomes of Sleep Questionnaire.

effects on sleepiness, the percentage of OSA group with an ESS score above 2 standard deviations of the mean of the control group was calculated. 45.9% and 5.4% of the OSA group (pre- and posttreatment) were found to have ESS scores above this age-corrected cut-off (16/17). These percentages are much less than those generated with the original cut-off score, which was based on a group of 72 healthy individuals in the age range of 22 to 59 [36]. Taken together, the sleepiness as shown in the OSA group posttreatment may not be much more than what one may expect from a healthy person in his/her 50s. Nevertheless, given the predictive power of posttreatment ESS on psychosocial outcomes in the OSA group found in this study, in addition to the rich literature on the associations between daytime somnolence and various health variables such as high blood pressure, obesity, coronary artery disease, and cerebrovascular disease [37, 38], which are very common in individuals with OSA, the issue of excessive sleepiness undoubtedly deserves more attention in this medically vulnerable group of patients. Optimizing treatment for individual patients whose excessive daytime sleepiness persists with compliant CPAP usage focusing on strategies for reducing and managing sleepiness is needed.

4.2. Are Sleep Quality, Functional Outcomes, and Psychosocial Outcomes Problems for Stably Treated OSA Individuals? A similar pattern of findings was shown in self-reported sleep quality, as the proportion of poor sleepers fell from 82% before treatment to 27% after treatment in the OSA group, as compared to 30% in the control group. As patients and controls did not differ on the PSQI (except for the trend for the OSA group having worse daytime dysfunction, which essentially taps into sleepiness), and the two groups were mostly comparable on PSG measures, it could be concluded that sleep quality of the OSA group was largely normalized.

No significant differences between the two groups were detected on the two mood measures, BDI and POMS. The percentages of people with clinical level of depressive symptoms were also comparable between individuals with OSA treated with CPAP and controls. These findings are in contrast with those reported by Vernet et al. in their recent study [4] as their healthy controls and treated OSA groups with and without residual sleepiness had higher BDI scores than our participants, ranging from 20 to 70% having elevated scores (adopted cut-off: >12), as compared to 0% and 8% in our control and OSA groups, respectively. These differences suggest that variability in psychosocial functioning across different patient samples may be noteworthy even when inclusion/exclusion criteria are similar. In view of the gender ratio difference between the two groups, BDI and POMS scores were regressed on gender in order to investigate the potential contribution of gender on mood or symptom reporting. Gender did not predict any mood measures ($P > .05$).

There was a trend toward individuals with OSA to have a reduced energy level even after treatment with CPAP, seen on subscales from both the POMS and the FOSQ. Thus, individuals with OSA seemed to continue to have a compromised level of energy and activity level after CPAP treatment. While exercise programs implemented in patients with untreated OSA have been found to be effective in reducing fatigue and depressive symptoms [39], such interventions should also be

TABLE 4: Prediction of Profile of Mood States subscales in participants with OSA treated with CPAP using stepwise regression.

Predictors	Tension anxiety	Depression dejection	Anger hostility	Vigor activity	Fatigue inertia	Confusion bewilderment
BMI						
β					0.38	
ΔR^2					.14	
t (df)					3.06 (26)	
P					.005	
ESS (post)						
β	0.48	0.39	0.46		0.47	0.47
ΔR^2	.23	.16	.21		.27	0.22
t (df)	2.83 (27)	2.23 (27)	2.70 (27)		3.06 (26)	2.78 (27)
P	.009	.035	.012		.005	.010
PSQI (post)						
β				−0.58		
ΔR^2				.33		
t (df)				−3.66 (27)		
P				.001		
Model R^2	.23	.15	.22	.33	.41	.22
Adjusted R^2	.20	.12	.18	.31	.37	.19
F (df)	7.99 (1, 27)	4.95 (1, 27)	7.28 (1, 27)	13.39 (1, 27)	9.14 (2, 26)	7.70 (1,27)
P	.009	.035	.012	.001	.001	.010

Nonsignificant predictor variables including age, education, diagnostic respiratory disturbance index (RDI), diagnostic peripheral oxygen saturation (SpO_2), and post-treatment sleep efficiency are not shown in the table.
BMI: body mass index; ESS: Epworth sleepiness scale; PSQI: Pittsburg sleep quality index.

TABLE 5: Prediction of Functional Outcomes of Sleep Questionnaire subscales in participants with OSA treated with CPAP using stepwise regression.

Predictors	Activity level	Vigilance	Intimate relationships	General productivity	Social outcomes
Age					
β	0.33				
ΔR^2	.12				
t (df)	2.31 (25)				
P	.030				
ESS (post)					
β	−0.032	−0.66			
ΔR^2	.09	.43			
t (df)	−2.12 (25)	−4.52 (25)	−2.30 (23)		
P	.044	.000	.031		
PSQI (post)					
β	−0.43			−0.40	−0.16
ΔR^2	.28			.16	0.37
t (df)	−2.86 (25)			−2.28 (27)	−3.95 (27)
P	.009			.031	.001
Model R^2	.49	.43	.19	.43	.37
Adjusted R^2	.43	.41	.15	.41	.34
F (df)	8.13 (3, 25)	20.41 (1, 27)	5.29 (1, 23)	20.41 (1, 27)	15.61 (1, 27)
P	.001	.000	.031	.000	.001

Non-significant predictor variables including education, diagnostic respiratory disturbance index (RDI), diagnostic peripheral oxygen saturation (SpO_2), and post-treatment sleep-efficiency are not shown in the table.
ESS: Epworth sleepiness scale; PSQI: Pittsburg sleep quality index.

considered for OSA-treated individuals with reduced energy level.

4.3. Predictors of Psychosocial Outcomes in Treated OSA Group.

Our data showed that self-reported sleepiness was a potent predictor of mood and functional outcomes, while subjective sleep quality predicted functional outcomes. Age was found to be a significant predictor of activity level, while BMI was associated with fatigue.

4.3.1. Emotional Functioning.

While the mean level of depressive symptoms (2.8) endorsed by patients on the BDI was well within the minimal range (i.e., 0 to 13) and the percentage of patients with BDI scores higher than the clinical cut-off was only 5%, our data showed that patients' mood was still associated with their daytime sleepiness. Our findings did not directly address the question regarding the association of OSA and mood as there was no pre-treatment mood measure. Nevertheless, the finding that mood was predicted by sleepiness suggests a relationship between daytime sleepiness associated with OSA and mood. This relationship is in keeping with the Wisconsin Sleep Cohort Study [7], which demonstrated a causal link between OSA and depression, although the current study does not address the directionality of the relationship. Significant correlations between ESS and POMS scores in the control group highlight the importance of daytime sleepiness in emotional functioning in a broad sense, above and beyond the OSA illness.

Several studies reported a lack of correlation between OSA and psychological functioning [40–42]. Some authors argue that sleepiness and fatigue are misinterpreted as depression [8], and yet others suggest that links between mood and OSA dissipate after controlling for covariates such as age, BMI, and hypertension in the analyses [9]. In this study, age and BMI were not significant predictors of BDI scores, suggesting that the association of sleepiness and mood is independent of these factors. In regard to the argument that sleepiness and fatigue in patients with OSA are misinterpreted as mood symptoms, our findings on the POMS may offer some insight. The total score and subscale scores separate out somatic symptoms (vigor, fatigue) from affective symptoms (anxiety, depression). We found that sleepiness (ESS) was associated with five of the six subscales, namely, tension anxiety, depression dejection, anger hostility, fatigue inertia, and confusion bewilderment, and, interestingly, not with vigor activity. The relationships with all the affective subscales, but not a physical scale (vigor activity), may suggest that the mood symptoms and their associations with sleepiness in patients with OSA are separable from the manifestations of fatigue.

4.3.2. Functional Outcomes.

Better functional outcomes were associated with less sleepiness and better subjective sleep quality; specifically, sleepiness predicted activity level and vigilance, while sleep quality predicted intimate relationships and sexual activity, general productivity, social outcome, and activity level. These findings concur with the finding that sleep quality is an independent predictor of daytime fatigue in untreated OSA [43]. Taken together and consistent with the findings on mood, current sleepiness and sleep quality play a crucial role in daytime functioning of individuals generally classified as "well treated." These relationships are not found in the healthy control group, despite the fact that the two groups seem to have comparable sleep quality, suggesting that the impact of the same level of quality of sleep may be different for individuals with and without a history of OSA and that there may be some specific factors that make an individual with OSA more susceptible to the adverse effects of poor sleep even after their OSA is well controlled by CPAP.

5. Conclusions

Previous studies of psychosocial functioning of individuals with OSA usually adopt one instrument to study one aspect of emotional functioning. We included multiple instruments for measuring mood and functional outcomes to more fully understand how OSA impacts the daily living of an individual who is compliant to the standard treatment of CPAP. Predictors of posttreatment psychosocial outcomes have not been adequately studied, and this study offers some preliminary evidence for future studies to build on; even though our sample size was only moderate, not many predictors could be included. Other caveats of this study were the baseline differences between gender ratio and the BMI of the two groups, although gender did not predict any outcomes and BMI was only associated with fatigue.

As found in this study, daytime sleepiness and subjective sleep quality are important predictors of functional outcomes and mood. It is pivotal to explore specific strategies targeting such factors [44]. For example, it would be valuable to study how interventions like sleep hygiene education and lifestyle management (e.g., controlling tobacco and alcohol use, weight control) affect sleep quality and daytime sleepiness and the respective impact on daytime functioning and emotional functioning. As most of these interventions as well as the CPAP usage itself involve drastic behavioral changes and adaptations, motivational interviewing techniques could be a valuable component in inducing and maintaining changes in OSA patients with persistent problems in sleep and psychosocial functioning [45].

Acknowledgments

This study was conducted at the Queen Elizabeth II Health Sciences Centre, Halifax, NS, Canada. This study was funded by a Health Research Project Grant from the Nova Scotia Health Research Foundation. These data form part of a doctoral thesis submitted by E. Y. Y. Lau. The authors are grateful to Drs. Ben Rusak, Ray Klein, and Penny Corkum for their comments on the original thesis. They appreciate the assistance of the sleep technologists at the Capital Health Sleep Disorders Laboratory with conducting and scoring sleep studies. E. Y. Y. Lau was supported by the Sir Edward Youde Memorial Overseas Fellowship, and G. A. Eskes was supported by a Dalhousie Faculty of Medicine Clinical Research Scholar Award. D. L. Morrison provides paid service to Vital Aire for reporting level III cardiorespiratory home studies. We would like to thank the anonymous reviewers and the editor, Dr. Marco Zucconi for their helpful comments on the manuscript.

References

[1] C. Guilleminault and A. G. Bassiri, "Clinical features and evaluation of obstructive sleep apnea-hypopnea syndrome and the upper airway resistance syndrome," in *Principles and Practice of Sleep Medicine*, M. H. Kryger, T. Roth, and W. C. Dement, Eds., pp. 1043–1052, Elsevier Saunders, Philadelphia, Pa, USA, 2005.

[2] H. M. Engleman and N. J. Douglas, "Sleep 4: sleepiness, cognitive function, and quality of life in obstructive apnoea/hypopnoea syndrome," *Thorax*, vol. 59, no. 7, pp. 618–622, 2004.

[3] M. Nowak, J. Kornhuber, and R. Meyrer, "Daytime impairment and neurodegeneration in OSAS," *Sleep*, vol. 29, no. 12, pp. 1521–1530, 2006.

[4] C. Vernet, S. Redolfi, V. Attali et al., "Residual sleepiness in obstructive sleep apnoea: phenotype and related symptoms," *European Respiratory Journal*, vol. 38, no. 1, pp. 98–105, 2011.

[5] M. M. Ohayon, "The effects of breathing-related sleep disorders on mood disturbances in the general population," *Journal of Clinical Psychiatry*, vol. 64, pp. 1195–1200, 2003.

[6] S. Mosko, M. Zetin, S. Glen et al., "Self-reported depressive symptomatology, mood ratings, and treatment outcome in sleep disorders patients," *Journal of Clinical Psychology*, vol. 45, no. 1, pp. 51–60, 1989.

[7] P. E. Peppard, M. Szklo-Coxe, K. M. Hla, and T. Young, "Longitudinal association of sleep-related breathing disorder and depression," *Archives of Internal Medicine*, vol. 166, no. 16, pp. 1709–1715, 2006.

[8] W. Cassel, "Sleep apnea and personality," *Sleep*, vol. 16, no. 8, pp. S56–S58, 1993.

[9] W. A. Bardwell, C. C. Berry, S. Ancoli-Israel, and J. E. Dimsdale, "Psychological correlates of sleep apnea," *Journal of Psychosomatic Research*, vol. 47, no. 6, pp. 583–596, 1999.

[10] K. Cheshire, H. Engleman, I. Deary, C. Shapiro, and N. J. Douglas, "Factors impairing daytime performance in patients with sleep apnea/hypopnea syndrome," *Archives of Internal Medicine*, vol. 152, no. 3, pp. 538–541, 1992.

[11] W. Yue, W. Hao, P. Liu, T. Liu, M. Ni, and Q. Guo, "A case-control study on psychological symptoms in sleep apnea-hypopnea syndrome," *Canadian Journal of Psychiatry*, vol. 48, no. 5, pp. 318–323, 2003.

[12] S. E. Martin, H. M. Engleman, I. J. Deary, and N. J. Douglas, "The effect of sleep fragmentation on daytime function," *American Journal of Respiratory and Critical Care Medicine*, vol. 153, no. 4, pp. 1328–1332, 1996.

[13] S. R. Patel, D. P. White, A. Malhotra, M. L. Stanchina, and N. T. Ayas, "Continuous positive airway pressure therapy for treating sleepiness in a diverse population with obstructive sleep apnea results of a meta-analysis," *Archives of Internal Medicine*, vol. 163, no. 5, pp. 565–571, 2003.

[14] Y. Nussbaumer, K. E. Bloch, T. Genser, and R. Thurnheer, "Equivalence of autoadjusted and constant continuous positive airway pressure in home treatment of sleep apnea," *Chest*, vol. 129, no. 3, pp. 638–643, 2006.

[15] A. I. Sánchez, G. Buela-Casal, M. P. Bermúdez, and F. Casas-Maldonado, "The effects of continuous positive air pressure treatment on anxiety and depression levels in apnea patients," *Psychiatry and Clinical Neurosciences*, vol. 55, no. 6, pp. 641–646, 2001.

[16] H. M. Engleman, R. N. Kingshott, P. K. Wraith, T. W. Mackay, I. J. Deary, and N. J. Douglas, "Randomized placebo-controlled crossover trial of continuous positive airway pressure for mild sleep apnea/hypopnea syndrome," *American Journal of Respiratory and Critical Care Medicine*, vol. 159, no. 2, pp. 461–467, 1999.

[17] M. Barnes, D. Houston, C. J. Worsnop et al., "A randomized controlled trial of continuous positive airway pressure in mild obstructive sleep apnea," *American Journal of Respiratory and Critical Care Medicine*, vol. 165, no. 6, pp. 773–780, 2002.

[18] M. J. Sateia, "Neuropsychological impairment and quality of life in obstructive sleep apnea," *Clinics in Chest Medicine*, vol. 24, no. 2, pp. 249–259, 2003.

[19] E. Y. Y. Lau, G. A. Eskes, D. L. Morrison, M. Rajda, and K. F. Spurr, "Executive function in patients with obstructive sleep apnea treated with continuous positive airway pressure," *Journal of the International Neuropsychological Society*, vol. 16, no. 6, pp. 1077–1088, 2010.

[20] A. Rechtschaffen and A. Kales, *A Manual of Standardized Terminology, Techniques and Scoring System for Sleep Stages of Human Subjects*, UCLA Brain Information Service/Brain Research Institute, Los Angeles, Calif, USA, 1968.

[21] M. W. Johns, "A new method for measuring daytime sleepiness: the Epworth sleepiness scale," *Sleep*, vol. 14, no. 6, pp. 540–545, 1991.

[22] M. W. Johns, "Reliability and factor analysis of the Epworth Sleepiness Scale," *Sleep*, vol. 15, no. 4, pp. 376–381, 1992.

[23] N. Hartenbaum, N. Collop, I. M. Rosen et al., "Sleep apnea and commercial motor vehicle operators: statement from the Joint Task Force of the American College of Chest Physicians, the American College of Occupational and Environmental Medicine, and the National Sleep Foundation," *Chest*, vol. 130, no. 3, pp. 902–905, 2006.

[24] F. M. Hardinge, D. J. Pitson, and J. R. Stradling, "Use of the Epworth Sleepiness Scale to demonstrate response to treatment with nasal continuous positive airways pressure in patients with obstructive sleep apnoea," *Respiratory Medicine*, vol. 89, no. 9, pp. 617–620, 1995.

[25] M. W. Johns, "Daytime sleepiness, snoring, and obstructive sleep apnea; The Epworth Sleepiness Scale," *Chest*, vol. 103, no. 1, pp. 30–36, 1993.

[26] S. Smith and K. A. Sullivan, "A reliable change index (RCI) for the Epworth sleepiness scale (ESS)," *Sleep Medicine*, vol. 9, no. 1, p. 102, 2007.

[27] D. J. Buysse, C. F. Reynolds, T. H. Monk, S. R. Berman, and D. J. Kupfer, "The Pittsburgh Sleep Quality Index: a new instrument for psychiatric practice and research," *Psychiatry Research*, vol. 28, no. 2, pp. 193–213, 1989.

[28] A. T. Beck, *Beck Depression Inventory*, The Psychological Corporation, San Antonio, Tex, USA, 1987.

[29] D. M. McNair, M. Lorr, and L. F. Druppleman, *EITS Manual for the Profile of Mood States*, Education and Industrial Test Services, San Diego, Calif, USA, 1971.

[30] W. A. Bardwell, S. Ancoli-Israel, and J. E. Dimsdale, "Comparison of the effects of depressive symptoms and apnea severity on fatigue in patients with obstructive sleep apnea: a replication study," *Journal of Affective Disorders*, vol. 97, no. 1–3, pp. 181–186, 2007.

[31] B.-H. Yu, S. Ancoli-Israel, and J. E. Dimsdale, "Effect of CPAP treatment on mood states in patients with sleep apnea," *Journal of Psychiatric Research*, vol. 33, no. 5, pp. 427–432, 1999.

[32] T. E. Weaver, A. M. Laizner, L. K. Evans et al., "An instrument to measure functional status outcomes for disorders of excessive sleepiness," *Sleep*, vol. 20, no. 10, pp. 835–843, 1997.

[33] M. R. M. Visser, F. J. Oort, and M. A. G. Sprangers, "Methods to detect response shift in quality of life data: a convergent validity study," *Quality of Life Research*, vol. 14, no. 3, pp. 629–639, 2005.

[34] M. J. Ramos Platón and J. Espinar Sierra, "Changes in psychopathological symptoms in sleep apnea patients after treatment with nasal continuous positive airway pressure," *International Journal of Neuroscience*, vol. 62, no. 3-4, pp. 173–195, 1992.

[35] J. Santamaria, A. Iranzo, J. Ma Montserrat, and J. de Pablo, "Persistent sleepiness in CPAP treated obstructive sleep apnea patients: evaluation and treatment," *Sleep Medicine Reviews*, vol. 11, no. 3, pp. 195–207, 2007.

[36] M. W. Johns, "Sensitivity and specificity of the multiple sleep latency test (MSLT), the maintenance of wakefulness test and the Epworth sleepiness scale: failure of the MSLT as a gold standard," *Journal of Sleep Research*, vol. 9, no. 1, pp. 5–11, 2000.

[37] J. Feng, Q. Y. He, X. L. Zhang, and B. Y. Chen, "Epworth Sleepiness Scale may be an indicator for blood pressure profile and prevalence of coronary artery disease and cerebrovascular disease in patients with obstructive sleep apnea," *Sleep and Breathing*, vol. 16, no. 1, pp. 31–40, 2011.

[38] S. M. H. A. Araujo, V. M. Bruin, E. F. Daher, C. A. Medeiros, G. H. Almeida, and P. F. Bruin, "Quality of sleep and day-time sleepiness in chronic hemodialysis: a study of 400 patients," *Scandinavian Journal of Urology and Nephrology*, vol. 45, no. 5, pp. 359–364, 2011.

[39] C. Kline, G. B. Ewing, J. B. Burch et al., "Exercise training improves selected aspects of daytime functioning in adults with obstructive sleep apnea," *Journal of Clinical Sleep Medicine*, vol. 8, no. 4, pp. 357–365, 2012.

[40] S. Lee, "Depression in sleep apnea: a different view," *Journal of Clinical Psychiatry*, vol. 51, no. 7, pp. 309–310, 1990.

[41] B. A. Phillips, D. T. R. Berry, and T. C. Lipke-Molby, "Sleep-disordered breathing in healthy, aged persons: fifth and final year follow-up," *Chest*, vol. 110, no. 3, pp. 654–658, 1996.

[42] G. Pillar and P. Lavie, "Psychiatric symptoms in sleep apnea syndrome: effects of gender and respiratory disturbance index," *Chest*, vol. 114, no. 3, pp. 697–703, 1998.

[43] C. J. Stepnowsky, J. J. Palau, T. Zamora, S. Ancoli-Israel, and J. S. Loredo, "Fatigue in sleep apnea: the role fo depressive symptoms and self-reported sleep quality," *Sleep Medicine*, vol. 12, no. 9, pp. 832–837, 2011.

[44] A. I. Sánchez, P. Martínez, E. Miró, W. A. Bardwell, and G. Buela-Casal, "CPAP and behavioral therapies in patients with obstructive sleep apnea: effects on daytime sleepiness, mood, and cognitive function," *Sleep Medicine Reviews*, vol. 13, no. 3, pp. 223–233, 2009.

[45] S. Rollnick, W. R. Miller, and C. C. Butler, *Motivational Interviewing in Health Care: Helping Patients Change Behavior*, Guilford Press, 2008.

5

Trait Hostility, Perceived Stress, and Sleep Quality in a Sample of Normal Sleepers

Nicholas D. Taylor,[1] Gary D. Fireman,[1] and Ross Levin[2]

[1] *Psychology Department, Suffolk University, 41 Temple Street, Boston, MA 02114, USA*
[2] *Independent Practice, 25 West 86th Street No. 3, New York, NY 10024, USA*

Correspondence should be addressed to Nicholas D. Taylor; taylornd55@gmail.com

Academic Editor: Giora Pillar

Objective. To date, no studies have directly examined the effects of cognitive trait hostility on prospectively assessed sleep quality. This is important as individuals with heightened trait hostility demonstrate similar patterns of reactivity to perceived stressors as is often reported by poor sleepers. The present study hypothesized that increased trait hostility is associated with poorer subjective sleep quality and that perceived stress mediates this relationship. *Methods.* A sample of 66 normal sleepers completed daily sleep and stress logs for two weeks. Trait hostility was measured retrospectively. *Results.* The cognitive dimension of trait hostility was significantly correlated with subjectively rated sleep quality indicators, and these relationships were significantly mediated by perceived daily stress. Individuals with higher levels of trait cognitive hostility reported increased levels of perceived stress which accounted for their poorer sleep ratings as measured by both retrospective and prospective measures. *Conclusions.* Overall, the findings indicate that high levels of cognitive hostility are a significant risk factor for disturbed sleep and suggest that this might be a fruitful target for clinical intervention.

1. Introduction

The relationship between trait hostility and sleep quality remains underexplored despite the empirical indications that individuals with increased hostility experience more stress, a factor known to degrade sleep quality [1–4]. Despite its widespread use as an outcome variable, there is no standard definition for sleep quality. Investigators frequently use both objective measures, such as total sleep duration, efficiency, and sleep onset latency, as well as subjective self-report measures to assess sleep quality [5]. While a number of variables can influence one's day-to-day sleep outcomes, stress is strongly associated with sleep disruption [1, 6]. Stress is thought to act on sleep primarily via increased cognitive and somatic arousal during the presleep period [7]. In a recent study, Morin et al. [6] confirmed that hyperarousal during the presleep period mediates the relationship between stress and sleep quality in normal and disordered sleepers alike. The study suggests that individual variation in stress reactivity determines the extent to which stress degrades sleep quality. Consistent with this finding, studies have demonstrated that

poor sleepers are characteristically hyperreactive to stress [1, 2, 6, 8].

Pronounced stress reactions are characteristic of individuals who score highly on measures of trait hostility [3]. The trait hostility construct is organized into three major components: cognitive, affective, and behavioral [9]. The cognitive components, cynicism and hostile attribution, reflect the extent to which negative beliefs about others are held and a tendency to interpret the antagonistic behavior of others as expressly directed at the self. The affective component of hostility consists of the tendency to experience several negative emotions including anger, annoyance, resentment, disgust, and contempt. The behavioral component of hostility reflects an individual's tendency to act aggressively. While the three components of hostility are interrelated, one does not necessitate the presence of the other, and measures of hostility that incorporate all three components often find only moderate intercorrelations [9].

Numerous studies [3, 10, 11] have found that individuals who report higher levels of trait hostility are highly reactive to and slower to recover from interpersonal stress. Although preliminary evidence suggests that individuals high in trait hostility report poorer sleep than controls [12–14], few studies have directly examined the relationship between hostility, stress, and sleep outcomes. The current study builds upon these preliminary findings by testing trait hostility's association with measures of retrospective and prospective sleep quality. Additionally, the current study examines whether the relationship between hostility and sleep quality is mediated by increased sensitivity to stress.

Stress is perhaps, the most studied psychosocial precipitant of sleep disturbance. Current models describe stress as a process with four basic aspects: the stress stimuli, perceived stress, the stress response (physiological, affective, and cognitive), and feedback from the stress response [15]. Thus, there are multiple ways in which stress may be measured, many of which address only a portion of the construct.

Observational and experimental studies link stress exposure to sleep quality, and it is widely acknowledged that stress plays a causal role in initiating sleep disruption and the onset of disordered sleeping [1, 6, 16]. However, the relationship between stress and sleep is complicated by individual variability in how intensely one experiences and responds to stress [2, 17]. The cognitive model of insomnia [7] emphasizes that some individuals are more prone to sleep disturbance and insomnia than others because of this variability in stress responding. In this model, individuals who are more affected by stress stimuli struggle with sleep because they have stronger or more frequent stress reactions and are more likely to engage in behaviors that exacerbate the impact of a stressor beyond the initial stress response, such as rumination or worry. The consequence is increased presleep arousal that is incompatible with sleep onset [7].

Morin et al. [6] tested this component of the cognitive model of insomnia. Participants completed measures of daily stress experience, presleep arousal, and sleep quality over the course of 21 days. Increased perceived stress was negatively associated with sleep quality across participants; however, poor sleepers were much more sensitive to stress events compared to normal sleepers. Poor sleepers rated major life events and daily stressors as more intense and more disruptive to their functioning than good sleepers. Further, presleep arousal mediated the relationship between stress experience and subsequent sleep quality. Consistent with the finding that poor sleepers are hyperaroused during the presleep period, poor sleepers also demonstrate signs of hyperarousal during the day [18, 19]. The findings suggest that groups that are characteristically sensitive to or more reactive to stress may also be at increased risk of sleep disturbance.

Individuals who score high on measures of trait hostility share a striking number of characteristics with poor sleepers, such as pronounced reactions to stress, increased negative affect, and ruminative tendencies which can prolong arousal following stress [8, 14, 20]. Further, trait hostility has been widely studied in connection to other outcomes related to pronounced stress and arousal, such as cardiovascular disease [4, 21, 22]. Such findings suggest that trait hostile individuals may be particularly vulnerable to stress-related-sleep disruption and the widespread consequences of poor sleep.

The psychophysiological reactivity model hypothesizes that hostile individuals experience anger more intensely and for longer periods than controls, causing more sustained and more intense activation of the sympathetic nervous system [23]. Additionally, hostility is associated with rumination, a likely mechanism through which daytime stress reactions are extended into the presleep period [24]. Empirical findings generally support the hyperreactivity hypothesis. The studies indicate that higher levels of hostility are associated with exaggerated cardiovascular reactivity (CVR) to stress [3, 11, 25] and that hostile individuals also take longer to recover from stressors compared to controls [26]. As such, a significant body of literature links hostility to pronounced stress reactions and pronounced stress reactions to poor sleep. Further, multiple studies have found associations between the behavioral and affective components of the hostility construct and sleep outcomes [10, 12, 27, 28]. Despite the relevance of stress to both sleep and hostility, research incorporating all three variables is virtually nonexistent.

To date, only one study has simultaneously examined sleep quality, hostility, and stress. Brissette and Cohen [14] examined a community sample of 47 adults over the course of 7 days. Across participants, increased interpersonal stress predicted to higher reported negative affect. This effect, however, was pronounced among individuals high in cynical hostility meaning they were more significantly impacted by conflict than other participants. Further, on days in which individuals experienced conflict, between-person differences in cynical hostility predicted the impact conflict had on sleep. This is consistent with the proposal that trait hostility influences individual reactivity to interpersonal stress, which subsequently impacts sleep quality. However, this study appeared to conflate self-report sleep duration with sleep quality and did not use a validated measure of stress, making the findings difficult to interpret and in need of replication.

Models of sleep disturbance emphasize the importance of individual differences in stress responding [7]. If individuals high in trait hostility are more reactive to stress than controls, and stress exposure is an established factor that degrades sleep quality, it follows that hostile individuals are likely to have poorer sleep compared to controls. Differences in stress responding likely mediate the relationship between trait hostility and sleep quality. This study tests these potential relationships. We hypothesize that self-reported daily sleep quality will be negatively associated with trait hostility such that poorer sleep quality will be associated with increased hostility. Second, we predict that perceived stress will be positively associated with trait hostility such that increased trait hostility will predict to increases in perceived stress. Third, we predict that stress exposure will be negatively associated with measures of sleep quality such that increased stress will predict reduced sleep quality. Finally, we predict that perceived stress will mediate any relationship between trait hostility and sleep quality.

A number of methodological improvements in the current study will extend previous work in this area. Specifically, this study utilizes multiple subscales of the Cook-Medley Hostility Scale [29] rather than the cynicism scale alone, allowing for a comparison of the cognitive components of hostility (cynicism, hostile attribution) and the behavioral component of hostility (aggressive responding). This study also utilized cross-sectional and prospective design elements over an extended time period (14 consecutive nights) to obtain more reliable estimates of perceived stress and sleep quality.

2. Method

2.1. Participants. A convenience sample of 73 undergraduate psychology students (26 men, 47 women) aged from 17 to 25 years ($M = 19.04$, SD = 1.57) was recruited from a university in the Northeast with 56 self identified as Caucasian, 3 as African American, 4 as Hispanic, 4 as Asian, 3 as mixed ethnicity, and 3 as Other Ethnicity. Individuals interested in participating signed up for the study via sign-up sheets placed in the psychology department of the university. Candidates were then contacted to ensure that they met inclusion criteria and to schedule a time to complete the initial surveys. The sample was intended to include a range of sleepers in order to generalize to the larger community, so only individuals that had a known condition affecting heart function or blood pressure, who took a medication that interfered with stress reactivity (such as benzodiazepines), or who used drugs or alcohol daily were excluded from participation. Of the original sample, 7 individuals failed to complete a minimum of ten daily surveys over the course of a two-week reporting period and were excluded from analysis for lack of sufficient data. There were no significant differences between individuals who completed the study and those lost to attrition. 92.4% of the sample completed 12 or more surveys out of a possible 14. The final sample consisted of 66 participants.

2.2. Cross-Sectional Measures

2.2.1. Demographics. This survey was created for the purposes of this investigation. It includes questions about gender, ethnic identification, living arrangements, a variety of health questions, and other health variables known to influence cardiovascular function and arousal.

2.2.2. Pittsburgh Sleep Quality Index (PSQI). The PSQI is one of the most widely used measures of subjective sleep quality. The PSQI is a retrospective, self-report inventory that asks participants to report on their subjectively experienced sleep quality and disturbances over the last month [30]. The index is composed of 19 items which compose seven component scores: subjective sleep quality, sleep latency, sleep duration, habitual sleep efficiency, sleep disturbances, use of sleep medication, and daytime dysfunction. A global score is derived by combining the composite scores and is the primary retrospective sleep quality variable used in our analysis. The index was normed with both good and poor sleepers that were slightly older than our sample (20–40 years old) and has proven useful as a clinical tool for identifying poor sleepers. Using a criterion score of five to identify poor sleepers, the sensitivity of the measure was 89.6% and specificity was reported at 86.5% (kappa = .75) [30]. In the current sample,

the average global PSQI score was 7.0 (SD = 3.13, range of 2 to 14). The scale was reverse coded for analyses to ease interpretation such that higher scores indicate better sleep.

2.2.3. Perceived Stress Scale (PSS). The PSS is a retrospective, self report measure of stress appraisal that asks about participants perceptions of stress over the previous month [31]. The scale has ten items from which a single perceived stress score is derived. This value is the primary indicator of retrospective perceived stress used in this study. Studies reporting psychometrics for the scale indicate good internal consistency ($\alpha = .84–.86$) in various samples and good test-retest reliability in a college sample ($r = .85$) [31]. The scale also demonstrates good discriminant validity with a measure of depression and daily life stress [32]. In the current sample, the scale displayed adequate internal reliability ($\alpha = .88$).

2.2.4. Cook-Medley Hostility Scale (CMHo). The CMHo Scale is a widely used 50 item self-report measure of trait hostility [29] with good discriminant and convergent validity [9, 33]. Factor analysis [9] revealed six subsets of items the authors categorized as cynicism, hostile attribution, aggressive responding, hostile affect, social avoidance, and others. Barefoot et al. [9] describes the measure as primarily cognitive, with some behavioral and affective loading items. This study used the cynicism and hostile attribution item subsets to reflect the cognitive component of the trait hostility construct and the aggressive responding item subset as an indication of the behavioral component of hostility. The other subscales were dropped to limit time burden. To identify a reliable subset of questions within the behavioral scale, a principal component analysis was completed and two components were retained. The component with the best reliability was composed of 4 questions ($\alpha = .5$) and was utilized in our analyses.

2.3. Prospective Self-Report Measures

2.3.1. The Sleep/Dream Checklist (SDC). The SDC, a 21 item self-report log, was developed by Levin and Fireman [34] to track various aspects of sleep quality and experience over time. It includes questions about total sleep time, sleep efficiency, sleep quality, disturbed dreaming, and affect. The measure has been associated with the Symptom Checklist-90-Revised, the State-Trait Anxiety Inventory, and the Beck Depression Inventory indicating good predictive validity [34].

Prospective daily sleep quality (DSQ) was measured by asking participants "What was the quality of your sleep last night?" Participants responded using a 9-point Likert scale. All daily ratings were averaged across the two-week reporting period for use in analyses.

2.3.2. Daily Stress Inventory (DSI). The DSI is a prospective, daily measure of the individualized impact of relatively minor stress events [35]. Participants indicate whether each of 58 events occurred for them within the preceding 24-hour period and then provide a severity rating for each event that occurred. For example, the inventory lists "Competed with someone" and "Criticized or verbally attacked" as possible events and asks participants to either mark that it did not occur or rate the severity of the stressor on a seven point Likert scale ranging from "1 = occurred but was not stressful" to "7 = caused me to panic." The measure has good convergent and divergent validity with other measures of stress and mood as well as sound internal validity (α = .83 to .87) [35].

To decrease the daily time commitment for participants, 19 items were eliminated that were likely to have a low occurrence among an undergraduate sample. The final measure included 39 events and two blank spaces for additional write-in events. The measure outcomes include the number of events that are endorsed as having occurred (stress events per day) and the sum total of the impact rating of these events (stress per day). These were used to calculate the average impact rating an individual endorses when experiencing a stress event (stress per event), our prospective estimate of perceived stress.

2.4. Procedure. The current study's design is correlation based and employed both cross-sectional and prospective measures [36]. Data collection occurred in two phases. Following recruitment, participants attended an initial 20-minute survey session. After informed consent was obtained, a brief demographic questionnaire designed for this study was completed, as well as the Pittsburgh Sleep Quality Index [30], Perceived Stress Scale [31], and the cynicism, hostile attribution, and aggressive responding subscales of the Cook-Medley Hostility Scale [9, 29]. Upon completing the initial surveys, participants were given instructions regarding the format and completion of the daily online surveys. Participants then completed the sleep/dream checklist [34] and the Daily Stress Inventory [35] online, daily, for two weeks. Participants received an email containing an internet link to that day's survey each day. The surveys were administered using an online hosting service (http://www.keysurvey.com/).

Data analyses were completing using a popular statistical software package. Initial analyses focused on establishing the psychometric properties of the collected data set. Internal consistency for measures was calculated using Cronbach's alpha. Variables were also examined to ensure they met assumptions of any statistical tests for which they were utilized. A series of Pearson's correlations describe the relationship between retrospective and prospective measures of sleep and stress to establish convergent validity. Convergent validity was also examined by replicating previously found associations between relevant variables. Examples include a positive association between cognitive hostility and some stress variables and negative associations between stress variables and sleep quality. A series of Pearson's correlations and regression analyses were used to test the studies main hypotheses. All mediation analyses were conducted using the process outlined in Baron and Kenny [37].

3. Results

3.1. Trait Hostility and Sleep Quality. The relationship between trait hostility and sleep quality was initially investigated using a series of Pearson's product-moment correlation coefficients. Cognitive hostility (as measured by the cynicism and hostile attribution subscales of the CMHo Scale) and behavioral hostility (as measured by the Aggressive Responding subscale) were correlated with the sleep quality component scores from the PSQI and the SDC.

Significant negative correlations were found between cognitive hostility and both measures of sleep quality such that increased hostility related to decreases in both retrospective sleep quality ($r(66)$ = −.43, P < .001) and prospectively measured sleep quality ($r(66)$ = −.26, P < .05). Behavioral hostility showed no meaningful association with the sleep quality variables.

3.2. Trait Hostility and Perceived Stress. The relationship between trait hostility and the three stress variables was investigated using Pearson's correlations. The cognitive and behavioral subscales of the Cook-Medley Hostility Scale were compared with a measure of retrospective perceived stress, the PSS, as well as the primary measures from the DSI: stress impact per event and stress events per day. There was a positive correlation between trait cognitive hostility and prospectively measured perceived stress, ($r(66)$ = .32, P < .01), as well as retrospective perceived stress ($r(66)$ = .36, P < .01). No relationship was found between cognitive hostility and the number of stress events experienced per day. No relationship was found between behavioral hostility and the stress measures.

3.3. Sleep Quality and Perceived Stress

3.3.1. Retrospective Sleep Quality. The sleep quality and stress variables were also compared using a series of Pearson's correlations. There was a strong negative correlation between the PSQI and PSS ($r(66)$ = −.584, P < .001) such that poorer sleep quality was associated with more perceived stress. PSQI scores were also moderately associated with the tendency to rate stress events as more severe ($r(66)$ = −.432, P < .001). The PSQI did not significantly relate to the average frequency of stress events per day.

3.3.2. Prospective Sleep Quality. Prospective measures of sleep were also associated with levels of daily and retrospective perceived stress such that increased stress experience predicted poorer sleep. DSQ was strongly associated with the average severity ratings per stress event ($r(66)$ = −.52, P < .001) and scores on the PSS ($r(66)$ = −.52, P < .001). However, daily sleep quality was not significantly correlated with the frequency of stress events per day.

3.4. Perceived Stress Mediates the Relationship between Hostility and Sleep Quality. To test our hypothesis that perceived stress mediates the relationship between trait hostility and self-reported sleep quality, a series of regression analyses were run using the procedure outlined by Baron and Kenny [37] as well as a bootstrapping method that tests for indirect effects.

3.4.1. Cognitive Hostility, Average Stress per Event, and Daily Sleep Quality. The first model examined whether the relationship between cognitive hostility and DSQ was mediated

TABLE 1: The pearson correlations.

Variable	PSQI	DSQ	CogHo	BHo	PSS
PSQI					
DSQ	.282*				
CogHo	−.421**	−.260*			
BHo	−.050	−.042	.208**		
PSS	−.584***	−.515***	.352*	−.104	
SPE	−.432***	−.517***	.321*	−.025	.613***

N = 66. PSQI: Pittsburg Sleep Quality Index; DSQ: daily sleep quality; CogHo: cognitive hostility subscales; BHo: aggressive responding subscale; PSS: perceived stress scale; SPE: stress per event.
*P < .05, **P < .01, ***P < .001.

TABLE 2: Cognitive hostility and daily SQ mediated by stress per event.

Step	IV	DV	B	SE	B	R^2	Adj R^2	sr^2
1	CogHo	DSQ	−.092	.043	−.290	.068	.053	.053*
2	CogHo	SPE	.092	.034	.321	.103	.089	.089*
3	CogHo	DSQ	−.037	.040	−.105	.277	.254	.010
	SPE	DSQ	−.596	.140	−.483	.277	.254	.210*
			Standardized indirect effect = −.0550, P < .001					
			95% CI = −.108; −.013					

N = 66. SPE: average stress severity rating per event; DSQ: daily sleep quality, CogHo: cognitive hostility.
*P < .05.

by the tendency to rate daily stress events as more severe. As can be seen in Table 1, cognitive hostility was significantly correlated with daily sleep quality. A series of regression analyses were employed to investigate average stress as a possible mediator. As shown in Table 2, the inclusion of the stress variable reduced the variance cognitive hostility explained in DSQ from 6.8% (sr^2 = .068) in the initial model to 1.0% (sr^2 = .010) in the final model. Bias-corrected confidence intervals further supported a significant indirect effect via stress per event (standardized indirect effect = −.0550, P < .001, 95% CI = −.108; −.013). The tendency to rate stress events as more severe partially mediated the relationship between cognitive hostility and daily subjective sleep quality.

3.4.2. Cognitive Hostility, Perceived Stress, and Retrospective Sleep Quality. The second mediation analysis examined whether the relationship between cognitive hostility and retrospective sleep quality (PSQI) is mediated by retrospective perceived stress. As seen in Table 3, the model was significant, with the PSS accounting for 37.4% of the variance in the PSQI. The addition of the mediator variable attenuated the impact of cognitive hostility on the IV, though hostility remained a significant predictor of the PSQI. The inclusion of the perceived stress variable reduced the amount of variance cognitive hostility explained in the PSQI from 17.7% (sr^2 = .177) in the first model to 5.3% (sr^2 = .053) in the final model. Bias-corrected confidence intervals further supported a significant indirect effect via perceived stress (standardized indirect effect = .1613, P < .001, 95% CI= .072; .279). Perceived stress partially mediated the relationship between cognitive hostility and sleep quality.

TABLE 3: Cognitive hostility and the PSQI mediated by PSS.

Step	IV	DV	B	SE	β	R^2	Adj R^2	sr^2
1	CogHo	PSQI	.388	.105	.421	.177	.164	.177*
2	CogHo	PSS	.718	.239	.352	.124	.110	.124*
3	CogHo	PSQI	.227	.097	.246	.393	.374	.053*
	PSS	PSQI	.225	.047	.497	.393	.374	.216*
			Standardized indirect effect = .1613, P < .001					
			95% CI = .072; .279					

PSS: Perceived Stress Scale; PSQI: Pittsburg Sleep Quality Index, CogHo: cognitive hostility.
*P < .05.

4. Discussion

The present study found that increased trait hostility is associated with decreased retrospective and prospectively measured sleep quality and that this relationship is significantly mediated by one's response to stress. Significantly, only the cognitive component of hostility was associated with heightened stress and sleep quality. This is consistent with previous studies which found differential associations between the components of hostility and both stress and sleep. For instance, Wilkinson [38] found no association between the aggressive responding subscale of the Cook-Medley Hostility Scale and coronary heart disease but did find the cynicism subscale to be predictive of health outcomes. Similarly, Ireland and Culpin [13] found that a measure of cynicism was a much stronger predictor of sleep quality than a measure of aggression.

Individuals who scored highly on cognitive hostility reported more daily and retrospective perceived stress compared to participants who scored low on the subscale. Importantly, while hostility was unrelated to stress event frequency, high hostility subjects reported heightened reactivity to their stressors and rated their stress as more severe than low hostile participants. This is consistent with Williams et al. [23] psychophysiological reactivity model, which predicts more intense cognitive and somatic reactions to stress events for high hostile individuals. The finding is also consistent with studies documenting hyperreactivity in hostile participants using measures of cardiovascular arousal [3, 10, 11].

Our study replicated previous findings associating increased stress with poor sleep quality [6, 18, 19, 39] utilizing both prospective and retrospective measures of stress and sleep. Generally, increased stress was associated with poorer sleep outcomes. Notably, just as stress event frequency did not relate to hostility, event frequency did not significantly relate to any sleep quality measure.

The subjective measures of sleep quality had a consistently strong, negative association with perceived stress. These data support earlier findings by Morin et al. [6] in which insomniacs and controls reported a similar number of stressful events over 21 days, but differed in their response to stress in that insomniacs rated their events as more intense and impactful. In addition, the data support earlier findings by Healey et al. [40] and Sadeh et al. [2] indicating that higher levels of perceived stress following a life event or lab induced stressor were associated with poorer subjective sleep quality.

The studies primary hypothesis was that increased reactivity to stress would account for a significant portion of the relationship between hostility and sleep quality. Consistent with the hypothesis, mediation analyses indicated that hostility is related to sleep primarily via increases in stress experience. This finding was true for both prospective and retrospectively measured sleep quality and perceived stress and indicates that trait hostility is a risk factor for stress-related sleep disruption.

This hypothesis was primarily based on two theories. The first theory, the psychophysiological reactivity model, asserts that individuals high in hostility are cognitively and somatically hyperreactive to stress [23]. The cognitive model of insomnia proposes that cognitive and somatic hyperarousal following stress is a major pathway through which sleep is degraded [7]. Together, the two models suggest that trait hostility is a possible risk factor for poor sleep to the extent that hostility results in increased arousal following stress. The current results are generally consistent with this logic in that more cognitive hostility was associated with poorer sleep quality by way of increased perceived stress. Previous studies have shown that perceived stress relates to sleep quality through increased cognitive and somatic arousal during the presleep period [6].

One possible explanation for these findings is that individuals high in cognitive hostility attend to and ruminate more on their internal responses to stress. The cognitive model of insomnia prioritizes this type of repetitive, negatively toned cognitive activity as a major pathway through which sleep can be disrupted [7]. These types of behaviors can result in a stronger cognitive and somatic response to stress and heightened presleep arousal, reducing sleep quality [7, 8]. Future studies should examine rumination and presleep arousal as possible mechanisms through which stress acts on sleep in this population.

While the behavioral component of trait hostility was unrelated to sleep quality, cognitive hostility was associated with subjective sleep quality. Previous studies have found similar associations [12–14]. In the current study, the strength of the association varied between sleep indicators. The PSQI for instance was moderately correlated with cognitive hostility while participant's daily ratings of their sleep quality were less closely associated with cognitive hostility.

Overall, the findings support our hypothesis that heightened trait hostility acts as a risk factor for poor sleep. However, behavioral hostility was not associated with any measure of sleep quality. Previous studies exploring aggression and sleep have generally reported a negative association between these two variables [13, 27, 28, 41, 42]. Interestingly, these studies looked primarily at objective measures of sleep such as sleep duration or the presence of a significant sleep disorder. Subjective sleep quality was not directly examined. In addition, these studies all utilized samples (incarcerated juveniles, adult sex offenders, children between the age of 2 and 14, clinically disturbed sleepers, and adolescent substance abusers) which may not be representative of the broader population. These measurement and sample differences may help clarify our null findings.

Causality cannot be directly addressed in the present study. The question of whether increased hostility leads to poor sleep, is caused by poor sleep, or some combination of the two will have to be resolved using a design appropriate for establishing causality. For instance, future investigators may attempt to manipulate levels of hostility and measure any subsequent changes in sleep quality. Studies already exist in which interventions targeting sleep quality impact variables associated with the hostility construct, such as aggression [14].

An interesting possibility is that the relationship between hostility and sleep is reciprocal. Trait hostility may actively degrade sleep via increased arousal as we suspect, and poor sleep may exacerbate hostile responding and stress responses. Conversely, good sleep might serve to diminish hostility, even in individuals who are high in trait hostility. Good sleep may therefore minimize the likelihood of negative outcomes associated with high trait hostility, such as coronary heart disease. Additionally, if arousal proves to be an important mechanism through which cognitive hostility impacts sleep and degrades health, then there are multiple points at which that process might be disrupted through intervention. One could actively target cognitive hostility or perceived stress through counseling.

A number of methodological and design issues in the present study suggest caution in interpreting our findings. The current study utilized self-report measures of hostility, stress, and sleep, which raises concerns of biased responding and shared method variance. Objective measures of sleep, hostility, and stress would be valuable supplements to any self-report instruments utilized in future studies. Additionally, the current study had a relatively small sample size consisting primarily of young, Caucasian college students. Future studies in this area should utilize broader samples. Last, we did not directly measure presleep arousal or utilize a design that allowed us to establish directionality. Important extensions of any subsequent studies will be to explicitly test for presleep arousal levels, establish causality, and look for the presence of proposed causal mechanisms such as rumination and possible moderators such as coping style.

Our findings suggest a number of fruitful avenues for clinical intervention. Interventions targeting at reducing hostile cognitions and behaviors thought to exacerbate stress responding in this group, such as rumination, might diminish the impact of hostility on sleep quality and health. Conversely, behavioral sleep interventions are generally low risk and highly effective. If poor sleep quality does exacerbate hostility, improving sleep quality might help to minimize some of the negative social and health effects trait hostility has been linked to. In conclusion, the current study provides evidence that increased trait cognitive hostility is associated with poorer subjective sleep via increases in perceived stress. Additional work is required to address issues of causality and directionality, as there are possible implications for the treatment and health of both poor sleepers and individuals high in hostility.

References

[1] S. Rubman, J. Brantley, W. Waters, G. Jones, J. Constans, and C. Findley, "Daily stress and insomnia," in *Proceedings of the Meeting of the Society of Behavioral Medicine*, Chicago, Ill, USA, 1990.

[2] A. Sadeh, G. Keinan, and K. Daon, "Effects of stress on sleep: the moderating role of coping style," *Health Psychology*, vol. 23, no. 5, pp. 542–545, 2004.

[3] E. C. Suarez and R. B. Williams, "Situational determinants of cardiovascular and emotional reactivity in high and low hostile men," *Psychosomatic Medicine*, vol. 51, no. 4, pp. 404–418, 1989.

[4] T. Q. Miller, T. W. Smith, C. W. Turner, M. L. Guijarro, and A. J. Hallet, "A meta-analytic review of research on hostility and physical health," *Psychological Bulletin*, vol. 119, no. 2, pp. 322–348, 1996.

[5] A. D. Krystal and J. D. Edinger, "Measuring sleep quality," *Sleep Medicine*, vol. 9, no. 1, pp. S10–S17, 2008.

[6] C. M. Morin, S. Rodrigue, and H. Ivers, "Role of stress, arousal, and coping skills in primary insomnia," *Psychosomatic Medicine*, vol. 65, no. 2, pp. 259–267, 2003.

[7] A. Harvey, "A cognitive model of insomnia," *Behaviour Research and Therapy*, vol. 40, no. 8, pp. 869–893, 2002.

[8] A. J. Guastella and M. L. Moulds, "The impact of rumination on sleep quality following a stressful life event," *Personality and Individual Differences*, vol. 42, no. 6, pp. 1151–1162, 2007.

[9] J. C. Barefoot, K. A. Dodge, B. L. Peterson, W. G. Dahlstrom, and R. B. Williams, "The Cook-Medley hostility scale: item content and ability to predict survival," *Psychosomatic Medicine*, vol. 51, no. 1, pp. 46–57, 1989.

[10] L. D. Jamner, D. Shapiro, I. B. Goldstein, and R. Hug, "Ambulatory blood pressure and heart rate in paramedics: effects of cynical hostility and defensiveness," *Psychosomatic Medicine*, vol. 53, no. 4, pp. 393–406, 1991.

[11] E. Brondolo, K. I. Grantham, W. Karlin et al., "Trait hostility and ambulatory blood pressure among traffic enforcement agents: the effects of stressful social interactions," *Journal of Occupational Health Psychology*, vol. 14, no. 2, pp. 110–121, 2009.

[12] N. Granö, J. Vahtera, M. Virtanen, L. Keltikangas-Järvinen, and M. Kivimäki, "Association of hostility with sleep duration and sleep disturbances in an employee population," *International Journal of Behavioral Medicine*, vol. 15, no. 2, pp. 73–80, 2008.

[13] J. L. Ireland and V. Culpin, "The relationship between sleeping problems and aggression, anger, and impulsivity in a population of juvenile and young offenders," *Journal of Adolescent Health*, vol. 38, no. 6, pp. 649–655, 2006.

[14] I. Brissette and S. Cohen, "The contribution of individual differences in hostility to the associations between daily interpersonal conflict, affect, and sleep," *Personality and Social Psychology Bulletin*, vol. 28, no. 9, pp. 1265–1274, 2002.

[15] H. Ursin and H. R. Eriksen, "The cognitive activation theory of stress," *Psychoneuroendocrinology*, vol. 29, no. 5, pp. 567–592, 2004.

[16] V. J. Fortunato and J. Harsh, "Stress and sleep quality: the moderating role of negative affectivity," *Personality and Individual Differences*, vol. 41, no. 5, pp. 825–836, 2006.

[17] S. Brand, M. Gerber, U. Pühse, and E. Holsboer-Trachsler, "Depression, hypomania, and dysfunctional sleep-related cognitions as mediators between stress and insomnia: the best advice is not always found on the pillow," *International Journal of Stress Management*, vol. 17, no. 2, pp. 114–134, 2010.

[18] A. N. Vgontzas, E. O. Bixler, H. M. Lin et al., "Chronic insomnia is associated with nyctohemeral activation of the hypothalamic-pituitary-adrenal axis: clinical implications," *Journal of Clinical Endocrinology and Metabolism*, vol. 86, no. 8, pp. 3787–3794, 2001.

[19] M. H. Burleson, K. M. Poehlmann, L. C. Hawkley et al., "Neuroendocrine and cardiovascular reactivity to stress in mid-aged and older women: long-term temporal consistency of individual differences," *Psychophysiology*, vol. 40, no. 3, pp. 358–369, 2003.

[20] J. F. Brosschot, S. Pieper, and J. F. Thayer, "Expanding stress theory: prolonged activation and perseverative cognition," *Psychoneuroendocrinology*, vol. 30, no. 10, pp. 1043–1049, 2005.

[21] J. F. Brosschot and J. F. Thayer, "Anger inhibition, cardiovascular recovery, and vagal function: a model of the link between hostility and cardiovascular disease," *Annals of Behavioral Medicine*, vol. 20, no. 4, pp. 326–332, 1998.

[22] M. F. Scheier and M. W. Bridges, "Person variables and health: personality predispositions and acute psychological states as shared determinants for disease," *Psychosomatic Medicine*, vol. 57, no. 3, pp. 255–268, 1995.

[23] R. Williams, J. Barefoot, and R. Shekell, "The health consequences of hostility," in *Anger and Hostility in Cardiovascular Disease and Behavioral Disorders*, M. Chesney and R. Rosenman, Eds., pp. 173–185, Hemisphere, Columbia, SC, USA, 1985.

[24] S. A. Neumann, S. R. Waldstein, J. J. Sollers, J. F. Thayer, and J. D. Sorkin, "Hostility and distraction have differential influences on cardiovascular recovery from anger recall in women," *Health Psychology*, vol. 23, no. 6, pp. 631–640, 2004.

[25] H. A. Demaree and D. E. Everhart, "Healthy high-hostiles: reduced parasympathetic activity and decreased sympathovagal flexibility during negative emotional processing," *Personality and Individual Differences*, vol. 36, no. 2, pp. 457–469, 2004.

[26] B. L. Fredrickson, K. E. Maynard, M. J. Helms, T. L. Haney, I. C. Siegler, and J. C. Barefoot, "Hostility predicts magnitude and duration of blood pressure response to anger," *Journal of Behavioral Medicine*, vol. 23, no. 3, pp. 229–243, 2000.

[27] R. D. Chervin, J. E. Dillon, K. H. Archbold, and D. L. Ruzicka, "Conduct problems and symptoms of sleep disorders in children," *Journal of the American Academy of Child and Adolescent Psychiatry*, vol. 42, no. 2, pp. 201–208, 2003.

[28] P. L. Haynes, R. R. Bootzin, L. Smith, J. Cousins, M. Cameron, and S. Stevens, "Sleep and aggression in substance-abusing adolescents: results from an integrative behavioral sleep-treatment pilot program," *Sleep*, vol. 29, no. 4, pp. 512–520, 2006.

[29] W. W. Cook and D. M. Medley, "Proposed hostility and Pharisaic-virtue scales for the MMPI," *Journal of Applied Psychology*, vol. 38, no. 6, pp. 414–418, 1954.

[30] D. J. Buysse, C. F. Reynolds, T. H. Monk, S. R. Berman, and D. J. Kupfer, "The Pittsburgh sleep quality index: a new instrument for psychiatric practice and research," *Psychiatry Research*, vol. 28, no. 2, pp. 193–213, 1989.

[31] S. Cohen, T. Kamarck, and R. Mermelstein, "A global measure of perceived stress," *Journal of Health and Social Behavior*, vol. 24, no. 4, pp. 385–396, 1983.

[32] S. Cohen, "Contrasting the Hassles scale and the perceived stress scale. Who's really measuring appraised stress?" *American Psychologist*, vol. 41, no. 6, pp. 716–718, 1986.

[33] K. Han, N. Weed, R. Calhoun, and J. Butcher, "Psychometric characteristics of the MMPI-2 cook-medley hostility scale," *Journal of Personality Assessment*, vol. 65, no. 3, pp. 567–585, 1995.

[34] R. Levin and G. Fireman, "Nightmare prevalence, nightmare distress, and self-reported psychological disturbance," *Sleep*, vol. 25, no. 2, pp. 205–212, 2002.

[35] P. J. Brantley, C. D. Waggoner, G. N. Jones, and N. B. Rappaport, "A daily stress inventory: development, reliability, and validity," *Journal of Behavioral Medicine*, vol. 10, no. 1, pp. 61–74, 1987.

[36] A. Kazdin, *Research Design in Clinical Psychology*, Allyn & Bacon, Boston, Mass, USA, 4th edition, 2002.

[37] R. M. Baron and D. A. Kenny, "The moderator-mediator variable distinction in social psychological research. Conceptual, strategic, and statistical considerations," *Journal of Personality and Social Psychology*, vol. 51, no. 6, pp. 1173–1182, 1986.

[38] R. G. Wilkinson, "Socioeconomic determinants of health: health inequalities: relative or absolute material standards?" *British Medical Journal*, vol. 314, no. 7080, pp. 591–595, 1997.

[39] R. T. Gross and T. D. Borkovec, "Effects of cognitive intrusion manipulation on the sleep-onset latency of good sleepers," *Behavior Therapy*, vol. 13, no. 1, pp. 112–116, 1982.

[40] E. S. Healey, A. Kales, and L. J. Monroe, "Onset of insomnia: role of life-stress events," *Psychosomatic Medicine*, vol. 43, no. 5, pp. 439–451, 1981.

[41] N. J. Ali, D. Pitson, and J. R. Stradling, "Sleep disordered breathing: effects of adenotonsillectomy on behaviour and psychological functioning," *European Journal of Pediatrics*, vol. 155, no. 1, pp. 56–62, 1996.

[42] B. D. Booth, J. Paul Fedoroff, S. D. Curry, and A. B. Douglass, "Sleep apnea as a possible factor contributing to aggression in sex offenders," *Journal of Forensic Sciences*, vol. 51, no. 5, pp. 1178–1181, 2006.

6

Sleep Lab Adaptation in Children with Attention-Deficit/Hyperactivity Disorder and Typically Developing Children

Meredith Bessey,[1] **Jennifer Richards,**[1] **and Penny Corkum**[1,2,3]

[1] Department of Psychology & Neuroscience, Dalhousie University, P.O. Box 15000, Halifax, NS, Canada B3H 4R2
[2] IWK Health Centre, 5850 University Avenue, Halifax, NS, Canada B3K 6R8
[3] Colchester East Hants ADHD Clinic, 600 Abenaki Road, Truro, NS, Canada B2N 5A1

Correspondence should be addressed to Penny Corkum; pvcorkum@dal.ca

Academic Editor: Marco Zucconi

Objectives. Research has shown inconsistencies across studies examining sleep problems in children with attention-deficit/hyperactivity disorder (ADHD). It is possible that these inconsistencies are due to sleep lab adaptation. The goal of the current study was to investigate the possibility that children with ADHD adapt differently to the sleep lab than do typically developing (TD) children. *Patients and Methods.* Actigraphy variables were compared between home and the sleep lab. Sleep lab adaptation reports from the parent and child were compared between children with ADHD ($n = 25$) and TD children ($n = 25$). *Results.* Based on actigraphy, both groups had reduced sleep duration and reduced wake after sleep onset in the sleep lab compared to home. The only interaction effect was that TD children had increased sleep efficiency in the sleep lab compared to home. *Conclusions.* The results of this study do not support the hypothesis that children with ADHD adjust to the sleep lab differently than their typically developing peers. However, both groups of children did sleep differently in the sleep lab compared to home, and this needs to be considered when generalizing research findings from a sleep lab environment to children's sleep in general.

1. Introduction

There have been growing research and clinical interest in the relationship between attention-deficit/hyperactivity disorder (ADHD) and sleep. Parent reports have consistently reported high rates of sleep problems in children with ADHD [1]; however, results from polysomnography (PSG) are inconsistent. There are several possibilities for these inconsistencies; for example, studies have often failed to match ADHD and typically developing (TD) groups on age and sex and lack control for stimulant medication use [2]. Another possibility is that sleep lab adaptation may be different for children with ADHD. The sleep lab is an unfamiliar environment that involves interacting with new people and sleeping with electrodes. This could lead to atypical sleep, helping to explain previous research inconsistencies.

The goal of the current study was to investigate sleep lab adaptation in children with ADHD and TD children, using actigraphy and parent- and child-completed questionnaires. It is hypothesized (a) that both groups of children will be negatively affected by the sleep lab environment, with children with ADHD possibly being more negatively affected, and (b) that parent and child reports will indicate that children with ADHD have more difficulty sleeping in the sleep lab than TD children.

2. Materials and Methods

2.1. Participants. A total of 50 children (25 with ADHD and 25 TD children), ages 6 to 12, participated in the study. All children with ADHD were recently rigorously diagnosed and medication naive. None of the participants had previous sleep lab experience or had comorbid, primary mental health, sleep, neurological, or genetic disorders.

2.2. Measures

2.2.1. Conners' Rating Scale-Revised Long Version (CRS-R:L [3]).
Both the Conners' Parent (CPRS) and Teacher (CTRS) were used as screening tools. The Conners' ADHD index was the only subscale analyzed.

2.2.2. Demographic Questionnaire.
This questionnaire was used to compare both groups on possible confounding variables [4].

2.2.3. Actigraphy.
Mini-Motionlogger Actigraphs (Ambulatory Monitoring Inc.) were used to collect data on four variables: (1) sleep duration, (2) sleep onset latency, (3) wake after sleep onset (WASO), and (4) sleep efficiency.

2.2.4. Sleep Lab Adaptation Questionnaire (SLAQ).
This investigator-developed measure includes five questions for parents and children. Questions focus on sleep onset, sleep duration, general sleep quality, overall sleep lab experience, and how child friendly the sleep lab appeared.

2.3. Procedure.
The study received ethical approval from the research ethics board at the hospital and ADHD clinic. First the child wore the actigraph for six nights. The parent and teacher completed the CTRS and CPRS. Then the overnight PSG study took place. Upon arrival at the sleep lab, the research assistant (RA) played a game with the child and the technician conducted the PSG hook-up, which took approximately one hour.

Once the hook up was complete, the child followed their usual weekday bedtime routine and an actigraph was placed on the child's wrist before bedtime. A technician monitored the child's sleep overnight. The following morning, upon waking at their usual weekday wake time, the electrodes and actigraph were removed from the child, and the parent and child completed the SLAQ. (The SLAQ was added to the study protocol following the beginning of this study, and therefore some SLAQ data was collected at a later time point for some of the participants.)

3. Results and Discussion

3.1. Sample Characteristics.
The two groups (TD and ADHD) did not differ on mean age ($t(48) = 0.10$, $P = .920$; ADHD = 106.10 months (SD = 22.47 months), TD children = 105.47 months (SD = 23.00 months)), sex ($P = 1.00$; 22 boys, 3 girls in each group), parental marital status ($P = 1.000$), SES ($t(48) = -0.75$, $P = .46$), or number of children in the home ($F(1, 48) = 1.438$, $P = .24$). Expectedly, the two groups differed significantly on the mean ADHD index t-score for the CTRS, $t(38) = 6.45$, $P < .001$ (ADHD = 68.54 (SD = 9.75), TD = 48.94 (SD = 7.95)), and the CPRS, $t(47) = 10.23$, $P < .001$ (ADHD = 70.36 (SD = 9.69), TD = 46.00 (SD = 6.57)).

3.2. Hypothesis 1.
Sleep latency of children with ADHD was 31.66 minutes (SD = 24.43) at home, versus 32.00 minutes (SD = 29.79) at the sleep lab. For TD children, latency was 22.05 minutes (SD = 16.82) at home, versus 24.28 minutes (SD = 18.10) in the sleep lab; neither the main effect ($F(1, 48) = 0.08$, $P = .78$) nor interaction ($F(1, 48) = 0.04$, $P = .84$) was significant. At home, sleep efficiency of children with ADHD was 83.35% (SD = 10.42%) and in the sleep lab 83.42% (SD = 10.01%). In TD children, sleep efficiency was 79.90% (SD = 10.76%) at home and 86.11% (SD = 7.25%) in the sleep lab; the main effect ($F(1, 48) = 5.79$, $P = .020$) and the interaction were significant ($F(1, 48) = 5.53$, $P = .023$). Sleep duration for children with ADHD was 571.03 minutes (SD = 42.23) at home versus 513.44 minutes (SD = 72.14) in the sleep lab. In TD children, sleep duration at home was 562.25 minutes (SD = 47.63) versus 525.84 minutes (SD = 62.58) in the sleep lab; the main effect was significant ($F(1, 48) = 21.34$, $P < .001$), but not the interaction ($F(1, 48) = 1.08$, $P = .30$). In children with ADHD, WASO was 95.27 minutes (SD = 57.80) at home and 86.08 minutes (SD = 55.50) in the sleep lab. In TD children, WASO was 111.47 minutes (SD = 58.31) at home and 73.52 minutes (SD = 41.28) in the sleep lab; again, the main effect was significant ($F(1, 48) = 10.03$, $P = .003$) but not the interaction ($F(1, 48) = 3.74$, $P = .059$).

3.3. Hypothesis 2.
Items on the SLAQ indicated no differences in sleep lab adaptation between children with ADHD and TD children (Table 1). Although the parents and children in both groups reported a positive experience in the sleep lab, they also reported that sleep was slightly worse than what was normal at home.

3.4. Discussion.
The goal of this study was to examine sleep lab adaptation in children with ADHD compared to TD children. Our results indicate that both groups of children slept approximately 50 minutes less while in the sleep lab and that both groups of children had fewer wake episodes in the sleep lab than at home. Interestingly, sleep efficiency of TD children improved by approximately 6% in the sleep lab, with no improvement in children with ADHD. Parents and children did not report significant differences between the two groups in terms of how the children adapted to sleeping in the sleep lab environment, and overall both groups of children were reported to have had a positive experience in the sleep lab, with sleep being slightly worse than sleep at home.

Based on our hypothesis that all children would be negatively affected by being in the sleep lab environment, the finding of reduced sleep duration in both groups is not surprising. The sleep lab is a novel environment that could be intimidating to the child, leading to shortened sleep. Therefore, generalization of data about sleep duration based on studies using PSG in a sleep lab should be interpreted with caution, as the data may not accurately represent the child's typical sleep. It is important that clinicians use judgement when using PSG parameters to make recommendations to their patients about sleep.

TABLE 1: Mean values on parent and child SLAQ.

Variable	ADHD (SD)	TD (SD)	P value
SLAQ Parent			
Do you think the PSG hook-up (e.g., wires, finger clip, chest bands) changed how long it took your child to *fall* asleep compared to his/her sleep at home?	2.44 (0.82)	2.64 (0.81)	.39
Do you think the PSG hook-up changed how long your child *slept for compared to home*?	2.28 (0.74)	2.48 (0.65)	.32
How was the Sleep Lab bedroom?	4.32 (0.75)	4.44 (0.82)	.59
How was your child's sleep in the Sleep Lab?	3.32 (0.90)	3.38 (0.78)	.80
Rate your child's over-all experience in the Sleep Lab.	4.52 (0.71)	4.44 (0.65)	.68
SLAQ Child			
Do you think the PSG hook-up (e.g., wires, finger clip, chest bands) changed how long it took you to *fall* asleep compared to your sleep at home?	2.16 (0.80)	2.70 (1.15)	.06
Do you think the PSG hook-up changed how long you *slept for compared to home*?	2.52 (0.83)	2.64 (1.04)	.65
How did you like the Sleep Lab bedroom?	4.32 (0.75)	4.28 (0.79)	.86
How was your sleep in the Sleep Lab?	3.56 (1.00)	3.92 (1.15)	.24
Rate your over-all experience in the Sleep Lab?	4.20 (0.96)	4.16 (0.99)	.88

Note: The SLAQ items were scored on a 1–5 scale, with 1 signifying a worse than typical sleep, 3 signifying no change and 5 signifying a better than typical sleep.

The finding of reduced WASO in the sleep lab was not consistent with our hypothesis of generally poorer sleep in the sleep lab. As discussed above, the sleep lab is a highly structured environment, with no siblings, pets, and so forth to disrupt the child's sleep. This may have reduced night waking in all children, regardless of whether the child has ADHD or not. Another possibility is that sleep efficiency improved given the shorter sleep duration.

The finding of improved sleep efficiency in TD children, but not in children with ADHD, was surprising. It suggests that perhaps the sleep lab is conducive to better sleep in TD children but not in children with ADHD, at least in terms of some sleep variables. The sleep lab tends to be a more organized and structured environment than the home environment, as there are no distractions (e.g., siblings, and noises from other rooms) to disrupt the child's sleep. Perhaps this highly structured environment promoted better sleep efficiency in TD children; however, it is unclear why children with ADHD did not benefit. It is possible that rather than being more negatively affected by the sleep lab, as hypothesized, children with ADHD are less able than their typically developing peers to benefit from the potentially sleep-promoting effects of the sleep lab.

4. Conclusion

Overall, this study provides interesting findings that are useful both clinically and in a research setting. Findings should be cautiously generalized from PSG to the home, as our results indicate that all children are affected by the sleep lab, with some sleep variables being negatively affected (i.e., sleep duration) and some being positively affected (i.e., WASO). In opposition to our hypothesis, it was found that children with ADHD were not differentially affected based on most variables analyzed in this study. Further research could investigate whether these findings extend to at-home PSG assessment. It is important to note that this study only

examined variables that could be assessed by both actigraphy and PSG, and therefore it is not possible to comment on how the sleep lab may affect sleep architecture or sleep movements. As the data for this study was drawn from a child's first night in the sleep lab, it would also be of interest to examine sleep lab adaptation over a number of nights in the sleep lab, during which the children would be expected to habituate to the environment.

Overall, it can be concluded that because the sleep of children with ADHD was not differentially affected by the sleep lab experience, it is unlikely that the sleep lab contributes to the inconsistencies in the literature regarding sleep problems in children with ADHD. Given that children with ADHD did not differ significantly from TD children in terms of adaptation to the sleep lab, it is likely that the differences we see in research are due to the heterogeneity of ADHD in terms of symptom presentation (e.g., hyperactivity, attention), comorbidities, and medication.

Acknowledgments

The authors would like to acknowledge the assistance of Andre Benoit, as well as of several research assistants (Ashton Parker, Melissa Gendron, Jaclyn Cappell, Tasha Cullingham, Anders Dorbeck, Shaune Ford, Katie Goodine, Melissa McGonnall, Sarah Melkert, Abbey Porier, Sunny Shaffner, Jillian Tonet, Nicolle Vincent, Jessica Waldon, and Lindsay Walker) in the Corkum lab, during the data collection process. This project was in part funded by the Canadian Institute of Health Research (CIHR).

References

[1] J. A. Owens, "The ADHD and sleep conundrum: a review," *Journal of Developmental and Behavioral Pediatrics*, vol. 26, no. 4, pp. 312–322, 2005.

[2] P. Corkum, H. Moldofsky, S. Hogg-Johnson, T. Humphries, and R. Tannock, "Sleep problems in children with attention-deficit/hyperactivity disorder: impact of subtype, comorbidity, and stimulant medication," *Journal of the American Academy of Child and Adolescent Psychiatry*, vol. 38, no. 10, pp. 1285–1293, 1999.

[3] C. K. Conners, *Conners-3: Conners' Rating Scales*, 3rd edition, 2008.

[4] Statistics Canada, "National Longitudinal Survey of Children and Youth (NLSCY)," 2006, http://www.statcan.gc.ca/cgi-bin/imdb/p2SV.pl?Function=getSurvey&SDDS=4450&lang=en&db=imdb&adm=8&dis=2.

7

The Effects of Acupuncture Treatment on Sleep Quality and on Emotional Measures among Individuals Living with Schizophrenia: A Pilot Study

Alon Reshef,[1,2] **Boaz Bloch,**[1,2] **Limor Vadas,**[1,3] **Shai Ravid,**[1]
Ilana Kremer,[2,4] **and Iris Haimov**[3]

[1] *Psychiatric Department, Emek Medical Center, Afula, Israel*

[2] *Technion—Israel Institute of Technology, Haifa, Israel*

[3] *Department of Psychology and the Center for Psychobiological Research, Yezreel Academic College, Emek Yezreel 19300, Israel*

[4] *Mazra Mental Health Center, Akko, Israel*

Correspondence should be addressed to Iris Haimov; i_haimov@yvc.ac.il

Academic Editor: Michel M. Billiard

Purpose. To examine the effects of acupuncture on sleep quality and on emotional measures among patients with schizophrenia. *Methods.* Twenty patients with schizophrenia participated in the study. The study comprised a seven-day running-in no-treatment period, followed by an eight-week experimental period. During the experimental period, participants were treated with acupuncture twice a week. During the first week (no-treatment period) and the last week of the experimental period, participants filled out a broad spectrum of questionnaires and their sleep was continuously monitored by wrist actigraph. *Results.* A paired-sample *t*-test was conducted comparing objective and subjective sleep parameters manifested by participants before and after sequential acupuncture treatment. A significant effect of acupuncture treatment was observed for seven objective sleep variables: sleep onset latency, sleep percentage, mean activity level, wake time after sleep onset, mean number of wake episodes, mean wake episode and longest wake episode. However, no significant effects of acupuncture treatment were found for subjective sleep measures. Likewise, the results indicate that acupuncture treatment improved psychopathology levels and emotional measures, that is, depression level and anxiety level. *Conclusions.* Overall, the findings of this pilot study suggest that acupuncture has beneficial effects as a treatment for insomnia and psychopathology symptoms among patients with schizophrenia.

1. Introduction

Schizophrenia is a mental disorder involving disturbances in basic mental functions, such as emotions, cognition, perception, and other aspects of behavior [1–3]. The clinical picture of schizophrenia is characterized by a mixture of two main categories of core symptoms: positive symptoms (i.e., delusions and hallucinations) and negative symptoms (i.e., apathy, flat affect, and lack of functioning) [4–6]. Its lifetime prevalence is about 1%, with equal distribution between men and women [4]. Schizophrenia is known to be one of the most debilitating and distressful mental disorders, and during its course the disease often deteriorates and becomes chronic [7–9]. Schizophrenia is responsible for tremendous emotional and economic burdens on patients, their families, and society as a whole [8, 10].

Further, it may be valuable to consider schizophrenia as a multidimensional disorder that includes several different domains, among them clinical, neurocognitive, occupational, familial, and societal, and perhaps most important subjective well-being and positive feelings [11]. Besides the core symptoms mentioned above, other clinical expressions of schizophrenia include depressive features, anxiety features and sleep disturbances, of which insomnia is most prevalent

[12–14]. The treatment of schizophrenia is complex and should be tailored to the patient, taking into consideration biopsychosocial components. Yet standard treatments, especially biological treatments, are only partially effective and have possible serious side effects.

Insomnia is the most common sleep disorder in psychiatry [15, 16]. Polysomnographic studies have shown that patients with schizophrenia exhibit increased sleep latency manifested by difficulties initiating or maintaining sleep, reduced sleep efficiency and total sleep time, reduced REM latency and REM density, and disturbed non-REM sleep architecture, specifically a decrease in SWS, especially in stage 4 [12, 17–21]. Among patients with schizophrenia, insomnia may precede relapse or appear during exacerbated schizophrenic episodes; it may even complicate schizophrenia to the degree that patients can exhibit suicidal behavior [22, 23].

Many studies have provided evidence showing that insomnia is not simply a typical symptom of depression or of other psychiatric disorders but may actually be a predictor (or an independent risk factor) for the development of such conditions [24, 25]. Further research has indicated that insomnia can be an important indicator in the diagnosis of mental disorder and can also play a role in the deterioration of existing mental disorders [25, 26]. Moreover, Kantrowitz et al. proposed in their study that sleep deficits reflect a core element of schizophrenia [20].

Among patients with schizophrenia, sleep disturbances and, specifically, changes in sleep architecture and sleep quality have an enormous impact on quality of life, level of functioning, and cognitive functioning [20]. Hence, preserving the integrity of sleep among such patients is an important health priority. The most prevalent treatment for insomnia in patients with schizophrenia involves pharmacotherapy. Medication has many disadvantages, among them side effects that add emotional, social, and economic burdens to the existing burden of the disease. For instance, one of the most common treatments for insomnia is the use of benzodiazepines, a heterogeneous class of anxiolytic drugs distinguished by their half-lives. At high doses, benzodiazepines result in across-the-board side effects, notably memory impairment, drowsiness, and increased likelihood of accidents [27]. Another common drug treatment is the use of imidazopyridines, whose effects have been found to resemble those of short-acting benzodiazepines [28–30] but with less influence on sleep architecture, cognitive behaviors, and withdrawal symptoms. In addition, antidepressants, antihistamines, and antipsychotics [31] have been mentioned as treatments for insomnia. Many of these have also been determined to have serious side effects, particularly during prolonged use [32]. Additionally, all drug treatments are relatively contraindicated in pregnancy, sleep apnea, liver or kidney dysfunction, prior history of substance abuse, or certain jobs requiring atypical shifts [27–32].

The disadvantages of drug treatment for insomnia in patients with schizophrenia underline the importance of seeking alternative nonpharmacological treatments, among them complementary medicine techniques such as shiatsu, reflexology, and acupuncture. Moreover, despite recent achievements in psychopharmacology, the pharmacological treatment for schizophrenia is far from satisfactory. Hence, additional treatment modalities are most welcome. Complementary therapies are widely used among psychiatric patients, including patients with schizophrenia. In the western world and in Israel, the most popular modality used for many somatic and mental disorders is acupuncture. Cumulative data suggest that complementary treatment strategies, including acupuncture, can be applied and carefully examined in schizophrenia [33–36].

Acupuncture is one of the oldest healing practices in the world. It is considered to be a safe and effective treatment modality which, according to Traditional Chinese Medicine (TCM), harmonizes the body's energies [37]. Acupuncture incorporates the use of ultrafine needles (0.15–0.30 mm diameter) inserted into specific points on the skin (acupoints). TCM teaches that the body's energy, or qi (pronounced chee), flows along a series of points called meridians. Each internal organ has a corresponding meridian, and the application of pressure (acupressure, shiatsu), heat (moxibustion), or needles (acupuncture) to the relevant acupoints is believed to have an impact upon the associated internal organs and thus to harmonize the body's qi [38]. The exact mechanism by which acupuncture induces physiological changes, relieves pain, and alleviates illness is still unclear. Research has shown that treatment with acupuncture results in nonspecific (placebo response) as well as specific effects such as local and systemic effects, among them an increase in the release of pituitary beta-endorphins and ACTH [38]. This release of endorphins may partly explain the analgesic effects of this treatment, whereas increased ACTH secretion—which leads to elevated serum cortisol levels—may account for its anti-inflammatory effects. Acupuncture can also cause accelerated synthesis and release of serotonin and noradrenaline into the central nervous system, thus activating descending antinociceptive pathways and deactivating multiple limbic areas that promote pain association [38].

Previous studies have demonstrated that acupuncture has a positive influence on a number of diseases and disorders, among them depression, chronic pain, and sleep disorders [39–41]. Nevertheless, tests of the use and effectiveness of acupuncture for mental disorders and sleep disturbances have yielded heterogeneous and inconclusive results [40, 42]. One explanation for these results may be the paucity of studies conducted so far, while another may be the lack of objective outcome measures. Objective sleep assessment may therefore be a preferable outcome measure, in addition to the usual clinical assessment tools. Another explanation may be the difficulty in testing Eastern treatments techniques using impeccable Western methodology.

The correlation between sleep difficulties and schizophrenia along with the data showing the beneficial effects of acupuncture for insomnia suggests that acupuncture may have a positive effect for patients with schizophrenia. Moreover, objective sleep measurement can be an excellent outcome measure and may help answer some validity issues concerning the effectiveness of TCM therapies in schizophrenia.

Accordingly, the current pilot study examines the effects of the acupuncture technique as a treatment for insomnia and as a possible treatment of core symptoms and emotional measures among patients with schizophrenia.

2. Method

The clinical experiment conformed to the principles outlined by the Declaration of Helsinki, and the complete study protocol was approved by the Helsinki Committee of the Haemek Medical Center (number 0015-08-EMC) and by the Institutional Ethics Committee of the Yezreel Academic College of Emek Yezreel (number 0028-YVC). After the study was completely described to all participants, their written informed consent was obtained.

2.1. Participants. Twenty individuals living with schizophrenia or schizoaffective disorder participated in the study (mean age = 43.15, SD = 9.42; 10 males and 10 females). All the patients were diagnosed as being on the schizophrenia spectrum (i.e., schizophrenia and schizoaffective disorder) (ICD-10 criteria) [43] and were treated with antipsychotic medications. In addition, some of them were treated with combinations of antidepressants and mood stabilizers along with anxiolytic medications, a common practice for the treatment of this clinical population [43].

Inclusion criteria included ICD-10 diagnosis of schizophrenia spectrum, clinical stability with no medication change during one month prior to study beginning.

Participants were ineligible for inclusion in the current study if they demonstrated symptomatic aggravation, suicidality (suicidal ideation or acts) during one month prior to study beginning, substance abuse, or physical or neurological unstable conditions [43].

All participants were recruited from the outpatient clinics of the Department of Psychiatry at Haemek Medical Center. Patients were recruited by a convenience sample since this was a naturalistic pilot design. Patients were consecutive and were not picked at certain days. All participants were living independently in the community or in rehabilitation settings (hostels). All of them had been stable in following their medication regimens for at least one month before the study began. All participants completed the study period; that is, the dropout rate was zero.

2.2. Procedure. The study began with a seven-day running-in, treatment-as-usual period, followed by an eight-week experimental period. During the experimental period, participants were treated with acupuncture twice a week, for a total sequential acupuncture treatment comprising 16 sessions. During the first week of the study (treatment-as-usual period) and the last week of the experimental period, participants' sleep was continuously monitored with a wrist actigraph, and participants completed a broad spectrum of questionnaires.

2.3. Measurements. General information was provided by a demographic questionnaire suitable for the study population. Evaluations included psychiatric clinical assessment, emotional condition assessment, sleep assessment, and Chinese medicine assessment.

2.3.1. Sleep Measurements. Sleep Questionnaires. All participants completed three questionnaires that subjectively evaluated their sleep patterns: (i) a qualitative questionnaire—the Mini Sleep Questionnaire (MSQ) [44, 45]; (ii) a quantitative informative questionnaire—the Technion Sleep Questionnaire [46]; (iii) a qualitative questionnaire—the Pittsburgh Sleep Quality Index Hebrew Translation (PSQI-H) [47].

Wrist Actigraph Recording. For the purposes of objectively evaluating sleep, each participant's sleep was continuously monitored over a one-week period by a miniature actigraph worn on the wrist (Mini Motionlogger, Ambulatory Monitoring, Inc., Ardsley, NY, USA). The wrist actigraph facilitates monitoring sleep under natural circumstances with minimal distortions. The actigraph measures wrist activity utilizing a piezoelectric element and translates wrist movements into an electrical signal that is digitized and memorized. Activity is recorded at 60-second intervals [48, 49]. The recordings were analyzed by an automatic algorithm (W2 scoring algorithm) provided by the manufacturer to determine time in bed (total number of minutes from bedtime to wake time), sleep onset latency (time taken to fall asleep from bedtime), sleep percentage (percentage of total sleep time out of total time in bed), mean activity level (mean activity score measured in counts/min), wake time after sleep onset (total number of wake minutes after sleep onset), mean number of wake episodes, mean wake episode (mean number of minutes participant is awake during waking episodes after initially falling asleep), and longest wake episode (number of minutes participant is awake during the longest waking episode after initially falling asleep).

2.3.2. Clinical and Emotional Assessment. Participants were interviewed by a psychiatrist and completed two questionnaires aimed at measuring their clinical morbidity.

(1) Brief Psychiatric Rating Scale (BPRS) [50, 51].

(2) Positive and Negative Syndrome Scale (PANSS) [51, 52] for schizophrenia and schizoaffective patients only.

Participants' level of depression was assessed through two subjective questionnaires.

(1) Beck Depression Inventory (BDI) [53, 54] is a 21-item self-report questionnaire. The 21 items correspond to symptoms such as mood, pessimism, and suicidal thoughts. The BDI is an internally consistent and valid measurement [55].

(2) Calgary Depression Scale for schizophrenia (CDSS) is a 9-item test that measures the severity of depression. The CDSS is used to assess depressive symptoms in people with schizophrenia, independent of their positive, negative, and general symptoms [56–58]. The questionnaire rates the severity of symptoms observed in depression, such as low mood, insomnia, agitation, anxiety and weight loss.

Anxiety level was assessed by two questionnaires.

(1) State-Trait Anxiety Inventory (STAI) [59–61] is a 40-item self-report measure comprising two 20-item scales. The first scale measures state anxiety, defined as a transitory emotional state or condition, and the second measures trait, character, and logical anxiety [60, 61].

(2) Hamilton Anxiety Rating Scale (HAS) is a 14-item test that measures the severity of anxiety symptoms in children and adults. It provides measures of overall anxiety, psychic anxiety (mental agitation and psychological distress), and somatic anxiety (physical complaints related to anxiety) [62, 63].

Hedonic state was assessed by the Snaith-Hamilton Pleasure Scale (SHAPS). The SHAPS questionnaire includes 14 items that indicate levels of hedonic states [64, 65].

The Quality of Life Enjoyment and Satisfaction Questionnaire (Q-LES-Q) [66, 67] was used to measure participants' general satisfaction with their life.

2.3.3. Chinese Medicine Assessment. All participants were interviewed by an acupuncture therapist at the beginning of each session (i.e., during the entire 16-session sequence) and answered a diagnostic Chinese medicine questionnaire to assess present diagnosis of physical and mental conditions from the perspective of TCM. This questionnaire assesses physical and mental morbidities, and primary and secondary complaints. In addition, at the beginning of each session, participants' pulse and tongue measurements were taken using Chinese medicine techniques.

2.4. Acupuncture Treatment. The treatment was acupuncture (needle acupuncture) using standard Chinese needles sized 0.15 mm × 0.18 mm, 0.22 mm × 0.30 mm, and 0.25 mm × 0.40 mm. The use of each size needle and the acupoint corresponding to it were determined by the guidelines set out in the *Manual of Acupuncture* [68]. Each treatment lasted 30 minutes. The acupoints selected by the practitioners were chosen for their compatibility with the practitioners' diagnosis of each patient. The treatment regimen and selected acupoints were determined by traditional Chinese medicine diagnosis of syndromes marked by complex sets of signs and symptoms. These syndromes do not fit Western diagnoses such as depression or schizophrenia. For example, the Western diagnosis of depression can be referred to as "liver qi stagnation" or "blood deficiency" or "heart fire" in traditional Chinese medicine. Certified acupuncturists gave the acupuncture treatments, and each patient had his own acupuncturist for all the sessions of this study. The treatment method and acupoints were chosen according to the patient's diagnosis in an attempt to address each and every patient's individual condition "as a whole" rather than aiming only at the patient's sleeping disorder by using a set of "protocol points."

2.5. Statistical Analysis. A paired sample *t*-test was conducted comparing psychopathology score, emotional measures, and objective and subjective sleep parameters manifested by participants before and after sequential acupuncture treatment.

3. Results

3.1. Objective and Subjective Sleep Measures. Actigraphic sleep measures included eight measures of sleep quality: time in bed, sleep onset latency, sleep percentage, mean activity level, wake time after sleep onset, mean number of wake episodes, mean wake episode, and longest wake episode. A paired sample *t*-test was conducted comparing objective sleep parameters manifested by participants before and after sequential acupuncture treatment. A significant effect of acupuncture treatment was observed for seven sleep variables (Table 1).

A significant difference was found in sleep latency ($t(16) = 2.21$, $P < 0.05$), indicating shorter sleep latency following acupuncture treatment (M = 14.32, SD = 12.81; M = 26.63, SD = 26.71, resp.) (Figure 1(a)). In addition, a significant difference was found in sleep percentage ($t(18) = 2.9$, $P < 0.01$), indicating higher sleep percentage following acupuncture treatment (M = 89.86, SD = 7.14) compared with baseline measures (M = 84.20, SD = 10.76) (Figure 1(b)). Likewise, a significant reduction was found in mean activity level ($t(18) = 3.2$, $P < 0.01$). Following acupuncture treatment, participants were less active during sleep compared to baseline measures (M = 13.26, SD = 7.63; M = 20.04, SD = 9.43, resp.) (Figure 1(c)).

A significant difference was also found in total wake minutes (Figure 1(d)) ($t(18) = 2.92$, $P < 0.01$), indicating fewer total wake minutes during sleep following acupuncture treatment (M = 46.58, SD = 32.64) compared to baseline measures (M = 67.43, SD = 45.86). Similarly, significant differences were found in mean wake episodes, long wake episodes, and longest wake episode ($t(18) = 2.26$, $P < 0.05$; $t(18) = 2.49$, $P < 0.05$; $t(18) = 2.87$, $P < 0.05$, resp.), revealing shorter mean wake episodes (M = 5.42, SD = 2.31), shorter long wake episodes (M = 2.85, SD = 1.54), and shorter longest wake episode (M = 18.16, SD = 11.55) following acupuncture treatment compared to baseline measures (M = 7.21, SD = 4.81; M = 3.76, SD = 1.62; M = 25.71, SD = 19.20, resp.). However, no significant effect of acupuncture treatment was found for total time in bed (n.s.).

A paired sample *t*-test was conducted comparing subjective sleep parameters manifested by participants before and after sequential acupuncture treatment. No significant effects of acupuncture treatment were found for subjective sleep measures (n.s.) (Table 1).

3.2. Objective and Subjective Emotional and Clinical Measures. A paired sample *t*-test was conducted comparing psychopathology score manifested by participants before and after sequential acupuncture treatment (Table 2).

Objective psychopathology levels were measured by the Brief Psychiatric Rating Scale (BPRS) and by the Positive and Negative Syndrome Scale (PANNS). A significant difference was found in psychopathology levels assessed by the Brief Psychiatric Rating Scale (BPRS), indicating that acupuncture

TABLE 1: Objective and subjective sleep measures (means and standard deviations) after each phase of the study and analysis of the comparisons between them.

Objective and subjective sleep measures	Baseline level Mean (SD)	Last week of acupuncture treatment Mean (SD)	t	P value
Total time in bed (minutes)	480.98 (±97.52)	475.39 (±96.82)	0.36	0.722
Sleep onset latency (minutes)	26.63 (±26.71)	14.32 (±12.81)	2.21	0.040
Sleep percentage (%)	84.20 (±10.76)	89.86 (±7.14)	2.90	0.010
Mean activity level	20.04 (±9.43)	13.26 (±7.63)	3.20	0.005
Wake time after sleep onset	67.43 (±45.86)	46.58 (±32.64)	2.92	0.009
Mean number of wake episodes	7.21 (±4.81)	5.42 (±2.31)	2.26	0.040
Mean wake episode (minutes)	3.76 (±1.62)	2.85 (±1.54)	2.49	0.023
Longest wake episode (minutes)	25.71 (±19.20)	18.16 (±11.55)	2.87	0.010
Subjective Sleep Quality (MSQ questionnaire)	3.64 (±1.15)	3.42 (±1.09)	2.152	0.187
Subjective Sleep Quality (PSQI questionnaire)	0.95 (±0.53)	0.80 (±0.54)	1.632	0.119

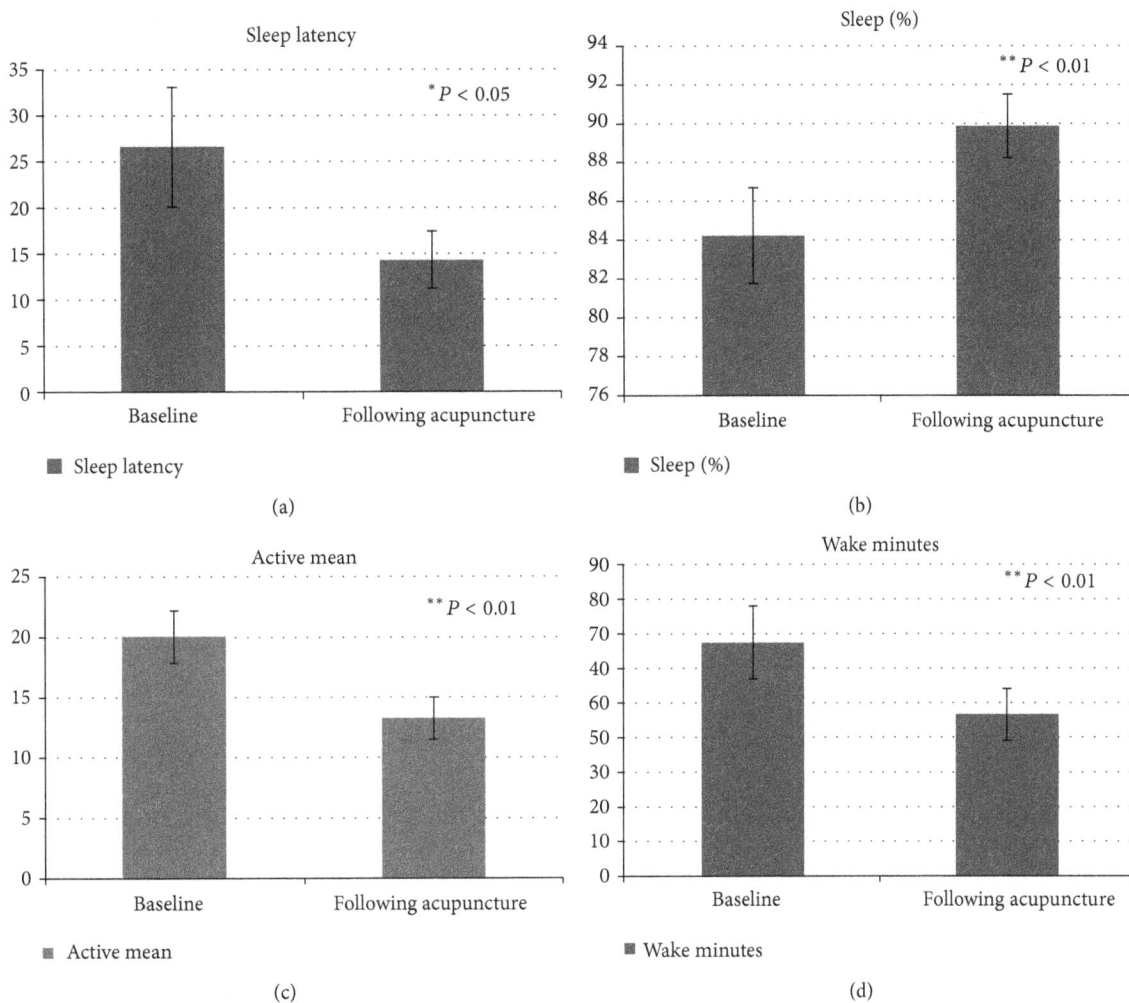

(a)

(b)

(c)

(d)

FIGURE 1: Objective measures of sleep as recorded by actigraph before and after acupuncture treatment: (a) sleep latency, (b) % of sleep percentage, (c) mean activity during sleep, and (d) total wake minutes during sleep.

TABLE 2: Emotional and clinical measures (means and standard deviations) after each phase of the study and analysis of the comparisons between them.

Emotional and clinical measures	Baseline level Mean (SD)	Last week of acupuncture treatment Mean (SD)	t	P value
Brief Psychiatric Rating Scale (BPRS)	2.49 (±0.81)	2.14 (±0.74)	6.67	0.001
Psychopathology score (PANSS)	2.96 (±0.98)	2.65 (±0.94)	8.26	0.001
Positive general symptoms (PANSS)	2.44 (±1.01)	2.04 (±0.88)	5.23	0.001
Negative general symptoms (PANSS)	3.62 (±1.20)	3.47 (±1.20)	2.97	0.008
General symptoms (PANSS)	2.83 (±0.95)	2.43 (±0.93)	7.96	0.001
Depression level (BDI questionnaire)	14.66 (±11.89)	12.01 (±11.61)	1.79	0.088
Depression level (CDSS questionnaire)	7.16 (±6.43)	4.21 (±4.90)	5.04	0.001
State Anxiety level (STAI questionnaire)	2.27 (±0.52)	2.12 (±0.48)	2.98	0.008
Anxiety level (HAS questionnaire)	1.21 (±0.68)	0.73 (±0.49)	5.96	0.001
Quality of Life level (QLESQ questionnaire)	3.60 (±0.58)	3.70 (±0.55)	−2.08	0.051
Anhedonia level (SHAPS questionnaire)	3.49 (±0.34)	3.41 (±0.45)	1.17	0.257

improved the general psychopathology score ($t(18) = 6.67$, $P < 0.01$), with a lower general psychopathology score following acupuncture treatment (M = 2.14, SD = 0.74) compared with the baseline score (M = 2.49, SD = 0.81) (Figure 2(a)).

Similarly, the results indicate that acupuncture improved the overall psychopathology score assessed by the Positive and Negative Syndrome Scale (PANNS) ($t(19) = 8.26$, $P < 0.01$), with a lower total psychopathology score following acupuncture treatment (M = 2.65, SD = 0.94) compared with the baseline measure (M = 2.96, SD = 0.98).

Likewise, significant differences were found for positive, negative, and general symptoms assessed by the Positive and Negative Syndrome Scale (PANNS) ($t(18) = 5.23$, $P < 0.01$; $t(18) = 2.97$, $P < 0.01$; $t(18) = 7.96$, $P < 0.01$, resp.), revealing lower positive, negative, and general symptoms following acupuncture treatment (M = 2.04, SD = 0.88; M = 3.47, SD = 1.20; M = 2.43, SD = 0.93, resp.) compared with baseline measures (M = 2.44, SD = 1.01; M = 3.62, SD = 1.20; M = 2.83, SD = 0.95, resp.) (Figures 2(b), 2(c), and 2(d)).

A paired sample t-test was conducted comparing emotional measures manifested by participants before and after sequential acupuncture treatment (Table 2).

A marginal significant difference was found in depression level as measured by the Beck Depression Inventory (BDI) questionnaire ($t(19) = 1.79$, $P = 0.088$), showing a reduced depression level following acupuncture treatment (M = 12.01, SD = 11.61) compared with the baseline depression level (M = 14.66, SD = 11.89). Moreover, a significant difference was found in depression level as measured by the Calgary Depression Scale for schizophrenia (CDSS) questionnaire ($t(18) = 5.04$, $P < 0.01$), revealing a lower depression level following acupuncture treatment (M = 4.21, SD = 4.90) compared to the baseline depression level (M = 7.16, SD = 6.43) (Figure 3(a)).

In addition, a significant difference was found in anxiety level as measured by the State-Trait Anxiety Inventory (STAI) and by the Hamilton Anxiety Rating Scale (HAS)

questionnaires ($t(19) = 2.98$, $P < 0.01$; $t(17) = 5.96$, $P < 0.01$, resp.), revealing a lower anxiety level following acupuncture treatment (M = 2.12, SD = 0.48; M = 0.73, SD = 0.49) compared with the baseline anxiety level (M = 2.27, SD = 0.52; M = 1.21, SD = 0.68) (Figure 3(b)).

A paired sample t-test was conducted comparing quality of life levels manifested by participants before and after sequential acupuncture treatment. The results revealed a marginal significant difference in quality of life level measured by the Quality of Life Enjoyment and Satisfaction Questionnaire (Q-LES-Q) ($t(19) = −2.08$, $P = 0.05$), showing a higher level of quality of life following acupuncture treatment (M = 3.70, SD = 0.55) compared with the baseline quality of life level (M = 3.60, SD = 0.58).

However, no significant effects of acupuncture treatment were found for depression level measured by the Beck Depression Inventory (BDI) or for hedonic level measured by the Snaith-Hamilton Pleasure Scale (SHAPS) (n.s.).

3.3. Traditional Chinese Medicine Assessments. The results of the traditional Chinese medicine assessments of patients from this study have been published previously [69].

4. Discussion

In the current pilot study we examined the efficacy of acupuncture treatment for patients with schizophrenia living in the community. Outcome measures included three different domains—sleep measures, clinical and emotional measures, and traditional Chinese medicine assessments. The results following acupuncture treatment indicate a significant improvement in objective sleep measures collected by actigraph device, among them sleep onset latency, sleep percentage, mean activity level, wake time after sleep onset, mean number of wake episodes, mean wake episode, and longest wake episode. The treatment made patients fall asleep faster. They slept better, with less wake time during sleep

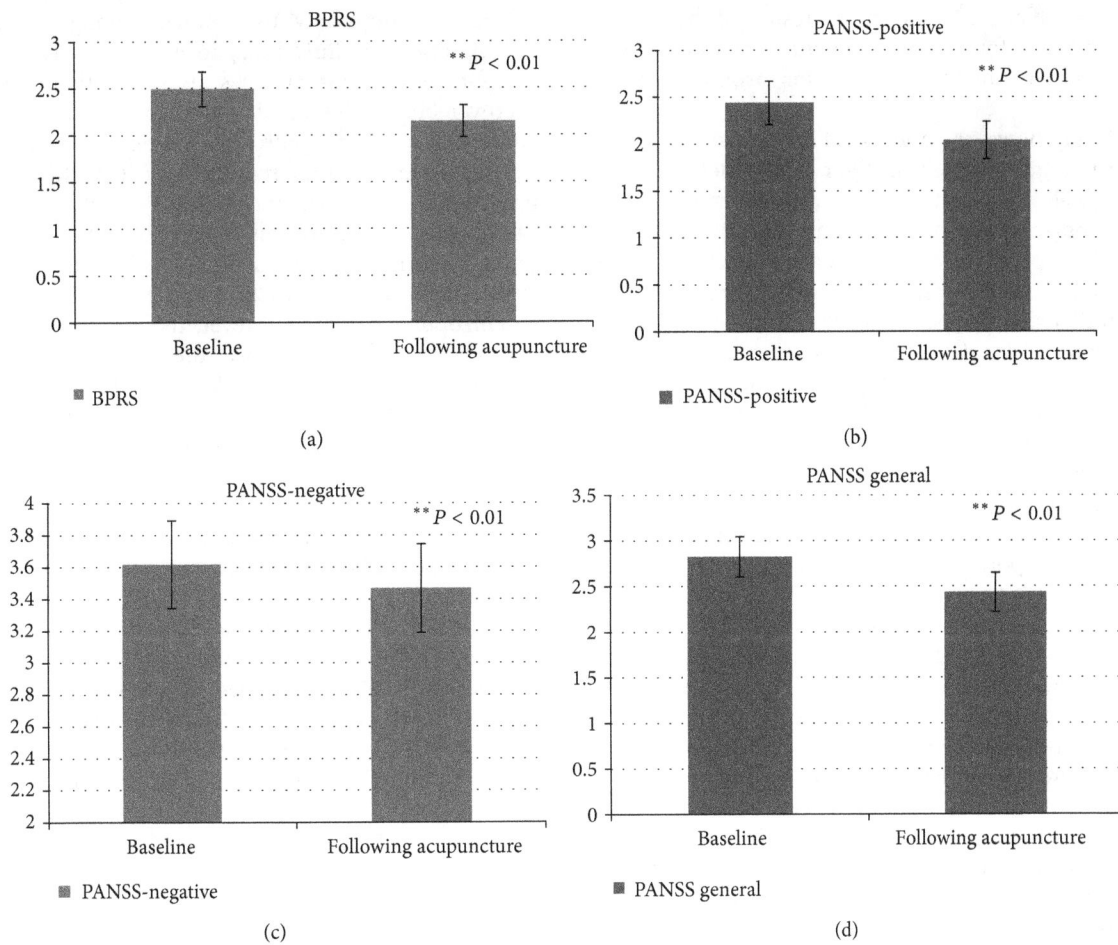

FIGURE 2: Objective psychopathology levels before and after acupuncture treatment: (a) general psychopathology score as recorded by the Brief Psychiatric Rating Scale (BPRS), (b) positive symptoms as measured by the Positive and Negative Syndrome Scale (PANSS), (c) negative symptoms as measured by the Positive and Negative Syndrome Scale (PANSS), and (d) general symptoms as measured by the Positive and Negative Syndrome Scale (PANSS).

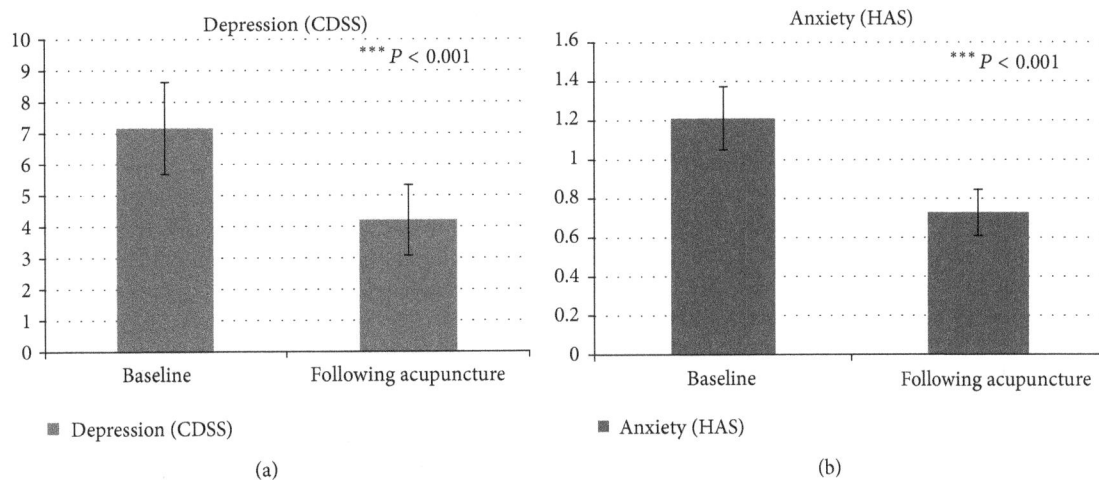

FIGURE 3: Emotional measures before and after acupuncture treatment: (a) depression level as measured by the Calgary Depression Scale for schizophrenia (CDSS), (b) anxiety level as measured by the Hamilton Anxiety Rating Scale (HAS).

and reduced activity level during sleep. As a result their sleep was more efficient. Moreover, the results of the current study revealed that, following acupuncture treatment, sleep percentage no longer met the criterion for insomnia (<85%) [70].

Interestingly, however, patients did not report any significant subjective improvement in their sleep. These findings raise the possibility of an optional discrepancy between subjective reported sleep measures and objective recorded measures. Many psychiatric disorders are evaluated both by objective and by subjective assessment tools to provide a general and multiangled perspective of the disorder examined. Yet, consistently arising discrepancies between different tools may suggest that these tools actually assess different phenomena. So the question is as follows: do subjective and objective sleep measures assess two distinct phenomena? In fact, several studies have shown that participant reports of their own sleep are only partly correlated to their objective sleep measures [46, 71–74]. The meaning of this difference between subjective sleep report and objective findings is far from being understood in terms of the biological factors involved, the clinical consequences, the treatment modality, and other factors as well. This subjective-objective discrepancy has been found repeatedly among different populations, such as posttrauma patients and elderly patients. Thus, findings revealing this discrepancy in patients with schizophrenia are in line with these studies. However, another explanation for this discrepancy of findings between objective and subjective assessments is the period of assessment of each measure. The objective measurements were taken over a brief period (one week at the end of the acupuncture treatment), while the patients may tend to subjectively assess their overall experience during the course of therapy, which they think may be ineffective. The subjective assessment results may also be heavily influenced by patients' own interpretation of their symptoms and experience as well as the wordings of the questionnaires.

Most importantly, these findings reinforce the influence of acupuncture on sleep measures, since the effect was found for the objective measures, implying that while the beneficial effect of acupuncture on sleep among patients with schizophrenia may exist, it may not be reportable. This makes the reliability of self-report with respect to sleep a questionable issue. These findings may be very important, since sleep difficulties are very common among patients with schizophrenia [19] and involve distress, malfunctioning, and impairment of quality of life, all directly related to sleep difficulties. Moreover, sleep difficulties and other domains of the psychopathology of schizophrenia, whether positive symptoms or symptoms such as anxiety and depression, have mutual and reciprocal relationships. Thus, sleep difficulties may play a crucial role in treatment resistance, partial remission, or relapse in schizophrenia.

Additionally, the results revealed an improvement in clinical and emotional assessments following acupuncture treatment. The core symptoms of schizophrenia, both positive and negative, as assessed by the Brief Psychiatric Rating Scale (BPRS) and by the Positive and Negative Syndrome Scale (PANSS), exhibited improvement compared to baseline following acupuncture treatments. Both the BPRS and the PANSS are commonly used scales among patients with schizophrenia for clinical diagnosis, for severity assessment, and for monitoring changes in the patient. Significant improvement on these scales shows a high correlation with clinical improvement, both objective and subjective.

This potential effect may be very important, especially in view of the unsatisfactory benefits of antipsychotic medications and the enormous burden of schizophrenia. This finding is concurrent with other studies that showed the beneficial effect of acupuncture on the core psychopathology of schizophrenia [36]. However, those studies had limited methodologies [36]. Likewise, the overall results of those studies are equivocal and insufficient [35].

Another clinical domain assessed was the domain of depression and anxiety. Depression and anxiety are very common in chronic schizophrenia and are connected with poor prognosis, greater distress, and higher rates of suicide [75–77]. It seems that acupuncture may not suffice as a sole treatment but rather can be used, as in this study, as an "add-on" for treating psychopathological domains other than the core domain of schizophrenia. Our study results revealed a significant beneficial effect of acupuncture on depression and anxiety levels, as assessed by the Calgary Depression Scale for schizophrenia (CDSS), by the State-Trait Anxiety Inventory (STAI), and by the Hamilton Anxiety Rating Scale (HAS). Because the symptoms of depression may overlap the negative symptoms of schizophrenia, we used the Calgary Depression Scale for schizophrenia (CDSS), which is used especially for assessing depression in the treatment of patients with schizophrenia. To summarize, the clinical outcome measures of the current study showed an overall improvement in depression, anxiety, and the core symptoms of schizophrenia.

In this study we chose to use acupuncture as an "add-on" treatment, and all of the patients continued their medication treatment as usual. The reason for not using acupuncture as a sole treatment was the unsatisfactory efficacy of acupuncture alone for schizophrenia in studies published so far. Moreover, schizophrenia is a complex disorder with multiple areas of distress and dysfunction, among them intrapsychic, interpersonal, and occupational, with long-term residual symptoms and rehabilitation difficulties. On the other hand, conventional treatment for schizophrenia, even at its best when combining pharmacotherapy, psychotherapy, and rehabilitation, achieves unsatisfactory results and only partial remission. All this suggests that supplemental treatments are of the utmost importance. Acupuncture as a supplementary treatment seems to be a promising option.

The study was carried out in the community with patients with schizophrenia living in hostels in "real life" situations with as few exclusion criteria as possible and without any limitations on the usual (pharmacotherapy, psychotherapy, and rehabilitation) treatment. There were no dropouts at any stage of the study. This zero dropout rate is unusual among general clinical studies and may signify high patient satisfaction with acupuncture treatment and low anxious or paranoid references, which would have been expected among patients with schizophrenia.

Altogether, this pilot study may suggest a good setting for evaluating an "add-on" treatment, and the results may have implications for real treatment choices. This is in contrast to rigorously designed studies, in which conclusions concerning "real life and real patients" are hard to obtain, or at least problematic.

This pilot study has several methodological limitations. Although the study used a within-subject design, it included a pre- and posttreatment evaluation but not a comparison with a control group, thus overlooking some other explanation for the effect. Therefore, the current study was vulnerable to placebo bias, either by participants or by therapists. Likewise, in this study, many statistical tests were performed, so there was a risk of committing type I errors.

Remarkably, we found a consistent and interesting change in many qualities that were not systematically assessed, such as changes in patients' voices, general appearance, posturing, pace and movement, and vitality. Since all of these and many more qualities are familiar to TCM therapists, and since TCM treatment aims at relieving a broad spectrum of symptoms and distress, new assessment tools should be developed for similar future studies. Furthermore, since all these qualities seem to be connected to different aspects of well-being and quality of life, it may be equally important to develop new assessment tools for conventional pharmacotherapeutic studies.

In summary, to the best of our knowledge this is the first study to evaluate the efficacy of acupuncture on sleep in patients with schizophrenia using actigraph sleep measurement as an objective efficacy measure. Our results suggest that, for patients with schizophrenia, acupuncture treatment may have a possible beneficial effect on clinical core schizophrenic symptoms and on depressive and anxiety symptoms. Moreover, for patients with schizophrenia the results suggest a possible beneficial effect of acupuncture treatment on objective sleep but not on the patients' subjective experience in the short term while the patients are undergoing eight weeks of therapy. These findings need to be validated in future studies; that is, large randomized controlled trials are required to assess the efficacy of acupuncture treatment for insomnia among patients with schizophrenia.

The results of the current study demonstrated the potential short-term benefits of acupuncture. Future studies should examine whether these benefits will be maintained after cessation of therapy or whether acupuncture must be continued forever to maintain the benefits. Therefore, future studies are needed to validate the benefits of long-term acupuncture treatment. Since the results of the current study revealed that no patient experienced any adverse effects throughout the course of therapy, there is definitely room to check the feasibility of long-term acupuncture treatment among patients with schizophrenia.

Conflicts of Interests

We declare that this was not an industry-supported study. This study was not supported by a grant or by funders. No conflict of interests exists in our research. None of the authors or our institutions has any financial or other relationship that might have inappropriately influenced our writing.

Authors' Contribution

Alon Reshef and Boaz Bloch contributed equally to this research.

Acknowledgments

The authors acknowledge the generous support of the participants and the generous assistance of several research assistants during the data collection process: Bendrihem Ronen, Levi Miri, Rabinovich Beeri, and Dvir Inbal.

References

[1] R. W. Heinrichs and K. K. Zakzanis, "Neurocognitive deficit in schizophrenia: a quantitative review of the evidence," *Neuropsychology*, vol. 12, no. 3, pp. 426–445, 1998.

[2] A. I. Green, M. S. Salomon, M. J. Brenner, and K. Rawlins, "Treatment of schizophrenia and comorbid substance use disorder," *CNS and Neurological Disorders—Drug Targets*, vol. 1, no. 2, pp. 129–139, 2002.

[3] P. F. Buckley, B. J. Miller, D. S. Lehrer, and D. J. Castle, "Psychiatric comorbidities and schizophrenia," *Schizophrenia Bulletin*, vol. 35, no. 2, pp. 383–402, 2009.

[4] American Psychiatric Association, *Diagnostic and Statistical Manual of Mental Disorders*, American Psychiatric Press, Washington, DC, USA, 4th edition, 1994.

[5] J. S. Brekke, J. D. Long, N. Nesbitt, and E. Sobel, "The impact of service characteristics on functional outcomes from community support programs for persons with schizophrenia: a growth curve analysis," *Journal of Consulting and Clinical Psychology*, vol. 65, no. 3, pp. 464–475, 1997.

[6] R. Hunter and S. Barry, "Negative symptoms and psychosocial functioning in schizophrenia: neglected but important targets for treatment," *European Psychiatry*, vol. 27, no. 6, pp. 432–436, 2012.

[7] E. Y. H. Chen, C. L. Kwok, J. W. Y. Au, R. Y. L. Chen, and B. S. T. Lau, "Progressive deterioration of soft neurological signs in chronic schizophrenic patients," *Acta Psychiatrica Scandinavica*, vol. 102, no. 5, pp. 342–349, 2000.

[8] A. Oni-Orisan, L. V. Kristiansen, V. Haroutunian, J. H. Meador-Woodruff, and R. E. McCullumsmith, "Altered vesicular glutamate transporter expression in the anterior cingulate cortex in schizophrenia," *Biological Psychiatry*, vol. 63, no. 8, pp. 766–775, 2008.

[9] G. Venkatasubramanian and M. S. Keshavan, "Early intervention in psychosis: perspectives on Asian studies," *Asian Journal of Psychiatry*, vol. 5, no. 1, pp. 1–2, 2012.

[10] K. T. Mueser, D. P. Valentiner, and J. Agresta, "Coping with negative symptoms of schizophrenia: patient and family perspectives," *Schizophrenia Bulletin*, vol. 23, no. 2, pp. 329–339, 1997.

[11] J. P. Lindenmayer, R. Bernstein-Hyman, and S. Grochowski, "Five-factor model of schizophrenia," *Journal of Nervous and Mental Disease*, vol. 182, no. 11, pp. 631–638, 1994.

[12] J. M. Monti and D. Monti, "Sleep in schizophrenia patients and the effects of antipsychotic drugs," *Sleep Medicine Reviews*, vol. 8, no. 2, pp. 133–148, 2004.

[13] S. Zisook, M. Nyer, J. Kasckow, S. Golshan, D. Lehman, and L. Montross, "Depressive symptom patterns in patients with chronic schizophrenia and subsyndromal depression," *Schizophrenia Research*, vol. 86, no. 1-3, pp. 226–233, 2006.

[14] K. Wulff, D. Dijk, B. Middleton, R. G. Foster, and E. M. Joyce, "Sleep and circadian rhythm disruption in schizophrenia," *The British Journal of Psychiatry*, vol. 200, no. 4, pp. 308–316, 2012.

[15] D. Riemann, "Insomnia and comorbid psychiatric disorders," *Sleep Medicine*, vol. 8, supplement 4, pp. S15–S20, 2007.

[16] W. Szelenberger and C. Soldatos, "Sleep disorders in psychiatric practice," *World Psychiatry*, vol. 4, no. 3, pp. 186–190, 2005.

[17] J. M. Kane and Z. A. Sharif, "Atypical antipsychotics: sedation versus efficacy," *Journal of Clinical Psychiatry*, vol. 69, supplement 1, pp. 18–31, 2008.

[18] J. Poulin, A. M. Daoust, G. Forest, E. Stip, and R. Godbout, "Sleep architecture and its clinical correlates in first episode and neuroleptic-naive patients with schizophrenia," *Schizophrenia Research*, vol. 62, no. 1-2, pp. 147–153, 2003.

[19] S. Cohrs, "Sleep disturbances in patients with schizophrenia: impact and effect of antipsychotics," *CNS Drugs*, vol. 22, no. 11, pp. 939–962, 2008.

[20] J. Kantrowitz, L. Citrome, and D. Javitt, "GABAB receptors, schizophrenia and sleep dysfunction: a review of the relationship and its potential clinical and therapeutic implications," *CNS Drugs*, vol. 23, no. 8, pp. 681–691, 2009.

[21] J. A. Costa e Silva, "Sleep disorders in psychiatry," *Metabolism: Clinical and Experimental*, vol. 55, supplement 2, pp. S40–S44, 2006.

[22] American Sleep Disorders Association, *International Classification of Sleep Disorders, Revised: Diagnostic and Coding Manual*, American Sleep Disorders Association, Rochester, Minn, USA, 1997.

[23] D. P. van Kammen, W. B. van Kammen, J. L. Peters et al., "CSF MHPG sleep and psychosis in schizophrenia," *Clinical Neuropharmacology*, vol. 9, no. 4, pp. 575–577, 1986.

[24] E. O. Johnson, T. Roth, and N. Breslau, "The association of insomnia with anxiety disorders and depression: exploration of the direction of risk," *Journal of Psychiatric Research*, vol. 40, no. 8, pp. 700–708, 2006.

[25] M. J. Peterson, M. E. Rumble, and R. M. Benca, "Insomnia and psychiatric disorders," *Psychiatric Annals*, vol. 38, no. 9, pp. 597–605, 2008.

[26] E. Collier, G. Skitt, and H. Cutts, "A study on the experience of insomnia in a psychiatric inpatient population," *Journal of Psychiatric and Mental Health Nursing*, vol. 10, no. 6, pp. 697–704, 2003.

[27] W. B. Mendelson, "Combining pharmacologic and nonpharmacologic therapies for insomnia," *Journal of Clinical Psychiatry*, vol. 68, no. 5, pp. 19–23, 2007.

[28] J. D. Hoehns and P. J. Perry, "Zolpidem: a nonbenzodiazepine hypnotic for treatment of insomnia," *Clinical Pharmacy*, vol. 12, no. 11, pp. 814–828, 1993.

[29] M. B. Scharf, T. Roth, G. W. Vogel, and J. K. Walsh, "A multicenter, placebo-controlled study evaluating Zolpidem in the treatment of chronic insomnia," *Journal of Clinical Psychiatry*, vol. 55, no. 5, pp. 192–199, 1994.

[30] S. H. Shaw, H. Curson, and J. P. Coquelin, "A double-blind, comparative study of zolpidem and placebo in the treatment of insomnia in elderly psychiatric in-patients," *Journal of International Medical Research*, vol. 20, no. 2, pp. 150–161, 1992.

[31] M. J. Sateia and P. D. Nowell, "Insomnia," *The Lancet*, vol. 364, no. 9449, pp. 1959–1973, 2004.

[32] W. V. McCall, "Pharmacologic treatment of insomnia," in *Sleep Medicine*, T. L. Lee-Ching, M. J. Satia, and M. A. Carskadon, Eds., pp. 169–176, Hanley and Blfus, Philadelphia, Pa, USA, 2002.

[33] J. Rathbone, L. Zhang, M. Zhang et al., "Chinese herbal medicine for schizophrenia: cochrane systematic review of randomised trials," *The British Journal of Psychiatry*, vol. 190, pp. 379–384, 2007.

[34] J. T. Shuval, N. Mizrachi, and E. Smetannikov, "Entering the well-guarded fortress: alternative practitioners in hospital settings," *Social Science and Medicine*, vol. 55, no. 10, pp. 1745–1755, 2002.

[35] J. Rathbone and J. Xia, "Acupuncture for schizophrenia," *Cochrane Database of Systematic Reviews*, no. 4, Article ID CD005475, 2005.

[36] M. S. Lee, B. C. Shin, P. Ronan, and E. Ernst, "Acupuncture for schizophrenia: a systematic review and meta-analysis," *International Journal of Clinical Practice*, vol. 63, no. 11, pp. 1622–1633, 2009.

[37] H. MacPherson, K. Thomas, S. Walters, and M. Fitter, "The York acupuncture safety study: prospective survey of 34 000 treatments by traditional acupuncturists," *The British Medical Journal*, vol. 323, no. 7311, pp. 486–487, 2001.

[38] C. M. H. Goertz, R. Niemtzow, S. M. Burns, M. J. Fritts, C. C. Crawford, and W. B. Jonas, "Auricular acupuncture in the treatment of acute pain syndromes: a pilot study," *Military Medicine*, vol. 171, no. 10, pp. 1010–1014, 2006.

[39] R. C. Kessler, J. Soukup, R. B. Davis et al., "The use of complementary and alternative therapies to treat anxiety and depression in the United States," *The American Journal of Psychiatry*, vol. 158, no. 2, pp. 289–294, 2001.

[40] D. K. Cheuk, W. F. Yeung, K. F. Chung, and V. Wong, "Acupuncture for insomnia," *Cochrane Database of Systematic Reviews*, no. 3, Article ID CD005472, 2007.

[41] W. F. Yeung, K. F. Chung, M. M. Poon et al., "Acupressure, reflexology, and auricular acupressure for insomnia: a systematic review of randomized controlled trials," *Sleep Medicine*, vol. 13, no. 8, pp. 971–984, 2012.

[42] M. D. Kutch, "Cost-effectiveness analysis of complementary and alternative medicine in treating mental health disorders," *Dissertation Abstracts International A*, vol. 71, no. 11, p. 4102, 2011.

[43] World Health Organisation, *International Statistical Classification of Diseases and Related Health Problems, 10th Revision (ICD-10)*, WHO, Geneva, Switzerland, 1992.

[44] J. Zomer, R. Peled, A. H. E. Rubin, and P. Lavie, "Mini Sleep Questionnaire (MSQ) for screening large populations for EDS complaints," in *Sleep 1984*, W. P. Koella, E. Ruther, and H. Schulz, Eds., pp. 467–469, Gustav Fischer, New York, NY, USA, 1985.

[45] O. Tzischinsky, A. Cohen, E. Doveh et al., "Screening for sleep disordered breathing among applicants for a professional driver's license," *Journal of Occupational and Environmental Medicine*, vol. 54, no. 10, pp. 1275–1280, 2012.

[46] I. Haimov, N. Breznitz, and S. Shiloh, "Sleep in healthy elderly: sources of discrepancy between self-report and recorded sleep," in *Clinical and Neurophysiological Aspects of Sleep*, V. M. Kumar and H. N. Mallick, Eds., pp. 145–148, Medimond, International Proceedings, 2006.

[47] T. Shochat, O. Tzischinsky, A. Oksenberg, and R. Peled, "Validation of the Pittsburgh sleep quality index hebrew translation (PSQI-H) in a sleep clinic sample," *Israel Medical Association Journal*, vol. 9, no. 12, pp. 853–856, 2007.

[48] J. O. Brooks III, L. Friedman, D. L. Bliwise, and J. A. Yesavage, "Use of the wrist actigraph to study insomnia in older adults," *Sleep*, vol. 16, no. 2, pp. 151–155, 1993.

[49] C. Mccall and W. V. Mccall, "Comparison of actigraphy with polysomnography and sleep logs in depressed insomniacs," *Journal of Sleep Research*, vol. 21, no. 1, pp. 122–127, 2012.

[50] J. E. Overall and D. E. Gorham, "The brief psychiatric rating scale," *Psychological Reports*, vol. 10, no. 3, pp. 799–812, 1962.

[51] M. Sherwood, A. E. Thornton, and W. G. Honer, "A quantitative review of the profile and time course of symptom change in schizophrenia treated with clozapine," *Journal of Psychopharmacology*, vol. 26, no. 9, pp. 1175–1184, 2012.

[52] S. R. Kay, L. A. Opler, and J. P. Lindenmayer, "Reliability and validity of the positive and negative syndrome scale for schizophrenics," *Psychiatry Research*, vol. 23, no. 1, pp. 99–110, 1988.

[53] A. T. Beck and R. A. Steer, *Beck Depression Inventory Manual*, The Psychological Corporation, San Antonio, Tex, USA, 1987.

[54] Y. J. Lee, S. J. Cho, I. H. Cho, J. H. Jang, and S. J. Kim, "The relationship between psychotic-like experiences and sleep disturbances in adolescents," *Sleep Medicine*, vol. 13, no. 8, pp. 1021–1027, 2012.

[55] A. T. Beck, R. A. Steer, and M. G. Garbin, "Psychometric properties of the beck depression inventory: twenty-five years of evaluation," *Clinical Psychology Review*, vol. 8, no. 1, pp. 77–100, 1988.

[56] M. J. Müller, H. Brening, C. Gensch, J. Klinga, B. Kienzle, and K. M. Müller, "The calgary depression rating scale for schizophrenia in a healthy control group: psychometric properties and reference values," *Journal of Affective Disorders*, vol. 88, no. 1, pp. 69–74, 2005.

[57] R. Schennach, M. Obermeier, F. Seemüller et al., "Evaluating depressive symptoms in schizophrenia: a psychometric comparison of the calgary depression scale for schizophrenia and the Hamilton depression rating scale," *Psychopathology*, vol. 45, no. 5, pp. 276–285, 2012.

[58] O. Schwartz-Stav, A. Apter, and G. Zalsman, "Depression, suicidal behavior and insight in adolescents with schizophrenia," *European Child and Adolescent Psychiatry*, vol. 15, no. 6, pp. 352–359, 2006.

[59] A. Okun, R. E. K. Stein, L. J. Bauman, and E. J. Silver, "Content validity of the psychiatric symptom index, CES-depression scale, and state-trait anxiety inventory from the perspective of DSM-IV," *Psychological Reports*, vol. 79, no. 3, pp. 1059–1069, 1996.

[60] C. D. Spielberger, R. L. Gorusch, and R. E. Lushene, *Manual for the State-Trait Inventory (Self-Evaluation Questionnaire)*, Consulting Psychologists Press, Palo Alto, Calif, USA, 1970.

[61] R. Meades and S. Ayers, "Anxiety measures validated in perinatal populations: a systematic review," *Journal of Affective Disorders*, vol. 133, no. 1-2, pp. 1–15, 2011.

[62] W. Maier, R. Buller, M. Philipp, and I. Heuser, "The Hamilton anxiety scale: reliability, validity and sensitivity to change in anxiety and depressive disorders," *Journal of Affective Disorders*, vol. 14, no. 1, pp. 61–68, 1988.

[63] M. Bellani, J. P. Hatch, M. A. Nicoletti et al., "Does anxiety increase impulsivity in patients with bipolar disorder or major depressive disorder?" *Journal of Psychiatric Research*, vol. 46, no. 5, pp. 616–621, 2012.

[64] R. P. Snaith, M. Hamilton, S. Morley, A. Humayan, D. Hargreaves, and P. Trigwell, "A scale for the assessment of hedonic tone. The Snaith-Hamilton pleasure scale," *The British Journal of Psychiatry*, vol. 167, no. 1, pp. 99–103, 1995.

[65] J. Thomas, M. Al Ali, A. Al Hashmi, and A. Rodriguez, "Convergent validity and internal consistency of an Arabic Snaith Hamilton pleasure acale," *International Perspectives in Psychology: Research, Practice, Consultation*, vol. 1, no. 1, pp. 46–51, 2012.

[66] J. Endicott, J. Nee, W. Harrison, and R. Blumenthal, "Quality of life enjoyment and satisfaction questionnaire: a new measure," *Psychopharmacology Bulletin*, vol. 29, no. 2, pp. 321–326, 1993.

[67] A. Luquiens, M. Reynaud, B. Falissard, and H. J. Aubin, "Quality of life among alcohol-dependent patients: How satisfactory are the available instruments? A systematic review," *Drug and Alcohol Dependence*, vol. 125, no. 3, pp. 192–201, 2012.

[68] P. Deadman and M. Al-Khafaji, *A Manual of Acupuncture*, Journal of Chinese Medicine Publications, England, UK, 1998.

[69] B. Bloch, S. Ravid, L. Vadas et al., "The acupuncture treatment of schizophrenia: a review with case studies," *Journal of Chinese Medicine*, no. 93, pp. 57–63, 2010.

[70] I. V. Zhdanova, R. J. Wurtman, M. M. Regan, J. A. Taylor, J. P. Shi, and O. U. Leclair, "Melatonin treatment for age-related insomnia," *Journal of Clinical Endocrinology and Metabolism*, vol. 86, no. 10, pp. 4727–4730, 2001.

[71] L. Zhang and Z. Zhao, "Objective and subjective measures for sleep disorders," *Neuroscience Bulletin*, vol. 23, no. 4, pp. 236–240, 2007.

[72] I. Kobayashi, J. M. Boarts, and D. L. Delahanty, "Polysomnographically measured sleep abnormalities in PTSD: a meta-analytic review," *Psychophysiology*, vol. 44, no. 4, pp. 660–669, 2007.

[73] E. Klein, D. Koren, I. Arnon, and P. Lavie, "Sleep complaints are not corroborated by objective sleep measures in post-traumatic stress disorder: a 1-year prospective study in survivors of motor vehicle crashes," *Journal of Sleep Research*, vol. 12, no. 1, pp. 35–41, 2003.

[74] M. Matousek, K. Cervena, L. Zavesicka, and M. Brunovsky, "Subjective and objective evaluation of alertness and sleep quality in depressed patients: correlation between the patients' statements and polygraphic findings," *BMC Psychiatry*, vol. 4, article 14, 2004.

[75] M. Pompili, X. F. Amador, P. Girardi et al., "Suicide risk in schizophrenia: learning from the past to change the future," *Annals of General Psychiatry*, vol. 6, article 10, 2007.

[76] R. A. Emsley, P. P. Oosthuizen, A. F. Joubert, M. C. Roberts, and D. J. Stein, "Depressive and anxiety symptoms in patients with schizophrenia and schizophreniform disorder," *Journal of Clinical Psychiatry*, vol. 60, no. 11, pp. 747–751, 1999.

[77] R. J. Bragaa, M. V. Mendlowicza, R. P. Marrocosd, and I. L. Figueiraa, "Anxiety disorders in outpatients with schizophrenia: prevalence and impact on the subjective quality of life," *Journal of Psychiatric Research*, vol. 39, no. 4, pp. 409–414, 2005.

8

Accuracy of Positive Airway Pressure Device—Measured Apneas and Hypopneas: Role in Treatment Followup

Carl Stepnowsky,[1,2] Tania Zamora,[1] Robert Barker,[3] Lin Liu,[4] and Kathleen Sarmiento[2,3]

[1] Health Services Research & Development Unit, Veterans Affairs San Diego Healthcare System, San Diego, CA 92161, USA
[2] Department of Medicine, University of California, San Diego, CA 92037, USA
[3] Pulmonary Service, Veterans Affairs San Diego Healthcare System, San Diego, CA 92161, USA
[4] Department of Family and Preventive Medicine, University of California, San Diego, CA 92037, USA

Correspondence should be addressed to Carl Stepnowsky; cstepnowsky@ucsd.edu

Academic Editor: Giora Pillar

Improved data transmission technologies have facilitated data collected from positive airway pressure (PAP) devices in the home environment. Although clinicians' treatment decisions increasingly rely on autoscoring of respiratory events by the PAP device, few studies have specifically examined the accuracy of autoscored respiratory events in the home environment in ongoing PAP use. "PAP efficacy" studies were conducted in which participants wore PAP simultaneously with an Embletta sleep system (Embla, Inc., Broomfield, CO), which was directly connected to the ResMed AutoSet S8 (ResMed, Inc., San Diego, CA) via a specialized cable. Mean PAP-scored Apnea-Hypopnea Index (AHI) was 14.2 ± 11.8 (median: 11.7; range: 3.9–46.3) and mean manual-scored AHI was 9.4 ± 10.2 (median: 7.7; range: 1.2–39.3). Ratios between the mean indices were calculated. PAP-scored HI was 2.0 times higher than the manual-scored HI. PAP-scored AHI was 1.5 times higher than the manual-scored AHI, and PAP-scored AI was 1.04 of manual-scored AI. In this sample, PAP-scored HI was on average double the manual-scored HI. Given the importance of PAP efficacy data in tracking treatment progress, it is important to recognize the possible bias of PAP algorithms in overreporting hypopneas. The most likely cause of this discrepancy is the use of desaturations in manual hypopnea scoring.

1. Introduction

Obstructive sleep apnea (OSA) is a chronic medical condition requiring nightly application of therapy to effectively limit the number of apneas and hypopneas that would occur without intervention. The gold-standard treatment for OSA is continuous positive airway pressure therapy (PAP), which provides a pneumatic splint of the soft tissue in the upper airway [1]. PAP devices can measure and record airflow and pressure levels whenever the device is worn. They contain internal, proprietary (i.e., differing by manufacturer) algorithms that identify breathing disturbances and whether these disturbances are due to persistent obstructive or nonobstructive events. Thus, PAP devices can provide a measure of "residual" Apnea-Hypopnea Index (AHI) and its components, the Hypopnea Index (HI) and Apnea Index (AI). Although not equivalent to the indices measured by polysomnography or

home sleep testing via Type III devices, the PAP terminology is nonetheless the same.

American Academy of Sleep Medicine practice parameters and clinical guidelines recommend routine monitoring of adherence and efficacy data provided by PAP devices as an indication of treatment progress [2, 3]. Because residual AHI is primarily used to inform pressure changes and because its measurement by the PAP device is different relative to polysomnography (PSG) or Type III devices, it requires further study. PAP-scored AHI is different from that scored by PSD for two main reasons: (1) PAP measures are based solely on an airflow signal, and (2) they are based on an automated, proprietary algorithm. Several studies have examined PAP-scored AHI but have primarily attempted to evaluate the ability of the PAP device (autoadjusting PAP, in particular) to provide an initial baseline AHI value. Most have reported a strong correlation between PAP-scored AHI and manual-scored AHI [4, 5]. However, a certain percentage of AHI values would have resulted in different classifications, which can affect clinical management decisions.

A related but different issue concerns the accuracy of the Apnea-Hypopnea Index (AHI), as measured by the PAP unit in the home environment for the purposes of treatment efficacy (i.e., after a period of use). AHI accuracy is particularly important, given the increasing use of and reliance upon PAP data by providers, patients, and intermediaries (i.e., durable medical equipment staff). Ambulatory models of OSA care are gaining popularity, particularly the use of autotitrating PAP devices in lieu of in-laboratory CPAP titrations. In contrast to fixed pressure devices, which simply count the number of apneas occurring while PAP is applied, autoadjusting devices can make pressure changes based on the identification of these disturbances. With an ever-increasing demand for sleep apnea care, the ability to identify patients who may not be therapeutic on their PAP devices is critical. Efficacy of therapy is also an important factor in patient adherence. New technologies allow for data transmission directly from the PAP device to software accessible to the provider and, more recently, to the patients themselves (e.g., SleepMapper, Philips Respironics, Murrysville, PA). A variety of data transmission methods are possible, including the use of a smartcard, wired modem (via telephone line), wireless modem (via cellular network), and, more recently, Bluetooth modems to connect directly into home computers, tablets, or Smartphones. Remote monitoring is a trend within healthcare that is clearly accelerating, and in the sleep field, it facilitates the evaluation of compliance and efficacy of PAP therapy [6].

Given the improved PAP data transmission technologies and resultant increased use of these data, we sought to investigate the accuracy of the PAP-measured AHI. We had the opportunity to conduct "PAP efficacy" studies in which participants wore PAP devices simultaneously with Type III cardiopulmonary recording equipment. Therefore, the goal of the present study was to specifically examine the accuracy of the identification of apneas and hypopneas by the PAP device.

2. Methods

2.1. Procedures. Twelve research participants from a larger trial evaluating a PAP adherence intervention were included in this study. The PAP adherence intervention study compared a usual care group to a group that was provided with extra education and clinical support via interactive website, phone calls, and in-person clinic visits [7]. They were also provided with daily access to their PAP data. Inclusion criteria for the study were purposefully broad and included those diagnosed with OSA (as defined by AHI >15 with predominately obstructive events) and prescribed PAP therapy. Participants who had a clinical indication for performing an efficacy study (e.g., either high residual PAP-measured AHI or subjective report that was inconsistent with PAP data) [3] were included. These participants underwent a home efficacy study, in which autoadjusting positive airway pressure therapy (APAP) devices was worn simultaneously with Embletta, a Type III cardiopulmonary recording device.

TABLE 1: Baseline characteristics.

	Mean ± SD	Range
Age	62.0 ± 12.3	46–78
Body Mass Index (BMI)	30.4 ± 5.9	21.5–41.7
Apnea-Hypopnea Index (AHI)	42.9 ± 21.5	11.3–76.9
Epworth Sleepiness Scale (ESS)	14.2 ± 3.9	8.0–19.0

2.2. Equipment Used. The Embletta (Embla, Inc., Broomfield, CO) was directly connected to the ResMed AutoSet S8 (ResMed, Inc., San Diego, CA) via a specialized cable that allowed for the direct recording of S8 data. Signals recorded include oximetry, chest effort, and body position. Airflow from the PAP device was used for scoring. RemLogic software was used for manual respiratory scoring. Apneas and hypopneas were manually scored according to the 2007 American Academy of Sleep Medicine guidelines, which included defining a hypopnea as being associated with a ≥4% oxygen desaturation [8]. AutoSet respiratory events were autoscored by the device, and summary statistics were obtained within RemLogic. Manual scoring was blind to the AutoSet-scored respiratory events.

2.3. Data Analysis. Descriptive statistics (mean, median, and standard deviation and range) were calculated for the AHI, HI, and AI data. Scatterplots were generated to show the relationship between PAP-scored and manual-scored indices and included the line of identity. Spearman correlation coefficient was calculated. Wilcoxon signed rank test was used to test mean difference between the indices, and concordance correlation coefficients [9, 10] with 95% confidence interval (CI) were used to assess the agreement between PAP-scored and manual-scored indices. The concordance correlation coefficient less than 0.90 is interpreted as poor agreement, 0.90–0.95 as moderate, 0.95–0.99 as substantial, and greater than 0.99 as almost perfect [11]. Bland-Altman plots were created to provide a visualization of the bias and limits of agreement [12]. Data were analyzed using R [13].

3. Results

Participants were primarily overweight, middle aged, and sleepy with moderate to severe OSA (see Table 1) who had been using PAP on average 84.8 days prior to the PAP efficacy study. There were 6 men and 6 women.

Mean PAP-scored AHI was 14.2 ± 11.8 (median: 11.7, range: 3.9–46.3) and mean manual-scored AHI was 9.4 ± 10.2 (median: 7.7, range: 1.2–39.3) (see Table 2). Paired sample means testing found differences between the PAP AHI and manual AHI (mean difference = 4.84, median difference = 4.25, $P < 0.001$) and between the PAP HI and manual HI (mean difference = 4.45, median difference = 3.5, $P < 0.001$), but not between PAP AI and manual AI (mean difference = 0.21, median difference = 0.4, $P = 0.53$). The correlation coefficient between PAP-scored and manual-scored AHI, AI, and HI was 0.93 ($P < 0.001$), 0.92 ($P < 0.001$), and 0.87 ($P < 0.001$), respectively.

TABLE 2: OSA variables measured on efficacy study.

	Manual scoring		Autoscoring	
	Mean ± SD	Range	Mean ± SD	Range
Apnea-Hypopnea Index (AHI)	9.4 ± 10.2	1.2–39.3	14.2 ± 11.8	3.9–46.3
Apnea Index (AI)	5.1 ± 7.9	0–28.4	5.3 ± 7.7	0.20–27.6
Central Apnea Index (CAI)	2.6 ± 6.6	0–23.5	—	—
Obstructive Apnea Index (OAI)	1.5 ± 2.3	0–7.7	—	—
Mixed Apnea Index (MAI)	0.9 ± 1.3	0–4.6	—	—
Hypopnea Index (HI)	4.3 ± 3.0	0.5–10.9	8.8 ± 4.9	3.1–18.7
Oxygen Desaturation Index (ODI)	7.7 ± 7.4	0.6–27.2	—	—

Concordance correlation coefficient is 0.87 (95% CI: 0.71–0.95) for AHI, 0.994 (95% CI: 0.98–0.998) for AI, and 0.50 (95% CI: 0.23–0.70) for HI. Based on published guidelines, the agreement between PAP and manual scoring is considered "poor" in AHI and HI and is "almost perfect" for AI.

Ratios between the mean indices were calculated. The PAP-scored HI was 2.0 times higher than the manual-scored HI, the PAP-scored AHI was 1.5 times higher than the manual-scored AHI, and the PAP-scored AI was 1.04 of the manual-scored AI. It appears that the PAP device evaluated in this study, relative to manual scoring, only slightly overscored the number of apneas but significantly overscored the number of hypopneas. The difference in scoring of hypopneas seems to be the main contributor to the different AHI values between the PAP device and manual scoring.

Two graphical displays of the data were created. Figures 1(a)–1(c) show the scatterplots for the three indices, including the line of identity. In each case, the PAP-scored index was higher than the corresponding manual-scored index. Figures 2(a)–2(c) show the Bland-Altman plots. The mean bias (95% limit of agreement) is 4.84 (−0.95 to 10.6) for AHI, 0.28 (−1.50 to 1.91) for AI, and 4.45 (−0.17 to 9.07) for HI.

4. Discussion

The practice of sleep medicine is evolving, and ambulatory models of sleep apnea management using home sleep testing and APAP therapy are not only noninferior to traditional evaluations but are also gaining wider acceptance by sleep providers [14]. Home sleep testing, or cardiorespiratory polygraphy, is indicated for the diagnosis of OSA in patients with a high pretest probability of moderate to severe OSA, to monitor efficacy of non-PAP therapies for OSA, and may be indicated in those who would otherwise not be recommended for home evaluation but who cannot undergo in-laboratory diagnostic testing [15]. Emphasis is placed on reviewing the raw data from home sleep tests to ensure accurate diagnoses. Similarly, review of downloaded data from PAP machines is of great importance in determining efficacy of therapy and should guide decisions to change PAP settings. Thus, in an era of increasing dependence on efficacy and compliance information in the clinical management of sleep apnea patients, a greater understanding of how to interpret this information is needed.

In this study of home-based PAP efficacy, as measured by the S8 APAP device, the PAP-scored HI was on average more than double the manual-scored HI. Given the importance of PAP efficacy data in tracking treatment progress, it is important to recognize that this particular APAP device may overscore hypopneas. The most likely causes of this discrepancy are (a) the use of a proprietary algorithm and (b) the use of desaturations in manual hypopnea scoring. Because the number of apneas was underscored relative to manual scoring, the overall AHI does not appear to be different from manual scoring. This study and the evolving literature in this area suggest that it is important to understand how a specific PAP device identifies both apneas and hypopneas.

One previous study that used the S8 device also found relatively good apnea measurement but an overscoring of hypopneas [16]. That study found that the PAP HI was 3.3 times higher than the manual HI, and the resulting AHI was just over two times greater. Those values are slightly higher than the values found in the present study, but both speak to the importance of understanding the scoring algorithms for apneas and hypopneas of a specific PAP device so that treatment decisions are well informed. If it is found that, on average, a specific PAP device scores hypopneas at a rate of 2.0 times greater than manual scoring, then an adjustment can be made by the provider. For example, in the case where the measured HI is 20, the adjustment can be made by dividing 20 by the factor of 2 or an HI of 10 (which would theoretically be comparable to manual scoring).

Other studies in this area have utilized the RemStar autoadjusting PAP device by Philips Respironics. These study results show a different pattern, specifically that respiratory event detection varies based on the number of events. For example, RemStar-measured AHI tended to overestimate the AHI at lower AHI levels but underestimate the AHI at higher AHI levels [5, 17]. In short, it appears that AHI measurement is dependent on the specific APAP device used.

If there are systematic differences between PAP devices, it is important for the field to request that the manufacturers provide clinicians and researchers with clear information regarding what level of adjustment is necessary to allow for the most accurate interpretation of the PAP-scored apneas and hypopneas. The PAP-scored AHI value is a useful data point for gathering information on therapeutic efficacy. Previous studies have examined the percentage of patients that continue to have residual OSA even while using a PAP device.

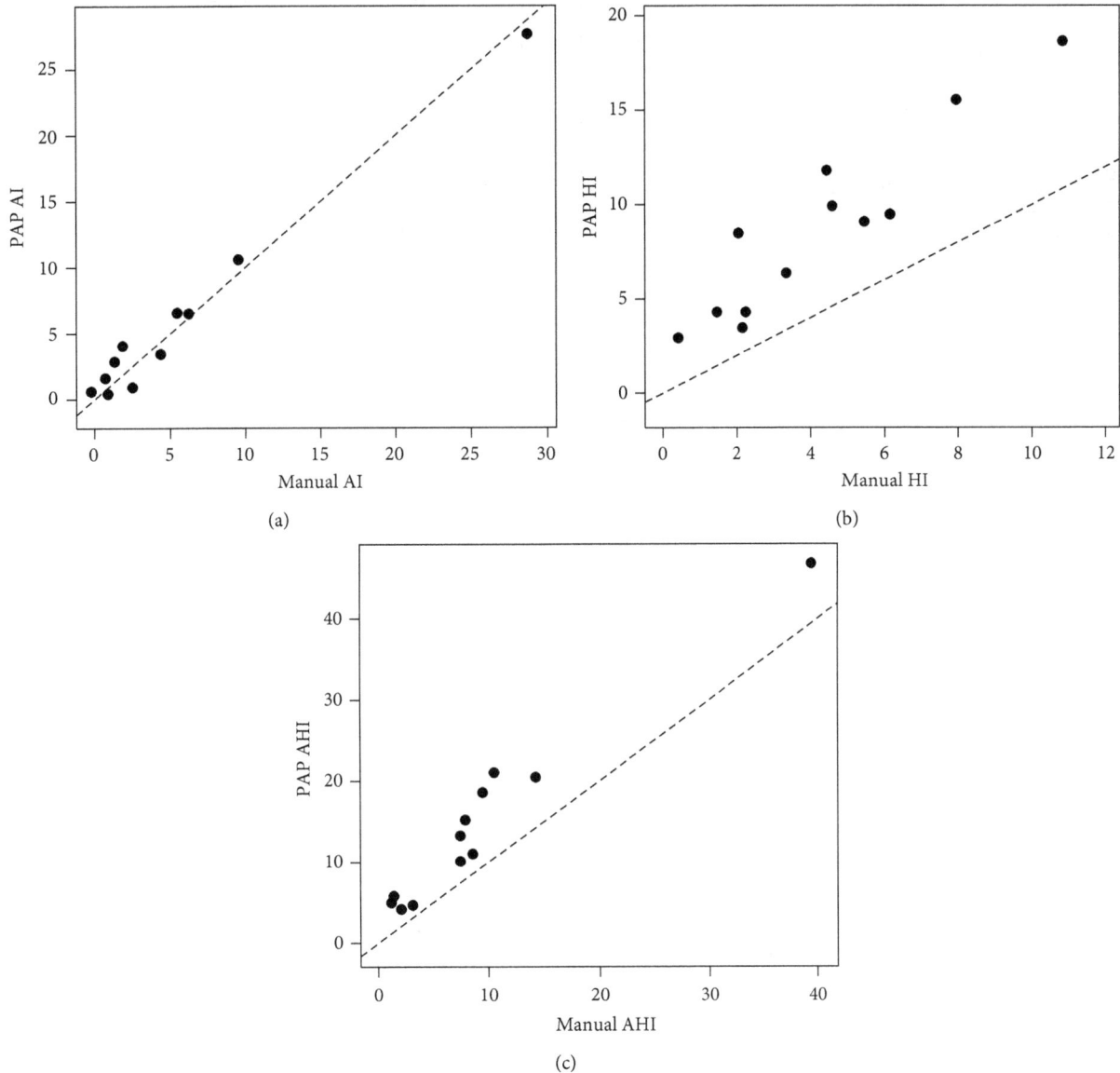

FIGURE 1: (a) Scatterplot of PAP-scored versus manual-scored Apnea Index. Each point represents one night. The diagonal line represents the line of identity. (b) Scatterplot of PAP-scored versus manual-scored Hypopnea Index. Each point represents one night. The diagonal line represents the line of identity. Note that all PAP HI values are greater than manual HI values. (c) Scatterplot of PAP-scored versus manual-scored Apnea-Hypopnea Index. Each point represents one night. The diagonal line represents the line of identity. Note that all values of PAP AHI are greater than manual AHI values.

In a study of patients using single-pressure CPAP, nearly 20% continued to have PAP AHI >10 after 3 months [18], while in another study of patients undergoing a home APAP trial, 29% had PAP AHI >10 [19]. The former study did not specify the CPAP device used, while the latter study used a ResMed AutoSet Spirit. Given the results of the current study and the associated literature, it would appear that the unique PAP device algorithms for automatic respiratory event detection affect the results of these and similar studies. Given the findings of the present study, it is possible that the study using the ResMed AutoSet has inflated AHI values, and therefore, the residual AHI in that study may be less than actually reported [19].

As per published clinical guidelines, the standard recommendation is that sleep monitoring is indicated for the assessment of treatment results on PAP therapy after (i) substantial weight loss (e.g., 10% of body weight) to ascertain whether PAP therapy is still needed at the prescribed pressure settings, (ii) substantial weight gain with return of symptoms (e.g., 10% of body weight) to ascertain whether pressure adjustments are needed, (iii) clinical response is insufficient (e.g., lack of symptom relief, above normal residual AHI, or poor adherence), or (iv) symptoms return despite a good initial response to CPAP [3, 20].

There are a number of potential study limitations. First, the number of participants is low relative to other studies

(a)

(b)

(c)

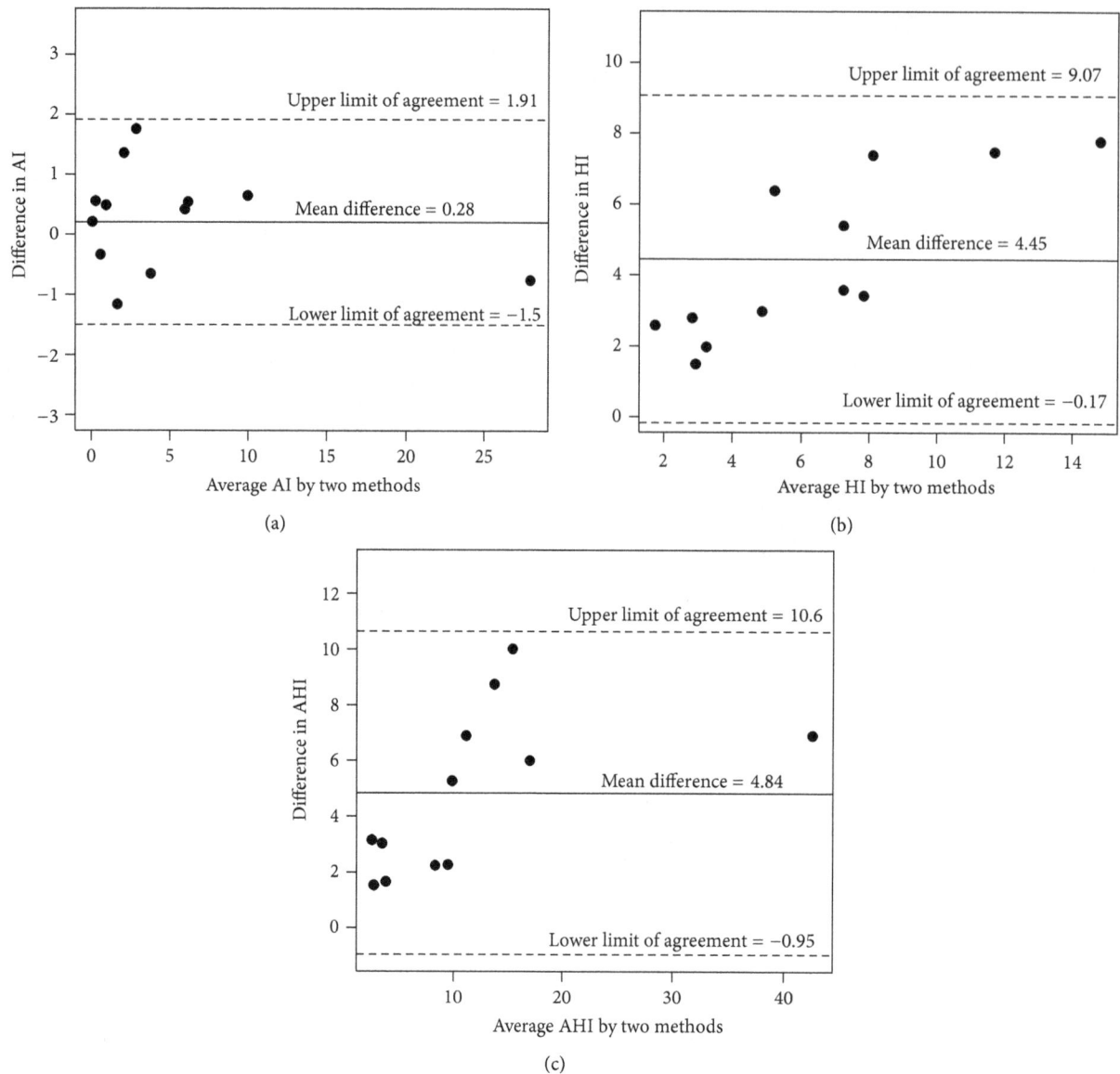

FIGURE 2: (a) Bland-Altman plot of PAP scoring versus manual scoring AI difference (PAP-scoring minus manual-scoring) by the mean. (b) Bland-Altman plot of PAP scoring versus manual-scoring HI difference (PAP scoring minus manual-scoring) by the mean. Note that all of the difference values were greater than 0, indicating that all PAP HI values were greater than the manual HI values. (c) Bland-Altman plot of PAP-scoring versus manual-scoring AHI difference (PAP scoring minus manual-scoring) by the mean. Note that all of the difference values were greater than 0, indicating that all PAP AHI values were greater than the manual AHI values.

in this area. That said, the results are consistent with the only other study that used the S8 APAP device. Second, the study was done in the home environment where there is less control than that in a laboratory environment. Third, there are limitations in scoring hypopneas with Type III home testing (events must meet flow and ≥4% saturation criteria but cannot be scored based on an arousal, as sleep is not measured). Finally, newer generation of PAP devices can distinguish central and obstructive events. Future studies can utilize this newer technology to see how well PAP algorithms can distinguish these events and what role they have in overall AHI values.

In summary, PAP devices have automated, proprietary algorithms for respiratory event detection. When event detection scoring is combined with PAP use duration in the denominator, a proxy AHI value is derived. Given the increased reliance on the PAP-scored events by both providers and patients, it is important to better understand the nuances of specific algorithms and how the PAP-scored AHI, HI, and AI values compare to those same values from manual scoring. Doing so is an important step toward making more informed treatment decisions.

Acknowledgments

This research was supported in part by the Department of Veterans Affairs, Veterans Health Administration, Office of Research and Development, and the Research Service of the San Diego Veterans Affairs Healthcare System (VA HSRD IIR 02-275 and 07-163 and AHRQ R18 017246).

References

[1] C. E. Sullivan, F. G. Issa, M. Berthon-Jones, and L. Eves, "Reversal of obstructive sleep apnoea by continuous positive airway pressure applied through the nares," *Lancet*, vol. 1, no. 8225, pp. 862–865, 1981.

[2] T. I. Morgenthaler, R. N. Aurora, T. Brown et al., "Practice parameters for the use of autotitrating continuous positive airway pressure devices for titrating pressures and treating adult patients with obstructive sleep apnea syndrome: an update for 2007. An American Academy of Sleep Medicine Report," *Sleep*, vol. 31, no. 1, pp. 141–147, 2008.

[3] L. J. Epstein, D. Kristo, P. J. Strollo Jr. et al., "Clinical guideline for the evaluation, management and long-term care of obstructive sleep apnea in adults," *Journal of Clinical Sleep Medicine*, vol. 5, no. 3, pp. 263–276, 2009.

[4] A. L. Denotti, K. K. Wong, G. C. Dungan II, J. W. Gilholme, N. S. Marshall, and R. R. Grunstein, "Residual sleep-disordered breathing during autotitrating continuous positive airway pressure therapy," *European Respiratory Journal*, vol. 39, pp. 1391–1397, 2012.

[5] R. B. Berry, C. A. Kushida, M. H. Kryger, H. Soto-Calderon, B. Staley, and S. T. Kuna, "Respiratory event detection by a positive airway pressure device," *Sleep*, vol. 35, no. 3, pp. 361–367, 2012.

[6] E. J. Topol, "Transforming medicine via digital innovation," *Science Translational Medicine*, vol. 2, no. 16, article 16cm4, 2010.

[7] C. Stepnowsky, C. Edwards, T. Zamora, R. Barker, and Z. Agha, "Patient perspective on use of an interactive website for sleep apnea," *International Journal of Telemedicine and Applications*, vol. 2013, Article ID 239382, 10 pages, 2013.

[8] C. Iber, S. Ancoli-Israel, A. Chesson, and S. F. Quan, *The AASM Manual for the Scoring of Sleep and Associated Events: Rules, Terminology, and Technical Specification*, American Academy of Sleep Medicine, Westchester, Ill, USA, 2007.

[9] L. I-Kuei Lin, "A concordance correlation coefficient to evaluate reproducibility," *Biometrics*, vol. 45, no. 1, pp. 255–268, 1989.

[10] L. I. K. Lin, "A note on the concordance correlation coefficient," *Biometrics*, vol. 56, pp. 324–325, 2000.

[11] G. B. McBride, "A proposal for strength-of-agreement criteria for Lin's Concordance Correlation Coefficient," NIWA Client Report, National Institute of Water & Atmospheric Research, Ltd, Hamilton, New Zealand, 2005.

[12] J. M. Bland and D. G. Altman, "Statistical methods for assessing agreement between two methods of clinical measurement," *Lancet*, vol. 1, no. 8476, pp. 307–310, 1986.

[13] R Development Core Team, *R: A Language and Environment For Statistical Computing*, R Foundation for Statistical Computing, Vienna, Austria, 2009.

[14] S. T. Kuna, I. Gurubhagavatula, G. Maislin et al., "Noninferiority of functional outcome in ambulatory management of obstructive sleep apnea," *American Journal of Respiratory and Critical Care Medicine*, vol. 183, no. 9, pp. 1238–1244, 2011.

[15] N. A. Collop, W. M. Anderson, B. Boehlecke et al., "Clinical guidelines for the use of unattended portable monitors in the diagnosis of obstructive sleep apnea in adult patients," *Journal of Clinical Sleep Medicine*, vol. 3, no. 7, pp. 737–747, 2007.

[16] K. Ueno, T. Kasai, G. Brewer et al., "Evaluation of the apnea-hypopnea index determined by the S8 auto-CPAP, a continuous positive airway pressure device, in patients with obstructive sleep apnea-hypopnea syndrome," *Journal of Clinical Sleep Medicine*, vol. 6, no. 2, pp. 146–151, 2010.

[17] A. Cilli, R. Uzun, and U. Bilge, "The accuracy of autotitrating CPAP-determined residual apnea-hypopnea index," *Sleep and Breathing*, pp. 1–5, 2012.

[18] M. A. Baltzan, I. Kassissia, O. Elkholi, M. Palayew, R. Dabrusin, and N. Wolkove, "Prevalence of persistent sleep apnea in patients treated with continuous positive airway pressure," *Sleep*, vol. 29, no. 4, pp. 557–563, 2006.

[19] L. Torre-Bouscoulet, M. S. Meza-Vargas, A. Castorena-Maldonado, M. Reyes-Zúñiga, and R. Pérez-Padilla, "Autoadjusting positive pressure trial in adults with sleep apnea assessed by a simplified diagnostic approach," *Journal of Clinical Sleep Medicine*, vol. 4, no. 4, pp. 341–347, 2008.

[20] C. A. Kushida, M. R. Littner, T. Morgenthaler et al., "Practice parameters for the indications for polysomnography and related procedures: an update for 2005," *Sleep*, vol. 28, no. 4, pp. 499–521, 2005.

9

The SomnuSeal Oral Mask Is Reasonably Tolerated by Otherwise CPAP Noncompliant Patients with OSA

N. Katz,[1] Y. Adir,[2] T. Etzioni,[3,4,5] E. Kurtz,[3] and G. Pillar[4,5]

[1] *Sleep Laboratory, Assuta Medical Services and Wolfson Hospital, 69710 Holon, Israel*
[2] *Pulmonary Unit, Carmel Hospital and Clalit Health Care, 34362 Haifa, Israel*
[3] *Sleep Clinic, Clalit Health Care, 34362 Haifa, Israel*
[4] *Sleep Laboratory, Rambam Health Care Campus, P.O. Box 9602, 31096 Haifa, Israel*
[5] *Department of Pediatrics, Carmel Hospital and Faculty of Medicine, Technion-Israel Institute of Technology, 34362 Haifa, Israel*

Correspondence should be addressed to G. Pillar; gpillar@tx.technion.ac.il

Academic Editor: Liborio Parrino

Compliance with CPAP is the major limiting factor in treating patients with OSA. The novel SomnuSeal mask is an oral self-adaptable mask located between the teeth and the lips ensuring that there are no air leaks or skin abrasions. Fifty patients with AHI > 20, who failed previous CPAP trials, were asked to sleep with the mask for one month. In all patients, the mask was connected to an AutoPAP machine with a heated humidifier. Efficacy, convenience, and compliance (average usage for 4 or more hours per night) were monitored. Fifty patients (41 m and 9 f, mean age 57 ± 12 years, BMI 33.6 ± 4.9 kg/m^2, and AHI 47 ± 23/h) participated. Eleven were classified as compliant (average mask usage of 26 nights, 4.7 hours per night), five were only partially compliant (average usage of 13 nights, 2.9 hours per night), and 34 could not comply with it. In all patients who slept with it, the efficacy (assessed by residual AHI derived from the CPAP device) was good with an AHI of less than 8/hour. Interestingly, the required optimal pressure decreased from an average of 9.3 cmH$_2$O to 4.6 cmH$_2$O. The SomnuSeal oral interface is effective and may result in converting noncompliant untreated patients with OSA into well-treated ones.

1. Introduction

Obstructive sleep apnea (OSA) is a common disorder characterized by recurrent hypoxemia, hypercapnia, and arousal from sleep and is associated with adverse neurocognitive and cardiovascular sequelae [1–6]. Application of continuous positive airway pressure (CPAP) leads to improvements in many of these adverse parameters [7–9], although residual sleep disordered breathing may still persist [10, 11].

The major limiting factor of CPAP treatment is compliance [12–14].

Some of the most important factors that have been reported as limiting compliance are skin abrasions or eruptions due to the pressure exerted by the mask, mask pressure on the ridge of the nose, claustrophobia, aerophagia, air leaks (eye irritation), dry mouth, dry nose, nasal stuffiness, epistaxis, sinusitis, facial pain or a noisy device, or pressure intolerance [15–21]. Other factors that have been identified as affecting compliance consist of disease severity, daytime sleepiness, motivation, age, socioeconomic status, education, race, marital status, spouse support, and copayment [12–31]. Even with the advanced and newer devices (such as the "C-Flex" CPAP device, BPAP, or automatic CPAP), data are not convincing for improved compliance [32–35].

Since CPAP treatment has a dramatic beneficial impact on patients [7–9, 23, 36–39], it is of great importance to seek interfaces that can improve compliance. The novel SomnuSeal mask (Figure 1) is an oral self-adaptable mask located between the teeth and the lips, ensuring that there are no air leaks or skin abrasions. It is more comfortable, adjusts better to the patient's specific anatomical structure, and potentially reduces rejection by claustrophobic patients. In a series of preliminary studies (published as abstracts [40, 41]), it has been shown to potentially improve compliance in struggling or otherwise CPAP noncompliant patients. These preliminary studies were conducted on a relatively small number of

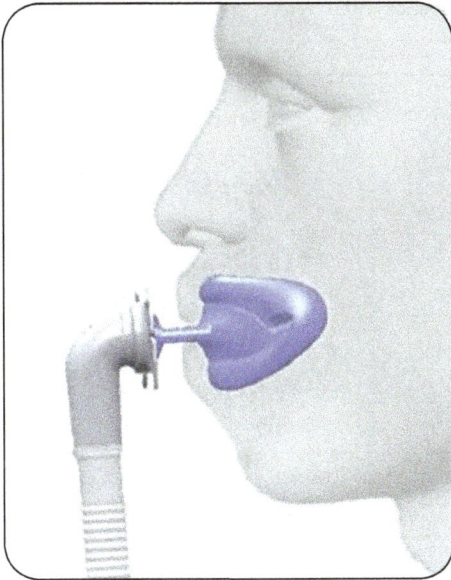

FIGURE 1: SomnuSeal mask.

patients and for relatively short periods of time (one night up to one week of use). However, the results were encouraging, indicating that up to 40% of patients with moderate-severe OSA may comply and tolerate the SomnuSeal mask. We speculated that the oral mask will be a second and not a first line of treatment, and therefore this study was planned to examine a longer period of efficacy and compliance with the SomnuSeal interface (one month of treatment), only in CPAP noncompliant patients with moderate-severe OSA.

2. Methods

2.1. Participants. Fifty patients were recruited with moderate-severe OSA (AHI > 20) who were otherwise untreated. All patients were established as noncompliant, having tried at least one CPAP mask previously and failed to comply with it or with any previous CPAP mask they had tried. Inclusion criteria consisted of a previous diagnosis of OSA with an AHI > 20/h, age above 18 years (males or females), failure of at least one CPAP mask in the past, not considering any other treatment (i.e., patients who are otherwise untreated), and consent to participate. All patients were recruited from the patients' registry (archives) of our sleep clinic and gave written informed consent prior to participation. The study was approved by the Rambam Health Care Campus Institutional Review Board (RMB-0010-11).

Exclusion criteria consisted of any unstable medical condition, active malignancy, age below 18 years, pregnant or lactating women, treatment for OSA other than CPAP (i.e., patients who use dental appliance or consider surgery), and periodontal diseases or mouth lesions according to the investigator's judgment.

2.2. Baseline Polysomnographic Study. All participants had a baseline full night sleep study using electroencephalogram, electrooculogram, submental electromyogram, bilateral anterior tibialis electromyography, electrocardiogram

(ECG), nasal-oral airflow (thermistors and nasal pressure), chest and abdominal wall motion (piezo- or impedance belts), body position, and arterial oxygen saturation (Embla, Broomfield, USA). Sleep staging and respiratory indices were scored by a trained technician. Apnea was defined as a ≥90% decrease in airflow persisting for at least 10 sec, while hypopnea was defined as a ≥50% decrease in the airflow amplitude (relative to baseline, persisting for at least 10 sec) with an associated ≥3% oxygen desaturation or an arousal. The apnea hypopnea index (AHI) was calculated as the number of respiratory events (apnea and hypopnea) divided by the total sleep time.

2.3. CPAP Devices and Interface. All participants were fitted in the clinic with CPAP and a SomnuSeal oral mask and were instructed to sleep with it on a nightly basis at home. In the clinic visit a trained sleep technician/respiratory therapist fitted them with the equipment. They were given two sizes of oral masks and were allowed to decide which one was more comfortable.

The SomnuSeal is an intraoral CPAP interface that provides the needed seal of the oral cavity from outside air (atmosphere) without the shortcomings of other intra- or extraoral masks (Figure 1). The mask is composed of a central part that delivers the compressed air directly to the oral cavity without impingement on intraoral tissues. This central part is surrounded by a special soft silicone part that can engage gently the delicate intraoral tissues in such a way as as to create a peripheral seal so that the intra-oral cavity is secluded from outside atmosphere. The interface is held in place by engagement of the central part with the lingual side of the lips. A nasal peg was not needed. After fitting the mask to a patient, it was connected to an AutoPAP machine (Winemann WM 27460/S). This is a CPAP with a heated humidifier and a usage meter which was reviewed after one month of participation (see below). In addition to hours of use, the device recorded the provided pressure, residual sleep disordered breathing events, and air leaks.

2.4. Study Design. The study consisted of two clinic visits and three telephone visits. In the first clinic visit, the selected patients reported to the clinic and signed an informed consent. A brief physical examination focusing on their oral cavity was then performed by a sleep physician. They were then fitted with the SomnuSeal mask, and, for about 30 minutes, they exercised breathing with it whilst being awake. They were trained for correct mask usage, how to connect it to the AutoPAP machine themselves, how to handle the mask and device in home, and how to wash the mask. They then took the equipment home and were instructed to use it every night for a one-month period.

During the month of the study, telephone visits were performed on a weekly basis. After one, two, and three weeks of use, a research assistant called each participant for an update. In the call, the participants reported their level of satisfaction and subjective tolerance of the mask. In cases when they needed some extra assistance with the interface or CPAP, the study technician discussed it with them, and upon their request they were also offered an actual meeting with him.

TABLE 1: Data categorized according to compliance with CPAP.

	Compliant	Strugglers	Noncompliant	All
N (% of all)	11 (22)	5 (10)	34 (68)	50 (100)
Number of males (%)	8 (73)	5 (100)	28 (82)	41 (82)
Age	61 ± 11	49 ± 9	56 ± 13	57 ± 12
BMI	32.3 ± 4.2	37.5 ± 4.8	33.3 ± 5.0	33.6 ± 4.9
Pretreatment AHI (/h)	40 ± 19	52 ± 34	49 ± 22	47 ± 23
Pretreatment minimal O2 Sat	74 ± 11	77 ± 4	77 ± 9	76 ± 9
Days of usage	26 ± 5	13 ± 7	5 ± 5	11 ± 10
Average usage per night (h)	4.7 ± 1.1	2.9 ± 1.1	1.8 ± 0.8	2.6 ± 1.5
Residual obstructive AHI (/h)	1.9 ± 4.1	1.2 ± 2.8	n/a	n/a
Average heart rate	65 ± 12	62 ± 14	67 ± 15	66 ± 14
Total sleep time (min)	346 ± 32	359 ± 39	332 ± 30	338 ± 32
Sleep efficiency	77 ± 9	81 ± 12	75 ± 10	76 ± 9
Stage 2 (% of TST)	66 ± 19	60 ± 15	64 ± 17	64 ± 17
Stage 3 (% of TST)	18 ± 6	22 ± 7	19 ± 5	19 ± 6
REM sleep (% of TST)	16 ± 4	18 ± 5	17 ± 4	17 ± 4

TABLE 2: Results from the satisfaction questionnaire. In all questions, scale runs between 1 (weak, bad) and 5 (strong, excellent).

	Compliant	Strugglers	Noncompliant	All
Air seal with the SomnuSeal	5 ± 0	5 ± 0	4.8 ± 0.6	4.9 ± 0.5
Quality of airflow	5 ± 0	5 ± 0	4.9 ± 0.2	4.9 ± 0.1
Excess salivation	1.5 ± 0.7	2.0 ± 1.0	3.9 ± 0.9	3.1 ± 1.4
Comparison with previous tried masks (higher is better)	4.6 ± 0.5	4.0 ± 0.8	2.2 ± 0.7	3.1 ± 1.3
Willingness to purchase (higher is better)	4.0 ± 1.0	3.0 ± 0.7	1.7 ± 0.7	2.5 ± 1.3

After one month of use, the second clinic visit (end of study visit) took place, in which another brief physical examination of the subjects was conducted (again focusing on the oral cavity). At that time the subjects were asked to complete a questionnaire evaluating their use of the mask, and the CPAP meter and output were downloaded and examined by the researcher. The outcome measures included the data retrieved from the CPAP objective usage meter so the actual time it was used by the patient was objectively quantified. In addition, efficacy was quantified based on the CPAP internal recorder (i.e., optimal pressure, residual AHI, and leaks). A subjective satisfactory questionnaire was completed by each participant at that visit. Data were collected regarding the convenience of using the mask, difficult/ease of using and handling it, changes in these parameters with time (from the first to last week of usage), potential side effects, self-assessment of usage, and free text of subjective judgment of the mask.

Data from the patients' charts, demographic data, usage meter data driven from the CPAP machine, and data from the satisfaction questionnaires were all collected in a data management sheet (Excel) for statistical analyses.

3. Results

Fifty patients participated in the study. Their mean age was 57 ± 12 years. Their average AHI was 47 ± 23/hour, and their average BMI (body mass index) was 33.6 ± 4.9 kg/m². Forty-one patients were males and 9 were females.

The patients were categorized into three subgroups according to their compliance with CPAP: compliant patients (usage of the CPAP for more than 70% of the nights, for four hours per night or more), struggling or partially compliant patients (who used it intermittently but in less than required to be considered as a compliant patient), and noncompliant patients (who could not tolerate the device). These results are summarized in Table 1.

The major results obtained from the satisfaction questionnaire are summarized in Table 2 (same classification as in Table 1). As can be seen (and expected), patients who complied with the SomnuSeal mask expressed it in their satisfaction, complained less of excess salivation, and indicated a high index of willingness to obtain the mask.

The two most importantly reported side effects were excess salivation and inconvenience of the mask in the mouth due to pressure on the lips. However, it should be stated that, in the physical examination at the end of the study, none had any ulcers or bruises on their lips or gingival.

Of note, the automated supplied air pressure provided by the autoPAP dramatically decreased with the SomnuSeal compared to the nasal mask. While with the nasal mask the average required pressure was 9.3 ± 1.8 cmH₂O, the pressure required with the SomnuSeal mask was 4.6 ± 0.9 cmH₂O.

4. Discussion

The major finding of our study is that 22% of patients with moderate-severe OSA, who failed any other treatment and were noncompliant to at least one CPAP mask which they tried and who otherwise remained untreated, managed to comply with the SomnuSeal oral mask for at least one month of use. They used it on average for 26 nights, with an average of 4.7 hours per night. This can potentially convert them from untreated to reasonably treated patients.

The advantages of CPAP treatment in patients with OSA are well documented. CPAP has been shown to reduce insulin resistance, improve blood pressure, reduce stroke, improve endothelial function, reduce health care utilization, reduce road accidents, improve cognition, improve mood, and improve quality of life [7–9, 23, 36–39]. Despite all of these factors, about 40% of patients who need CPAP remain untreated. The leading cause for CPAP failure is that the device is not tolerated by patients. There are many reported reasons for this noncompliance [15–21, 42]. Since the SomnuSeal mask is placed in the mouth and not on the nose, it eliminates potential limiting factors such as skin abrasions or eruptions due to pressure exerted by nasal masks, mask pressure on the ridge of the nose, eye irritation due to air leaks, dry nose, nasal stuffiness, epistaxis, and potentially sinusitis. It is less cumbersome so even claustrophobia may not be as dramatic as it is with nasal mask. Thus, it is plausible that, in the 22% of patients who complied with the oral SomnuSeal mask and not with nasal mask, these were the limiting factors. Obviously, 22% of patients are not enough, but it should be kept in mind that the participants in this study were otherwise not treated at all! Thus, 22% is a substantially positive number.

The finding that a lower pressure is required for the SomnuSeal mask compared to the nasal mask is very interesting and not intuitive. Potential explanations for this finding consist of stabilizing respiration, and maybe even more relevant, a forward displacement of the lower jaw as occurs with oral appliances [43]. In the current study we did not perform PSG studies on the treated patients and did not assess hypercapnia or respiratory control variables. As a result, we can only speculate that respiratory stabilization had occurred. In addition, we have not assessed anatomical changes of jaw position, and thus the potential anterior mandibular displacement with the SomnuSeal mask is just a speculation. Regardless of the reason for improvement in respiration with relatively low pressure, it may have beneficial effects on the cardiovascular system. Bradley et al. [44], in a study of CPAP in congestive heart failure, showed that, at a CPAP of $5\,\mathrm{cmH_2O}$, the cardiac index and stroke volume indices were increased in the subgroup with poor baseline hemodynamics and higher LV diastolic pressures [44]. Clearly, long-term studies to show any difference in cardiac function with differing CPAP pressures are needed, but it is reasonable to believe that reduction in the required optimal CPAP pressure as observed with the SomnuSeal mask may be beneficial for patients with OSA, especially those with cardiac dysfunction.

Our study has several limitations. Firstly, from the efficacy point of view, our study was a home and not a lab study. Although not tested with oral masks, but with nasal masks, there are very strong data indicating that the automatic algorithm of the CPAP is very accurate and that most patients sleeping with autoPAP have an AHI of less than 10/h. In order to reduce costs, we conducted our study in home and relied on the residual respiratory event counter of the CPAP itself. Obviously, this is a limitation, and future studies will need to be conducted in the lab. Secondly, we did not quantify outcome measures such as vigilance, mood, cognitive function, or medical outcome such as blood pressure or glucose control. This was beyond the scope of our study. The primary aim was to examine the tolerability and compliance of treated patients with this oral mask. Future studies will have to deal with behavioral medical and cognitive outcome with this interface. Thirdly, as with many previous CPAP compliance studies, this was a specific clinical study and not a field study. It is plausible that some of our patients may have made an extra effort to tolerate the SomnuSeal and it does not guarantee that they would have complied with this device in a real-life field setting. Such a study would be possible only if patients start using the SomnuSeal interface on a clinical basis. Finally, the n of this study is not huge. For a CPAP compliance study, more than 11 users (of 50 potential users) would be needed. We consider this study as a preliminary study with encouraging results.

In conclusion, despite these limitations, this prospective open study of 50 noncompliant patients demonstrated that a new self-adapting mask has encouraging results in this challenging group of patients. The finding of lower than average CPAP pressures may confer important long-term cardiovascular benefits.

Conflict of Interests

G. Pillar was a consultant for DMD. The other authors have no financial conflict of interests.

Acknowledgment

This study was supported by a nonrestricted Grant from DMD (Discover Medical Devices), the manufacturer of the SomnuSeal mask.

References

[1] J. E. Remmers, W. J. deGroot, E. K. Sauerland, and A. M. Anch, "Pathogenesis of upper airway occlusion during sleep," *Journal of Applied Physiology Respiratory Environmental and Exercise Physiology*, vol. 44, no. 6, pp. 931–938, 1978.

[2] P. Lavie, P. Herer, and V. Hoffstein, "Obstructive sleep apnoea syndrome as a risk factor for hypertension: population study," *British Medical Journal*, vol. 320, no. 7233, pp. 479–482, 2000.

[3] P. E. Peppard, T. Young, M. Palta, and J. Skatrud, "Prospective study of the association between sleep-disordered breathing and hypertension," *The New England Journal of Medicine*, vol. 342, no. 19, pp. 1378–1384, 2000.

[4] J. Hung, E. G. Whitford, R. W. Parsons, and D. R. Hillman, "Association of sleep apnoea with myocardial infarction in men," *The Lancet*, vol. 336, no. 8710, pp. 261–264, 1990.

[5] M. E. Dyken, V. K. Somers, T. Yamada, Z. Ren, and M. B. Zimmerman, "Investigating the relationship between stroke and obstructive sleep apnea," *Stroke*, vol. 27, no. 3, pp. 401–407, 1996.

[6] U. Leuenberger, E. Jacob, L. Sweer, N. Waravdekar, C. Zwillich, and L. Sinoway, "Surges of muscle sympathetic nerve activity during obstructive apnea are linked to hypoxemia," *Journal of Applied Physiology*, vol. 79, no. 2, pp. 581–588, 1995.

[7] J. Hedner, B. Darpo, H. Ejnell, J. Carlson, and K. Caidahl, "Reduction in sympathetic activity after long-term CPAP treatment in sleep apnoea: cardiovascular implications," *European Respiratory Journal*, vol. 8, no. 2, pp. 222–229, 1995.

[8] K. Narkiewicz, M. Kato, B. G. Phillips, C. A. Pesek, D. E. Davison, and V. K. Somers, "Nocturnal continuous positive airway pressure decreases daytime sympathetic traffic in obstructive sleep apnea," *Circulation*, vol. 100, no. 23, pp. 2332–2335, 1999.

[9] J. M. Marin, S. J. Carrizo, E. Vicente, and A. G. N. Agusti, "Long-term cardiovascular outcomes in men with obstructive sleep apnoea-hypopnoea with or without treatment with continuous positive airway pressure: an observational study," *The Lancet*, vol. 365, no. 9464, pp. 1046–1053, 2005.

[10] D. P. White and T. J. Gibb, "Evaluation of the Healthdyne NightWatch system to titrate CPAP in the home," *Sleep*, vol. 21, no. 2, pp. 198–204, 1998.

[11] A. I. Pack, J. E. Black, J. R. L. Schwartz, and J. K. Matheson, "Modafinil as adjunct therapy for daytime sleepiness in obstructive sleep apnea," *American Journal of Respiratory and Critical Care Medicine*, vol. 164, no. 9, pp. 1675–1681, 2001.

[12] M. R. DiMatteo, "Variations in patients' adherence to medical recommendations: a quantitative review of 50 years of research," *Medical Care*, vol. 42, no. 3, pp. 200–209, 2004.

[13] N. B. Kribbs, A. I. Pack, L. R. Kline et al., "Objective measurement of patterns of nasal CPAP use by patients with obstructive sleep apnea," *American Review of Respiratory Disease*, vol. 147, no. 4, pp. 887–895, 1993.

[14] T. E. Weaver, N. B. Kribbs, A. I. Pack et al., "Night-to-night variability in CPAP use over the first three months of treatment," *Sleep*, vol. 20, no. 4, pp. 278–282, 1997.

[15] H. M. Engleman, N. Asgari-Jirhandeh, A. L. McLeod, C. F. Ramsay, I. J. Deary, and N. J. Douglas, "Self-reported use of CPAP and benefits of CPAP therapy: a patient survey," *Chest*, vol. 109, no. 6, pp. 1470–1476, 1996.

[16] J. Strollo Jr., M. H. Sanders, and C. W. Atwood, "Positive pressure therapy," *Clinics in Chest Medicine*, vol. 19, no. 1, pp. 55–68, 1998.

[17] J. L. Pepin, P. Leger, D. Veale, B. Langevin, D. Robert, and P. Levy, "Side effects of nasal continuous positive airway pressure in sleep apnea syndrome: study of 193 patients in two French sleep centers," *Chest*, vol. 107, no. 2, pp. 375–381, 1995.

[18] G. N. Richards, P. A. Cistulli, R. G. Ungar, M. Berthon-Jones, and C. E. Sullivan, "Mouth leak with nasal continuous positive airway pressure increases nasal airway resistance," *American Journal of Respiratory and Critical Care Medicine*, vol. 154, no. 1, pp. 182–186, 1996.

[19] S. A. Herrejon, A. I. Inchaurraga, and M. Gonzalez, "Spontaneous pneumothorax associated with the use of nighttime BiPAP with a nasal mask," *Archivos de Bronconeumología*, vol. 34, no. 10, p. 512, 1998.

[20] R. Alvarez-Sala, S. Diaz, C. Prados, C. Villasante, and J. Villamor, "Increase of intraocular pressure during nasal CPAP," *Chest*, vol. 101, no. 5, p. 1477, 1992.

[21] N. N. Jarjour and P. Wilson, "Pneumocephalus associated with nasal continuous positive airway pressure in a patient with sleep apnea syndrome," *Chest*, vol. 96, no. 6, pp. 1425–1426, 1989.

[22] N. McArdle, G. Devereux, H. Heidarnejad, H. M. Engleman, T. W. Mackay, and N. J. Douglas, "Long-term use of CPAP therapy for sleep apnea/hypopnea syndrome," *American Journal of Respiratory and Critical Care Medicine*, vol. 159, no. 4 I, pp. 1108–1114, 1999.

[23] A. Tarasiuk, G. Reznor, S. Greenberg-Dotan, and H. Reuveni, "Financial incentive increases CPAP acceptance in patients from low socioeconomic background," *PLoS ONE*, vol. 7, no. 3, Article ID e33178, 2012.

[24] F. Campos-Rodriguez, N. Peña-Griñan, N. Reyes-Nuñez et al., "Mortality in obstructive sleep apnea-hypopnea patients treated with positive airway pressure," *Chest*, vol. 128, no. 2, pp. 624–633, 2005.

[25] T. E. Weaver, "How much is enough CPAP?" *Sleep Medicine*, vol. 4, article S52, 2003.

[26] L. E. Burke and I. S. Ockene, *Compliance in Healthcare and Research*, Futura Publishing, Armonk, NY, USA, 2001.

[27] H. M. Engleman, S. E. Martin, and N. J. Douglas, "Compliance with CPAP therapy in patients with the sleep apnoea/hypopnoea syndrome," *Thorax*, vol. 49, no. 3, pp. 263–266, 1994.

[28] T. Simon-Tuval, H. Reuveni, S. Greenberg-Dotan, A. Oksenberg, A. Tal, and A. Tarasiuk, "Low socioeconomic status is a risk factor for CPAP acceptance among adult OSAS patients requiring treatment," *Sleep*, vol. 32, no. 4, pp. 545–552, 2009.

[29] C. A. Massie, R. W. Hart, K. Peralez, and G. N. Richards, "Effects of humidification on nasal symptoms and compliance in sleep apnea patients using continuous positive airway pressure," *Chest*, vol. 116, no. 2, pp. 403–408, 1999.

[30] M. E. Billings, D. Auckley, R. Benca et al., "Race and residential socioeconomics as predictors of CPAP adherence," *Sleep*, vol. 34, no. 12, pp. 1653–1658, 2011.

[31] L. Ye, A. I. Pack, G. Maislin et al., "Predictors of continuous positive airway pressure use during the first week of treatment," *Journal of Sleep Research*, vol. 21, no. 4, pp. 419–426, 2012.

[32] J. Bakker, A. Campbell, and A. Neill, "Randomized controlled trial comparing flexible and continuous positive airway pressure delivery: effects on compliance, objective and subjective sleepiness and vigilance," *Sleep*, vol. 33, no. 4, pp. 523–529, 2010.

[33] J. Pépin, J. Muir, T. Gentina et al., "Pressure reduction during exhalation in sleep apnea patients treated by continuous positive airway pressure," *Chest*, vol. 136, no. 2, pp. 490–497, 2009.

[34] D. C. Dolan, R. Okonkwo, F. Gfullner, R. J. Hansbrough, R. J. Strobel, and L. Rosenthal, "Longitudinal comparison study of pressure relief (C-Flex) versus CPAP in OSA patients," *Sleep and Breathing*, vol. 13, no. 1, pp. 73–77, 2009.

[35] N. S. Marshall, A. M. Neill, and A. J. Campbell, "Randomised trial of compliance with flexible (C-Flex) and standard continuous positive airway pressure for severe obstructive sleep apnea," *Sleep and Breathing*, vol. 12, no. 4, pp. 393–396, 2008.

[36] S. K. Sharma, S. Agrawal, D. Damodaran et al., "CPAP for the metabolic syndrome in patients with obstructive sleep apnea," *The New England Journal of Medicine*, vol. 365, no. 24, pp. 2277–2286, 2011.

[37] I. H. Iftikhar, M. F. Khan, A. Das, and U. J. Magalang, "Meta-analysis: continuous positive airway pressure improves insulin resistance in patients with sleep apnea without diabetes," *Annals of the American Thoracic Society*, vol. 10, no. 2, pp. 115–120, 2013.

[38] M. A. Martínez-García, F. Campos-Rodríguez, P. Catalán-Serra et al., "Cardiovascular mortality in obstructive sleep apnea in the elderly: role of long-term continuous positive airway pressure treatment: a prospective observational study," *American*

Journal of Respiratory and Critical Care Medicine, vol. 186, no. 9, pp. 909–916, 2012.

[39] T. G. Weinstock, X. Wang, M. Rueschman et al., "A controlled trial of CPAP therapy on metabolic control in individuals with impaired glucose tolerance and sleep apnea," *Sleep*, vol. 35, no. 5, pp. 617–625, 2012.

[40] G. Pillar, S. Suraiya, A. Segev, and M. Majdob, "A novel oral mask improve convenience in CPAP treated OSA patients," *Sleep*, vol. 33, article A168, 2010.

[41] G. Pillar, A. Segev, and E. Kurtz, "The SomnuSeal oral mask is reasonably tolerated by otherwise CPAP non compliant patients with OSA," *Sleep*, vol. 35, article A164, 2012.

[42] J. C. Borel, R. Tamisier, S. Dias-Domingos et al., "Type of mask may impact on continuous positive airway pressure adherence in apneic patients," *PLoS ONE*, vol. 8, no. 5, Article ID e64382, 2013.

[43] V. K. Somers, D. P. White, R. Amin et al., "Sleep Apnea and Cardiovascular Disease: an American Heart Association/American College of Cardiology Foundation scientific statement from the American Heart Association Council for High Blood Pressure Research Professional Education Committee, Council on Clinical Cardiology, Stroke Council, and Council on Cardiovascular Nursing," *Circulation*, vol. 118, no. 10, pp. 1080–1111, 2008.

[44] T. D. Bradley, R. M. Holloway, P. R. McLaughlin, B. L. Ross, J. Walters, and P. P. Liu, "Cardiac output response to continuous positive airway pressure in congestive heart failure," *American Review of Respiratory Disease*, vol. 145, no. 2, part 1, pp. 377–382, 1992.

10

A Preliminary Evaluation of the Physiological Mechanisms of Action for Sleep Restriction Therapy

Annie Vallières,[1,2,3] Tijana Ceklic,[1,2] Célyne H. Bastien,[1,2] and Colin A. Espie[4]

[1] École de psychologie, Université Laval, Québec, QC, Canada G1V A06
[2] Centre d'étude des troubles du sommeil, Centre de recherche de l'institut universitaire en santé mentale de Québec, Québec, QC, Canada G1J 2G3
[3] Centre de recherche du centre hospitalier universitaire en santé mentale du Québec, Québec, QC, Canada G1V 4G2
[4] Nuffield Department of Clinical Neurosciences, Sleep & Circadian Neuroscience Institute, University of Oxford, Oxford OX3 9DU, UK

Correspondence should be addressed to Annie Vallières; annie.vallieres@psy.ulaval.ca

Academic Editor: Marco Zucconi

Our objective was to investigate the physiological mechanisms involved in the sleep restriction treatment of insomnia. A multiple baseline across subjects design was used. Sleep of five participants suffering from insomnia was assessed throughout the experimentation by sleep diaries and actigraphy. Ten nights of polysomnography were conducted over five occasions. The first two-night assessment served to screen for sleep disorders and to establish a baseline for dependent measures. Three assessments were undertaken across the treatment interval, with the fifth and last one coming at follow-up. Daily cortisol assays were obtained. Sleep restriction therapy was applied in-lab for the first two nights of treatment and was subsequently supervised weekly. Interrupted time series analyses were computed on sleep diary data and showed a significantly decreased wake time, increased sleep efficiency, and decreased total sleep time. Sleepiness at night seems positively related to sleep variables, polysomnography data suggest objective changes mainly for stage 2, and power spectral analysis shows a decrease in beta-1 and -2 powers for the second night of treatment. Cortisol levels seem to be lower during treatment. These preliminary results confirm part of the proposed physiological mechanisms and suggest that sleep restriction contributes to a rapid decrease in hyperarousal insomnia.

1. Introduction

Sleep restriction therapy for insomnia was developed by Spielman et al. in 1987 [1]. This behavioral intervention consists of restricting the time spent in bed to correspond to the estimated amount of time spent asleep by the patient [1]. Weekly changes are made to the time spent in bed as a function of the patient's clinical response. Since this first publication, sleep restriction therapy has been frequently included in cognitive-behavioral therapy for insomnia (CBT-I). Meta-analyses of nonpharmacological treatments of insomnia have shown that sleep restriction can be effective in decreasing sleep-onset latency and greatly increasing sleep efficiency in a relatively short time [2–4]. Another meta-analysis has shown that sleep restriction, applied with other behavioral treatment, benefits sleep of adults and older adults, with the exception of total sleep time [5]. Sleep restriction efficacy is well acknowledged by sleep clinicians and researchers [6, 7] who consider it an essential therapeutic component.

Sleep restriction mechanisms are seen as involving physiological and psychological processes of sleep. Despite the effectiveness attributed to sleep restriction, little is known about how or why it improves sleep. From a physiological point of view, it is suggested that the prescribed total time spent in bed entrains the biological clock and produces a mild sleep-deprived state that increases daytime wakefulness and thus the sleep homeostatic drive [1, 8, 9]. This in turn increases sleepiness at night that facilitates falling asleep, sleep consolidation, decreases rapid cortical activity, and increases slow wave sleep during early sleep cycles. In this sense, sleepiness at night and the cortical activity changes are markers of the physiological process of sleep restriction.

Sleepiness has been seen as an inevitable part of treatment that appears in the first weeks of treatment [10, 11] but is known to diminish by the follow-up assessment. Two recent studies evaluated sleep restriction alone and focus on sleepiness and vigilance [11, 12]. One evaluated daytime functioning of nine participants with chronic insomnia who received three sessions of sleep restriction [12]. This study demonstrated that sleep restriction immediately resulted in an impaired vigilance and an increased sleepiness at night. The second study [10] evaluated 16 participants with insomnia who received 4 weeks of sleep restriction and showed that sleep restriction therapy is associated with an elevated daytime sleepiness and impaired vigilance in the first three weeks of treatment. Although there is evidence of elevated sleepiness during the first week of sleep restriction, it is still uncertain how that could negatively affect treatment compliance as previously suggested [2, 4, 7] or how this sleepiness is related to cortical activity and to subjective sleep.

A few studies have investigated cortical activity with PSG and power spectral analysis (PSA) before and after CBT-I [9, 13, 14]. One study evaluated cortical activity in the presleep period before and after a combined sleep restriction, stimulus control, and relaxation treatment of insomnia [13]. Twelve participants with insomnia received 5 treatment sessions over 10 weeks of sleep restriction and stimulus control combined to relaxation and were compared to 14 normal sleepers. This study observed a decrease in the beta percent total power in the presleep period after treatment of insomnia, suggesting that these participants had, after treatment, less rapid cortical activity before going to bed. The second study investigated nine people suffering from chronic mixed-type insomnia [14]. Participants received eight weeks of CBT-I including sleep restriction therapy. Their PSG results showed a decrease in stage 2 sleep and an increase in both slow wave sleep (SWS) and REM sleep. The PSA showed a reduction in the beta activity during NREM sleep and an increase in SWS after CBT-I. Another study evaluated 16 participants with chronic insomnia and compared them to a placebo control group [9]. Participants in the treatment group received 8 weeks CBT-I including sleep restriction therapy. These authors found that CBT-I led to a greater rate of exponential decline in delta power over NREM sleep periods. No other frequency band changes were found to be significant after CBT-I. Therefore, there is some evidence that treatment of insomnia can produce a change in the rapid cortical activity of people with insomnia. However, because these studies used either a relaxation or a multicomponent treatment, it is not known whether these changes are due to sleep restriction therapy. Moreover, because PSG nights were done before and after treatment, they do not inform how and when sleep restriction works.

Cortisol is another possible physiological marker of sleep restriction, as it is a marker of the hypothalamus-pituitary-adrenal axis activity [15, 16]. Cortisol is associated with stress, cortical activity, and physiological hyperarousal. Therefore, according to the hyperarousal model of insomnia, cortisol should be higher in insomnia than in good sleepers. A few studies investigated the cortisol cycle in insomnia. People with insomnia were found to have a higher cortisol level in both the morning [15, 16] and evening [16] compared to good sleepers. Other studies have shown that relaxation may reduce overall cortisol level [17]. Therefore, it is likely that effective sleep restriction therapy that produces a decrease in total wake time could also lead to a decrease in cortisol levels.

In summary, although sleep restriction is currently recommended as a treatment of insomnia and frequently included in CBT-I, very few studies have evaluated sleep restriction therapy mechanisms, other than the seminal work by Spielman and colleagues [1]. The present study tests a methodology that would be useful in evaluating sleep restriction physiological mechanisms in a larger program. A single-case design is used to explore the physiological mechanisms using continuous data collection throughout the treatment. The main goal of the present study is to explore the physiological mechanisms of sleep restriction: these mechanisms are explored using several measures of objective sleep, perceived sleepiness and alertness, and morning and evening cortisol levels. In addition, the study evaluates the efficacy of sleep restriction specifically, using data gathered daily in order to more closely follow the links between the treatment effects observed and the mechanisms under study.

2. Methodology

2.1. Participants. Participants were recruited by physician referrals in the Greater Glasgow area. Inclusion criteria were as follows: (a) being between 18 and 65 years old; (b) presenting insomnia according to DSM-IV-TR [18] criteria; (c) reporting significant distress or daytime impairments (item 6 score of 2 or higher) as evaluated by the Insomnia Severity Index [19]; (d) cessation, at least one month prior to experimentation, of any sleep or other psychotropic medication that could alter sleep; (e) a baseline sleep efficiency lower than 75%; and (f) reporting a BDI score between "0" and "15." Exclusion criteria were as follows: (a) presence of sleep state misperception insomnia defined as a marked discrepancy between subjective complaint and objective measure of total sleep time; (b) presence of another sleep disorder (apnoea and hypopnoea index > 15; periodic limb movement index > 15); (c) evidence that insomnia was related to a medical condition; (d) presence of major depression, anxiety disorder, alcohol/substance abuse, or any other psychopathology as diagnosed with the SCID-IV [20]; (e) being currently in psychotherapy; (f) regular use of medication interfering with sleep; and (g) use of antibiotics two weeks prior to the onset of the study or steroids within six months prior to study, which could affect cortisol level. Inclusion and exclusion criteria aimed at selecting severe insomnia in order to favor clear changes in the time in bed (TIB) from the beginning of treatment. The study was approved by the Research Ethics Committee of Greater Glasgow Health Board, at the Southern General Hospital (ethics reference number: 05/S0701/45).

Twenty-one eligible participants responded to the advertisement and underwent telephone screening. Sixteen were then excluded for the following reasons: sleep improved before the interview ($n = 5$); use of medication interfering with sleep or hypnotics ($n = 6$); the baseline sleep efficiency was higher than 75% ($n = 4$); and participants were no longer interested in the study ($n = 1$). Subsequent assessments included a semistructured sleep history interview [19] and a SCID-IV evaluation [20]. Thus, the final sample included five participants (1 male and 4 females) meeting DSM-IV-TR [18] criteria for primary insomnia. Only these five participants completed the experimentation from the beginning. Four participants completed the treatment and the whole experimentation while one completed the treatment but not the entire protocol. Their mean age was 41.1 years (ranging from 22 to 62) with an average education level of 15.2 years (ranging from 10 to 19). The average insomnia duration was 12.6 years (SD = 6.7). One participant presented sleep-onset insomnia only, and four presented mixed insomnia (sleep-onset, sleep maintenance, and/or terminal insomnia). Participants were free of any sleep medication for at least one month before entering the study.

2.2. Design and Procedures

2.2.1. Design. A single-case design called multiple baseline across subjects design [21] was used to evaluate the impact of sleep restriction on physiological variables. This particular single-case design provides a controlled investigation of treatment mechanisms [22]. Baseline length has to be different for each participant to ensure that the introduction of the experimental treatment (here, the sleep restriction therapy) occurs at a different time for each participant. This particularity of the present design provides a control for possible maturation. Maturation refers to natural changes over time of a participant's sleep that occur without treatment. Figures 1 and 2 illustrate the design by showing that each participant has a different baseline length.

2.2.2. Procedure. After the screening procedure, participants began a baseline with varying lengths before treatment. At baseline and throughout the experimentation, participants completed continuous assessments of their sleep, cortisol, sleepiness, and alertness. They also wore an actigraph from baseline until the end of treatment. Participants completed the Insomnia Severity Index at three assessment periods: baseline, posttreatment, and 3-month follow-up. At five occasions, they also spent two consecutive weekday nights of in-lab PSG, with the first two being at the first baseline week and for which the very first night served as a screening night for other sleep disorders. The following three occasions of PSG nights were scheduled during the treatment interval: (a) two nights at the first sleep restriction therapy session, (b) two nights when sleep was considered stabilized, and (c) two nights after three weeks of sleep stabilization. The remaining two PSG nights were at a 3-month follow-up.

Sleep was considered stabilized when sleep efficiency (SE) reached 85% or more, night-to-night variability was visually observed to have reduced relative to SE baseline, and a clinical judgment of progress was made. Night-to-night variability in sleep is an important feature of insomnia that is suggested to be an indicator of treatment responsiveness [23]. Moreover, the criteria used are closed to the clinical context in which the therapy takes place.

2.2.3. Treatment. The sleep restriction administered in this study is outlined in a treatment manual [24] and follows reviewed recommendations [25]. The content and aim of each sleep restriction session are summarized in Table 1. The manual includes also answers to frequently asked questions (FAQ) in order to standardize answers given to participants and avoid delivering cognitive therapy or stimulus control therapy for insomnia (FAQ are available upon request from the first author). The first two nights of treatment were supervised and spent in laboratory as training for the sleep restriction procedures. Sleep restriction therapy consists of curtailing the time spent in bed to conform to the reported amount of time asleep. A sleep window is determined using the average of total sleep time reported by participants in their two baseline weeks of sleep diaries. The sleep window is increased by 15 minutes, contingent upon reaching a SE of 85% or more. When SE is between 80% and 85%, the sleep window is kept stable and when SE is lower than 80%, the sleep window is decreased to correspond to the total sleep time estimated. The lower limit of the sleep window is five hours. An educational component including basic facts about sleep is included in the treatment in order to give a more reliable treatment rationale to participants.

Sleep restriction therapy was introduced following each baseline period for four to six individual treatment sessions of 50 minutes. The first sessions are performed weekly until sleep is stabilized as previously described. Then, one more session is planned three weeks after sleep stabilization. Participants are instructed to increase their sleep window according to the same rules based on SE during weeks without a therapy session and at posttreatment after the supervised treatment periods. Also, they are invited to increase the sleep window by modifying their bedtimes to keep the lower limit constant throughout the treatment.

Treatment Fidelity. Several methodological strategies were used to monitor treatment fidelity. First, the multiple-baseline design controlled the beginning of the treatment, assuring that sleep restriction began only as previously determined. Second, the use of the manual facilitates treatment standardization and replication. Third, the two-night in-lab training of sleep restriction assured appropriate treatment application by participants. Finally, actigraph measures provided objective confirmation of treatment fidelity.

Therapist. A graduate student in psychology performed telephone screening. Treatment sessions and assessment interviews were led by a licensed clinical psychologist (AV) who had several years of experience in sleep restriction therapy.

2.3. Measures

2.3.1. Initial Screening and Evaluation. Initial screening included a 20-minute telephone interview to determine

TABLE 1: Summary content of the sleep restriction therapy.

Sleep restriction procedures
(i) Sleep diaries used to estimate total sleep time (TST) and sleep efficiency (SE)
(ii) Sleep window length = the average of the two last baseline weeks of TST
(iii) The minimum sleep window duration is five hours
(iv) Sleep window respected every night
(v) Alarm clock used to ensure arising
(vi) The sleep window
(a) is increased for 15–20 minutes if SE ≥ 85%
(b) is kept stable if SE is between 80% and 85%
(c) is decreased to correspond to the total sleep time estimated if SE < 80%
Session 1: sleep information and sleep restriction
Aim: to transmit information about normal sleep, sleep disorders, and their effects and to begin sleep restriction therapy
(i) Basic facts about sleep: sleep architecture, circadian rhythm and sleep homeostasis as regulators of sleep, and changes in sleep patterns over the life span
(ii) Nature and causes of insomnia
(iii) Introduction of sleep restriction therapy and determination of the first sleep window
Session 2: sleep restriction
Aim: to restructure sleep so that it meets individual needs and develops a stable pattern
(i) Review previous week
(ii) Continue sleep restriction
(iii) Teach participants to modify their own sleep window
(iv) Clarify the distinction between sleepiness and fatigue
Session 3 and following ones until sleep stabilization: sleep restriction, developing natural sleep patterns
Aim: same goal. In addition, teach participants to use sleep restriction
(i) Continue sleep restriction
(ii) Teach participants to modify their own sleep window
(iii) Encourage fidelity to the new sleep schedule
Last session: sleep restriction and therapeutic gain maintenance
Aim: same goal. In addition, focus on further improvement and therapeutic gain maintenance
(i) Continue sleep restriction
(ii) Teach participants to modify their own sleep window
(iii) Encourage fidelity to the new sleep schedule
(iv) Review the concept of homeostatic pressure and more generally of the sleep restriction rationale
(v) Maintain therapeutic gains and/or keep improving after treatment

participant eligibility. Subsequently, a multimeasure pretreatment evaluation was conducted, comprised of a semistructured sleep history interview to diagnose insomnia and the SCID-IV [20] to evaluate the presence of psychopathology.

2.3.2. Sleep Assessment

Sleep Diaries. Participants completed sleep diaries each morning upon rising throughout the experiment. From these diaries, total wake time (TWT; summation of time awake in bed including sleep-onset latency), total sleep time (TST), and SE were derived. Participants also monitored their sleepiness and alertness levels in the morning and evening using a "0" to "4" Likert scale as well as recording their saliva sample time.

Polysomnography (PSG). Participants underwent a total of 10 nights of sleep laboratory assessment (see Section 2.2). The PSG montage included electroencephalographic (EEG; including C3, C4, O1, and O2), electromyographic (EMG; chin), and electro-oculographic (EOG; left and right: supraorbital ridge of one eye and the infraorbital ridge of the other) monitoring. Electrodes were referred to linked mastoids with a forehead ground, and interelectrode impedance was maintained below 5 kOhms. A Lifelines Trackit Recorders Mark 1 were used for data acquisition using Trackit software (hardware gain 500 +/− 2%; bandwidth 0.16–70 Hz) and PSG signals were digitized at a sampling rate of 256 Hz of 512 Hz using commercial software product (Harmonie, Stellate System, Montreal, Canada). Sleep recordings and limb movements were scored visually (Luna, Stellate System, Montreal, Canada) by qualified technicians using standardized criteria [26]. Recordings were made over 30-second epochs, and an independent scorer conducted reliability checks to insure a minimum of 85% interscorer agreement. Participants diagnosed with any other sleep disorder were excluded and referred to an appropriate sleep specialist. Respiration (airflow, tidal volume, and oxygen saturation) and anterior tibialis EMG readings were monitored during the first night of PSG recording in order to eliminate recordings made during sleep apnoea or periodic limb movements. Although sleep scoring was done before publication of the most recent guidelines [27], we chose to conserve the original scoring method, since it is more appropriate for research involving quantitative analyses of the EEG or finer techniques of EEG analyses (e.g., event-related potentials; ERPs).

Outcome measures (sleep-onset latency (SOL), wake after sleep onset (WASO), TST, and SE) were based on the average of baseline nights (BN1 and BN2: nights 1 and 2), first treatment nights (TR3 and TR4: nights 3 and 4), sleep stabilized nights (TR5 and TR6: nights 5 and 6), posttreatment nights (TR7 and TR8: nights 7 and 8), and follow-up nights (FUN9 and FUN10: nights 9 and 10).

Power Spectral Analysis (PSA). PSA was conducted on EEG at C3 site only by computing fast Fourier transforms. EMG artefacts were detected automatically and rejected from the spectral analyses [28]. Further artefacts were eliminated by visual detection. Manual selection of periods of the night for PSA included all NREM and REM sleep as well as parts of each NREM sleep stage (1 to 4) of each sleep cycle (when available), excluding miniarousals (0.1–7 seconds), microarousals (7.1–14.9 seconds), arousals (15 seconds and longer), movement time, movements or artefacts, and the five minutes before and after a stage shift. Within a cycle, if no uninterrupted period of a specific sleep stage lasted longer than 10 minutes, a portion of this sleep stage was selected while excluding the first and last 40 seconds (two epochs) so not to include stage shifts in the analysis.

A comparison between baseline and the introduction of treatment permits study of homeostatic processes occurring at the beginning of treatment. It is also possible that sleep recuperation occurs after the introduction of treatment. Clinical sleep data were derived from PSG night 2 (BN2), night 3 (TR3), and night 4 (TR4) only. PSA was computed for consecutive 4-second epochs, with a resolution of 0,25 Hz and an EEG segment length of 30 seconds. Data were cosine tapered, and fast Fourier transform windows were nonoverlapping. Frequencies were defined as follows: slow waves (0–1 Hz), delta (1–4 Hz), theta (4–7 Hz), alpha (7–11 Hz), sigma (11–14 Hz), beta-1 (14–20 Hz), beta-2 (20–35 Hz), gamma (35–60 Hz), omega (60–125 Hz), and total (0–125 Hz). Absolute power spectral values (μV^2) of REM and NREM sleep were log transformed to normalize the distributions.

Actigraphy. The actigraph is a watch-like device which records movement information over short periods by means of an accelerometer/microprocessor link. Presence of movement was interpreted as wake time and absence of movement as sleep time. The actigraphs used are from Cambridge Neurotechnology, AW-4. An algorithm (maximum sampling frequency 32 Hz, recording all movements over 0.05 g., filters set 3–11 Hz) enabled Sleepwatch software to estimate the sleep parameters using 1-minute epochs.

2.3.3. Cortisol Assessment. Salivary cortisol samples were drawn using a plastic tube. Each sample contained approximately 2 mL of saliva. Throughout the experimentation, samples were drawn 10 minutes before going to bed as well as 10 minutes after awakening. For home assessment, a kit of 14 plastic tubes was supplied weekly to each participant, who was instructed to collect salivary samples twice a day, not to eat or brush their teeth during the hour before collection, and to rinse their mouth with water 10 minutes before sampling. Then, they were instructed to put it in the appropriate plastic tube and to store it in their own refrigerator. Participants returned their 14 samples when they came to treatment sessions. In-lab and home salivary samples were stored at the Department of Biochemistry at the Glasgow Royal Infirmary and analyzed by an experienced biomedical technologist. When analyzed, samples were centrifuged (2500 rpm) for 10 minutes and the supernatant was frozen at −20c until assayed in the laboratory. These supernatants were radio immunoassayed using microencapsulated antibody and I-cortisol as a tracer. Cortisol level is expressed in nmol/mL.

2.3.4. Insomnia Measure. Insomnia Serverity Index (ISI) [19] includes seven items. Ratings on a "0" to "4" point scale were obtained on the perceived severity of sleep-onset, sleep maintenance, and early morning awakening problems, satisfaction with current sleep patterns, interference with daily functioning, noticeable impairments attributed to sleep problems, and level of distress. The ISI score ranges from "0" to "28" with higher scores indicating more severe insomnia. This index has adequate psychometric properties and has been shown to be sensitive to changes in clinical trials of insomnia [29–31].

2.3.5. Compliance Measures. Adherence to treatment protocol was evaluated with sleep diaries and actigraphy. A daily percentage of adherences to the prescribed time to go to bed as well as to arising time were computed separately for each participant and assessment device. Going to bed more than 15 minutes earlier and getting out of bed more than 15 minutes later than the prescribed sleep window was considered as nonadherence to the respective element of the sleep restriction procedure. A daily average in minutes of nonadherence time was also computed for each participant and assessment device.

2.3.6. Treatment Response. Clinical judgments of treatment response were made according to the following criteria: (a) having a marked decreased in ISI score from baseline to posttreatment, (b) having sleep stabilized during treatment, and (c) presenting a significant increase in SE during treatment. Participants' responses were recorded as responder (meeting three of the above criteria), moderate responder (two criteria), or minimal responder (one criterion).

2.4. Data Analysis. Sleep diary data for four dependent variables (i.e., SOL, TWT, TST, and SE) were divided into consecutive series according to each period (i.e., baseline, treatment, and posttreatment) for each participant. An interrupted time series analysis (ITSA) [32] was conducted to statistically test whether the treatment was associated with a gradual (slope) or abrupt (level) change in the data series. Two comparisons of adjacent experimental periods were completed: (a) baseline versus treatment and (b) treatment versus posttreatment. To perform these analyses, ITSA models were developed using the AUTOREG procedure of SAS 9.1.3 [33], which uses a generalized least-squares regression method with residuals corrected for autocorrelation (serial dependency). Missing data were estimated within the model. Time, level, and slope effects were estimated following the recommendations of Huitema and McKean [34]. Autocorrelation of observations was studied for the first 12 lags. Final residuals were inspected to ensure that they were normally distributed and that they exhibited homogenous variance as well as no significant autocorrelation.

To study the physiological mechanisms of sleep restriction, statistical analyses were chosen as a function of (a) the objective, that is, to document the effect of sleep restriction on objective sleep, on subjective sleepiness and alertness, and on morning and evening cortisol levels, and (b) the nature of available data for each participant. For example, few data points are available for PSG, given the limited number of nights that each participant spent in the lab, while series of daily data are available from sleep diaries.

Descriptive statistics were computed and visually inspected for PSG data for each two-night period spent in the laboratory except for the baseline nights where data were taken only for the second night because of a possible first night effect. For the PSA, statistical analyses were performed separately for participants who responded to treatment and for those who did not. Considering the small sample sizes, nonparametric statistics were used. The Friedman test evaluated potential statistical differences between the second baseline night (BN2) and the two first treatment nights (TR3 and TR4) for power spectral analysis variables of responders. In case of a significant Friedman test, post hoc analyses were performed using the Wilcoxon signed-rank test and a Bonferroni correction was applied, which resulted in a significance level of $P < 0.017$. The lack of data for some variables justified the direct use of the Wilcoxon test since the Friedman test could not be performed. In that case, the Bonferroni correction resulted in a significance level set at $P < 0.025$. This was the case for a few variables: NREM, REM, and stage 2 of the third cycle, stages 1 and 2 of the fourth cycle, and all variables for the minimal responder.

To study the longitudinal association between alertness, sleepiness, and sleep, Spearman correlations were calculated between subjective levels of alertness and sleepiness in the morning and the previous night's sleep variables (SOL, WASO, TWT, TST, and SE). Similar correlations were calculated between sleepiness at night and sleep variables. Finally, daily morning and evening cortisol levels were measured to ensure the reliability of these data, and z-scores were derived to facilitate comparisons between participants. Weekly means of standard scores were computed. Given the small sample size, no inferential analysis was performed.

3. Results

3.1. Sleep Restriction Efficacy. Figures 1 and 2 show daily changes in SE and TWT for all participants throughout the experiment. Visual inspection of both SE and TWT over time shows extensive variability over nights in the sleep patterns of participants during baseline and no sleep improvement before treatment introduction. ITSA were performed on SOL, TWT, TST, and SE separately for each participant to determine if there was significant improvement after introducing treatment. The statistical modeling of these series explained an average of 79.6% of variance for SOL (R^2 range from 56.9% to 93.9%), 66.0% of variance for TWT (R^2 range from 47.7% to 90.0%), 50.4% of variance for TST (R^2 range from 24.8% to 77.5%), and 60.0% of variance for SE (R^2 range from 35.5% to 89.9%).

Results for the nature and direction of change for each sleep variable and participant are presented in Table 2. Four out of five participants presented a significantly decreased level of SOL from baseline to treatment (an average of 30 minutes). Moreover, all of them presented a significant decrease in TWT (an average of 96 minutes). Sleep efficiency increased significantly for three participants (an average of 15.9%) during treatment. Meanwhile, TST decreased significantly for three participants (an average of 56 minutes).

3.1.1. Insomnia Severity. Data presented in Table 3 indicated a decrease in severity from baseline to posttreatment for participants 1, 2, 3, and 5. Improvements were maintained at the 3-month follow-up although participant 2 was by then showing mild clinical insomnia. Participant 4 presented a severe insomnia at each assessment period.

3.1.2. Course of Sleep Restriction. Sleep restriction was adapted as a function of individual response to treatment. Accordingly, the first sleep window length and its modification during treatment varied for each participant (see Table 3). Along with sleep window modifications, varied sleep restriction courses can be observed as sleep stabilization was attained: participants 1 and 2 presented the shortest time to stabilization and participant 3 took 16 days while the two other participants barely reached stabilization.

3.1.3. Compliance. Percentages of adherence varied greatly across individuals and weeks. Moreover, the adherence rate was lower when assessed using the actigraph than using the sleep diary. Deviations from the sleep window were different for each participant. The data show that four participants modified their sleep window during the week (see Table 3). According to actigraph measurements, participant 1 shortened his sleep window while participant 3 delayed his sleep window for an average of half an hour compared to the prescribed duration. Deviations of participant 4 indicated an increase in its sleep window length of about 90 minutes.

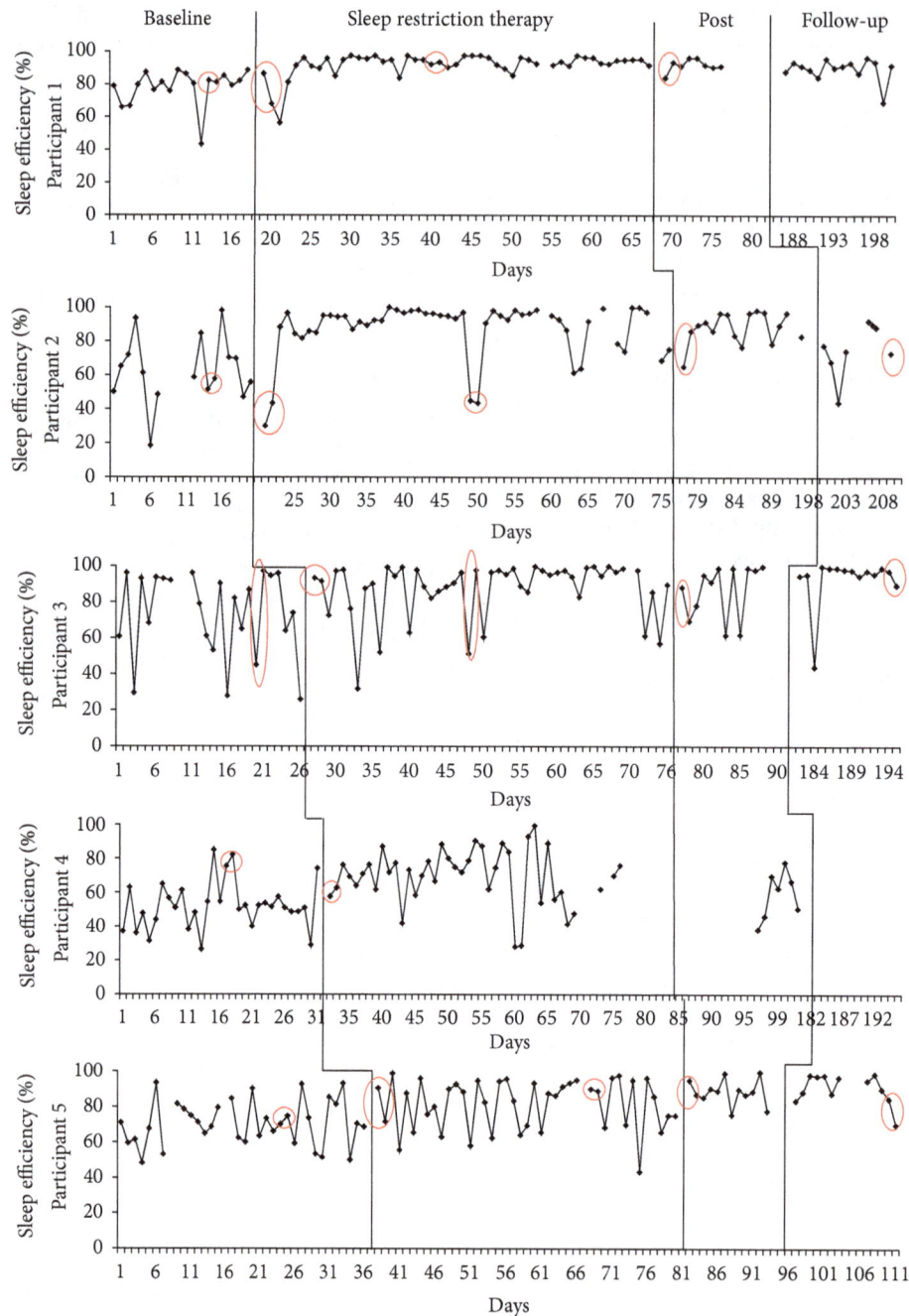

FIGURE 1: Daily sleep efficiency course for each participant. Circled data correspond to PSG nights.

Finally, participant 5 increased his sleep window in the morning.

3.1.4. Treatment Response.

Based on the clinical criteria described in the Data Analysis section, three participants responded to treatment (participants 1, 2, and 3), one had a minimal treatment response (participant 5), and one dropped out of treatment (participant 4). Therefore, participants 1, 2, and 3 were considered as being treatment responders and participants 4 and 5 as nonresponders.

3.2. Physiological Mechanisms of Sleep Restriction

3.2.1. Objective Sleep.

Means and standard deviations for PSG variables are presented in Table 4 for each assessment period. Objective data support ITSA of the sleep diary for most of the sleep variables in participants. Indeed, visual inspection of PSG data reveals a decrease in SOL and an increase in SE from the first nights of treatment spent in the laboratory to posttreatment. WASO seemed to improve similarly except at posttreatment. TST seemed to decrease during the first two nights of treatment but increased once

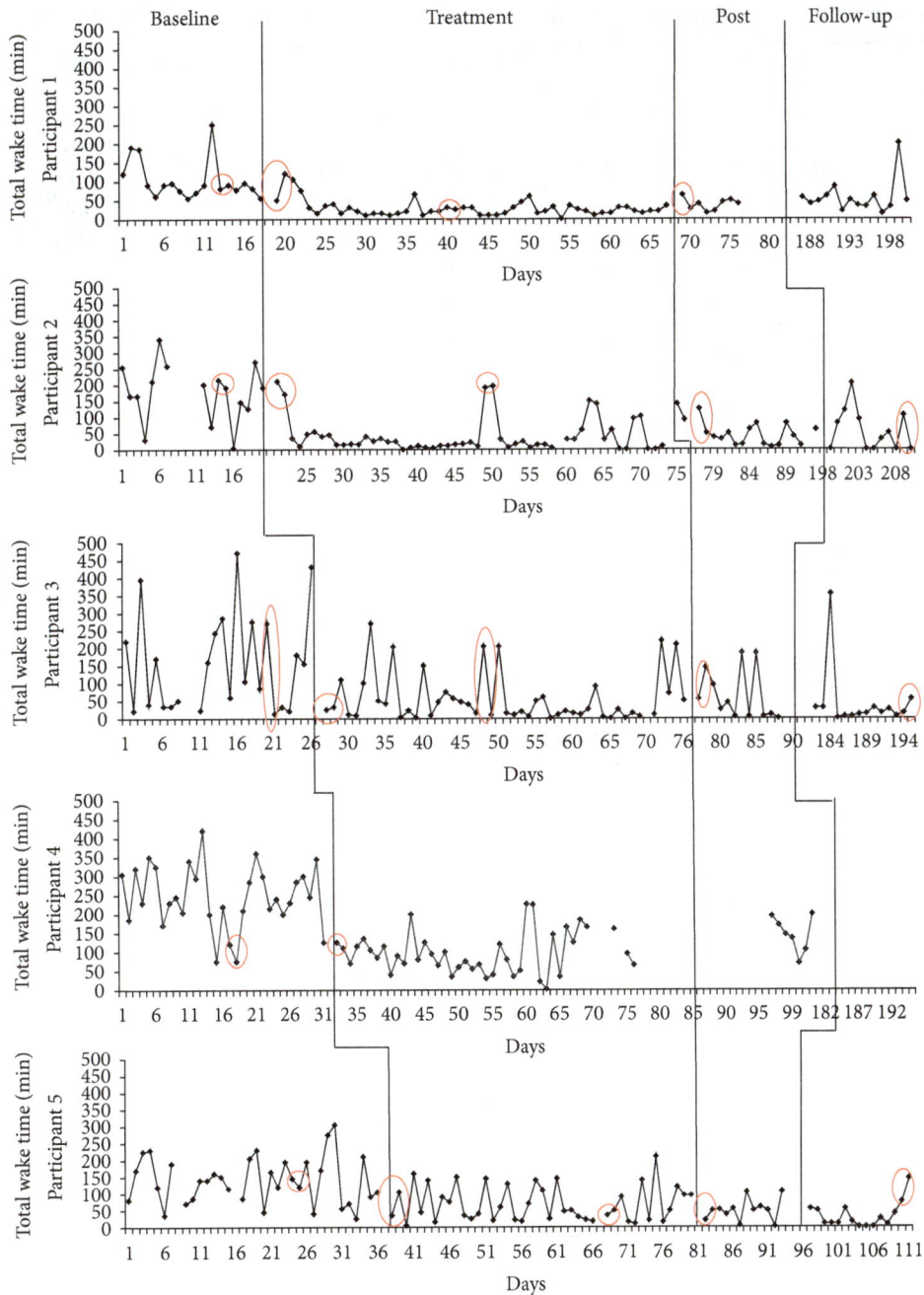

FIGURE 2: Daily total wake time course for each participant. Circled data correspond to PSG nights.

sleep was considered stabilized and at posttreatment. For participants who had minimal treatment response, objective sleep measures indicate that both wake time and sleep time decreased from the very beginning of treatment. However, wake time remained superior to the clinical threshold of 30 minutes.

Results for sleep stages indicate that the percentage of stage 2 sleep decreased slightly while the percentage of time asleep in stages 3 and 4 seemed to increase slightly between baseline and the first two nights of sleep restriction. REM sleep seemed to show the most marked increase at that time.

These changes seemed to remain stable when sleep became stabilized. At posttreatment, percentage of time spent asleep in stage 2 appeared to return to baseline level while percentage of stages 3 and 4 decreased beneath the baseline level. For minimal responders, sleep stage changes were similar during the first night of in-lab treatment. Afterwards, stage 2 increased and stages 3-4 decreased drastically. Moreover, the proportion of REM sleep increased to 32% of the night for one participant.

Median power values for band frequencies from the second baseline night (BN2) and the two first treatment

TABLE 2: Nature and direction of change between baseline, treatment, and post-treatment for each sleep variable and participant.

Sleep variables/participants	DFE	R^2	Treatment			Posttreatment		AR	AO
			Time	Level	Slope	Level	Slope		
Sleep-onset latency									
1	64	91.04	-0.56^{ns}	-34.28^{***}	0.30^{ns}	7.27^{ns}	1.52^{ns}	1, 11	2
2	70	93.89	-0.65^{**}	3.07^{ns}	0.46^{ns}	4.99^{ns}	0.10^{ns}	7	4
3	74	56.90	2.09^{ns}	-69.77^{*}	-2.72^{ns}	37.23^{ns}	-2.22^{ns}	1	3
4	67	83.01	-0.18^{ns}	-31.35^{***}	0.38^{ns}	-71.90^{**}	33.30^{***}	9	5
5	74	72.97	-0.28^{ns}	-18.93^{*}	0.34^{ns}	-15.86^{ns}	0.43^{ns}	6, 10, 11	5
Mean	n/a	79.56	0.08	-30.25	-0.25	-7.65	6.63	n/a	n/a
Total wake time									
1	63	89.99	-0.71^{ns}	-46.30^{***}	0.52^{ns}	21.22^{ns}	-0.43^{ns}	4	5
2	73	73.08	0.75^{ns}	-155.94^{***}	-0.38^{ns}	8.22^{ns}	-3.15^{ns}	14	5
3	72	59.70	1.89^{ns}	-87.79^{**}	-1.94^{ns}	43.12^{ns}	-3.46^{ns}	3, 9	4
4	72	59.34	-1.04^{ns}	-140.16^{***}	1.35^{ns}	60.47^{ns}	-6.89^{ns}	8	0
5	79	47.73	-0.58^{ns}	-50.56^{*}	0.30^{ns}	-37.65^{ns}	5.17^{ns}	9, 13	1
Mean	n/a	69.97	0.06	-96.15	-0.03	19.08	-1.75	n/a	n/a
Total sleep time									
1	62	77.54	0.77^{ns}	-65.55^{**}	0.48^{ns}	-41.98^{ns}	14.89^{*}	14	5
2	71	61.44	-4.57^{ns}	-0.31^{ns}	6.19^{*}	-109.06^{*}	9.09^{ns}	1, 10, 11	3
3	72	57.33	-0.44^{ns}	-134.33^{***}	2.41^{ns}	-63.32^{ns}	5.14^{ns}	1	5
4	71	24.79	1.15^{ns}	-60.08^{*}	-1.43^{ns}	-41.27^{ns}	10.94^{ns}	6, 12	0
5	79	30.95	0.43^{ns}	-17.26^{ns}	-0.39^{ns}	35.12^{ns}	5.41^{ns}	5	2
Mean	n/a	50.41	-0.53	-55.51	1.45	-44.10	9.09	n/a	n/a
Sleep efficiency									
1	61	89.89	0.20^{ns}	7.10^{**}	-0.13^{ns}	-3.83^{ns}	0.18^{ns}	0	5
2	71	71.57	-0.28^{ns}	36.08^{***}	0.13^{ns}	-6.46^{ns}	1.03^{ns}	1, 10	4
3	72	50.96	-0.30^{ns}	10.49^{ns}	0.37^{ns}	-9.83^{ns}	0.80^{ns}	1, 9	4
4	68	51.79	0.06^{ns}	18.60^{**}	-0.10^{ns}	-20.02^{ns}	2.55^{ns}	12, 14	3
5	79	35.47	0.12^{ns}	7.19^{ns}	-0.05^{ns}	8.02^{ns}	-0.61^{ns}	1, 9, 13	0
Mean	n/a	59.94	-0.04	15.89	0.04	-6.42	0.79	n/a	n/a

DFE: degree of freedom; AR: autocorrelation; AO: number of outliers; ns: not significant.
$^{*}P < 0.05$; $^{**}P < 0.01$; $^{***}P < 0.001$.

nights (TR3 and TR4) are presented in Table 5. PSA showed that, for cycles 1 and 2, all statistically significant Friedman test results were observed in the beta-1 and beta-2 band frequencies and appeared mainly during the first cycle. For beta-1, significant differences were observed for beta-1 in stages 2 ($\chi^2(2) = 6.00$, $P = 0.05$) and 3 ($\chi^2(2) = 6.00$, $P = 0.05$) of the first cycle. Only beta-1 had a significant decrease for the second cycle across the three nights during NREM ($\chi^2(2) = 6.00$, $P = 0.05$). Altogether, there seems to be an overall decrease across the three nights in beta-1 power during stages 2 and 3 of sleep of the first cycle and NREM sleep of the second cycle. For beta-2, significant differences were observed during NREM ($\chi^2(2) = 6.00$, $P = 0.05$) and stage 4 ($\chi^2(2) = 6.00$, $P = 0.05$) of the second stage. The medians seem to indicate a slight increase from BN2 to TR3 in beta-2 power followed by a decrease at TR4, which resulted in less power values at TR4 than at BN2 during stage 4 and NREM. However, post hoc analyses did not reveal

any significant differences across nights and the Z value was similar in all comparisons. Due to the treatment procedure of restricting the time in bed, TR4 data were missing for cycles 3, 4, and 5 and TR3 data for cycle 5. Therefore, BN2 and TR3 data were compared using a Wilcoxon signed-rank test and on REM, NREM, and stage 2 only. No significant results emerged.

Overall, a variable representing the mean power value of all the cycles was computed for each band frequency and sleep stage. As documented in Table 5, a few significant results were observed. During stage 2 of sleep, both beta bands ($\chi^2(2) = 6.00$, $P = 0.05$) significantly differed across the three nights. A slight increase appears from BN2 to TR3 in beta-2 power followed by a decrease at TR4, which resulted in less power values at TR4 than at BN2. On the other hand, beta-1 power seems to decrease from BN2 to TR4. Beta-1 also significantly differed across nights during stage 3 ($\chi^2(2) = 6.00$, $P = 0.05$) and NREM ($\chi^2(2) = 6,00$, $P = 0.05$).

TABLE 3: Descriptive information of participants and treatment course.

	Age	Insomnia duration (Years)	ISI			Sleep window		Sleep stabilisation (days)	Respect to time off bed (min)		Respect to arising time (min)	
			B	Post	Fu3	Duration of the 1st	Modification		Actigraph M (SD)	Sleep diary M (SD)	Actigraph M (SD)	Sleep diary M (SD)
P1	22	17	11	6	7	6:30	Weekly ↑ by 15 min	6	16.4 (16.7)	18.3 (34.5)	−8.9 (17.7)	0.9 (28.4)
P2	36	6	18	10	10	5:00	Weekly ↑ by 15 min until week 6	9	4.4 (11.4)	−0.6 (14.1)	7.7 (11.1)	13.6 (15.7)
P3	62	5	17	13	8	6:40	↑ by 15 min at weeks 3, 5, and 6	16	24.1 (24.2)	−1.6 (2.7)	23.8 (19.8)	13.4 (11.8)
P4	36	15	15	0	0	6:00	↑ by 15 min at weeks 3 and 4	n/a	−21.2 (0.0)	−9.5 (19.2)	72.2 (0.0)	5.38 (18.6)
P5	53	20	11	6	7	6:15	Weekly ↓ by 15 min for 3 weeks; then ↑ by 15 min	25	−1.98 (17.9)	13.5 (11.8)	46.0 (25.0)	29.0 (15.8)

ISI: Insomnia Severity Index; B: baseline; Post: posttreatment; Fu3: 3-month follow-up; ↑: increase; ↓: decrease; min: minute; Respect to time off bed: a score of "0" means a perfect respect of the time off bed. A positive score means going to bed later than the prescribed time while a negative score means going to bed earlier; Respect to arising time: a score of "0" means a perfect respect of the prescribed time to get out bed in the morning. A positive score means getting out of bed later than prescribed time in the morning while a negative score means getting out of bed earlier than prescribed.

Thus, beta-1 power seems to decrease across nights in stages 2, 3, and NREM among responders. Again, post hoc analyses revealed no significant results.

For minimal responders, BN2 data were missing for all the variables for the cycles from 1 to 5. Therefore, statistical analyses were performed only on TR3 and TR4. Results for the first 2 cycles and all cycles combined are shown in Table 5. In all analyses, no significant results could be observed. Again, because of the sleep restriction procedures, many data were missing from cycles 3 to 5.

3.2.2. Perceived Sleepiness and Alertness in Relation with Sleep. Longitudinal associations between sleepiness and alertness in the morning, sleepiness at night, and sleep variables were assessed with correlational analyses. Table 6 shows correlational coefficients between each variable for each participant during treatment. During baseline, there are only a few significant correlations, mainly between sleepiness at night and TWT and WASO ($Ps < 0.01$). During treatment, participants 1, 2, and 3, who responded to treatment, presented several significant positive correlations between morning sleepiness and both SOL and TWT ($Ps < 0.0001$ and 0.01, resp.) and TST and SE were negatively associated with sleepiness in the morning ($Ps < 0.01$). These results show that greater sleepiness at night is associated with higher SE and shorter wake time during the night. Participant 2 presented significant associations as well between alertness in the morning and sleep variables ($Ps < 0.01$, 0.05, and 0.001, resp.), showing that a high wake time was associated with a low level of alertness and a high sleep time was associated with a high level of alertness. Participant 3 had only a few significant associations. Participants 4 and 5, who did not respond well to treatment, had a few significant associations during treatment, mainly between sleepiness at night and WASO ($P < 0.01$) or TWT ($P < 0.01$). None of them presented significant associations with alertness in the morning.

3.2.3. Morning and Evening Cortisol Levels. The mean morning cortisol level for the participants was 22.4 nmol/mL (SD = 11.4) and the evening level was 4.3 (SD = 5.1), which are within the normal range for these times of day. Overall, 69 of 262 evening saliva samples and 62 of 262 morning saliva samples were missing or unessayable, with saliva being contaminated before reaching the lab. Most of the missing saliva samples are from participant 4 who did not complete the experiment. Higher cortisol levels are associated with higher wake times. Figure 3 showed the weekly mean morning and evening cortisol levels in standard scores for the three participants with an excellent response to sleep restriction. Visual inspection of these data suggests a tendency for both levels of cortisol to decrease before treatment. By the second week of treatment, both levels seemed lower than baseline as reflected by each participant's personal average which is represented by a standard score of 0. After treatment, both cortisol levels showed a tendency to increase. Participants 4 and 5 showed a similar trend in their cortisol levels in the morning. However, their cortisol levels in the evening tended to be higher, reaching an average of 0.35 by the end of treatment compared to a baseline level of −0.32. This trend is opposite to that seen in treatment responder.

TABLE 4: Means (M) and standard deviations (SD) of polysomnographic data.

Sleep variables	Baseline (BN2) M (SD)	1st nights (TR3, TR4) M (SD)	Sleep stabilized M (SD)	Posttreatment M (SD)	Follow-up M (SD)
			Evaluation periods		
		Treatment			
Treatment responders ($n = 3$, except at follow-up $n = 2$)					
SOL (min)	51.8 (69.9)	13.0 (15.5)	7.7 (7.6)	14.8 (11.1)	46.0 (65.0)
WASO (min)	55.1 (25.9)	26.2 (14.3)	17.5 (17.5)	42.0 (56.9)	32.5 (29.9)
TST (min)	330.1 (80.5)	306.7 (32.6)	348.5 (18.6)	350.9 (37.3)	371.5 (29.4)
SE (%)	74.8 (16.3)	88.2 (4.4)	92.5 (4.6)	86.3 (11.6)	85.2 (14.5)
% stage 2	52.1 (6.4)	49.9 (6.9)	46.5 (4.9)	55.3 (6.8)	54.7 (8.1)
% stages 3-4	21.9 (5.1)	23.7 (7.5)	24.6 (3.9)	14.0 (19.8)	15.6 (8.1)
% REM	17.8 (5.0)	22.7 (5.5)	25.2 (2.8)	27.5 (4.2)	26.1 (2.4)
Nonresponders ($n = 2$ for baseline and 1st nights, then, $n = 1$)					
SOL (min)	17.1 (13.0)	18.0 (7.7)	6.3 (6.7)	5.3 (0.4)	28.0 (24.5)
WASO (min)	115.5 (73.6)	26.3 (8.5)	64.3 (27.9)	55.8 (2.5)	64.8 (15.2)
TST (min)	302.4 (85.1)	289.1 (39.2)	285.0 (25.5)	312.8 (1.1)	385.8 (40.7)
SE (%)	68.8 (14.9)	86 (3.5)	79.5 (6.4)	83.0 (0.0)	80.0 (8.5)
% stage 2	56.0 (5.3)	54.8 (8.7)	70.1 (1.6)	56.0 (4.9)	63.0 (1.8)
% stages 3-4	15.8 (4.4)	18.7 (10.2)	2.0 (1.7)	10.5 (3.6)	6.2 (5.1)
% REM	21.9 (8.0)	21.2 (5.3)	24.9 (0.3)	32.2 (2.0)	27.7 (6.9)

BN2: baseline night 2; TR3: the third night in lab and the first of treatment; TR4: the fourth night in lab and the second of treatment; SOL: sleep-onset latency; WASO: wake time after sleep-onset; TST: total sleep time; SE: sleep efficiency; REM: rapid eye movement; min: minutes.

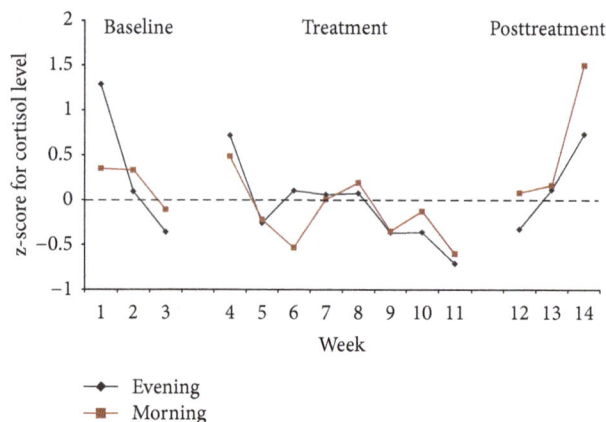

FIGURE 3: Evening and morning cortisol levels compared to their respective average for participants 1, 2, and 3. 0 as z-score means participant's average of cortisol levels. A negative z-score means a cortisol level lower than participant's average while a positive z-score means a cortisol level higher than participant's average of cortisol levels.

4. Discussion

Our study illustrates that physiological mechanisms of sleep restriction therapy could be evaluated using an appropriate methodological strategy. By beginning measurements on the first night of treatment, it was revealed that sleep restriction might have a rapid impact on subjective sleep and on the physiological markers of sleep. First, the results showed that sleep restriction decreased total wake time sleep-onset latency and increased sleep efficiency. Second, these results showed that the subjective total sleep time is decreased by about one hour during the first week of treatment. Visual inspection of PSG data suggests that stage 2 decreases when introducing the treatment, while stage 3 seems to increase. An increase in REM sleep can also be observed. PSA indicated a change in beta-1 and -2 beginning with the second treatment night. Third, the results illustrated a potential action of sleep restriction on cortisol levels as both morning and evening cortisol levels seem to decrease during treatment. Fourth, with respect to sleepiness, the results show that greater sleepiness at night is associated with higher sleep efficiency and shorter wake time during the night. They also suggest that alertness in the morning is associated with previous sleep time. Finally, the results on sleepiness indicate that these associations were not present before treatment, suggesting that they are induced by sleep restriction.

Objective sleep data obtained in the present study present similarities and divergences with results from other studies. They are similar to Cervena and colleagues [14] except that the increase in SWS in their study was clearer. PSA suggest that, when treatment is effective, beta-1 power decreases from baseline to the introduction of sleep restriction therapy. On the second night of treatment, both beta bands' powers seem to decrease. These PSA results converge with other studies [13, 14] that found a decrease after treatment in beta-1 and -2 while they diverge from the Krystal and Edinger study [9] that did not find a decrease in beta bands after CBT-I. Regarding powers of lower frequency bands (slow or delta), our study

TABLE 5: Median (range) power values for responders for beta-1 and beta-2 band frequencies.

	Sleep stages	BN2		TR3		TR4	
		Median	Range	Median	Range	Median	Range
		Beta-1					
Cycle 1	NRem	2.41	1.62–12.14	2.09	1.92–9.06	1.48	1.13–2.98
	Rem	1.83	0.78–5.93	1.88	0.89–6.37	2.45	0.58–3.11
	1	3.01	1.06–7.54	2.93	2.93-2.93	1.80	1.14–2.45
	2*	4.27	2.99–13.88	3.29	2.22–11.89	3.15	1.31–5.13
	3*	2.30	2.10–9.09	1.91	1.59–6.97	1.34	1.29–3.95
	4	1.53	1.40–7.45	1.62	1.48–5.09	3.02	2.90–4.64
Cycle 2	NRem*	3.86	1.72–11.04	3.44	1.33–4.75	1.81	1.14–2.55
	Rem	1.65	0.73–5.28	1.11	0.98–6.34	1.33	0.66–2.86
	1	1.40	1.40-1.40	1.55	1.55-1.55	1.88	1.40–2.36
	2	8.45	2.31–14.80	3.44	2.31–6.78	2.79	1.67–5.13
	3	2.02	1.42–8.16	5.10	1.15–9.04	1.75	1.28–3.83
	4	3.37	1.27–5.47	2.44	0.95–3.92	1.44	0.76–1.56
All cycles	NRem*	3.21	1.76–11.99	2.77	1.69–7.43	2.38	1.19–4.22
	Rem	1.57	0.77–5.78	1.52	1.02–6.36	1.67	0.61–3.04
	1	3.46	1.14–7.05	2.71	1.33–7.25	2.39	0.95–3.19
	2*	3.53	2.23–14.64	3.30	2.18–10.10	3.19	1.51–5.77
	3*	2.09	1.51–8.47	1.91	1.34–6.79	1.57	1.33–3.87
	4	1.53	1.37–5.96	1.62	1.22–4.14	1.38	0.92–1.62
		Beta-2					
Cycle 1	NRem	0.75	0.56–3.27	1.01	0.92–4.08	0.51	0.51–1.10
	Rem	1.13	0.86–4.01	1.04	0.89–5.29	0.98	0.60–1.64
	1	1.43	0.87–5.64	1.08	1.08-1.08	1.16	0.93–1.38
	2	1.25	0.89–3.13	1.39	1.31–5.82	1.19	0.66–2.09
	3	0.67	0.63–2.25	0.80	0.58–2.46	0.48	0.47–1.15
	4	0.56	0.50–2.17	0.84	0.59–2.48	1.18	0.96–1.61
Cycle 2	NRem*	1.78	0.67–2.51	1.00	0.47–1.89	0.67	0.42–0.93
	Rem	1.11	0.79–3.24	0.95	0.84–5.70	0.86	0.53–1.55
	1	1.43	1.43-1.43	1.35	1.35-1.35	1.00	0.92–1.07
	2	3.01	0.75–4.51	1.00	0.78–5.43	0.70	0.55–1.41
	3	0.68	0.53–2.18	1.49	0.48–2.50	0.60	0.45–1.14
	4*	1.09	0.47–1.71	1.04	0.49–1.59	0.53	0.32–0.75
All cycles	NRem	1.14	0.77–3.01	0.96	0.90–2.76	0.75	0.52–1.36
	Rem	1.11	0.82–3.59	1.00	0.88–5.72	0.92	0.58–1.80
	1	1.39	1.25–5.09	1.27	1.15–9.01	1.06	1.03–2.78
	2*	1.10	0.75–3.07	1.29	1.18–3.73	0.85	0.58–1.64
	3	0.66	0.54–2.20	0.80	0.52–2.35	0.55	0.47–1.14
	4	0.56	0.49–1.82	0.84	0.54–1.75	0.51	0.35–0.77

BN2: baseline night 2; TR3: the third night in lab and the first of treatment; TR4: the fourth night in lab and the second of treatment; NREM: nonrapid eye movement; REM: rapid eye movement. *Significant results at $P \leq 0.05$ between nights for the sleep stages targeted.

is more similar to Krystal and Edinger's findings [9] than to Cervena et al.'s finding [14]; the latter found an increase in SWS after treatment. Given that sleep restriction is used alone in our study while it is included in a multicomponent treatment in other studies, similarities between studies can be interpreted as being due to sleep restriction. Divergences might reflect an effect of another component of the CBT-I that was used in other studies. Nevertheless, our results support the assessment of beta-1 and -2 separately as it has been done in our previous studies [35, 36]. Cautiously, it could be suggested that this decrease in beta powers might also be an indicator of treatment efficacy or at least reflect a positive response to treatment.

Our results reporting an increase in REM sleep are similar to those of other studies reporting PSG data after treatment [14, 37]. However, our results make a further contribution

TABLE 6: Correlation coefficients between subjective sleepiness, alertness, and sleep variables for each participant during treatment.

Participants/alertness and sleepiness	Sleep variables				
	SOL	WASO	TWT	TST	SE
Participant 1					
Alertness	−0.30*	0.13	−0.07	0.19	0.12
Sleepiness	0.51***	0.01	0.35**	−0.37**	−0.42
Sleepy at night	−0.39**	−0.29*	−0.39**	−0.02	0.32
Participant 2					
Alertness	−0.41**	−0.28*	−0.32*	0.53***	0.35**
Sleepiness	−0.01	0.26	0.28*	−0.17	−0.28*
Sleepy at night	−0.29*	−0.07	−0.07	−0.07	0.01
Participant 3					
Alertness	−0.02	−0.28	−0.22	0.25	0.21
Sleepiness	−0.02	0.32*	−0.02	−0.16	0.01
Sleepy at night	−0.16	0.31*	0.05	−0.08	−0.04
Participant 4					
Alertness	0.01	−0.27	0.08	0.29	0.03
Sleepiness	0.13	0.55***	0.17	−0.52***	−0.28
Sleepy at night	−0.30	−0.16	−0.05	0.18	0.09
Participant 5					
Alertness	−0.13	−0.44**	−0.28	0.29	0.31*
Sleepiness	−0.07	0.39**	0.17	−0.17	−0.19
Sleepy at night	−0.25	−0.27	−0.38**	0.24	0.36*

SOL: sleep-onset latency; WASO: wake after sleep-onset; TWT: total wake time including SOL, WASO, and early morning awakening; TST: total sleep time.
$^*P < 0.05$; $^{**}P < 0.01$; $^{***}P < 0.001$.

by indicating that REM sleep begins to increase from the beginning of sleep restriction therapy and further increases during and after treatment. Based on the idea that REM sleep in insomnia is unstable and may contribute to sleep misperception [38], the increase in REM sleep observed during sleep restriction therapy could be interpreted as showing that sleep restriction consolidates REM sleep. Furthermore, one previous study found that REM sleep contributes to disrupt subjective perceptions of sleep and waking time [39]. Therefore, when the amount of REM sleep is increased and consolidated, it could contribute to the improvement of the subjective perception of sleep and wake time. However, the two participants who had a minimal response to sleep restriction treatment had an increase in REM sleep in the first nights. This suggests that other mechanisms are involved during treatment. The mechanisms underlying the increase in REM sleep seen during sleep restriction should be further investigated in larger studies.

Contrary to expectations, PSA do not indicate increase in SWS during sleep restriction therapy. This surprising result diverges from other studies [9, 14] that found an increase in SWS after CBT-I or that CBT-I led to a more rapid decline in delta power during NREM sleep. These two studies used a multicomponent treatment, while the methodology used in the present study isolated the effect of sleep restriction

therapy. Therefore, one can argue that the SWS increase is not due to sleep restriction. Clearly, further studies will be needed to investigate the physiological mechanisms of action for other components of CBT-I. Nevertheless, because the sample of the present study is small, our results could also reflect a subsample of insomnia sufferers who happened to present an altered SWS.

The cortisol results seem congruent with an improvement in sleep during our sleep restriction treatment. Indeed, cortisol levels (evening and morning) are lower during treatment than at baseline for participants who had a treatment response. Moreover and most importantly, the decrease in cortisol levels can be detected very early in treatment. Cortisol levels are known to be higher for people with insomnia than for good sleepers [15, 16]. Thus, our results indicate that the use of sleep restriction alone, since it impacts cortisol levels, is a beneficial avenue for treating insomnia. Cortisol levels should thus be further evaluated during CBT-I.

In addition to the physiological sleep restriction therapy mechanisms, the findings highlight the rapid change observed in subjective sleep. Indeed, sleep restriction provides a rapid and marked decrease in wake time that is sustained during treatment. The findings also confirm a previously observed decrease in TST, quantifying that decrease at about an hour. Interestingly, these benefits in sleep were observed in spite of variations in the compliance data. It seems that individuals cope differently with difficulties encountered during treatment; some delayed their sleep window while some others shortened or changed the timing of the sleep window. Therefore, it appears that sleep restriction can be effective without a full application by the participant of the sleep restriction procedure.

Taken together, the data on PSG, sleepiness, and cortisol provide indications that sleep restriction decreases hyperarousal and cortical activity while increasing sleepiness to facilitate sleep. It is not clear, however, if these involve an increase of the homeostatic drive for all participants. The decrease in beta powers and in cortisol levels during treatment might reflect a decrease in hyperarousal. Contrary to both expectations and visual inspection of PSG, no increase in powers of lower frequency bands (slow or delta) indicative of greater homeostatic pressure was observed across nights. This, along with an increase in REM sleep, could reflect a malfunction of the homeostatic drive, implying that a decrease in wake time and sleep time will not generate the expected homeostatic sleep drive effect as previously suggested [8, 40]. Nevertheless, the sleepiness results suggest a relationship between sleep restriction and an increase in sleepiness at night, facilitating falling sleep and confirming a previous clinical report [41]. These data on perceived sleepiness are consistent with those of two studies [10, 12] as well as with the hypothesis that sleep restriction increases the homeostatic drive. Therefore, a strong and complete evaluation of the sleep restriction effect on homeostatic drive is warranted to more fully understand the sleep restriction mechanism.

These preliminary results possess some methodological limitations, although they are promising as a further step toward understanding sleep restriction mechanisms. A first limit concerns the small sample size that precludes obtaining strong statistical evidence of the mechanisms. Second, the procedure of daily assessing several variables during 10 to 12 weeks could have rendered the participants' tasks onerous, thus affecting data reliability. For this reason, sleep diary data were analyzed using ITSA. Third, cortisol data itself has several limitations: the trend for cortisol levels to decrease during baseline precludes definitive statements. The weekly adjustment of the sleep window might also have affected the evening cortisol level. However, although the time of going to bed differed for participants, the results followed a similar pattern. Moreover, both evening and morning cortisol levels were within the normal range for the time of day and the saliva methodology replicated that used in another study [34]: we see no reason to doubt the reliability of our cortisol results. Fourth, the fact that the first sleep restriction nights are spent in the laboratory might have influenced sleep data reported afterwards compared to other studies that did not use this strategy. On the other hand, this procedure has the advantage of standardizing the implementation of sleep restriction instructions by providing training for the procedure.

5. Conclusion

This research evaluated the impact of sleep restriction on physiological markers of sleep, thus allowing a description of the putative physiological mechanisms for this treatment. The PSG and PSA results of the present study are innovative. They illustrate how a more in-depth investigation of the physiological variables related to sleep restriction could enlighten the knowledge on how sleep restriction works and on cortical activity in insomnia. The methodology used should be taken as a guideline for future studies. These findings illustrated the relevance of dismantling CBT-I to understand each component of treatment mechanism and enhance treatment efficacy. Future studies should investigate if the REM sleep increase observed with sleep restriction contributes to the improvement of sleep perception in insomnia. Circadian timing of sleep restriction and of other CBT-I components should also be further investigated in other studies. In addition, the sleepiness results, along with results obtained for TST, suggest that more attention should be given to the relationship between these two variables over the course of sleep restriction to evaluate a potential acute negative effect of sleep restriction. Finally, future studies should focus on empirically identifying sleep restriction mechanisms of action in order to increase efficacy and make relevant clinical recommendations concerning this promising form of therapy.

Acknowledgments

This research was supported by a studentship from the Canadian Institutes of Health Research awarded to the first author and by grants from The Welcome Trust, Chief Scientist Office (Section Government Hewett Department), and the Dr. Mortimer and Theresa Sackler Foundation awarded to the second author. The authors wish to thank Dr. Maria Gardani for her work during the experimentation, Dr. Simon Kyle for his helpful comments on the paper, and Dr. James Everett for English revision.

References

[1] A. J. Spielman, P. Saskin, and M. J. Thorpy, "Treatment of chronic insomnia by restriction of time in bed," *Sleep*, vol. 10, no. 1, pp. 45–56, 1987.

[2] C. M. Morin, J. P. Culbert, and S. M. Schwartz, "Nonpharmacological interventions for insomnia: a meta-analysis of treatment efficacy," *American Journal of Psychiatry*, vol. 151, no. 8, pp. 1172–1180, 1994.

[3] D. R. R. Murtagh and K. M. Greenwood, "Identifying effective psychological treatments for insomnia: a meta-analysis," *Journal of Consulting and Clinical Psychology*, vol. 63, no. 1, pp. 79–89, 1995.

[4] M. T. Smith, M. L. Perlis, A. Park et al., "Comparative meta-analysis of pharmacotherapy and behavior therapy for persistent insomnia," *American Journal of Psychiatry*, vol. 159, no. 1, pp. 5–11, 2002.

[5] M. R. Irwin, J. C. Cole, and P. M. Nicassio, "Comparative meta-analysis of behavioral interventions for insomnia and their efficacy in middle-aged adults and in older adults 55+ years of age," *Health Psychology*, vol. 25, no. 1, pp. 3–14, 2006.

[6] T. Morgenthaler, M. Kramer, C. Alessi et al., "Practice parameters for the psychological and behavioral treatment of insomnia: an update. An American Academy of Sleep Medicine Report," *Sleep*, vol. 29, no. 11, pp. 1415–1419, 2006.

[7] C. M. Morin, R. R. Bootzin, D. J. Buysse, J. D. Edinger, C. A. Espie, and K. L. Lichstein, "Psychological and behavioral treatment of insomnia: update of the recent evidence (1998-2004)," *Sleep*, vol. 29, no. 11, pp. 1398–1414, 2006.

[8] W. R. Pigeon and M. L. Perlis, "Sleep homeostasis in primary insomnia," *Sleep Medicine Reviews*, vol. 10, no. 4, pp. 247–254, 2006.

[9] A. D. Krystal and J. D. Edinger, "Sleep EEG predictors and correlates of the response to cognitive behavioral therapy for insomnia," *Sleep*, vol. 33, no. 5, pp. 669–677, 2010.

[10] S. D. Kyle, C. B. Miller, Z. Roger, M. Siriwardena, K. M. Mac Mahon, and C. A. Espie, "Sleep restriction therapy for insomnia is associated with reduced objective total sleep time, increased daytime somnolence, and objectively-impaired vigilance: implications for the clinical management of insomnia disorder," *Sleep*. In press.

[11] S. D. Kyle, K. Morgan, K. Spiegelhalder, and C. A. Espie, "No pain, no gain: an exploratory within-subjects mixed-methods evaluation of the patient experience of sleep restriction therapy (SRT) for insomnia," *Sleep Medicine*, vol. 12, no. 8, pp. 735–747, 2011.

[12] C. B. Miller, S. D. Kyle, N. S. Marshall, and C. A. Espie, "Ecological momentary assessment of daytime symptoms during sleep restriction therapy for insomnia," *Journal of Sleep Research*, vol. 22, pp. 266–272, 2013.

[13] G. D. Jacobs, H. Benson, and R. Friedman, "Home-based central nervous system assessment of a multifactor behavioral intervention for chronic sleep-onset insomnia," *Behavior Therapy*, vol. 24, no. 1, pp. 159–174, 1993.

[14] K. Cervena, Y. Dauvilliers, F. Espa et al., "Effect of cognitive behavioural therapy for insomnia on sleep architecture and

sleep EEG power spectra in psychophysiological insomnia," *Journal of Sleep Research*, vol. 13, no. 4, pp. 385–393, 2004.

[15] J. Backhaus, K. Junghanns, and F. Hohagen, "Sleep disturbances are correlated with decreased morning awakening salivary cortisol," *Psychoneuroendocrinology*, vol. 29, no. 9, pp. 1184–1191, 2004.

[16] A. N. Vgontzas, E. O. Bixler, H.-M. Lin et al., "Chronic insomnia is associated with nyctohemeral activation of the hypothalamic-pituitary-adrenal axis: clinical implications," *Journal of Clinical Endocrinology and Metabolism*, vol. 86, no. 8, pp. 3787–3794, 2001.

[17] P. Tucker, A. Dahlgren, T. Akerstedt, and J. Waterhouse, "The impact of free-time activities on sleep, recovery and well-being," *Applied Ergonomics*, vol. 39, no. 5, pp. 653–662, 2008.

[18] American Psychiatric Association, Ed., *Diagnostic and Statistical Manual of Mental Disorders*, American Psychiatric Association, Washington, DC, USA, 4th edition, 2000.

[19] C. M. Morin, *Insomnia: Psychological Assessment and Management*, The Guilford Press, New York, NY, USA, 1993.

[20] M. B. First, R. L. Spitzer, M. Gibbon, and J. B. W. Williams, *Structured Clinical Interview for DSM-IV Axis I Disorders, Clinical Version (SCID-IV)*, American Psychiatric Association, Washington, DC, USA, 1997.

[21] D. H. Barlow and M. Hersen, *Single-Case Experimental Designs: Strategies for Studying Behavior Change*, Pergamon Press, New York, NY, USA, 2nd edition, 1984.

[22] A. E. Kazdin, *Methodological Issues & Strategies in Clinical Research*, American Psychological Association, Washington, DC, USA, 3rd edition, 2003.

[23] M. M. Sánchez-Ortuño and J. D. Edinger, "Internight sleep variability: its clinical significance and responsiveness to treatment in primary and comorbid insomnia," *Journal of Sleep Research*, vol. 21, pp. 527–534, 2012.

[24] C. M. Morin and C. A. Espie, *Insomnia: a Clinical Guide to Assessment and Treatment*, Kluwer Academic, Plenum Press, New York, NY, USA, 2003.

[25] J. D. Edinger and M. K. Means, "Cognitive-behavioral therapy for primary insomnia," *Clinical Psychology Review*, vol. 25, no. 5, pp. 539–558, 2005.

[26] A. Rechtschaffen and A. Kales, *A Manual of Standardized Terminology, Techniques and Scoring System for Sleep Stages of Human Subjects*, Brain Information Service/Brain Research Institute, UCLA, Los Angeles, Calif, USA, 1968.

[27] C. Iber, S. Ancoli-Israel, A. Chesson, and S. F. Quan, *The AASM Manual For the Scoring of Sleep and Associated Events: Rules, Terminology and Technical Specifications*, American Academy of Sleep Medicine, Westchester, Ill, USA, 2007.

[28] D. P. Brunner, R. C. Vasko, C. S. Detka, J. P. Monahan, C. F. Reynolds III, and D. J. Kupfer, "Muscle artifacts in the sleep EEG: automated detection and effect on all-night EEC power spectra," *Journal of Sleep Research*, vol. 5, no. 3, pp. 155–164, 1996.

[29] C. H. Bastien, A. Vallières, and C. M. Morin, "Validation of the insomnia severity index as an outcome measure for insomnia research," *Sleep Medicine*, vol. 2, no. 4, pp. 297–307, 2001.

[30] S. Smith and J. Trinder, "Detecting insomnia: comparison of four self-report measures of sleep in a young adult population," *Journal of Sleep Research*, vol. 10, no. 3, pp. 229–235, 2001.

[31] C. M. Morin, G. Belleville, L. Bélanger, and H. Ivers, "The insomnia severity index: psychometric indicators to detect insomnia cases and evaluate treatment response," *Sleep*, vol. 34, no. 5, pp. 601–608, 2011.

[32] B. S. Gorman and D. B. Allison, "Statistical alternatives for single-case designs," in *Design and Analysis of Single-Case Research*, R. D. Franklin, D. B. Allison, and B. S. Gorman, Eds., Lawrence Erlbaum Associates, Hillsdale, NJ, USA, 1996.

[33] SAS Institute, *SAS/STAT 9.1.3 USer'S Guide*, vol. 1–7, SAS Institute, Cary, NC, USA, 2005.

[34] B. E. Huitema and J. W. McKean, "Design specification issues in time-series intervention models," *Educational and Psychological Measurement*, vol. 60, no. 1, pp. 38–58, 2000.

[35] G. St-Jean, I. Turcotte, and C. H. Bastien, "Cerebral asymmetry in insomnia sufferers," *Frontiers in Neurology* , vol. 3, article 47, 2012.

[36] G. St-Jean, I. Turcotte, A. D. Perusse, and C. H. Bastien, "REM and NREM power spectral analysis on two consecutive nights in psychophysiological and paradoxical insomnia sufferers, International," *Journal of Psychophysiology*, vol. 89, no. 2, pp. 181–194, 2013.

[37] C. M. Morin, A. Vallières, B. Guay et al., "Cognitive behavioral therapy, singly and combined with medication, for persistent insomnia: a randomized controlled trial," *The Journal of the American Medical Association*, vol. 301, no. 19, pp. 2005–2015, 2009.

[38] D. Riemann, K. Spiegelhalder, C. Nissen, V. Hirscher, C. Baglioni, and B. Feige, "REM sleep instability—a new pathway for insomnia?" *Pharmacopsychiatry*, vol. 45, pp. 167–176, 2012.

[39] B. Feige, A. Al-Shajlawi, C. Nissen et al., "Does REM sleep contribute to subjective wake time in primary insomnia? A comparison of polysomnographic and subjective sleep in 100 patients," *Journal of Sleep Research*, vol. 17, no. 2, pp. 180–190, 2008.

[40] A. Besset, E. Villemin, M. Tafti, and M. Billiard, "Homeostatic process and sleep spindles in patients with sleep—maintenance insomnia: effect of partial (21 h) sleep deprivation," *Electroencephalography and Clinical Neurophysiology*, vol. 107, no. 2, pp. 122–132, 1998.

[41] T. J. Hoelscher and J. D. Edinger, "Treatment of sleep-maintenance insomnia in older adults: sleep period reduction, sleep education, and modified stimulus control," *Psychology and Aging*, vol. 3, no. 3, pp. 258–263, 1988.

11

Sleep Quality among Female Hospital Staff Nurses

Pei-Li Chien,[1] Hui-Fang Su,[2] Pi-Ching Hsieh,[2] Ruo-Yan Siao,[1]
Pei-Ying Ling,[3] and Hei-Jen Jou[3,4]

[1] Department of Preventive Medicine, Taiwan Adventist Hospital, No. 424, Section 2, Bade Road, Songshan District,
Taipei 105, Taiwan
[2] Department of Health Care Management, National Taipei University of Nursing and Health Sciences, No. 89,
Nei-Chiang Street, Wanhua District, Taipei 10845, Taiwan
[3] Department of Obstetrics and Gynecology, Taiwan Adventist Hospital, No. 424, Section 2, Bade Road, Songshan District,
Taipei 105, Taiwan
[4] Department of Obstetrics and Gynecology, National Taiwan University Hospital, No. 7, Zhongshan S. Road, Zhongzheng District,
Taipei 100, Taiwan

Correspondence should be addressed to Hei-Jen Jou; jouheijen@gmail.com

Academic Editor: Michel M. Billiard

Purpose. To investigate sleep quality of hospital staff nurses, both by subjective questionnaire and objective measures. *Methods.* Female staff nurses at a regional teaching hospital in Northern Taiwan were recruited. The Chinese version of the pittsburgh sleep quality index (C-PSQI) was used to assess subjective sleep quality, and an electrocardiogram-based cardiopulmonary coupling (CPC) technique was used to analyze objective sleep stability. Work stress was assessed using questionnaire on medical worker's stress. *Results.* A total of 156 staff nurses completed the study. Among the staff nurses, 75.8% (117) had a PSQI score of ≥5 and 39.8% had an inadequate stable sleep ratio on subjective measures. Nurses with a high school or lower educational degree had a much higher risk of sleep disturbance when compared to nurses with a college or higher level degree. *Conclusions.* Both subjective and objective measures demonstrated that poor sleep quality is a common health problem among hospital staff nurses. More studies are warranted on this important issue to discover possible factors and therefore to develop a systemic strategy to cope with the problem.

1. Introduction

Poor sleep quality among hospital stuff nurses is a critical issue for healthcare system. It not only leads to health problems of the nurses, but it is also associated with a lower work performance and a higher risk of medical errors which may jeopardize patient's safety [1]. The incidence of sleep disturbance among general Asian population ranged from 26.4% to 39.4% [2, 3]. Most previous studies on sleep quality of nurses focused on the effect of shift work on subjective sleep perception using self-report questionnaire and revealed that up to 57% of shift-working nurses had sleep disturbance [4]. It is therefore warranted to find out possible factors associated with sleep disturbance of working nurses.

The perception of sleep quality is complex and associated with various subjective factors such as fatigue, work stress, or other emotional factors in addition to objective sleep quality. However, limited study of objective sleep quality of hospital nurses provides little information for better understanding of sleep disturbance among this population.

The current methods used to assess objective sleep physiology primarily rely on polysomnography (PSG) which is based on the analysis of signals of electroencephalography (EEG), electrooculography, electromyography, and electrocardiography (ECG). Although PSG is the gold standard for objective sleep quality assessment, the cost and technical complexity of PSG limit its use as a routine screening tool. In addition, it has been noted that PSG measurement may have been largely affected by "first-night effect" from an unfamiliar laboratory environment and discomfort from PSG sensors and equipment [5]. In addition, sleep pattern of subjects at home may be quite different when compared with that in the laboratory room. Previous studies have also demonstrated inconsistency between subjective sleep perception and PSG staging [6–8].

Recently, an alternative method term cardiopulmonary coupling (CPC) analysis has been developed to quantify sleep stability. The technique is based on analysis of continuous ECG signals using take-home ECG devices [9]. This novel technology is less expensive and is more convenient since the measures do not require subjects to sleep in a laboratory room. Therefore the study does not interrupt the daily work of the nurses.

The purpose of this study was to assess the sleep quality of hospital stuff nurses, including subjective sleep perception by self-report questionnaire and objective sleep stability by CPC method. We also tried to identify possible demographic, lifestyle, and work factors for poor sleep quality among hospital working nurses.

2. Methods

2.1. Subjects. A cross-sectional study was conducted from March 1, 2009 to September 30, 2009 to investigate the subjective sleep perception, objective sleep stability, and the possible factors associated with poor sleep quality among staff nurses at a regional teaching hospital with 389 nurses. One hundred and seventy-five subjects from the hospital, including nurses and nurse managers, were randomly selected by computer chaos generator with an approximate nurse/nurse manager ratio of 3 : 1 and study subjects comprising about half of the total hospital nursing staff and nursing managers. Male nurses were excluded from the study because of their small proportion among the nursing staff. Written informed consent from each subject was obtained after the study's approval by the Institutional Review Board of the study hospital.

The authors developed a detailed questionnaire according to the literature, which included demographic information (age, gender, education level, marital status, etc.) and associated factors such as regular exercise, managerial position, and work shift. Regular exercise was defined as a regular exercise habit of ≥3 exercise per week with duration of ≥30 minutes every time. Work shift was defined as >1 work shift per week during last month.

2.2. Assessment of Work Stress. Questionnaire on medical worker's stress (QMWS) (Cronbach alpha coefficient 0.84) was used to assess the subjects' work stress [10]. There are eight questions in the QMWS, including stress from (1) running the hospital, (2) preparing the accreditation of the hospital, (3) the stability of the patients' condition, (4) the relationship with patients, (5) medical dispute or lawsuits, (6) salary, (7) personal assessment, and (8) position upgrade or academic research. Each item scored from 1 (very sure not to be a stress factor) to 6 (very sure to be a stress factor) with a total score ranging from 8 to 48. The subjects were subdivided into

two groups: the higher stress group (HSG) with a score of >32 and the lower stress group (LSG) with a stress score of ≤32.

2.3. Assessment of Subjective Sleep Quality. The Chinese edition Pittsburgh sleep quality index (C-PSQI) was used to assess subjective sleep quality [11]. Subjects were asked to assess their sleep condition in the previous month. The PSQI is a self-rated questionnaire and comprises 18 questions to assess seven domains of sleep, including subjective sleep quality, sleep latency, sleep duration, habitual sleep efficiency, sleep disturbances, use of sleeping medication, and daytime dysfunction. Each domain is rated on a 4-point scale (0–3), which generates a total score ranging between 0 and 21. Poor sleepers had a total score of 5 or above, while good sleepers had a score of less than 5. The Cronbach's α values were 0.83 for the original PSQI instrument [12] and 0.77 for C-PSQI [11], respectively.

2.4. Assessment of Objective Sleep Quality. A take-home Holter ECG SD-100 portable recorder (Microstar Inc., Taipei, Taiwan) was used to obtain continuous ECG signals of the subjects during their time in bed with only 4 leads attached to the trunk of the subjects. All subjects received ECG recording at home after a detailed demonstration of the recording process by the researcher. The ECG recording was collected on the second day and then uploaded to a central laboratory. The signals were automatically processed and analysed to generate a sleep pictogram using an ECG-based CPC (cardiopulmonary coupling analysis) technique [9]. Three physiological sleep states were classified based on CPC analysis: stable sleep, unstable sleep, and REM/wakeful (awake/dream) states [9], as expressed by both absolute time duration and ratio of time in bed. A stable sleep ratio ≥41% was regarded as adequate sleep "stability", while inadequate sleep stability indicated a stable sleep ratio of <41%. Recorded data also included total sleep time, sleep latency duration, and apnea/hypopnea index (AHI).

In addition to the three physiological sleep patterns, the machine also records sleep apnea/hypopnea of the subjects. The AHI represents an index of apnea/hypopnea per hour of time in bed. An AHI of 5 to 15 was defined as mild apnea/hypopnea, an AHI between 16 and 30 meant moderate apnea/hypopnea, and an AHI of greater than 30 signified severe apnea/hypopnea.

2.5. Statistic Analysis. Descriptive analysis was used to analyze basic characteristics of the subjects with mean values ± standard deviation (*SD*). Comparison between groups was done with Student's *t*-test for continuous variables and χ^2 test for discrete variables. Multiple variable logistic regression was used to calculate the odds ratios of variant demographic factors on subjective perception and objective sleep stability. Linear regression was used to identify the association between PSQI and parameters of objective measures. We considered the differences were significant at $P < 0.05$ for all statistical tests. All analyses were performed with the SPSS 17.0. (Allyn & Bacon, Inc., Needham Heights, MA, USA).

3. Results

3.1. Subjects. During the study period, 19 subjects dropped out, including 6 of 44 nurse managers and 13 of 131 first-line staff nurses, which resulted in a response rate of 89.1% (156/175). The reasons for the dropout included, worrying about sleep interruption by the equipment (10), unwillingness to do the test (6), and personal issues (3). There were two subjects who failed their initial CPC recording, and a second test was performed.

3.2. Demographic Data and Sleep Assessment. The subjects' mean age and years of nursing work experience were 34.6±8.1 and 7.9 ± 7.2 years, respectively. Half of the subjects (50.0%) were single. Nurse managers had a higher percentage of college or higher level of education when compared with that of nonmanager nurses (68% versus 37%, $P = 0.01$). Table 1 summarized basic characteristics of the subjects. Forty-five percent of the nurses had less five years of nursing experience, and 50.6% had a QMWS score of >32. Table 2 demonstrated subjective and objective sleep measures of the subjects. Mean PSQI score was 7.34 ± 2.94. Objective measures showed a mean stable sleep ratio of 46.62 ± 17.26% and a mean AHI of 4.32 ± 7.68.

A comparison among variable factors with sleep measures by logistic regression is summarized in Table 3. Sleep assessments revealed that 75.0% (117/156) of subjects had a total PSQI score of 5 or above, which indicated a significant sleep problem, and 39.7% of subjects (62/156) had inadequate sleep stability according to CPC records. Comparison between the basic characteristics and the sleep measures showed that years of nursing work experience, age, marital status, number of child, habit of regular exercise, work position, work shift, and work stress were not significantly related to a poor subjective sleep perception or an inadequate stable sleep ratio. However, there was significant relationship between the education levels and both subjective sleep perception and objective sleep stability. Nurses with educational level of high school or under had odds ratios of 2.69 to be a poor sleeper ($P = 0.02$) and of 2.71 to have an inadequate sleep stability ($P = 0.01$).

Linear correlation analysis revealed that PSQI score was weakly but significantly correlated with the unstable sleep duration ($r = 0.20$, $P = 0.01$), unstable sleep ratio ($r = 0.22$, $P = 0.006$), and AHI frequency ($r = 0.25$, $P = 0.002$) (Table 4). A significant reverse correlation between stable sleep ratio and PSQI score ($r = 0.17$, $P = 0.03$) was observed as well. There were no significant correlations between PSQI score and awake/dream duration ($r = 0.04$, $P = 0.58$), awake/dream ratio ($r = 0.02$, $P = 0.89$), and sleep latency duration ($r = 0.04$, $P = 0.59$).

4. Discussion

The present study has demonstrated that nurses working in a hospital setting had a high prevalence of sleep disturbance. Most previous studies were based on subjective questionnaire. However, our data provided objective evidence, which

TABLE 1: Basic characteristics of the subjects.

Variable	N	%
Total	156	100
Nursing experience		
<5 years	70	44.9
≥5 year	86	55.1
Age		
<40 years	115	73.7
≥40 years	41	26.3
Education level		
College or higher degree	70	44.9
High school or lower degree	86	55.1
Marital status		
Married	78	50.0
Single	78	50.0
Number of children		
≥1	63	40.4
None	93	59.6
Regular exercise		
Yes	77	47.8
No	79	50.6
Nurse manager		
Yes	38	24.4
No	118	75.6
Work shift		
Yes	49	32.3
No	107	67.7
Working pressure		
Lower (8–32)	79	50.6
Higher (33–48)	77	49.4

Note. * Work pressure: measured by questionnaire of medical worker's stress (QMWS): lower work pressure: score 8–32; higher work pressure: 33–48.

TABLE 2: Subjective and objective sleep measures of the subjects.

Sleep indices	Mean	SD
PSQI (score)	7.34	2.94
Subject sleep quality (score)	1.25	0.77
Sleep latency (minute)	18.33	13.09
Sleep duration (hours)	6.11	1.22
Sleep efficiency (%)	83.20	13.81
Sleep disturbance (score)	6.54	3.41
Use of sleep medications (score)	0.23	0.63
Daytime dysfunction (score)	1.91	1.43
CPC		
Sleep latency (minute)	26.79	43.80
Stable sleep ratio (%)	46.62	17.26
Unstable sleep ratio (%)	29.78	13.34
Awake/dream sleep (%)	22.26	8.01
AHI	4.32	7.68

Note. PSQI: Pittsburgh sleep quality index; CPC: cardiopulmonary coupling analysis, AHI: apnea/hypopnea index.

TABLE 3: The relationship between variable factors in subjective or objective poor sleep quality.

Variable	PSQI*				CPC**			
	Poor sleeper	Good sleeper	OR	P	Inadequate sleep stability	Adequate sleep stability	OR	P
N (total = 156)	117	39			62	94		
Working years								
<5 years	56	14			26	44		
≥5 year	61	25	0.40	0.06	36	50	0.81	0.63
Age								
<40 years	85	30			41	74		
≥40 years	32	9	1.64	0.34	21	20	0.91	0.85
Education level								
College or higher degree	47	23			34	36		
High school or lower degree	70	16	2.69	0.02	28	58	2.71	0.01
Marital status								
Married	58	20			32	46		
Single	59	19	0.67	0.60	30	48	0.78	0.71
Number of Children								
≥1	46	17			26	37		
None	71	22	0.60	0.49	36	57	0.98	0.97
Regular exercise								
Yes	56	21			27	50		
NO	61	18	1.08	0.85	35	44	0.72	0.38
Nurse manager								
Yes	28	10			14	24		
No	89	29	0.67	0.43	48	70	0.53	0.17
Work shift								
Yes	36	13			17	32		
No	81	26	0.90	0.82	45	62	1.90	0.16
AHI								
≦15	109	38			53	94		
>15	8	1	2.34	0.45	9	0	NA	NA
Working pressure#								
Lower (8–32)	56	21			25	52		
Higher (33–48)	61	18	1.68	0.21	37	42	0.49	0.07

Note. PSQI: pittsburgh sleep quality index, good sleeper had a PSQI <5 and a poor sleeper had a PSQI ≥5; CPC: cardiopulmonary coupling analysis, a stable sleep ratio ≥41% indicates adequate sleep stability and a stable sleep ratio <41% indicates inadequate sleep stability; #Work pressure measured by questionnaire of medical worker's stress (QMWS). Multiple variable logistic regression was used for statistical analysis.

TABLE 4: Correlation between objective sleep indices and PSQI score.

	PSQI score		
	β	r	P
Sleep latency duration (minute)	0.003	0.04	0.59
Stable Sleep ratio (%)	−0.03	0.17	0.03
Unstable Sleep duration	1.26	0.20	0.01
Unstable Sleep ratio (%)	0.05	0.22	0.006
Awake/Dream duration	0.26	0.04	0.58
Awake/Dream ratio (%)	−0.004	0.01	0.89
AHI frequency	0.09	0.25	0.002

PSQI: pittsburgh sleep quality index; CPC: cardiopulmonary coupling analysis; AHI: Apnea-hyponea Index.

is less affected by chronic fatigue or subjective perception on this important issue. In addition, the present study revealed that nurses with educational level of high school or under had a much higher risk of sleep disturbance when compared with nurses with a college or higher degree. There were no significant associations between sleep disturbance and years of nursing experience, age, marital status, number of children, regular exercise habit, manager position, work shift, or work stress.

The present study revealed that neither subjective nor objective sleep quality was related to shift work. Although some previous studies have revealed that shift work schedule contributed one of the major causes of subjectively poor sleep quality of nurses [4, 13], the conclusions were inconsistent. The study by Sveinsdóttir failed to show such relationship using a questionnaire called "Women's Health" [14]. It has been proposed that adequate shift assignment and stress reduction can prevent pathologically disrupt circadian cycle and sleep disturbance [14], but further studies are needed to clarify this hypothesis.

Only limited number of studies has examined the relationship between sleep disturbance and educational level of nursing staff. The present study demonstrated that nurses with an educational level of high school or under had two times higher incidence of poor sleep quality when compared with nurses with an educational level of college or higher degree. These results were compatible with previous studies [15, 16], in which the authors proposed that nurses with higher educational level had a less work-related stress [15] and less emotional exhaustion [16]. But the present study failed to show the association between work stress and poor sleep quality.

Hospital staff nurses with moderate/severe sleep apnea/hypopnea did not have significantly higher incidence of poor sleep perception when compared with nurses with less AHI. To our best knowledge, no previous study investigated the incidence of sleep apnea/hypopnea among hospital staff nurses. The results of the present study were compatible with previous studies on subjects with severe obstructive sleep apnea (OSA) [17–19]. Possible explanations for failure of association between the degree of AHI and subjective sleep perception might include the factors other than OSA affect subjective sleep quality. Additionally, AHI scoring was based on the frequency of apnea/hypopnea instead of severity of OSA, but poor sleep perception was more related to the frequency of arousal caused by OSA. However, only nine nurses had an AHI > 15 in the present study. Study on a larger population is needed to get further conclusion on this issue.

Objective measurement may be affected by instruments, resulting in differences of sleep condition between test days and ordinary days. This was the reason for which this study opted to use home instruments. However, although the prevalence of the "first-night effect" caused by environmental changes may be prevented, sleep may be disturbed by electrodes being stuck to their bodies. The present study demonstrated that the ECG-based measures were likely to prevent the first-night effect because only two subjects reported that their sleep was bothered by the devices and needed a second measurement. Further studies comparing the positive and the negative predictive value of the CPC against the PSG measures may be helpful on this issue.

The present study revealed that the relationship was weak, though being significant, between PSQI score and variant objective parameters by CPC measures. The results indicate that the two measures may get different results, and that they cannot be substituted for each other. This study used PSQI questionnaires to investigate the sleep conditions of subjects over the previous month, and therefore special events or differing sleep perceptions may influence the test results. The objective measurement conducted by this study can only present the sleep conditions on the day of testing. Although the results showed decreased stable sleep ratio, increased unstable sleep duration, increased unstable ratio, and higher AHI frequency may be indicators for a poor subjective sleep quality, gaps are found in terms of objective and subjective

sleep evaluations. Nurses had higher incidence of poor PSQI than of inadequate objective sleep stability. Factors other than poor objective sleep stability may also contribute to a poor PSGI score, which can explain the discrepancy between objective and subjective measures.

Several limitations of this study need to be taken into account when making conclusions. First of all, there is no data from a nonmedical general population as a control group in the study design to compare the difference of sleep disturbance between hospital staff nurses and the general population. Secondly, survey from one hospital would limit the applicability and generalization of study findings to other hospitals with different level. Furthermore, the study did not clarify the type of work shift and did not include possible factors such as chronic fatigue or other emotional factors. It is very difficult to assess all possible factors in one single study. Further studies are needed on this issue. However, the present study did reveal that it can be very helpful when used as an objective measure as an adjuvant of self-report questionnaire to assess sleep quality in spite of the difference in the nature of the two tests.

In conclusion, the present study showed that poor subjective sleep quality and poor objective sleep stability both occur frequently among hospital nursing staff. Some objective measures that are easily applicable can be used to assist the interpretation of subjective data. Educational level of high school or lower degree is the only predictor for poor sleep quality of the nurses in the present study. This finding provides important information for hospitals in Taiwan. Poor sleep quality remains a vital health issue for hospital staff nurses, and in-service education may be helpful for reducing sleep disturbance in this population. However, further research on this subject using larger populations is needed to reach an appropriate conclusion.

Conflict of Interests

The authors declare that they have no conflict of interests.

References

[1] D. M. Gaba and S. K. Howard, "Fatigue among clinicians and the safety of patients," *The New England Journal of Medicine*, vol. 347, no. 16, pp. 1249–1255, 2002.

[2] Y. Doi, M. Minowa, M. Uchiyama, and M. Okawa, "Subjective sleep quality and sleep problems in the general Japanese adult population," *Psychiatry and Clinical Neurosciences*, vol. 55, no. 3, pp. 213–215, 2001.

[3] W. S. Wong and R. Fielding, "Prevalence of insomnia among Chinese adults in Hong Kong: a population-based study," *Journal of Sleep Research*, vol. 20, no. 1, part 1, pp. 117–126, 2011.

[4] M. F. Shao, Y. C. Chou, M. Y. Yeh, and W. C. Tzeng, "Sleep quality and quality of life in female shift-working nurses," *Journal of Advanced Nursing*, vol. 66, no. 7, pp. 1565–1572, 2010.

[5] J. Mendels and D. R. Hawkins, "Sleep laboratory adaptation in normal subjects and depressed patients ("first night effect")," *Electroencephalography and Clinical Neurophysiology*, vol. 22, no. 6, pp. 556–558, 1967.

[6] D. A. Conroy, J. Todd Arnedt, K. J. Brower et al., "Perception of sleep in recovering alcohol-dependent patients with insomnia: relationship with future drinking," *Alcoholism*, vol. 30, no. 12, pp. 1992–1999, 2006.

[7] B. Feige, A. Al-Shajlawi, C. Nissen et al., "Does REM sleep contribute to subjective wake time in primary insomnia? A comparison of polysomnographic and subjective sleep in 100 patients," *Journal of Sleep Research*, vol. 17, no. 2, pp. 180–190, 2008.

[8] C. A. Kushida, A. Chang, C. Gadkary, C. Guilleminault, O. Carrillo, and W. C. Dement, "Comparison of actigraphic, polysomnographic, and subjective assessment of sleep parameters in sleep-disordered patients," *Sleep Medicine*, vol. 2, no. 5, pp. 389–396, 2001.

[9] R. J. Thomas, J. E. Mietus, C. K. Peng, and A. L. Goldberger, "An electrocardiogram-based technique to assess cardiopulmonary coupling during sleep," *Sleep*, vol. 28, no. 9, pp. 1151–1161, 2005.

[10] L. C. See, H. J. Chang, M. J. Liu, and H. K. Cheng, "Development and evaluation of validity and reliability of a questionnaire on medical workers' stress," *Taiwan Journal of Public Health*, vol. 26, no. 6, pp. 452–461, 2007.

[11] P. S. Tsai, S. Y. Wang, M. Y. Wang et al., "Psychometric evaluation of the Chinese version of the Pittsburgh Sleep Quality Index (CPSQI) in primary insomnia and control subjects," *Quality of Life Research*, vol. 14, no. 8, pp. 1943–1952, 2005.

[12] D. J. Buysse, C. F. Reynolds, T. H. Monk, S. R. Berman, and D. J. Kupfer, "The Pittsburgh Sleep Quality Index: a new instrument for psychiatric practice and research," *Psychiatry Research*, vol. 28, no. 2, pp. 193–213, 1989.

[13] T. Rutledge, E. Stucky, A. Dollarhide et al., "A real-time assessment of work stress in physicians and nurses," *Journal of Health Psychology*, vol. 28, no. 2, pp. 194–200, 2009.

[14] H. Sveinsdóttir, "Self-assessed quality of sleep, occupational health, working environment, illness experience and job satisfaction of female nurses working different combination of shifts," *Scandinavian Journal of Caring Sciences*, vol. 20, no. 2, pp. 229–237, 2006.

[15] H. Lu, A. E. While, and K. Louise Barriball, "A model of job satisfaction of nurses: a reflection of nurses' working lives in Mainland China," *Journal of Advanced Nursing*, vol. 58, no. 5, pp. 468–479, 2007.

[16] M. K. Alimoglu and L. Donmez, "Daylight exposure and the other predictors of burnout among nurses in a University Hospital," *International Journal of Nursing Studies*, vol. 42, no. 5, pp. 549–555, 2005.

[17] E. J. Kezirian, S. L. Harrison, S. Ancoli-Israel et al., "Behavioral correlates of sleep-disordered breathing in older men," *Sleep*, vol. 32, no. 2, pp. 253–261, 2009.

[18] P. M. Macey, M. A. Woo, R. Kumar, R. L. Cross, and R. M. Harper, "Relationship between obstructive sleep apnea severity and sleep, depression and anxiety symptoms in newly-diagnosed patients," *PLoS ONE*, vol. 5, no. 4, Article ID e10211, 2010.

[19] S. Naismith, V. Winter, H. Gotsopoulos, I. Hickie, and P. Cistulli, "Neurobehavioral functioning in obstructive sleep apnea: differential effects of sleep quality, hypoxemia and subjective sleepiness," *Journal of Clinical and Experimental Neuropsychology*, vol. 26, no. 1, pp. 43–54, 2004.

12

Daytime Sleepiness in Parkinson's Disease: Perception, Influence of Drugs, and Mood Disorder

M. Ataide,[1] **C. M. R. Franco,**[2] **and O. G. Lins**[1]

[1] *Pós-Graduação em Neuropsiquiatria e Ciências do Comportamento, Universidade Federal de Pernambuco, Recife, PE, Brazil*
[2] *Hospital das Clinicas, Universidade Federal de Pernambuco, Recife, PE, Brazil*

Correspondence should be addressed to M. Ataide; marceloataideneuro@gmail.com

Academic Editor: Diego Garcia-Borreguero

Parkinson's disease (PD) is associated with sleep complaints as excessive daytime sleepiness (EDS) and several factors have been implicated in the genesis of these complaints. *Objective.* To correlate the subjective perception of EDS with variables as the severity of the motor symptoms, medications, and the presence of depressive symptoms. *Materials and Methods.* A cross-sectional study, using specific scales as Epworth sleepiness scale (ESS), Beck depression inventory (iBeck) and Hoehn and Yahr (HY), in 42 patients with PD. *Results.* The patients had a mean age of 61.2 ± 11.3 years and mean disease duration of 4.96 ± 3.3 years. The mean ESS was 7.5 ± 4.7 and 28.6% of patients reached a score of abnormally high value (>10). There was no association with gender, disease duration, and dopamine agonists. Patients with EDS used larger amounts of levodopa (366.7 ± 228.0 versus 460.4 ± 332.25 mg, $P = 0.038$), but those who had an iBeck > 20 reached lower values of ESS than the others (5.9 ± 4.1 versus 9.3 ± 4.8, $P = 0.03$). *Conclusions.* EDS was common in PD patients, being related to levodopa intake. Presence of depressed mood may influence the final results of self-assessment scales for sleep disorders.

1. Introduction

Parkinson's disease (PD) is a leading progressive neurodegenerative disease, with prevalence estimated 1-2% of the population above 55 years. Sleep-related complaints are frequent in this population and, in some cases, may be the initial manifestation of the disease. Around 60 to 90% of PD patients affected by sleep disorders suffer negative impact on their quality of life [1]. A population study, which evaluated 245 patients with Parkinson's disease, showed that more than two-thirds of them had complaints about sleep disturbances and complaints of the same type are found in 46% of diabetic patients and 33% of control patients [2].

Excessive daytime sleepiness (EDS) has an estimated prevalence from 15.5 to 74% of PD patients [1]. Clinical evidence support the hypothesis of EDS being a particular symptom of PD and its potential association with disease progression [2–4]. However, there are studies that contradict this association [5–7]. The EDS can also arise as a secondary symptom nighttime sleep deprivation or other sleep disorders such as sleep apnea (present in 20–30% of PD patients). Patients with REM sleep behavior disorders did not show greater EDS, even if REM sleep is interrupted by violent dreams [8]. Finally, the association between the dopamine replacement therapy and the EDS has been described [1]. Although there are reports that the dopamine agonists cause drowsiness as a class effect [9], in many studies, the main predictive factor is the total amount of the dose dopamine [10, 11].

Several subjective measures have been proposed to assess EDS in PD. By using the Epworth sleepiness scale (ESS) [12], patients with scores higher than 7 show a sensitivity of 75% risk of road accidents [4]. Some studies have indicated that the ESS shows a correlation with objective tests, such as the Multiple Sleep Latency Test (MSLT) [5, 10, 13], while others did not show this correlation [14, 15]. Nevertheless, the ESS is recommended, by the Movement Disorders Society, for the evaluation of EDS in patients with PD and it has been proposed that the cut-off of 10/11 is indicative of pathological sleepiness [16].

In relation to mood disorders, depression is very common in PD patients and it is a major cause of insomnia in this population [17], but its relationship with EDS is questionable.

The objective of this study is to evaluate, through a subjective measure of the level of daytime sleepiness, the characteristics and determinants of EDS in patients with PD, including the influence of depressive symptoms.

2. Materials and Methods

This is an observational study conducted in the outpatient clinic of Neurology, in the Hospital das Clinicas of Universidade Federal de Pernambuco, Brazil, from January 2011 to August 2012. All patients gave their written informed consent to participate in the study, which was approved by the ethics committee in research involving humans at the Center for Health Sciences of Universidade Federal de Pernambuco.

Forty-two patients fulfilling clinical criteria of PD (the United Kingdom Parkinson's Disease Society Brain Bank clinical diagnostic criteria) were included in the study. Cognition was evaluated by Mini-Mental State Examination (MMSE). Patients had to have an MMSE score equal to or above 24.

Patients in the study answered a questionnaire that includes disease duration and drug record. To compare different medications directly at dosages of equivalent efficacy, we converted the dosages into levodopa dosage equivalents (LDEs) [18]. The following formula was used: LDE = (regular levodopa dose × 1) + (levodopa controlled release dose × 0.75) + (pramipexole dose × 67) + (ropinirole dose × 16.67) + (pergolide dose × 100) + (bromocriptine dose × 10) + {[regular levodopa dose + (levodopa controlled release dose × 0.75)] × 0.25 if taking tolcapone}. PD symptoms were evaluated using Hoehn and Yahr modified version (HY). To assess depressive symptoms we used the Beck depression inventory (iBeck). In the subjective assessment of daytime sleepiness, we used ESS, considering cut-off from 10 points as the presence of pathological sleepiness.

The *Statistica* (data analysis software system) for Windows version 8.0 (2007) was used for all analyses. Descriptive statistics were used as required. Since most parameters did not follow a normal distribution, nonparametric tests were applied, such as the Mann-Whitney test. Spearman's rank correlation coefficients were used to determine the association between ESD and other variables, such as disease duration, motor and depression symptoms, and use of antiparkinsonian medications. Fisher's exact test was used for dichotomous variables. Significance was defined as $P < 0.05$.

3. Results

Of a total of 65 patients interviewed, seven were excluded because they did not meet the diagnostic criteria for idiopathic PD and sixteen, because they had cognitive impairment that would hinder the completion of the scales and questionnaire. Demographic and clinical characteristics are shown in Table 1. The duration of parkinsonian symptoms

TABLE 1: Descriptive statistics ($n = 42$).

Measure	Mean ± SD
Age (years)	61.2 ± 11.3
Gender (masculine/feminine)	25/17[*]
Duration of disease (years)	4.96 ± 3.3
Hoehn and Yahr modified stage	2.1 ± 0.98
Mini-Mental State Examination	26.7 ± 2.6
Epworth sleepiness scale	7.5 ± 4.7
Beck depression inventory	18.7 ± 10.7
Levodopa dosage (mg)	393.45 ± 261.4
Levodopa dosage equivalents (mg)	441.3 ± 272.5

[*]Total of patients.

was 4.96 ± 3.3 (mean ± standard deviation) years (range: 1–14). The scores of motor symptoms, according to the H&Y, were 2.1 ± 0.98 points (range: 1–4). Twelve patients were in advanced stages of PD (HY ≥ 3) and five were in stage 4. The mean Mini-Mental State Examination was 26.7 ± 2.6 points (range: 24–30). All patients were taking antiparkinsonian drugs: levodopa ($n = 37$), pramipexole ($n = 23$), amantadine ($n = 8$), and biperiden ($n = 7$). The mean levodopa equivalent dose (LED) was 441.3 ± 272.5 mg. Ten patients (24%) were taking benzodiazepines and/or antidepressants. Regarding depressive symptoms, the average score was 18.7 ± 10.7 points (range = 0–42) and 22 (52.4%) patients had moderate to severe depressive symptoms.

The mean ESS was 7.5 ± 4.7 points (range = 0–19), with a median of 7 points. Twelve (28.6%) patients had excessive daytime sleepiness (ESS score > 10 points). There were not significant differences in age, gender, disease duration, motor symptoms, and levodopa equivalent dose between patients with and without EDS. The patients with EDS showed use of higher doses of levodopa than the patients without EDS (460.4 ± 332.25 versus 366.7 ± 228.0 mg, $P = 0.038$). However, when evaluating patients using levodopa alone and levodopa with pramipexole, there was not increase in sleepiness with the addition of dopamine agonist (Fisher's exact test, $P = 0.50$). To the remaining variables, we did not observe any association with pathological sleepiness, including the use of benzodiazepines and antidepressants, where increased drowsiness with use of these medications was not observed (Fisher's exact test, $P = 0.20$) (Table 2).

There was a trend for lower depressive symptoms scores, through iBeck, in patients with EDS than those without (13.8 ± 9 versus 20.6 ± 10.9, $P = 0.056$), showing a weak association between these two variables ($r_s = -0.32$). Twenty-two patients had scores iBeck > 20. These patients with more depressive symptoms had lower levels of ESE compared to patients with iBeck scores ≤ 20 (5.9 ± 4.1 versus 9.3 ± 4.8, $P = 0.03$) (Figure 1).

4. Discussion

The data demographic of this study is presented in accordance with those found in world literature. Thus, although the males have predominated in the screening evaluation, the females

TABLE 2: Comparison of variables scores according to excessive daytime sleepiness.

	Epworth < 10 ($n = 30$) Mean ± SD	Epworth ≥ 10 ($n = 12$) Mean ± SD	P (value)
Age (years)	61.5 ± 11.8	60.5 ± 10.4	0.327
Gender (male/female)	11/19[*]	9/3[*]	0.594
Duration of disease (years)	5.05 ± 3.1	4.75 ± 3.9	0.157
Hoehn and Yahr modified version	2.1 ± 1.0	2.1 ± 1.0	0.428
Mini-Mental State Examination	26.6 ± 2.8	27.1 ± 2.2	0.089
Beck depression inventory	20.6 ± 10.9	13.8 ± 9.1	0.056
Levodopa dosage (mg)	366.7 ± 228.0	460.4 ± 332.25	0.038
Levodopa dosage equivalents (mg)	410.8 ± 235.1	517.6 ± 348.2	0.46

[*]Total of patients.

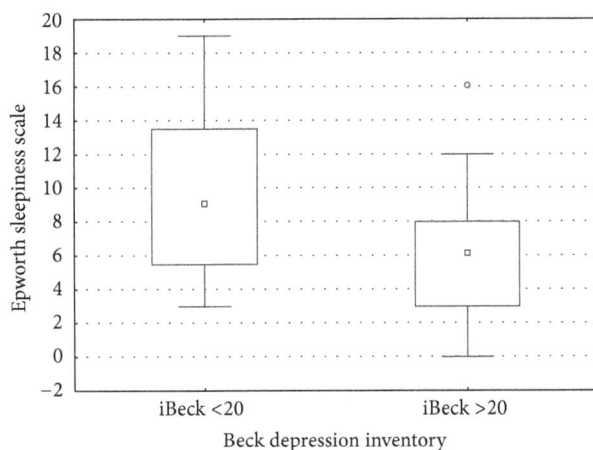

FIGURE 1: Association of daytime sleepiness, by the Epworth sleepiness scale, and depressive symptoms, as the Beck depression inventory.

have prevailed in the interviews, a fact possibly related to increased attendance and interest in participating in this gender.

Excessive daytime sleepiness occurred in 28.2% of patients with a mean score of ESS similar to those found in other studies, within an interval ranging from 4.9 ± 3.6 [19] to 11.1 ± 5.9 [20]. Margis et al., in a study in the Brazilian population, found a mean score of 7.74 ± 4.82 [21]. However, some considerations must be made when using the ESS. To be a self-assessment scale, the interpretation of the items is linked with the sociocultural and linguistic characteristics of each population, so that the comparison between studies is valid, but the comparison within the same population may be more realistic. Santamaria already commented on the ambiguity of some items of ESS [22]. Study objectives, such as the MSLT, can provide more concrete and less risk of bias on this aspect.

In this study, EDS was associated with the total amount of levodopa. One of the first studies that evaluated the chronic use of levodopa showed that daytime sleepiness was disabling adverse effects in 13.7% of patients [23] and that the patients became sleepy more after one year of drug treatment [24]. Kaynak et al., who used the MSLT for evaluation of EDS, have

shown that daytime sleepiness was not present in untreated patients but appeared later during dopaminergic treatment and that high dose of levodopa was a strong predictor of EDS [25].

However, in our study it was not observed significant association between EDS and the dopamine agonist utilized (pramipexole) or between EDS and the levodopa equivalent dose. The Cochrane database collects somnolence as a side-effect in placebo-controlled trials of the antiparkinsonian effect of various dopamine agonists, where the somnolence occurred in 21% of patients in the pramipexole group compared with 10% in the placebo group. Other dopaminergic agonists also showed the SED as a side-effect: somnolence occurred in 13% of patients in the pergolide group compared with 4% in the placebo group and in 28% patients in the ropinirole group compared with 6% in the placebo group [26]. However, there are studies that question this symptom, not finding this association of sleepiness with specific drug class [4, 10, 11]. Razmy et al. showed that the mean ESS score did not differ as a function of treatment group, like mean MSLT [11]. The contradiction of these claims justifies the multifactorial nature of EDS. Although an association between the severity of the parkinsonian motor symptoms and pathological somnolence has not been demonstrated, the patients in advanced stages of disease (in clinical status where there is greater structural impairment of the mechanisms responsible for controlling the sleep-wake cycle, involving dopaminergic, noradrenergic, cholinergic, serotonergic, histaminergic, and hypocretinergic neurons) used higher doses and associations of antiparkinsonian medications and they are subject to more adverse effects. Thus, the attempt to define the impact of antiparkinsonian medication isolated on EDS becomes a task more abstract than real.

Moreover, the perception of the nap may be altered in these patients. In an interesting study, Razmy et al. observed patients using high doses of dopaminergic medications, that theoretically had a higher risk for the development of EDS, did not report accurately the presence or absence of daytime sleepiness [11]. The anosognosia of daytime nap is common in patients with PD and in those with disorders of EDS, and it seems to be more severe in patients with PD [27]. These data suggest a more careful evaluation of the ESS scores in this subgroup of patients.

We also observed a considerable amount of patients who met criteria for depression where more than half of the patients have major depressive symptoms. The results are well above the data presented by Brazilian researchers, as Silberman et al., who found a prevalence of depression of 39.1% [28], but within the wide variations in prevalence when using self-assessment questionnaires (27.3 to 76%) [29]. Furthermore, there was a negative correlation between the intensity of depressive symptoms and the presence of excessive sleepiness, where patients with more depressive symptoms were less sleepy. PD patients who may have depressive symptoms that differ from the general population showed significantly less anhedonia but more concentration problems than depressed control subjects [30]. Thus, as the perception of sleep disorders, including excessive daytime sleepiness, may be impaired in depressed PD patients, we should be more careful in evaluating sleep disorders in clinical situations involving high levels of depression. The use of scales for the identification and ranking of depressive symptoms seems to be very valuable in the clinical evaluation of the presence of sleep-related symptoms.

Some limitations were observed in the study. The first is the small number of patients interviewed, which can lead to a restricted analysis of variables related to sleep. The second is the predominance of patients with mild to moderate motor symptoms, with small numbers of patients most severely affected, which may not be representative of the whole. Third, by socioeconomic conditions, objective measures to quantify sleep parameters via polysomnographic have not been carried out. It has been admitted that nocturnal sleep deprivation may contribute to EDS and sleep disorders such as sleep fragmentation, periodic limb movements during sleep and obstructive sleep apnea may contribute to daytime sleepiness in PD. And finally, a specific scale for assessing insomnia was not use. This could be an aid in determining whether the inverse association between excessive daytime sleepiness and depressive symptoms is attributed to greater impact of insomnia in depression or whether there is more misperception of sleep disturbance in more depressed patients. Further studies, using objective measurements of EDS such MSLT, may shed light into this issue.

5. Conclusions

Despite these limitations, we conclude that the excessive daytime sleepiness is a common symptom in patients with PD, being more closely associated with the amount of ingested levodopa, and that the presence of depressive symptoms may have a significant impact on the results of self-assessment scales. Therefore, we recommend the assessment of mood changes and the more careful analysis of the results obtained in this specific population of patients with Parkinson's disease.

Conflict of Interests

The authors declare that there is no conflict of interests regarding the publication of this paper.

References

[1] A. Iranzo, "Parkinson's disease and sleepiness," *Sleep Medicine Clinics*, vol. 1, no. 1, pp. 127–137, 2006.

[2] E. Tandberg, J. P. Larsen, and K. Karlsen, "A community-based study of sleep disorders in patients with Parkinson's disease," *Movement Disorders*, vol. 13, no. 6, pp. 895–899, 1998.

[3] M. D. Gjerstad, D. Aarsland, and J. P. Larsen, "Development of daytime somnolence over time in Parkinson's disease," *Neurology*, vol. 58, no. 10, pp. 1544–1546, 2002.

[4] D. E. Hobson, A. E. Lang, W. R. Wayne Martin, A. Razmy, J. Rivest, and J. Fleming, "Excessive daytime sleepiness and sudden-onset sleep in Parkinson disease: a survey by the Canadian Movement Disorders Group," *Journal of the American Medical Association*, vol. 287, no. 4, pp. 455–463, 2002.

[5] I. Arnulf, E. Konofal, M. Merino-Andreu et al., "Parkinson's disease and sleepiness: an integral part of PD," *Neurology*, vol. 58, no. 7, pp. 1019–1024, 2002.

[6] M. A. Brodsky, J. Godbold, T. Roth, and C. W. Olanow, "Sleepiness in Parkinson's disease: a controlled study," *Movement Disorders*, vol. 18, no. 6, pp. 668–672, 2003.

[7] P. Braga-Neto, F. Pereira Da Silva-Júnior, F. Sueli Monte, P. F. C. de Bruin, and V. M. S. de Bruin, "Snoring and excessive daytime sleepiness in Parkinson's disease," *Journal of the Neurological Sciences*, vol. 217, no. 1, pp. 41–45, 2004.

[8] V. C. De Cock, M. Vidailhet, S. Leu et al., "Restoration of normal motor control in Parkinson's disease during REM sleep," *Brain*, vol. 130, no. 2, pp. 450–456, 2007.

[9] I. Schlesinger and P. D. Ravin, "Dopamine agonists induce episodes of irresistible daytime sleepiness," *European Neurology*, vol. 49, no. 1, pp. 30–33, 2003.

[10] S. Stevens, C. L. Comella, and E. J. Stepanski, "Daytime sleepiness and alertness in patients with Parkinson disease," *Sleep*, vol. 27, no. 5, pp. 967–972, 2004.

[11] A. Razmy, A. E. Lang, and C. M. Shapiro, "Predictors of impaired daytime sleep and wakefulness in patients with Parkinson disease treated with older (Ergot) vs newer (Nonergot) dopamine agonists," *Archives of Neurology*, vol. 61, no. 1, pp. 97–102, 2004.

[12] M. W. Johns, "A new method for measuring daytime sleepiness: the Epworth sleepiness scale," *Sleep*, vol. 14, no. 6, pp. 540–545, 1991.

[13] R. Poryazova, D. Benninger, D. Waldvogel, and C. L. Bassetti, "Excessive daytime sleepiness in parkinson's disease: characteristics and determinants," *European Neurology*, vol. 63, no. 3, pp. 129–135, 2010.

[14] I. Shpirer, A. Miniovitz, C. Klein et al., "Excessive daytime sleepiness in patients with parkinson's disease: a polysomnography study," *Movement Disorders*, vol. 21, no. 9, pp. 1432–1438, 2006.

[15] J. Bušková, J. Klempíř, V. Majerová et al., "Sleep disturbances in untreated Parkinson's disease," *Journal of Neurology*, vol. 258, no. 12, pp. 2254–2259, 2011.

[16] B. Högl, I. Arnulf, C. Comella et al., "Scales to assess sleep impairment in Parkinson's disease: critique and recommendations," *Movement Disorders*, vol. 25, no. 16, pp. 2704–2716, 2010.

[17] M. Menza, R. D. Dobkin, H. Marin, and K. Bienfait, "Sleep disturbances in Parkinson's disease," *Movement Disorders*, vol. 25, supplement 1, pp. S117–S122, 2010.

[18] D. E. Hobson, A. E. Lang, W. R. Wayne Martin, A. Razmy, J. Rivest, and J. Fleming, "Excessive daytime sleepiness and

sudden-onset sleep in Parkinson disease: a survey by the Canadian Movement Disorders Group," *Journal of the American Medical Association*, vol. 287, no. 4, pp. 455–463, 2002.

[19] S. Kumar, M. Bhatia, and M. Behari, "Excessive daytime sleepiness in Parkinson's disease as assessed by Epworth Sleepiness Scale (ESS)," *Sleep Medicine*, vol. 4, no. 4, pp. 339–342, 2003.

[20] W. G. Ondo, K. D. Vuong, H. Khan, F. Atassi, C. Kwak, and J. Jankovic, "Daytime sleepiness and other sleep disorders in Parkinson's disease," *Neurology*, vol. 57, no. 8, pp. 1392–1396, 2001.

[21] R. Margis, K. Donis, S. V. Schinwald et al., "Psychometric properties of the Parkinson's Disease Scale—Brazilian version," *Parkinsonism & Related Disorders*, vol. 15, pp. 495–499, 2008.

[22] J. Santamaria, "How to evaluate excessive daytime sleepiness in Parkinson's disease," *Neurology*, vol. 63, no. 8, supplement 3, pp. S21–S23, 2004.

[23] R. P. Lesser, S. Fahn, and S. R. Snider, "Analysis of the clinical problems in parkinsonism and the complications of long-term levodopa therapy," *Neurology*, vol. 29, no. 9, pp. 1253–1260, 1979.

[24] G. Fabbrini, P. Barbanti, C. Aurilia, C. Pauletti, N. Vanacore, and G. Meco, "Excessive daytime somnolence in Parkinson's disease. Follow-up after 1 year of treatment," *Neurological Sciences*, vol. 24, no. 3, pp. 178–179, 2003.

[25] D. Kaynak, G. Kiziltan, H. Kaynak, G. Benbir, and O. Uysal, "Sleep and sleepiness in patients with Parkinson's disease before and after dopaminergic treatment," *European Journal of Neurology*, vol. 12, no. 3, pp. 199–207, 2005.

[26] R. G. Holloway, I. Shoulson, S. Fahn et al., "Pramipexole vs levodopa as initial treatment for Parkinson Disease: a 4-year randomized controlled trial," *Archives of Neurology*, vol. 61, no. 7, pp. 1044–1053, 2004.

[27] M. Merino-Andreu, I. Arnulf, E. Konofal, J. P. Derenne, and Y. Agid, "Unawareness of naps in Parkinson's disease and in disorders with excessive daytime sleepiness," *Neurology*, vol. 60, no. 9, pp. 1553–1554, 2003.

[28] C. D. Silberman, J. Laks, C. F. Capitão, C. S. Rodrigues, I. Moreira, and E. Engelhardt, "Recognizing depression in patients with Parkinson's Disease," *Arquives of Neuropsiquiatry*, vol. 64, no. 2, pp. 407–411, 2006.

[29] J. S. A. M. Reijnders, U. Ehrt, W. E. J. Weber, D. Aarsland, and A. F. G. Leentjens, "A systematic review of prevalence studies of depression in Parkinson's disease," *Movement Disorders*, vol. 23, no. 2, pp. 183–189, 2007.

[30] U. Ehrt, K. Brønnick, A. F. G. Leentjens, J. P. Larsen, and D. Aarsland, "Depressive symptom profile in Parkinson's disease: a comparison with depression in elderly patients without Parkinson's disease," *International Journal of Geriatric Psychiatry*, vol. 21, no. 3, pp. 252–258, 2006.

13

The Epidemiology of Sleep Quality and Consumption of Stimulant Beverages among Patagonian Chilean College Students

Juan Carlos Vélez,[1] **Aline Souza,**[2] **Samantha Traslaviña,**[2] **Clarita Barbosa,**[1]
Adaeze Wosu,[2] **Asterio Andrade,**[1] **Megan Frye,**[1] **Annette L. Fitzpatrick,**[3]
Bizu Gelaye,[2] **and Michelle A. Williams**[2]

[1] *Centro de Rehabilitación Club de Leones Cruz del Sur, Punta Arenas, Suiza 01441, Chile*
[2] *Department of Epidemiology, Multidisciplinary International Research Training Program, Harvard University School of Public Health,*
  Boston, MA 02131, USA
[3] *Departments of Epidemiology and Global Health, University of Washington, Seattle, WA 98195, USA*

Correspondence should be addressed to
Bizu Gelaye; bgelaye@hsph.harvard.edu

Academic Editor: Diego Garcia-Borreguero

Objectives. (1) To assess sleep patterns and parameters of sleep quality among Chilean college students and (2) to evaluate the extent to which stimulant beverage use and other lifestyle characteristics are associated with poor sleep quality. *Methods.* A cross-sectional study was conducted among college students in Patagonia, Chile. Students were asked to complete a self-administered questionnaire to provide information about lifestyle and demographic characteristics. The Pittsburgh Sleep Quality Index (PSQI) was used to evaluate sleep quality. In addition, students underwent a physical examination to collect anthropometric measurements. *Results.* More than half of students (51.8%) exhibited poor sleep quality. Approximately 45% of study participants reported sleeping six hours or less per night and 9.8% used medications for sleep. In multivariate analysis, current smokers had significantly greater daytime dysfunction due to sleepiness and were more likely to use sleep medicines. Students who reported consumption of any stimulant beverage were 1.81 times as likely to have poor sleep quality compared with those who did not consume stimulant beverages (OR:1.81, 95% CI:1.21–2.00). *Conclusions.* Poor sleep quality is prevalent among Chilean college students, and stimulant beverage consumption was associated with the increased odds of poor sleep quality in this sample.

1. Introduction

Insufficient sleep is a major public health concern and a common medical condition with serious adverse consequences. The recommended durations of sleep are 8.5–9.5 hours for adolescents (10–17 years old) and 7–9 hours for persons ≥18 years of age [1]. Yet many college students do not reach these recommendations and many sleep <6 hours per night. Insufficient sleep has been implicated to affect endocrine, immune, and nervous systems and cardiometabolic risk including obesity, diabetes, impaired glucose tolerance, and hypertension [2]. Additionally, insufficient sleep has been

reported as an important factor influencing the regulation of body weight and metabolism [3]. Sufficient sleep enhances memory and has been associated with good academic performance [4, 5]. Sufficient sleep has also been associated with self-rated happiness as was observed in a cross-sectional study of 3,461 Chilean college students [6].

Short sleep duration has been associated with poor academic performance, use of cigarettes, marijuana, and alcohol, mood disorders, physical inactivity, and excessive use of internet [7, 8]. Additionally, investigators have noted that short sleep may contribute to frequent use of medications and alcohol as sleep aids and stimulants use to increase daytime alertness [9]. Consumption of stimulants (e.g., coffee, caffeine shots, and energy drinks) has increased in recent years. Studies have shown that stimulant use among healthy adolescents may be associated with feelings of jitteriness and nervousness, difficulty in sleeping, loss of appetite, and stomach discomfort [10]. Higher doses of energy drink consumption have been implicated in liver damage, chest discomfort, heart rhythm irregularities, increased blood pressure, electrolyte disturbance, kidney failure, heart failure, and death [11, 12]. However, few studies have examined the relationship between energy drink consumption and sleep quality [13, 14].

Since their introduction in 2001, energy drinks have steadily grown in popularity in Chile. Reports indicate that Latin America was the region of the world where energy drinks consumption grew the most, with 31% between 2004 and 2010, while globally the increase was 14.1%. In the same period, energy drinks consumption in Chile increased by 26.7% [15]. These drinks, typically high in caffeine and sugar content, may be particularly appealing to youth and young adults due to marketing efforts. Many energy drink producers advertise their products as performance enhancements for athletics, school, and social situations.

In this cross-sectional study, we assessed sleep patterns and sleep quality among Patagonian, Chilean college students. We also evaluated the extent to which stimulant beverage use and other lifestyle characteristics are associated with poor sleep quality in this population.

2. Methods

2.1. Study Setting and Sample. This cross-sectional study was conducted at four universities in the Magallanes region of Chile (Patagonia): Universidad de Magallanes, Universidad Tecnologica de Chile (INACAP), Universidad del Mar, and Universidad Santo Tomas between December 2010 and June 2011. Universidad de Magallanes is a research and training university and has more than 160 faculty members and over 4,000 students enrolled in engineering, humanities, social sciences, and health fields. The INACAP is the largest educational community in Chile with 25 campuses from Arica to Punta Arenas, Chile. The Punta Arenas campus has more than 2,000 pre- and postgraduate students. Universidad del Mar is a private institution with about 14,000 students and 15 campuses in 8 regions of Chile. Universidad Santo Tomas is private and has over 18,000 students.

Flyers were posted in each department to invite participants. Students who expressed an interest in participating in the study were invited to meet in a large classroom or an auditorium where they were informed about the purpose of the study and were invited to participate in the survey. Students consenting to participate were asked to complete self-administered individual surveys. There was no time limit for completing the survey. Vision impaired students and those who could not read the consent and questionnaire forms were not eligible to participate. Those enrolled in correspondence, extension, or night school programs were not included as well since their experience might be different from regular time students.

A total of 994 undergraduate students participated in the study. For the present analysis, we excluded subjects over the age of 35 and subjects with incomplete information on sleep quality ($n = 162$). The final analyzed sample included 832 students (241 males and 590 females). All completed questionnaires were anonymous, and no personal identifiers were collected. Given the minimum risk of the study and use of anonymous questionnaire, waiver of documentation of written consent form was approved by the ethics committees. The procedures used in this study were approved by the institutional review boards of Centro de Rehabilitación Club de Leones Cruz del Sur, Punta Arenas, Chile, and the University of Washington, USA. The Harvard School of Public Health Office of Human Research Administration, USA, granted approval to use the anonymised data set for analysis.

2.2. Data Collection and Variable Specification. A self-administered questionnaire was used to collect information for this study. The questionnaire ascertained demographic information including age, sex, and education level. Questions were also included regarding behavioral risk factors such as smoking, energy drinks, caffeinated beverages, and alcohol consumption.

Participants were first asked if they consumed more than one energy drinks or caffeinated beverages per week each month during the current academic semester/quarter. Participants who answered "yes" were then asked to identify the specific type of energy or caffeinated drinks. Energy drinks included international and local brands such as Red Bull, Dark Dog, Burn, Shark, Red Devil, and Battery. Caffeinated beverages included coffee, tea, yerba mate, and cola drinks such as Coca Cola and Pepsi Cola. We summed the number of different stimulant drinks to estimate the variety of different energy drinks or stimulants consumed per week. We use the term stimulant drinks to describe both energy drinks as well as other caffeinated beverages consumed per week.

Sleep quality was evaluated using the Pittsburgh Sleep Quality Index (PSQI) [16]. The PSQI is a 19-item self-reported questionnaire that evaluates sleep quality over the past month. The PSQI yields seven sleep components related to sleep habits including duration of sleep, sleep disturbance, sleep latency, estimates of habitual sleep efficiency, use of sleep medicine, daytime dysfunction due to sleepiness, and overall sleep quality. Each sleep component yielded a score ranging from 0 to 3, with three indicating the greatest dysfunction [16]. Subsequently, the sleep component scores are summed to yield a global sleep quality score (range 0 to 21) with higher scores indicating poor sleep quality during the previous month. Based on the prior literature, participants with a global score of greater than 5 were classified as poor sleepers. Those with a score of 5 or less were classified as good sleepers. This classification is consistent with prior studies of college students [17].

In accordance with PSQI for sleep quality subscales, subjective sleep efficiency, sleep latency, sleep medication use, and daytime dysfunction due to sleepiness, we computed a dichotomous variable of optimal and suboptimal sleep quality. Specific categories were long sleep latency ($\geq$30 versus

<30 minutes); estimates of poor sleep efficiency (<85% versus ≥85%); daytime dysfunction due to sleepiness (≥ once per week versus <once a week); and sleep medication use during the past month (≥once per week versus <once a week). Sleep duration was assessed using the PSQI questionnaire which queried how many hours per night the participants slept during the previous month. Given the lack of prior data on cutoffs for defining "short sleep duration" among college students, we used quartiles. The following quartiles were used to define sleep duration: ≤6.0 hours, 6.1–7.0 hours, ≥7.1–8.0 hours, and >8.0 hours. The group with the lowest quartile of sleep duration (≤6 hours) was defined as having short sleep duration.

We defined alcohol consumption as low (0–4 alcoholic beverages a month), moderate (5–15 alcoholic beverages a month), and high to excessive consumption (≥16 alcoholic beverages a month). Other variables were categorized as follows: age (years), sex, smoking history (never, former, current), and engaging in moderate or vigorous physical activity (no versus yes). Body mass index (BMI) was calculated as weight (kg)/height squared (m^2). Thresholds of BMI were set according to the World Health Organization (WHO) protocol (underweight: <18.5 kg/m^2; normal: 18.5–24.9 kg/m^2; overweight: 25.0–29.9 kg/m^2; and obese ≥30 kg/m^2) [18].

2.3. Statistical Analysis. We examined frequency distributions of sociodemographic and behavioral characteristics of study participants by quality of sleep. Characteristics were summarized using means (±standard deviation) for continuous variables and counts and percentages for categorical variables. Chi-square test and Student's t-test were used to determine bivariate differences for categorical and continuous variables, respectively. The distributions of PSQI scores among male and female students, as well as the sex-specific prevalence of poor sleep quality across age groups, were also estimated. Multivariable logistic regression estimated the odds ratios (OR) and 95% confidence intervals (95% CI) for the associations between poor sleep quality and sociodemographic and behavioral factors in unadjusted and adjusted models. Forward logistic regression modeling procedures combined with the change-in-estimate approach were used to select the final models reported in this research [19]. Prevalence estimates and risk of suboptimal dichotomous sleep quality subscales were also evaluated in relation to stimulant drinks and lifestyle characteristics adjusted for age and gender. All analyses were performed using IBM's SPSS Statistical Software for Windows (IBM SPSS Version 19, Chicago, Illinois, USA). All reported P values are two-sided and deemed statistically significant at $\alpha = 0.05$.

3. Results

Characteristics of the 832 study participants included in the analysis are summarized in Table 1. Approximately 71% of participants were females and the overall mean age was 21.9 ± 3.4 years. Overall, 44.2% of the study population reported being current smokers, 22.5% reported consuming ≥16 alcoholic beverages per month, and 52.0% reported

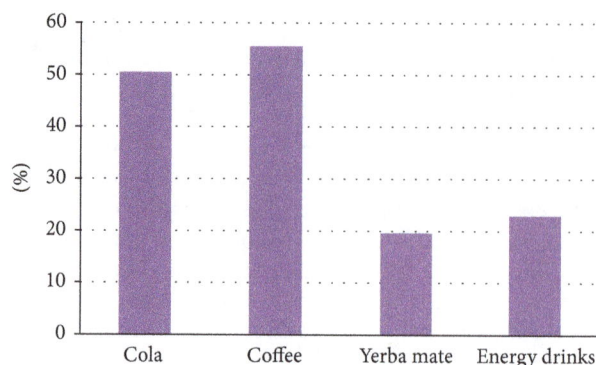

FIGURE 1: Frequency of stimulant beverages consumed.

weekly consumption of caffeinated or stimulant beverages. Obesity (14.9%) and physical inactivity (33.5%) were also common in this study population. More than half of the study population (51.8%) was classified as having poor sleep quality. The prevalence of poor sleep quality was higher in females than males for all age groups. Additionally, students with poor sleep quality were more likely to be weekly consumers of stimulant beverages (59.9% versus 49.7%, P value = 0.004). The most common types of stimulant beverages consumed were colas and coffee (Figure 1). Approximately 55% of students reported coffee drinking while 50% of them consuming caffeinated cola products (Pepsi/Coke).

Table 2 summarizes the distribution of PSQI sleep components subscales for the entire study population and for male and female students, respectively. More females (54.4%) than males (45.6%) were found to have poor sleep quality (P value = 0.022). Overall, 45.1% of the study cohort reported sleeping ≤6 hours per day. Approximately 41.4% of the cohort reported longer sleep latency (≥31 minutes), and 22.3% reported having daytime dysfunction due to sleep loss at least once per week. A total of 30.4% were classified as having poor sleep efficiency (<85%), and 3.8% reported using sleep medicine at least once per week. Sleep latency was the only sleep quality component that differed by sex, with 81.2% of females versus 71.0% of males (P value = 0.007) requiring more than 15 minutes in bed before falling asleep (Figure 2).

We evaluated the odds of poor sleep quality according to participants' demographic and behavioral characteristics. Female students were almost 50% more likely to have poor sleep quality compared with males, after adjusting for all demographic and behavioral covariates listed in Table 3 (OR = 1.48; 95% CI 0.97–2.25), though this association did not reach statistical significance. Adjusting for age and sex, consumers of any stimulant beverages were found to have higher odds of poor sleep quality (OR = 1.52; 95% CI 1.14–2.02) compared with nonconsumers. Further adjustments for cigarette smoking, alcohol consumption, and physical activity strengthened the association. In this larger multivariable model we found that consumers of any stimulant beverage were 80% more likely to have reported poor sleep quality than their counterparts who were nonconsumers (OR = 1.81; 95% CI 1.21–2.73). Physical activity, smoking, and alcohol

TABLE 1: Characteristics of the study population.

Characteristics	All $N = 832$ n (%)	Good sleep quality $N = 401$ n (%)	Poor sleep quality $N = 431$ n (%)	P value
Age (mean ± SD, years)	21.9 ± 3.4	21.6 ± 3.2	22.2 ± 3.5	0.231
Age (years)				
18	91 (10.9)	48 (12.0)	43 (10.0)	0.373
19	132 (15.9)	64 (16.0)	68 (15.8)	
20	121 (14.5)	63 (15.8)	58 (13.5)	
21	99 (11.9)	52 (13.0)	47 (10.9)	
≥22	388 (46.6)	173 (43.2)	215 (49.9)	
Sex				
Male	241 (29.0)	131 (32.8)	110 (25.5)	0.022
Female	590 (71.0)	269 (67.2)	321 (74.5)	
Cigarette smoking status				
Never	325 (39.1)	172 (45.6)	153 (38.9)	0.159
Former	77 (9.3)	37 (9.8)	40 (10.2)	
Current	368 (44.2)	168 (44.6)	200 (50.9)	
Alcohol consumption				
Low (0–4 drinks/month)	167 (20.1)	78 (32.5)	89 (32.7)	0.966
Moderate (5–15 drinks/month)	158 (19.0)	73 (30.4)	85 (31.2)	
High (≥16 drinks)	187 (22.5)	89 (37.1)	98 (36.0)	
Weekly consumption of stimulants				
No	356 (42.8)	196 (50.3)	160 (40.1)	
Yes	433 (52.0)	194 (49.7)	239 (59.9)	0.004
Body mass index (kg/m^2)				
Underweight (<18.5)	10 (1.2)	3 (0.8)	7 (1.7)	
Normal (18.5–24.9)	444 (53.4)	225 (57.8)	219 (52.6)	0.300
Overweight (25.0–29.9)	227 (28.2)	101 (26.0)	126 (30.3)	
Obese (≥30.0)	124 (14.9)	60 (15.4)	64 (15.4)	
Any physical activity				
No	279 (33.5)	140 (38.3)	139 (37.5)	0.826
Yes	458 (55.0)	226 (61.7)	232 (62.5)	

*Due to missing data, percentages may not add up to 100%; physical activity includes moderate and vigorous physical activity.

consumption were not associated with sleep quality in this sample.

We next explored the relationships of specific types of stimulant beverages with poor sleep quality. As shown in Figure 3, the prevalence of poor sleep quality was highest among participants who reported consuming energy drinks (including Red Bull, Dark Dog, Battery, Red Devil, Shark, and Turbo Energy) (P value = 0.002). Prevalence estimates were lower for participants who consumed coffee, yerba mate, and cola. The prevalence of poor sleep quality was higher among participants who reported consuming three or more stimulant beverages per week (57.9% versus 42.1%, P value = 0.073) although this association did not reach statistical significance (data not shown).

The distribution of stated reasons for consuming energy drinks is summarized in Figure 4. Of the stated reasons for consuming energy drinks, approximately 18.5% of participants reported using energy drinks as a consequence of sleep deprivation, and an additional 27.3% cited energy drink consumption to offset a general need for energy and 29.5% in order to study. Approximately 11.3% of participants reported combining energy drinks with alcohol consumption at parties.

Table 4 summarizes the distribution of stimulant and caffeine use in relation to sleep quality. There was a statistically significant association between poor sleep quality and the consumption of any stimulant beverages (P value < 0.001); those who reported using Red Bull, coffee, and/or tea were more likely to be classified as having poor sleep quality. There was no significant difference in sleep quality between those who consumed coffee/tea with sugar and without sugar.

We next examined the prevalence of specific sleep quality components in relation to demographic and lifestyle characteristics (Table 5). Compared with those who reported never smoking, former and current smokers were more likely to report daytime dysfunction due to sleep loss (OR = 1.72; 95% CI 1.17–2.53) and more likely to use sleep medicines (OR = 2.55; 95% CI 1.40–4.63). Compared with those who

TABLE 2: PSQI sleep quality patterns by sex.

Characteristics	All N = 832	Male N = 241	Female N = 590	P value
Sleep duration (hours)				
≤6.0	375 (45.1)	114 (47.3)	261 (44.2)	0.584
6.1–7.0	167 (20.1)	51 (21.2)	116 (19.7)	
7.1–8.0	161 (19.4)	40 (16.6)	121 (20.5)	
≥8.1	129 (15.5)	36 (14.9)	92 (15.6)	
Sleep latency (minutes)				
≤15	181 (21.8)	70 (29.0)	111 (18.8)	0.007
16–30	306 (36.8)	78 (32.4)	228 (38.6)	
31–60	220 (26.4)	64 (26.6)	155 (26.3)	
≥60	125 (15.0)	29 (12.0)	96 (16.3)	
Daytime dysfunction due to sleep loss				
Never	197 (23.7)	66 (27.4)	130 (22.0)	0.066
<once a week	450 (54.1)	135 (56.0)	315 (53.4)	
1-2 times per week	156 (18.8)	34 (14.1)	122 (20.7)	
≥3 times per week	29 (3.5)	6 (2.5)	23 (3.9)	
Sleep efficiency (%)				
≥85	579 (69.6)	176 (73.0)	402 (68.1)	0.431
75–84	127 (15.3)	31 (12.9)	96 (16.3)	
65–74	63 (7.6)	19 (7.9)	44 (7.5)	
<65	63 (7.6)	15 (6.2)	48 (8.1)	
Sleep medicine use				
Not during the past month	758 (91.2)	222 (92.1)	536 (90.8)	0.262
<once a week	41 (4.9)	12 (5.0)	29 (4.9)	
1-2 times per week	17 (2.0)	6 (2.5)	11 (1.9)	
≥3 times per week	15 (1.8)	1 (0.4)	14 (2.4)	
Sleep quality (a priori groupings)				
Good	401 (48.2)	131 (54.4)	269 (45.6)	0.022
Poor	431 (51.8)	110 (45.6)	321 (54.4)	

TABLE 3: Odds ratio (OR) and 95% confidence intervals (CI) for poor sleep quality.

Characteristic	Unadjusted OR (95% CI)	Age and sex adjusted OR (95% CI)	Multivariate *adjusted OR (95% CI)
Sex			
Male	1.00 (Reference)	1.00 (Reference)	1.00 (Reference)
Female	1.42 (1.05–1.92)	1.39 (1.03–1.89)	1.48 (0.97–2.25)
Smoking status			
Never	1.00 (Reference)	1.00 (Reference)	1.00 (Reference)
Former	1.22 (0.74–2.0)	1.24 (0.75–2.05)	1.08 (0.55–2.13)
Current Smoker	1.34 (0.99–1.81)	1.26 (0.93–1.71)	0.93 (0.61–1.43)
Alcohol consumption			
Low (0–4 drinks/m)	1.00 (Reference)	1.00 (Reference)	1.00 (Reference)
Moderate (5–15 drinks/m)	1.02 (0.66–1.58)	1.07 (0.68–1.66)	1.15 (0.71–1.87)
High (≥16 drinks/m)	0.97 (0.64–1.47)	1.06 (0.69–1.63)	0.99 (0.61–1.60)
Stimulant beverage consumption			
No	1.00 (Reference)	1.00 (Reference)	1.00 (Reference)
Yes	1.51 (1.14–2.00)	1.52 (1.14–2.02)	1.81 (1.21–2.73)
Physical activity			
No	1.00 (Reference)	1.00 (Reference)	1.00 (Reference)
Yes	1.03 (0.77–1.39)	1.08 (0.80–1.47)	0.96 (0.64–1.43)

*Multivariate includes age and all other covariates listed in the table. For alcohol, the total number of drinks per month was used and the total number of stimulant drinks was also used.

TABLE 4: Consumption of energy drinks, caffeinated beverages and stimulants in relation to sleep quality status.

Exposure	Good sleep quality (N = 401) n (%)	Poor sleep quality (N = 431) n (%)	P value
Any stimulant beverages			
No	200 (50.4)	171 (41.2)	<0.01
Yes	197 (49.6)	244 (58.8)	
Type of beverage			
Coke/Pepsi with sugar	178 (44.4)	193 (44.8)	0.910
Coke/Pepsi sugar-free	17 (4.2)	32 (7.4)	0.051
Red Bull	65 (16.2)	108 (25.1)	<0.01
Dark Dog	31 (7.7)	53 (12.3)	0.029
Other energy drinks*	11 (2.7)	22 (5.1)	0.081
Coffee			
No	188 (46.9)	179 (41.5)	0.120
Yes	213 (53.1)	252 (58.5)	
With sugar	140 (34.9)	147 (34.1)	0.807
Sugar-free	73 (18.2)	105 (24.4)	0.031
Tea			
No	328 (81.8)	341 (79.1)	0.331
Yes	73 (18.2)	90 (20.9)	
With sugar	4 (1.0)	5 (0.6)	0.821
Sugar-free	69 (17.2)	85 (19.7)	0.351
Number of stimulant beverages/week			
0	141 (35.2)	121 (28.1)	0.073
1	64 (16.0)	76 (17.6)	
2	106 (26.4)	110 (25.5)	
≥3	90 (22.4)	124 (28.8)	

*Other energy drinks include the following: Burn, Shark, Red Devil, and Battery.

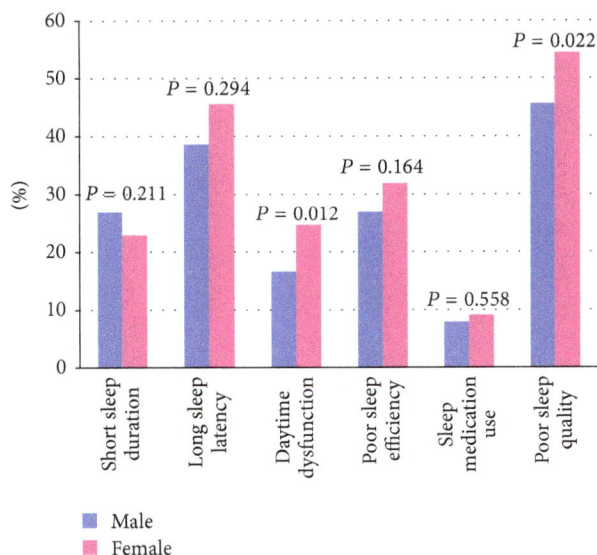

FIGURE 2: Sleep quality and sleep quality patterns according to gender.

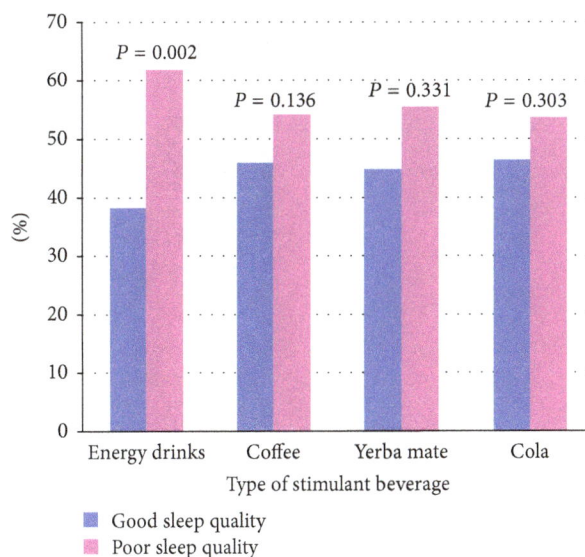

FIGURE 3: Sleep quality according to types of stimulant beverage consumed.

consumed <1 alcoholic beverage per month, those who reported consuming ≥16 alcoholic beverages per month had 55% lower odds of poor sleep efficacy (OR = 0.45; 95% CI 0.28–0.72) but increased odds of short sleep duration (OR = 1.42; 95% CI 0.91–2.21), long sleep latency (OR = 1.19; 95% CI

TABLE 5: Prevalence and odds ratios for sleep quality parameters in relation to lifestyle characteristics.

Sleep quality parameters	All (N = 832) n	Short sleep duration (<6 hours) (N = 457) %	OR (95% CI)	Long sleep latency (>30 min) (N = 345) %	OR (95% CI)	Day dysfunction due to sleep loss (N = 185) %	OR (95% CI)	Poor sleep efficiency (<85%) (N = 253) %	OR (95% CI)	Sleep medicine use (N = 73) %	OR (95% CI)
Smoking status											
Never	325	55.4	1.00 (Reference)	36.6	1.00 (Reference)	16.0	1.00 (Reference)	31.7	1.00 (Reference)	4.9	1.00 (Reference)
Former	77	57.1	1.17 (0.70–1.97)	45.4	1.40 (0.84–2.32)	28.6	2.23 (1.24–3.99)	24.7	0.73 (0.41–1.29)	9.1	1.92 (0.70–4.87)
Current	368	54.6	1.14 (0.83–1.56)	44.0	1.32 (0.97–1.80)	24.7	1.72 (1.17–2.53)	31.2	0.98 (0.71–1.36)	12.2	2.55 (1.40–4.63)
P value for trend			*0.416*		*0.100*		*0.007*		*0.47*		*0.003*
Alcohol consumption											
Low	167	46.7	1.00 (Reference)	38.3	1.00 (Reference)	22.7	1.00 (Reference)	39.5	1.00 (Reference)	10.2	1.00 (Reference)
Moderate	158	55.7	1.50 (0.96–2.37)	40.5	1.11 (0.71–1.74)	23.4	1.09 (0.65–1.84)	28.5	0.61 (0.38–0.97)	8.9	0.90 (0.42–1.91)
High	187	54.0	1.42 (0.91–2.21)	40.6	1.19 (0.77–1.85)	26.2	1.35 (0.82–2.23)	23.0	0.45 (0.28–0.72)	10.7	1.19 (0.59–2.4)
P value for trend			*0.127*		*0.89*		*0.232*		*0.003*		*0.85*
Any stimulant beverages											
No	356	58.4	1.00 (Reference)	37.9	1.00 (Reference)	17.4	1.00 (Reference)	31.2	1.00 (Reference)	8.4	1.00 (Reference)
Yes	433	51.7	0.72 (0.53–0.96)	42.7	1.21 (0.91–1.62)	24.7	1.53 (1.08–2.18)	30.5	0.96 (0.71–1.30)	7.9	0.93 (0.56–1.56)
Physical activity											
No	279	59.1	1.00 (Reference)	39.4	1.00 (Reference)	21.1	1.00 (Reference)	31.2	1.00 (Reference)	8.6	1.00 (Reference)
Yes	458	51.1	0.74 (0.51–0.96)	41.0	1.12 (0.82–1.52)	21.4	1.07 (0.74–1.55)	29.7	0.94 (0.68–1.31)	7.9	0.94 (0.55–1.62)

* Adjusted for age and gender; * all frequencies in the table (except for those of all subjects) indicate percentages within the lifestyle characteristics; † low (0–4 drinks/month); moderate (5–15 drinks/month); high (≥16 drinks/month).

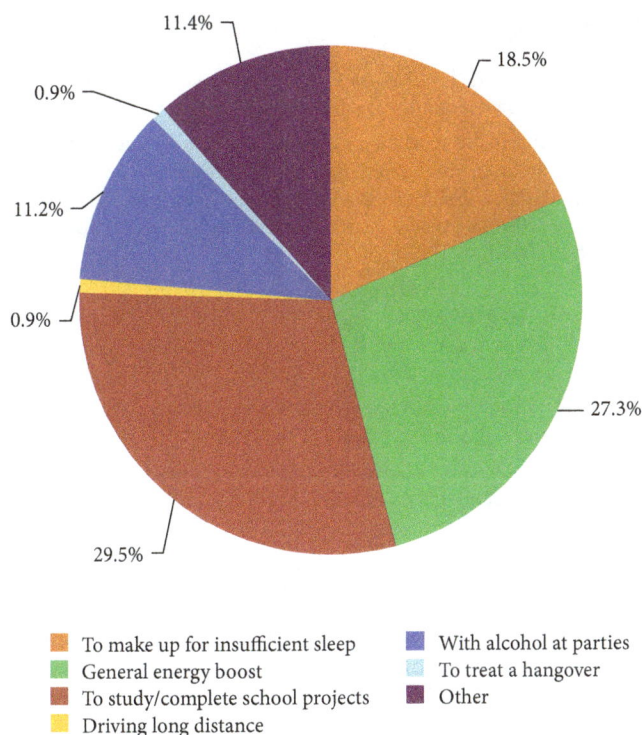

FIGURE 4: Motivations for consuming energy drinks.

0.77–1.85), daytime dysfunction due to sleep loss (OR = 1.35; 95% CI 0.82–2.23), and increased sleep medication use (OR = 1.19; 95% CI 0.59–2.4)) although statistical significance was not reached. Engaging in any physical activity was associated with reduced odds of short sleep duration (OR = 0.74; 95% CI 0.51–0.96). Any stimulant use was associated with a 50% increased odds of increased daytime dysfunction due to sleep loss (OR = 1.53; 95% CI 1.08–2.18).

Because energy drinks were more strongly associated with poor sleep quality than other caffeinated beverages, we conducted sensitivity analyses that specifically evaluated odds of subjective sleep efficiency, sleep latency, sleep medication use, and daytime dysfunction due to sleep loss in relation to energy drink consumption. In these analyses we found that students who consumed energy drinks had an 80% increased odds of overall poor sleep quality (OR = 1.83; 95% CI 1.29–2.60) as compared with students who did not use any caffeinated beverages. Students who consumed energy drinks were almost twice as likely to report short sleep duration (OR = 1.93; 95% CI 1.33–2.81) compared with those who did not use any caffeinated beverages (data not shown). The magnitude and direction of associations for other sleep quality parameters were largely similar to those reported in Table 5.

4. Discussion

The high prevalence of poor sleep quality among Patagonian Chilean college students is consistent with results from sleep studies among college students in the US and in other countries. We note that consumption of stimulant beverage was associated with increased odds of poor sleep quality and that associations were stronger for those who reported using energy drinks. Although caffeine is the primary ingredient in energy drinks, many include additional ingredients that may have a stimulating effect. The plant Guarana, for example, contains additional caffeine. The amino acid, taurine, a frequent ingredient in energy drinks, is thought to increase the effects of caffeine [20]. Although the absolute amounts of these individual ingredients in energy drinks typically fall below the levels thought to promote adverse effects, little is known about their possible synergistic effects [21].

Available evidence suggests that, when consumed in high amounts or mixed with alcohol, energy drinks may contribute to increased risks of arrhythmia, elevated blood pressures, and psychological symptoms [22]. The stimulatory effect of energy drinks has also been shown to negatively influence sleep quality [23]. Overall, sleep problems are common among college students and are important correlates of significant adverse behavioral and health outcomes including driving while drowsy, reduced cognitive function and productivity, increased interpersonal problems, and lower academic performance [9, 24, 25]. A study conducted in large state university in southeastern United States noted that college students who are at risk for sleep disorders were more likely to have an academic failure (GPA < 2.0) [24]. Another study conducted in the US found that college students with later bed times and wake-up times were more likely to have lower academic performance [26]. The authors estimated that GPAs (provided by the university registrar office) would have been expected to decrease by 0.13 points on a scale of 0–4 for each hour delay in rising time [24, 27]. Possible wellness and health promotion strategies designed to offset these adverse health consequences include circadian rhythm management, sleep hygiene education, and use of sleep stimulants such as white noise [28].

Our results are largely consistent with results from previous studies [29]. For example, in a study of over 40,000 men and women from eight Asian and African countries, investigators reported higher prevalence estimates of sleep problems in female versus male participants. In our study, poor sleep quality was more prevalent among female students. Our findings are also in general agreement with some previous studies that have documented associations of poor sleep quality with increased consumption of caffeinated beverages [30]. For instance, Hindmarch et al. have shown that caffeinated beverages had a dose-dependent negative effect on sleep onset, sleep time, and sleep quality [30]. However, we did not have information concerning frequency and dose of caffeine consumption in the present study to confirm these findings.

Our study has several limitations. First, given the cross-sectional nature of our study, it is difficult to determine whether poor sleep quality is a result of lifestyle factors including stimulant beverage consumption or whether these behaviors resulted as a coping mechanism for the effects of poor sleep. Second, our use of a self-administered survey that relied on subjective measures of sleep quality and other covariates may have introduced some degree of error, and the period of the semester when the survey was administered could have influenced the sleep quality. Third, sleep quality was determined using the PSQI, which relates good sleep quality to global scores of ≤ 5 and poor sleep quality with scores 6–21. With this broad grouping, there could be substantial heterogeneity among subjects deemed to be poor sleepers, potentially masking important associations. Fourth, we did not have information concerning frequency, timing, and dose of energy drinks consumption in the present study. As a result, it is possible that the binary grouping of energy drinks consumption attenuated the magnitude of association towards null. Fifth, although we adjusted for several potential confounders, we cannot exclude the possibility of residual confounding due to misclassification of adjusted variables or confounding by other unmeasured variables. Finally, our sample was not a random selection which may limit generalizability.

In summary, poor sleep quality is highly prevalent among Patagonian Chilean college students, and consumption of stimulant beverages, particularly energy drinks, is associated with increased odds of poor quality sleep. College students in Chile, and possibly other parts of South America, should be made aware of the impact caffeine beverage consumption has on sleep quality and patterns. Improved sleep quality benefits college students in their daily activities and academic performance and also improves their health status [31, 32]. The college environment and academic demands provide increased exposure to sleep-inhibiting factors, like psychological stress and increased opportunities for social engagements. Avoiding the build-up of a chronic sleep debt during early adulthood through awareness, education, and effective management of sleep disorders may be important in enhancing the academic performance during their college stay and in reducing the development of psychiatric and cardiometabolic disorders later in life.

Authors' Contribution

A. Souza and S. Traslaviña contributed equally to this work.

Conflict of Interests

The authors declare that they have no conflict of interests.

Acknowledgments

This research was completed while A. Souza and S. Traslaviña were research training fellows with the Harvard School of Public Health Multidisciplinary International Research Training (HSPH MIRT) Program. The HSPH MIRT Program is supported by an award from the National Institute for Minority Health and Health Disparities (T37-MD000149). The authors thank the Centro de Rehabilitación Club de Leones Cruz del Sur for providing facilities and logistic support throughout the research process. The authors also thank the participating universities for supporting the conduct of this study.

References

[1] CDC, *Centers For Disease Control, Sleep and Sleep Disorders*, Geneva, Switzerland, 2012, http://www.cdc.gov/features/sleep/.

[2] IOM and Institute of Medicine, "Committee on sleep medicine and research," in *Sleep Disorders and Sleep Deprivation: An Unmet Public Health Problem*, R. H. Colten and M. B. Altevogt, Eds., National Academy of Sciences Press, Washington, DC, USA, 2006.

[3] J. P. Chaput, J. P. Després, C. Bouchard, and A. Tremblay, "Short sleep duration is associated with reduced leptin levels and increased adiposity: results from the Québec family study," *Obesity*, vol. 15, no. 1, pp. 253–261, 2007.

[4] G. Ficca and P. Salzarulo, "What is sleep is for memory," *Sleep Medicine*, vol. 5, no. 3, pp. 225–230, 2004.

[5] S. Diekelmann, I. Wilhelm, and J. Born, "The whats and whens of sleep-dependent memory consolidation," *Sleep Medicine Reviews*, vol. 13, no. 5, pp. 309–321, 2009.

[6] J. A. Piqueras, W. Kuhne, P. Vera-Villarroel, A. Van Straten, and P. Cuijpers, "Happiness and health behaviours in Chilean college students: a cross-sectional survey," *BMC Public Health*, vol. 11, article no. 443, 2011.

[7] L. R. McKnight-Eily, D. K. Eaton, R. Lowry, J. B. Croft, L. Presley-Cantrell, and G. S. Perry, "Relationships between hours of sleep and health-risk behaviors in US adolescent students," *Preventive Medicine*, vol. 53, no. 4-5, pp. 271–273, 2011.

[8] A. H. Eliasson and C. J. Lettieri, "Early to bed, early to rise! Sleep habits and academic performance in college students," *Sleep and Breathing*, vol. 14, no. 1, pp. 71–75, 2010.

[9] D. J. Taylor and A. D. Bramoweth, "Patterns and consequences of inadequate sleep in college students: substance use and motor vehicle accidents," *Journal of Adolescent Health*, vol. 46, no. 6, pp. 610–612, 2010.

[10] J. R. Hughes and K. L. Hale, "Behavioral effects of caffeine and other methylxanthines on children," *Experimental and Clinical Psychopharmacology*, vol. 6, no. 1, pp. 87–95, 1998.

[11] S. M. Seifert, J. L. Schaechter, E. R. Hershorin, and S. E. Lipshultz, "Health effects of energy drinks on children, adolescents, and young adults," *Pediatrics*, vol. 127, no. 3, pp. 511–528, 2011.

[12] D. Bunka, "The drink of athletics, rock stars, college students…and your twelve year old! RxFiles," Saskatoon Health Region, 2011, http://www.rxfiles.ca/rxfiles.

[13] G. E. McIlvain, M. P. Noland, and R. Bickel, "Caffeine consumption patterns and beliefs of college freshmen," *American Journal of Health Education*, vol. 42, no. 4, pp. 235–244, 2011.

[14] B. M. Malinauskas, V. G. Aeby, R. F. Overton, T. Carpenter-Aeby, and K. Barber-Heidal, "A survey of energy drink consumption patterns among college students," *Nutrition Journal*, vol. 6, article no. 35, 2007.

[15] Estudios Cd, "Centro de Estudios en Retail," Facultad de Ingeniería Universidad de Chile, Geneva, Switzerland, 2012, http://www.ceret.cl/noticias/america-latina-lidera-consumo-de-bebidas-energeticas/.

[16] D. J. Buysse, C. F. Reynolds, T. H. Monk, S. R. Berman, and D. J. Kupfer, "The Pittsburgh sleep quality index: a new instrument for psychiatric practice and research," *Psychiatry Research*, vol. 28, no. 2, pp. 193–213, 1989.

[17] C. E. Carney, J. D. Edinger, B. Meyer, L. Lindman, and T. Istre, "Daily activities and sleep quality in college students," *Chronobiology International*, vol. 23, no. 3, pp. 623–637, 2006.

[18] WHO, "Physical status: the use and interpretation of anthropometry," Report of A WHO Expert Committee, Organization WHO, Geneva, Switzerland, 1995.

[19] K. J. Rothman, S. Greenland, and T. L. Lash, *Modern Epidemiology*, Lippincott Williams & Wilkins, Philadelphia, Pa, USA, 2008.

[20] M. Rath, "Energy drinks: what is all the hype? The dangers of energy drink consumption," *Journal of the American Academy of Nurse Practitioners*, vol. 24, no. 2, pp. 70–76, 2012.

[21] K. A. Clauson, K. M. Shields, C. E. McQueen, and N. Persad, "Safety issues associated with commercially available energy drinks," *Journal of the American Pharmacists Association*, vol. 48, no. 3, pp. e55–e64, 2008.

[22] M. Cote-Menendez, C. X. Rangel-Garzon, M. Y. Sanchez-Torres, and A. Medina-Lemus :, "Bebidas energizantes: hidratantes o estimulantes?" *Revista Facultad de Medicina*, vol. 59, no. 3, pp. 255–266, 2011.

[23] C. J. Calamaro, T. B. A. Mason, and S. J. Ratcliffe, "Adolescents living the 24/7 lifestyle: effects of caffeine and technology on sleep duration and daytime functioning," *Pediatrics*, vol. 123, no. 6, pp. e1005–e1010, 2009.

[24] J. F. Gaultney, "The prevalence of sleep disorders in college students: impact on academic performance," *Journal of American College Health*, vol. 59, no. 2, pp. 91–97, 2010.

[25] A. A. Gomes, J. Tavares, and M. H. de Azevedo, "Sleep and academic performance in undergraduates: a multi-measure, multi-predictor approach," *Chronobiology International*, vol. 28, no. 9, pp. 786–801, 2011.

[26] M. T. Trockel, M. D. Barnes, and D. L. Egget, "Health-related variables and academic performance among first-year college students: implications for sleep and other behaviors," *Journal of American College Health*, vol. 49, no. 3, pp. 125–131, 2000.

[27] G. Curcio, M. Ferrara, and L. De Gennaro, "Sleep loss, learning capacity and academic performance," *Sleep Medicine Reviews*, vol. 10, no. 5, pp. 323–337, 2006.

[28] L. M. Forquer, A. E. Camden, K. M. Gabriau, and C. M. Johnson, "Sleep patterns of college students at a public university," *Journal of American College Health*, vol. 56, no. 5, pp. 563–565, 2008.

[29] S. Stranges, W. Tigbe, F. X. Gomez-Olive, M. Thorogood, and N. B. Kandala :, "Sleep problems: an emerging global epidemic? Findings from the INDEPTH WHO-SAGE Study among more than 40, 000 older adults from 8 countries across Africa and Asia," *Sleep*, vol. 35, no. 8, pp. 1173–1181, 2012.

[30] I. Hindmarch, U. Rigney, N. Stanley, P. Quinlan, J. Rycroft, and J. Lane, "A naturalistic investigation of the effects of day-long consumption of tea, coffee and water on alertness, sleep onset and sleep quality," *Psychopharmacology*, vol. 149, no. 3, pp. 203–216, 2000.

[31] W. Buboltz, S. M. Jenkins, B. Soper, K. Woller, P. Johnson, and T. Faes, "Sleep habits and patterns of college students: an expanded study," *Journal of College Counseling*, vol. 12, no. 2, pp. 113–124, 2009.

[32] K. Vail-Smith, W. M. Felts, and C. Becker, "Relationship between sleep quality and health risk behaviors in undergraduate college students," *College Student Journal*, vol. 43, no. 3, pp. 924–930, 2009.

14

The Association between Sleep and Injury among School-Aged Children in Iran

Forugh Rafii,[1] Fatemeh Oskouie,[1] and Mahnaz Shoghi[2]

[1] *Center for Nursing Care Research and School of Nursing and Midwifery, Iran University of Medical Sciences, Rashid Yasemi Street, Valiasr Avenue, P.O. Box 19395-4798, Tehran 19964, Iran*
[2] *School of Nursing and Midwifery, Iran University of Medical Sciences, Rashid Yasemi Street, Valiasr Avenue, P.O. Box 19395-4798, Tehran 19964, Iran*

Correspondence should be addressed to Mahnaz Shoghi; m-shoghi@razi.tums.ac.ir

Academic Editor: Pillar Giora

Background. A good night's sleep plays a key role in diseases resistance, injury prevention, and mood stability. The objective of this study was to examine relationship between sleep problems and accidental injury occurrences in school-aged children. *Method.* A retrospective study was conducted for comparing two groups of children. Children who have experienced injuries for at least two times during an academic year are the participants in the injury group (IG) and those who have not experienced any kind of injuries are placed in the noninjury group (NIG). Data was collected through parent-reported sleep patterns and problems using Children's Sleep Habits Questionnaire (CSHQ). *Findings.* The findings showed that global sleep problems were more in the IG than in the NIG. Multivariate logistic regression analysis showed that the daytime sleepiness and sleep duration are the two major reasons for accidental injury. In addition, significant difference was seen between the sleep patterns of the two groups. Sleep duration was also shorter in the IG, and this group had a greater percentage (63% versus 41.1%) of "short sleepers" (<9 h). *Conclusion.* There is a significant relationship between injury occurrence and sleep problems and sleep duration in Iranian school-aged children.

1. Background

Adequate sleep with regard to both quality and quantity is among the basic needs of human beings and plays a significant role in the physical, emotional, and cognitive development of children [1]. Sleep is regulated by complex and interacting biological and circadian processes, and sleep patterns also depend on physical, psychological, and environmental factors [2, 3]. Children's sleep patterns and habits in particular are influenced by external factors such as culture, health-related behaviors, parenting practices, and social interactions within the family. For example, caregivers' beliefs and their understanding of the meaning and importance of sleep may not only have direct effects on children's sleep patterns but may also impact parents' interpretation of sleep behaviors and their willingness to address problematic behaviors with their healthcare providers [2, 4, 5].

Sleep disturbances and irregular sleep patterns in childhood often lead to daytime sleepiness and short- and long-term consequences [2, 6], including somatic complaints such as headaches [7] and mood and neurobehavioral problems such as irritability, hyperactivity, and inattention [8–10]. The psychological and behavioral consequences may in turn result in increase in family and peer conflicts and parenting stress. Cognitive sequelae including poor impulse control and increased distractibility not only have potentially profound effects on academic achievement but may also have impacts on their life quality [11].

Many studies have been carried out regarding the relationship between sleep disturbance and injury in adults. for example, a number of studies have examined the relationship between insomnia and occupational [12–14] and driving accidents [15, 16] in adults. However, similar empirical evidence remains sparse for children [17–20]. In a study conducted in a pediatric emergency department, Valent et al. [20] reported a correlation between injury rates and sleep duration. In another emergency room study, Owens et al. [18] reported an relationship among accidental injuries, increased injury risk behaviors, and sleep problems in children [18].

Li et al. reached the same result in school-aged children [17]. Schwebel and Brezausek [19] study showed a relationship between the trauma occurrences and sleep disorders and night waking in toddlers [19].

Studies show that over the past twenty two years, deaths from accidents have been the second leading cause of death in Iranian children [21–23]. Iranian children were found to have more sleep problems compared to the American children and their sleep duration on average was 1.5 hour shorter than that of their American counterparts across all age groups. School start time is 8 a.m. in Iran and often children go to bed in irregular time at nights. Sleep time of children often is not very important for parents. Normally children and parents donot have different bed times and they usually sleep at the same time.

If sleep disturbance is associated with an increased risk of accidental injuries as the previous studies have shown, the increased rates of sleep problems in Iranian children may be one of the factors contributing to these high injury rates. Because little work has been conducted with respect to this potentially important and modifiable relationship between sleep behavior and injury in Iran, we conducted this study to explore the relationship between sleep problems and injuries in school-aged children from an urban area of Iran.

The aim of this retrospective case-control study was to examine the association between parent-reported sleep problems and accidental injuries in a sample of school-aged children in Iran. Our hypotheses were (1) children who have experienced accidental injuries at school will be more likely to have reported daytime sleepiness compared to children without injuries and (2) children who have experienced accidental injuries will have more parent-reported sleep problems compared to the noninjured group.

2. Methods

2.1. Subjects. All subjects were recruited from 17 elementary schools serving approximately 5000 students in Tehran, Iran. Participants were 400 school-aged children of 6–11 years old who live in a two-parent household in Tehran. Psychological disorders, chronic disease, ADHD, consumption of sedative or opioids/benzodiazepines/psychotropic drugs by children, and history of head trauma were considered as excluded criteria. In case of having any of the mentioned conditions in the child's health report in school or parents' reports during filling out the questionnaire, that specific child was not considered as a participant anymore.

All Iranian children go through a medical test before they start any academic year and the report will be recorded and kept in the school. Children are insured at the beginning of the academic year. In case of any injury incidence in school, primary therapeutic actions will be performed by school nurses and in case of more serious injuries, the school authorities will inform the child parents and the child will be sent to the clinics under contract with the school for further treatments. Since the information just related to major injuries which is needed for referral is recorded in the children's health reports, minor injuries and harms that were not reported by the child have not been considered in this study.

The injury group includes those children who have reports about accidental injuries at school and who have faced accidental injuries for at least two times or more in the school during one educational year and have been sent to clinic for basic treatments by the school nurse. The noninjury group includes those children who are at the same age and they do not have any report concerning the injuries at school until the day of the administration of the questionnaires.

2.2. Instruments Procedure. Two survey questionnaires were used in this study. The first questionnaire consists of two parts: a demographic section which includes variables such as child characteristics (age, gender, …) and parent characteristics (job, education, …). The second questionnaire deals with the questions about children's sleep problems and sleep patterns. The Children's Sleep Habits Questionnaire (CSHQ) is a validated parent-reported scale that assesses sleep behavior over a typical week and consists of 33 items grouped into eight subscales that reflect a variety of sleep domains: bedtime resistance, sleep-onset delay, sleeps duration, sleep anxiety, night awakenings, parasomnias, sleep-disordered breathing, and day-time sleepiness [24]. The CSHQ items are rated on a three-point scale: (1) "usually" if the sleep behavior occurred 5–7 times per week; (2) "sometimes" for 2–4 times per week; and (3) "rarely" for 0–10 time per week, with a higher score indicating more sleep problems. In addition, three questions regarding sleep patterns were asked about bedtime, morning wake-up time, and duration of daytime naps. Sleep duration was calculated by subtracting the reported bedtime and wake-up time, while nap duration was an actual time. Nine hours was used as a cutoff point for sleep duration in accordance to pediatric text books' recommendation of a minimum 9 h of sleep per night for this age group [25, 26].

This questionnaire was translated in to Persian previously and has been used in several studies concerning sleep habits in school-aged children in Iran. Content validity was used to estimate the scientific validity of this instrument. The reliability of the Persian version of this questionnaire was estimated as $r = 0.87$ using test-retest reliability coefficient [27–29].

Procedure. Receiving the letter of introduction from university and getting approval letter from Tehran Ministry of Education and Training, the researcher was introduced to public schools by this center. Having gone to the schools and having studied the children's health reports at the end of the educational year (June 2011), the researcher prepared a list of children who faced injuries for at least two times and were taken to clinics for further treatments (from September 23, 2010, to June 21, 2012). Those children who have experienced injuries which have happened within the last 15 days were considered as participants. After calling their mothers for a written permission, the researcher asked them to fill out the questionnaire in the school where both mothers and the child were present. The mothers were asked to fill out the questionnaire by focusing on the last time that their child had an injury and they also were asked to report the sleep patterns of their child one week before the occurrence of the injury. The injury group included 218 children. Ten mothers did not fill out the questionnaire and eight questionnaires were discarded due to incompleteness. All in all, 200 questionnaires have been left for analysis.

In order to avoid selection bias, the researcher chose stratified random sampling. The populations of boys or girls were chosen in the same age group and they were matched regarding their gender and age to compromise the noninjured (NIG). The questionnaires were administered and filled out in this group just like the previous group. The mothers were asked to fill out the questionnaire by focusing on the last time that their child had an injury and they also were asked to report the sleep patterns of their child one week before the occurrence of the injury.

2.3. Statistical Analysis. SPSS (version 15) was used for statistical analyses. The t-test analysis was used to determine the differences in sleep problem rates and daytime sleepiness between the two groups. Multivariate logistic regression analyses were conducted to examine the association between sleep problems (independent variable) and injury (dependent variable). Odds ratios (OR) and 95% confidence intervals (95% CI) were calculated. All statistical significance was set at $P < 0.05$.

3. Results

200 children in the case group (62 girls, 138 boys) and 200 in the control group (78 girls, 122 boys) took part in this study. Gender distribution was similar across groups ($\chi^2 = 2.83$, $P = 0.93$); the average ages of the control and case groups were 8.6 ± 1.73 and 8.4 ± 1.73, respectively, and not significantly different ($\chi^2 = 2.21$, $P = 0.89$). Parental occupations were also similar. 81% of mothers were housewives in both groups and 35.7% of case group's fathers and 37.5% of control group's fathers were self-employed. Comparing two groups of case and control, using χ^2 test, the researcher did not find any difference regarding their age grade ($\chi^2 = 0.871$, $P = 1.83$), mothers' education ($\chi^2 = 12.1$, $P = 1.17$), fathers' education ($\chi^2 = 11.539$, $P = 0.061$), mothers' jobs ($\chi^2 = 0.0$, $P = 1$), and fathers' jobs ($\chi^2 = 12.11$, $P = 1.17$).

3.1. Sleep/Wake-up Patterns. Mean bedtime at night for the total sample was 22 : 38 (standard deviation (SD): 1.57), mean morning wake-up time was 7.55 (SD: 1.07), and mean nocturnal sleep duration was 9.45 h (SD: 1.55).

For the IG children, mean bedtime at night was 10 : 61 (SD: 1.98 h), mean morning wake-up time was 7.19 a.m. (SD: 1.13 h), and mean nocturnal sleep duration was 8.98 h (SD: 1.36 h). Sleep duration was calculated by subtracting the reported bedtime and wakeup time. For the control children, mean bedtime at night was 10.14 (SD: 0.94 min), mean morning wake-up time was 7.22 (SD: 0.88 min), and mean nocturnal sleep duration was 9.91 h (SD: 1.06 h). Of all three indices of sleep patterns, mean bed time at night ($t = -5.68$, $P = 0.03$), mean morning wakeup time ($t = 6.56$,

$P = 0.00$), and nocturnal sleep duration ($t = -6.23$, $P = 0.00$) differed significantly between IG and NIG. Furthermore, 63.5% ($n = 127$) of children in the IG slept less than 9 h during the night, while only 41.1% ($n = 87$) of NIG children were reported to sleep less than 9 h ($\chi^2 = 20.29$, $P = 0.00$). ($^*P < 0.05$).

3.2. Comparisons of CSHQ. Regarding the second research hypothesis (children in IG would have a higher rate of sleep problems than children in NIG), the results were shown in Table 1.

3.3. Association of Injury with Sleep Problems in Injury Group. First, multivariate logistic regression analysis was conducted to examine the association between each subscale of the 8 individual sleep problems and injury. The results were shown in Table 2.

According to the findings of this study, these five categories of sleep problems have relationship with injury occurrence. The higher they go, the higher the probability of injury occurrence will be. Based on this model, the three categories of night waking, sleep duration, and daytime sleepiness have the greatest impact on injury occurrences (exep B).

4. Discussion

Comparing the sleep patterns of the two groups, one can conclude that the children in IG sleep less than control group on average. They go to bed later than control group for various reasons and wake up earlier in the morning compared to control group. In addition, the number of short sleeper children (sleep < 9 hours) in IG was significantly greater than that of the children in NIG. Several studies have supported the mentioned results [17, 19, 20]; however Owens et al. [18], who did a research concerning children of 3–7 years old who had trauma, didn't find any significant relationship between the number of trauma occurrence and sleep duration [18].

The current study also suggests an association between sleep-onset delay, sleep duration, sleep anxiety, night wakenings, parasomnias, sleep-disordered breathing, day-time sleepiness, CSHQ total score, and accidental injuries. Li et al. [17] with similar results in their study showed that those kids with trauma experience in comparison with the ones without any experience suffer more from parasomnias, daytime sleepiness, sleep anxiety, and irregular sleep duration [17]. According to Owens et al. [18] sleep disturbance has significant relationship with the number of trauma occurrences and those children with more trauma experience suffer more from sleep disturbances such as bedtime resistance, sleep anxiety, and sleep-disordered breathing, compared to the children with less trauma experience [18]. This study supports other studies and shows that sleep anxiety is related more to trauma occurrence in school-aged children rather than other variables. Owens et al. [18] and Li et al. [17] reached similar results regarding this issue [17, 18].

The results of the current study support the existence of the relationship between sleep problems and injury occurrence in school-aged children. Perhaps exhaustion followed

TABLE 1: Comparison of CSHQ scale scores between the IG and NIG means ± SD.

Sleep problems variables	IG ($n = 200$)	NIG ($n = 200$)	t	P
Bedtime resistance	11.88 ± 2.64	8.49 ± 2.08	14.23	0/00*
Sleep-onset delay	1.9 ± 0.78	1.32 ± 0.57	8.90	0/00*
Sleep duration	5.81 ± 1.48	4.11 ± 1.15	13.62	0/00*
Sleep anxiety	7.83 ± 1.97	5.38 ± 1.60	13.62	0/00*
Night waking	5.29 ± 1.44	3.69 ± 1.03	12.66	0/00*
Parasomnias	10.48 ± 2.33	8.09 ± 1.48	12.23	0/00*
Sleep-disordered breathing	4.46 ± 1.67	3.30 ± 0.8	8.79	0/00*
Daytime sleepiness	14.59 ± 3.26	10.45 ± 2.30	14.66	0/00*
Total scores	58.24 ± 9.84	41.99 ± 6.55	19.42	0/00*

*$P < 0.05$.

TABLE 2: Association of accidental injuries with sleep problem: multivariate logistic regression.

Sleep problem	B	SE	Wald	P	Exep (B)	95% C.I. for EXP (B)	
						Upper	Lower
Daytime sleepiness	−0.181	0.067	7.266	0.00	0.834	0.952	0.731
Bedtime resistance	−0.282	0.122	5.350	0.00	0.754	0.958	0.594
Parasomnias	−0.307	0.123	6.197	0.00	0.736	0.937	0.578
Night waking	−0.219	0.082	7.150	0.006	0.803	0.943	0.684
Sleep duration	−0.199	0.055	12.812	0.021	0.820	0.914	0.735

Daytime sleepiness entered on step 1; bedtime resistance entered on step 2; parasomnias entered on step 3; night waking entered on step 4; sleep duration entered on step 5.
*$P < 0.05$.

by parasomnias or the decrease of sleep quality was the reason concerning this issue [30]. Maybe decrease in the sleep quality and quantity could cause day-time sleepiness which would result in concentration loss, carelessness, and aggressiveness. Perhaps these conditions increased the risk of injury occurrence in school-aged children [6]. These findings do not appear to support cause-and-effect relationship between injuries and sleep problems.

It should be said that this study has some limitations. The mothers were asked to remember the sleep patterns of the week before the child's last injury while 15 days have passed since the last injury and this resulted in recall bias. Among the other factors that may have impacts on sleep pattern, one can refer to time of year. The concept of injury may vary among the parents and this should be considered as a factor as well. Since parents' definition may vary concerning the concept "injury," their reports are very subjective and what one parent may consider as a minor injury may have been considered as major by another mother. Other factors such as parenting practices, family composition, and the environment should also be considered in future studies as influential variables.

Sleep patterns may also vary in relationship to other factors, such as time of year. Variability in individual parent's thresholds for concern about injury may have also been a confounding factor in the analysis. Sleep information was based on subjective parental report. We lost data about minor and nonreported injuries. Finally, other factors such as family composition, household environment, and parenting practices may also play an important role in increased risk for injury and should be considered in future studies.

Despite its preliminary nature, the results of this study support an association between sleep disturbance and injury, among children in an urban area of Iran. Additional research is needed to further corroborate this relationship, using prospective designs, multiple observer reports of injuries and behavior, more detailed injury descriptions (e.g., time of day), and more objective and varied measures of daytime sleepiness. Our results underscore the need for screening and identification of sleep problems in children by healthcare providers and suggest that attention should be paid to sleep disturbance as a potential risk factor in children with increased injury rates. Both parents and school nurse should also be made aware of the possible association between sleep problems and injury risk as another potential consequence of inadequate and disturbed sleep.

Acknowledgments

The authors' special thanks go to Owens for giving them the permission to use the questionnaire and for her enormous help and Neda Khodaverdi for English editing of this paper. They wish to thank all the mothers and children who took part in this study.

References

[1] L. B. C. Carvalho, L. B. Do Prado, L. Silva et al., "Cognitive dysfunction in children with sleep disorders," *Arquivos de Neuro-Psiquiatria A*, vol. 62, no. 2, pp. 212–216, 2004.

[2] J. C. Blader, H. S. Koplewicz, H. Abikoff, and C. Foley, "Sleep problems of elementary school children: a community survey," *Archives of Pediatrics and Adolescent Medicine*, vol. 151, no. 5, pp. 473–480, 1997.

[3] J. A. Owens, "Introduction: culture and sleep in children," *Pediatrics*, vol. 115, supplement 1, pp. 201–203, 2005.

[4] O. G. Jenni and B. B. O'Connor, "Children's sleep: an interplay between culture and biology," *Pediatrics*, vol. 115, supplement 1, pp. 204–216, 2005.

[5] X. Liu, L. Liu, J. A. Owen, and D. L. Kaplan, "Sleep patterns and sleep problems among schoolchildren in the United States and China," *Pediatrics*, vol. 115, supplement 1, pp. 241–249, 2005.

[6] G. Fallone, J. A. Owens, and J. Deane, "Sleepiness in children and adolescents: clinical implications," *Sleep Medicine Reviews*, vol. 6, no. 4, pp. 287–306, 2002.

[7] O. Bruni, P. M. Russo, R. Ferri, L. Novelli, F. Galli, and V. Guidetti, "Relationships between headache and sleep in a non-clinical population of children and adolescents," *Sleep Medicine*, vol. 9, no. 5, pp. 542–548, 2008.

[8] M. A. Carskadon, A. R. Wolfson, C. Acebo, O. Tzischinsky, and R. Seifer, "Adolescent sleep patterns, circadian timing, and sleepiness at a transition to early school days," *Sleep*, vol. 21, no. 8, pp. 871–881, 1998.

[9] R. Epstein, N. Chillag, and P. Lavie, "Starting times of school: effects on daytime functioning of fifth-grade children in Israel," *Sleep*, vol. 21, no. 3, pp. 250–256, 1998.

[10] A. R. Wolfson and M. A. Carskadon, "Sleep schedules and daytime functioning in adolescents," *Child Development*, vol. 69, no. 4, pp. 875–887, 1998.

[11] C. Drake, C. Nickel, E. Burduvali, T. Roth, C. Jefferson, and P. Badia, "The pediatric daytime sleepiness scale (PDSS): sleep habits and school outcomes in middle-school children," *Sleep*, vol. 26, no. 4, pp. 455–458, 2003.

[12] N. T. Ayas, L. K. Barger, B. E. Cade et al., "Extended work duration and the risk of self-reported percutaneous injuries in interns," *Journal of the American Medical Association*, vol. 296, no. 9, pp. 1055–1062, 2006.

[13] T. Bunn, S. Slavova, T. Struttmann, and S. R. Browning, "Sleepiness/fatigue and distraction/inattention as factors for fatal versus nonfatal commercial motor vehicle driver injuries," *Accident Analysis and Prevention*, vol. 37, no. 5, pp. 862–869, 2005.

[14] A. P. J. de Vries, N. Kassam-Adams, A. Cnaan, E. Sherman-Slate, P. R. Gallagher, and F. K. Winston, "Looking beyond the physical injury: posttraumatic stress disorder in children and parents after pediatric traffic injury," *Pediatrics*, vol. 104, no. 6, pp. 1293–1299, 1999.

[15] C. C. Caruso, "Possible broad impacts of long work hours," *Industrial Health*, vol. 44, no. 4, pp. 531–536, 2006.

[16] J. Connor, G. Whitlock, R. Norton, and R. Jackson, "The role of driver sleepiness in car crashes: a systematic review of epidemiological studies," *Accident Analysis and Prevention*, vol. 33, no. 1, pp. 31–41, 2001.

[17] Y. Li, H. Jin, J. A. Owens, and C. Hu, "The association between sleep and injury among school-aged children in rural China: a case-control study," *Sleep Medicine*, vol. 9, no. 2, pp. 142–148, 2008.

[18] J. A. Owens, S. Fernando, and M. Mc Guinn, "Sleep disturbance and injury risk in young children," *Behavioral Sleep Medicine*, vol. 3, no. 1, pp. 18–31, 2005.

[19] D. C. Schwebel and C. M. Brezausek, "Nocturnal awakenings and pediatric injury risk," *Journal of Pediatric Psychology*, vol. 33, no. 3, pp. 323–332, 2008.

[20] F. Valent, S. Brusaferro, and F. Barbone, "A case-crossover study of sleep and childhood injury," *Pediatrics*, vol. 107, no. 2, p. E23, 2001.

[21] F. Amani and A. Kazemnejad, "Changing pattern of mortality trends in Iran, south, south-west Asia and world, 1970-2010," *Iranian Journal of Public Health*, vol. 39, no. 3, pp. 20–26, 2010.

[22] A. Khosravi, R. Taylor, M. Naghavi, and A. D. Lopez, "Mortality in the Islamic Republic of Iran, 1964–2004," *Bulletin of the World Health Organization*, vol. 85, no. 8, pp. 607–614, 2007.

[23] P. Yavari, A. Abadi, and Y. Mehrabi, "Mortality and changing epidemiological trends in Iran during 1979–2001," *Hakim*, vol. 6, pp. 7–14, 2003.

[24] J. A. Owens, A. Spirito, and M. McGuinn, "The Children's Sleep Habits Questionnaire (CSHQ): psychometric properties of a survey instrument for school-aged children," *Sleep*, vol. 23, no. 8, pp. 1043–1051, 2000.

[25] M. J. Hockenberry and D. Wilson, *Wong's Nursing Care of Infants and Children*, Mosby/Elsevier, Orlando, Fla, USA, 2007.

[26] M. J. Hockenberry, D. Wilson, and D. L. Wong, *Wong's Essentials of Pediatric Nursing: Mosby Incorporated*, Mosby/Elsevier, Orlando, Fla, USA, 2012.

[27] M. Shoghi, S. Khanjari, F. Farmani, and F. Hossaini, "Parasomnias in school-age children," *Iran Journal of Nursing*, vol. 18, no. 41-42, pp. 153–159, 2005.

[28] M. Shoghi, S. Khanjari, F. Farmani, and F. Hossaini, "Sleep pattern in school-age children, residents of the West Area in Tehran," *Iran Journal of Nursing*, vol. 18, no. 43, pp. 83–89, 2005.

[29] M. Shoghi, S. Khanjari, F. Farmani, and F. Hosseini, "Sleep habits of school age children," *Iran Journal of Nursing*, vol. 18, no. 41-42, pp. 131–138, 2005.

[30] U. Brook and M. Boaz, "Children hospitalized for accidental injuries: Israeli experiences," *Patient Education and Counseling*, vol. 51, no. 2, pp. 177–182, 2003.

15

Validation of the CPAP Habit Index-5: A Tool to Understand Adherence to CPAP Treatment in Patients with Obstructive Sleep Apnea

Anders Broström,[1,2] **Per Nilsen,**[3] **Benjamin Gardner,**[4] **Peter Johansson,**[5] **Martin Ulander,**[2,6] **Bengt Fridlund,**[7] **and Kristofer Årestedt**[8,9,10]

[1] *Department of Nursing Science, School of Health Sciences, Jönköping University, 551 11 Jönköping, Sweden*
[2] *Department of Clinical Neurophysiology, Linköping University Hospital, 581 85 Linköping, Sweden*
[3] *Division of Health Care Analysis, Faculty of Health Sciences, Department of Health and Society, Linköping University, 581 83 Linköping, Sweden*
[4] *Health Behaviour Research Centre, Department of Epidemiology and Public Health, University College London, London, WC1E 6BT, UK*
[5] *Department of Cardiology, Linköping University Hospital, 581 85 Linköping, Sweden*
[6] *Departement of Clinical and Experimental Medicine, Division of Clinical Neurophysiology, Faculty of Health Sciences, Linköping University, 581 83 Linköping, Sweden*
[7] *School of Health Sciences, Jönköping University, 551 11 Jönköping, Sweden*
[8] *Faculty of Health and Life Sciences, Linnaeus University, 391 82 Kalmar, Sweden*
[9] *Department of Medicine and Health Sciences, Linköping University, 581 83 Linköping, Sweden*
[10] *Palliative Research Centre, Ersta Sköndal University College and Ersta Hospital, 100 61 Stockholm, Sweden*

Correspondence should be addressed to Anders Broström; anders.brostrom@hhj.hj.se

Academic Editor: Giora Pillar

Long-term adherence to continuous positive airway pressure (CPAP) is low among patients with obstructive sleep apnea (OSA). The potential role of "habit" in sustaining adherence to CPAP use has not been studied. This study aimed to establish the relevance of habit to CPAP adherence, via validation of an adaptation of the Self-Report Habit Index (the CPAP Habit Index-5; CHI-5). Analyses focused on the homogeneity, reliability, and factor structure of the CHI-5 and, in line with theoretical predictions, its utility as a predictor of long-term CPAP adherence in middle-aged patients with OSA. A prospective longitudinal design was used. 117 patients with objectively verified OSA intended for CPAP treatment were recruited. Data was collected via clinical examinations, respiratory recordings, questionnaires, and CPAP devices at baseline, 2 weeks, 6 months, and 12 months. The CHI-5 showed satisfactory homogeneity interitem correlations (0.42–0.93), item-total correlations (0.58–0.91), and reliability (α = 0.92). CHI-5 data at 6 months showed a one-factor solution and predicted 63% of variance in total CPAP use hours after 12 months. Based on the satisfactory measurement properties and the high amount of CPAP use variance it explained, the CHI-5 can be seen as a useful tool in clinical practice.

1. Introduction

Obstructive sleep apnea (OSA) is a common sleep-related breathing disorder where repeated episodic collapses of the upper airways during sleep cause apneas and/or hypopneas. The resulting sleep fragmentation can cause daytime symptoms, including sleepiness, headaches, and cognitive dysfunction. This condition is termed obstructive sleep apnea syndrome (OSAS) [1]. Apart from the short-term negative consequences due to disturbed breathing, a growing body of evidence indicates that OSAS is also a risk factor for hypertension, cardiac failure, stroke [2, 3], and occupational accidents due to sleepiness. The current treatment of choice is continuous positive airway pressure (CPAP) [4]. Adherence to CPAP treatment is important since sufficient use can eliminate apneas completely and improve sleep quality, excessive daytime sleepiness, and quality of life for both patients and partners. Furthermore, CPAP treatment can reduce morbidity and mortality in cardiovascular diseases, as well as consumption of health care resources [2].

Despite the documented beneficial effects of CPAP treatment, adherence rates tend to be low [5–7]. Initial refusal to engage in CPAP treatment ranges from 8% to 15% and the long-term usage is reported to be between 65% and 80%. In a study by Kribbs et al. [8], less than 50% of patients were considered adherent (i.e., measured as use of CPAP for at least 4 hours per night). Explanations of low and varying degrees of adherence have predominantly focused on technical and physiological aspects [7]. Side effects from treatment, such as dry throat, nasal congestion, and mask leaks tend to be common and are believed to reduce adherence [9–12]. Several technical solutions have been proposed to overcome these problems, such as air humidifiers and different types of devices, yet the increase in adherence has not been proportional to the reduction in side effects offered by these solutions [13]. Objective measures of disease severity are only weakly to moderately associated with CPAP adherence [7].

The difficulties in explaining low CPAP adherence rates have led to calls for more research on the influence of psychological factors on CPAP adherence [6, 9, 14–16]. A few studies have examined psychological factors such as risk perception, attitudes to treatment, outcome expectancies, and self-efficacy [7, 17, 18], which are important constructs in many social-cognitive theories such as the theory of planned behaviour, the theory of reasoned action, and the social cognitive theory [19]. These theories tend to position intention, which summarises various motivational concepts such as attitudes and self-efficacy, as the key determinant of behaviour. However, findings in various fields indicate a rather substantial intention-behaviour gap that implies that behaviour is not consistently guided by motivation [20]. Intentions tend to predict initiation of behaviour but are less predictive of maintenance over time [21]. Within health psychology, "habit" is increasingly attracting interest as a potential mechanism for the maintenance of behaviour [22, 23].

Habitual behaviours are automatic, impulse-driven responses to contextual cues, acquired through repetition of behaviour in the presence of these cues [22]. The context is the environment in which behaviour takes place; the features or cues that trigger action can be anything from physical location, time, and preceding actions to emotions or people [24]. Habit formation offers a useful goal for behaviour change interventions: automatically initiated behaviours may persist over time, even when conscious motivation erodes, which will aid maintenance. As habits form, control over the behaviour is transferred from conscious motivation to environmental cues [25]. Maintenance of the behaviour becomes less reliant on conscious attention and memory processes and instead becomes automatic and "second nature," proceeding without forethought [25]. Theory predicts that people with stronger habits will be more likely to perform the (habitual) behaviour [26]. CPAP adherence is likely to have the potential to become habitual, given that CPAP is (or should be) used frequently (nightly) in similar settings (the bedroom) [27].

Identifying "habit"—or its absence—in CPAP patients requires a robust and reliable measure of habit strength. The self-report habit index (SRHI) is the most widely applied generic habit strength measure [22, 28, 29]. It has been used with numerous behaviours, including snacking, fruit consumption, engaging in exercise and active sports, watching television, and using a bicycle as a means of transportation [22], but also in adherence to medication [19]. However, no previous study has investigated its usefulness for understanding adherence to CPAP treatment. It would be valuable from a clinical perspective to adapt to the SRHI for a CPAP context, for the purposes of describing the automaticity with which CPAP is used, tracking the formation of CPAP-use habits over time, and predicting long-term CPAP adherence.

Accordingly, the aim of this study was to validate an adapted version of the SRHI called the CPAP Habit Index-5 (CHI-5) in a population of middle-aged patients with OSA. To this end, we sought to establish the internal consistency of the CHI-5, its underlying factor structure, and, in an illustrative application, its utility as a predictor of long-term CPAP adherence. We hypothesised that the CHI-5 would be a homogeneous, reliable, and unidimensional measure predictive of long-term CPAP adherence.

2. Materials and Methods

2.1. Description of the SRHI. The SRHI is comprised of 12 items concerning three characteristics of habit: 8 items relating to aspects of automaticity (e.g., "Behaviour X is something I do without thinking"), 3 items concerning frequency (e.g., "Behaviour X is something I do frequently"), and 1 item that focuses on the relevance of the habit to self-identity (e.g., "Behaviour X is typically 'me'") [29]. A 5- or 7-point Likert-type scale is typically used. Several shorter versions of SRHI have been used with no apparent losses in reliability or predictive validity [30], suggesting that some items may be redundant.

2.2. Development of the CPAP Habit Index-5. Three of the authors (AB, PN, and MU) reduced the 12-item SRHI to 5 items for the purposes of achieving a pragmatic tool for potential use in CPAP treatment practice. The selected items were then discussed by a multiprofessional expert panel consisting of three physicians specialized in sleep medicine, three nurses working primarily with CPAP treatment, and a behavioural scientist, as well as two nurse researchers with experience of OSAS. The aim of this discussion was to establish face and content validity of the items. After a consensus decision it was determined to use the 5 items (3 automaticity items and 2 frequency items) in the CHI-5. Previous work has shown that self-identity is not a necessary component of a habit, and so the self-identity item was excluded from our six-item index. A five-point Likert-type

TABLE 1: A description of the CPAP Habit Index-5.

(1) Using the CPAP nightly is part of my routines a normal week	Strongly agree 1	Agree 2	Undecided 3	Disagree 4	Strongly disagree 5
(2) A special reason is needed if I'm not going to use the CPAP during a normal night	Strongly agree 1	Agree 2	Undecided 3	Disagree 4	Strongly disagree 5
(3) I have used the CPAP nightly for a long time	Strongly agree 1	Agree 2	Undecided 3	Disagree 4	Strongly disagree 5
(4) It feels weird not to use the CPAP during a normal night	Strongly agree 1	Agree 2	Undecided 3	Disagree 4	Strongly disagree 5
(5) I use the CPAP more or less automatically during a normal night	Strongly agree 1	Agree 2	Undecided 3	Disagree 4	Strongly disagree 5

scale (1–5) was applied for each item, yielding a possible range for the CHI-5 of 5–25, with a lower score indicating a stronger habit of wearing the CPAP. To strengthen face validity, a group consisting of 20 patients with OSAS answered 5 open-ended questions and was interviewed after performing a pilot test during follow-up visits at the CPAP clinic regarding readability, clarity, and layout with satisfactory results during the development phase.

To secure equivalence when translating the CHI-5 into English all steps in Brislin's model [31] were followed. First two external bilingual adult individuals (i.e., one healthcare professional and one lay person) examined and approved the conceptual structure of the Swedish text. Then two of the authors (AB and PN) translated the scale into English. The English translation was examined by a behavioural scientist with English as a first language (Benjamin Gardner.) and a bilingual group consisting of three sleep experts (i.e., physician, nurse, and technician), as well as two bilingual patients with OSAS, who proposed only a few minor modifications of the wording. One of the authors (Per Nilsen and an external bilingual individual then translated the scale back into Swedish. Finally, the back translation of CHI-5 was carefully examined by the external bilingual group and determined to be equivalent to the original text. The CHI-5 questions are presented in Table 1.

2.3. Design and Setting. A prospective longitudinal design was used. One hundred and seventeen eligible patients 18–65 yrs with objectively verified OSA (i.e., based on six channel polygraphy recordings scored according to the American Academy of Sleep Medicines criteria [4]) referred to for CPAP treatment at an Ear Nose and Throat clinic at a county hospital in the southeast of Sweden were recruited. CPAP initiation followed clinical routines and Auto-CPAP, humidifier, and a nasal or full face mask (ResMed; Sweden) were used with the intention to treat during all hours of sleep. There was an initial visit to a physician and thereafter four visits to a nurse during the first year (i.e., initiation meeting and followup after 2 weeks, 6 months, and 12 months.) Exclusion criteria were terminal disease, severe psychiatric disease, dementia, alcohol/drug abuse, or difficulties reading and understanding the Swedish language. The study, following the Helsinki declaration, was approved by the ethics committee (study code M29-07) at the University of Linköping, Sweden, and all participants provided informed consent.

2.4. Data Collection

2.4.1. Clinical Variables. At baseline a physician examined the patient and data regarding sleep related symptoms, body composition, blood pressure, medication, and comorbidities were collected. Diagnosis of diabetes mellitus was based on history, current treatment (oral therapy or insulin), or repeated fasting blood glucose values ≥7 mmol/L. Ischemic heart disease was defined as a history of angina pectoris and/or myocardial infarction and/or coronary angioplasty and/or coronary bypass surgery. Respiratory disease was defined as a history of asthma or chronic obstructive pulmonary disease or current treatment with β^2 agonists and/or inhaled corticosteroids. Objective adherence to CPAP treatment (minutes/night) was obtained from the CPAP device after 12 months. A cutoff of CPAP use >4 h/night was also used to establish adherence.

2.4.2. Self-Rating Scales. The CHI-5 was administered after 6 months. Three other measures were used, for sample description purposes.

The well-validated Epworth Sleepiness Scale (ESS) was used at baseline to measure excessive daytime sleepiness [32]. The eight items (i.e., different daily situations in which the subjects are asked to rate the likeliness of dozing or falling asleep) are rated on a scale of 0–3, where high scores indicate a greater propensity of falling asleep. The total score ranges from 0 to 24 points, with a cut-off of >10 indicating excessive daytime sleepiness.

The side effects to CPAP inventory (SECI) was used after 6 months to measure CPAP side effects [12]. A five-point Likert-type scale, with scores ranging from 1 to 5, is used for frequency, magnitude, and perceived impact on adherence of a list of 15 different side effects. The total score for each SECI scale ranges from 15 to 75 with a higher score indicating a higher frequency, a higher magnitude, and a stronger impact on adherence.

The attitudes to CPAP inventory (ACTI) was used after two weeks to measure attitudes to CPAP treatment [17]. The five items are rated on a scale of 1–5 giving a total score ranging from 5 to 25 with a higher score indicating a more negative attitude to CPAP treatment.

2.4.3. Statistical Processing and Analysis. Normally distributed clinical variables on an interval scale were analysed with parametric statistics. The homogeneity of the items was evaluated by calculating item-total correlations for overlap. Correlations above 0.3 were defined as satisfactory. In addition, Cronbach's alpha if item deleted was evaluated [33]. Ceiling and floor effects were evaluated by inspection of frequency of endorsement for the item response alternatives. The D'Agostino-Pearson test was applied to test the normality distribution of the CHI-5 [34].

Exploratory factor analysis (principal component factoring) was performed on 6-month data to investigate the dimensionality among the items [35]. Data were first examined with Bartlett's test of sphericity ($\chi^2(10) = 510.1$, $P < 0.001$) and with Kaiser-Meyer Olkin measure (KMO) in each item (0.79–0.96) and all items together (0.86). All these examinations indicated great sampling adequacy. Horn's parallel analysis (1000 repetitions) was conducted to decide number of factors.

Nested linear regression models were conducted to explore if habits could predict long-term CPAP adherence. In an initial model, total hours of CPAP use and days of CPAP use >4 h/night were regressed by habits (CHI-5). To control for theoretically sound predictors of adherence [5], OSA severity (AHI), excessive daytime sleepiness (ESS score), attitudes to CPAP (ACTI), and side effects of CPAP (SECI) were included as covariates in a full model.

All statistical analyses were performed with STATA 13.1 (StataCorp LP, College Station, TX, USA).

3. Results

3.1. Description of Study Population. Table 2 shows demographic and clinical data of the study population. The mean age of the population was 57.8 (SD 6.7) years and 56% were males. Ischemic heart disease and hypercholesterolemia were the most common comorbidities and occurred among 75% and 34% of the participants, respectively. Mean AHI was 26.7 (SD 19.8). After the six-month follow-up was done 29 patients (i.e., 25% of the initial patients) decided to stop using the CPAP. Before the 12-month follow-up 16 additional patients (i.e., 18% of the remaining patients) decided to drop out. At the 12-month follow-up 20 of the remaining CPAP users did not have data regarding CHI-5 and were therefore not included in the linear regression models. Thus, 52 patients (i.e., 44% of the included patients) remained after 12 months. Table 2 shows CPAP use after 2 weeks, 6 months, and 12 months. The mean CHI-5 score (11.04; SD 5.53) was around the scale midpoint, indicating moderate typical habit strength among the sample.

3.2. Is the CHI-5 Internally Consistent? There was a cumulative, but consistent response pattern for the five CHI items, with the majority of patients scoring strongly agree or agree. No response alternative had a greater frequency of endorsement than 48%. According to the coefficient of variation, the greatest variability was demonstrated for item 3, CV = 0.61 (Table 3). The CHI-5 total score showed a positively skew distributed and deviated significantly from a normal distribution ($\chi^2(2) = 9.49$, $P = 0.009$).

TABLE 2: Characteristics of the population before treatment initiation ($n = 117$).

Variables	Total ($n = 117$)
Age, m (sd)	57.8 (6.7)
Gender, n (%)	
Male	66 (56)
Female	51 (44)
Education, n (%)	
6 years	28 (24)
9 years	28 (24)
15 years	32 (27)
>15 years	24 (21)
Unknown	5 (4)
Marital status, n (%)	
Married	92 (79)
Divorced/living alone	18 (15)
Widow/widower	6 (5)
Unknown	1 (1)
Body composition, m (sd)	
Body mass index	30.6 (5.1)
Blood pressure, m (sd)	
Systolic blood pressure	143.4 (18.6)
Diastolic blood pressure	87.8 (11.2)
Comorbidities, n (%)	
IHD	88 (75)
Hypercholesterolemia	40 (34)
Diabetes	20 (17)
Respiratory disease	6 (5)
Smoking, n (%)	
Smoking	16 (14)
Exsmoker	26 (22)
Nonsmoker	75 (64)
Obstructive sleep apnea, m (sd)	
AHI	26.7 (19.8)
ODI	24.8 (19.2)
Mean saturation	93.3 (1.7)
Self-rated sleep, m (sd)	
Sleep duration, hours	6.8 (1.1)
Daytime sleepiness	
Total ESS score, m (sd)	8.1 (4.4)
ESS ≥ 10, n (%)	40 (34)
CPAP use	
Hours/night after 2 weeks ($n = 117$), m (sd)	4.92 (2.3)
>4 hours/night after 2 weeks ($n = 117$), n (%)	74 (63)
Hours/night after 6 months ($n = 117$), m (sd)	4.63 (2.9)
>4 hours/night after 6 months ($n = 117$), n (%)	87 (74)
Hours/night after 12 months ($n = 72$), m (sd)	5.75 (1.6)
>4 hours/night after 12 months ($n = 72$), n (%)	61 (85)

Key: AHI: apnea-hypopnea index; ESS: Epworth sleepiness scale; IHD: ischaemic heart disease; ODI: oxygen desaturation index.

The homogeneity of items was satisfactory with significant ($P < 0.001$) interitem correlations between 0.42 and 0.93 (Table 4) and item-total correlations between 0.58 and 0.91

TABLE 3: Item analysis of the CPAP Habit Index-5 after 6 months of CPAP use ($n = 116$)[1].

Items	Item statistics			Item score distribution				
	Mean (SD)	CV	ITC	1	2	3	4	5
(1) Using the CPAP nightly is part of my routines a normal week	2.02 (1.22)	0.603	0.881	56 (48.3)	25 (21.6)	17 (14.7)	13 (11.2)	5 (4.3)
(2) A special reason is needed if I'm not going to use the CPAP during a normal night	2.16 (1.32)	0.614	0.580	49 (42.2)	34 (29.3)	9 (7.8)	14 (12.1)	10 (8.6)
(3) I have used the CPAP nightly for a long time	2.28 (1.28)	0.561	0.855	46 (39.7)	23 (19.8)	21 (18.1)	21 (18.1)	5 (4.3)
(4) It feels weird not to use the CPAP during a normal night	2.50 (1.33)	0.534	0.716	37 (31.9)	25 (21.6)	23 (19.8)	21 (18.1)	10 (8.6)
(5) I use the CPAP more or less automatically during a normal night	2.09 (1.25)	0.597	0.913	53 (45.7)	25 (21.6)	18 (15.5)	14 (12.1)	6 (5.2)
Total score	11.04 (5.53)	0.501						

CV: coefficient of variation; ITC: item total correlations.
[1]One participant excluded according to missing data in item no 3.

TABLE 4: Homogeneity and factor structure among items of the CPAP Habit Index-5 after 6 months of CPAP use ($n = 116$)[1].

Items	Interitem correlations					Factor analysis	
	1	2	3	4	5	Factor	Uniqueness
(1) Using the CPAP nightly is part of my routines a normal week	0.818[b]					0.936	0.124
(2) A special reason is needed if I'm not going to use the CPAP during a normal night	0.585***	0.955[b]				0.700	0.511
(3) I have used the CPAP nightly for a long time	0.887***	0.591***	0.918[b]			0.918	0.157
(4) It feels weird not to use the CPAP during a normal night	0.696***	0.421***	0.710***	0.896[b]		0.822	0.324
(5) I use the CPAP more or less automatically during a normal night	0.929***	0.593***	0.846***	0.753***	0.792[b]	0.955	0.088
Explained variance						0.759	
Kaiser-Meyer-Olkin						0.859	
Bartlett test of sphericity						$\chi^2 (10) = 510.1, <0.001$	
Cronbach's α						0.915	
Cronbach's α 95% CI[a]						0.878/0.941	

[a]Bias-corrected (based on bootstrapping with 1000 replications)
[b]Measure of sampling adequacy.
[1]One participant excluded according to missing data in item no 3.
***$P < 0.001$.

(Table 3). Internal consistency, measured with Cronbach's alpha, was 0.92 (95% CI = 0.88–0.94) (Table 4).

3.3. Does the CHI-5 Have a Unidimensional Factor Structure? Horn's parallel analysis supported a one-factor solution which was in congruence with the Kaiser criteria with eigenvalues >1. The one factor structure based on data after 6 months explained 76% of the total variance (Table 4). The factor loadings were strong for all items (0.70–0.96) and the uniqueness was in general low and did not exceed the common and critical rule of >0.7 (0.09–0.51).

3.4. Does the CHI-5 Predict Long-Term Adherence to CPAP Treatment? A significant association ($P < 0.001$) was shown between habit strength after 6 months and CPAP adherence after 12 months, for both total CPAP use in hours and

days of CPAP use >4 h/night (Table 5). These associations remained when covariates (i.e., OSA severity and excessive daytime sleepiness at baseline, attitudes to CPAP treatment after 2 weeks, and side effects of CPAP treatment after 6 months) were included in the full models. Habit strength after 6 months explained 63% of the variance in total CPAP use in hours after 12 months. The corresponding figure concerning days of CPAP use >4 h/night was 60%. None of the covariates were significantly associated with any of the dependent variables in the full models.

4. Discussion

This study aimed to validate an index tapping the habitual nature of CPAP use among CPAP treated patients with OSA. The index, an adapted version of the SRHI called the CHI-5, showed satisfactory validity and reliability, and CHI-5 data at

TABLE 5: The association between habits after 6 months and CPAP adherence at 12 months ($n = 52$).

Dependent variable	Independent variables	Initial model		Full model	
		B (se)	95% CI	B (se)	95% CI
Total hours of CPAP use $n = 52$	(i) Habits	-132.3 (14.3)***	$-161.1/-103.5$	-141.9 (15.6)***	$-173.3/-110.5$
	(ii) OSA severity at baseline			-4.0 (2.7)	$-9.5/1.5$
	(iii) Excessive daytime sleepiness at baseline			-11.7 (15.5)	$-42.8/19.4$
	(iv) Attitudes to CPAP treatment after 2 weeks			5.8 (21.0)	$-36.4/48.1$
	(v) Side effects of CPAP treatment after 6 months			15.6 (10.6)	$-6.0/37.2$
	Model statistics	$F(1, 50) = 85.10, P < 0.001, R^2 = 0.63$		$F(5, 46) = 18.94, P < 0.001, R^2 = 0.67$	
Days of CPAP use over 4 h/night $n = 52$	(i) Habits	-18.4 (2.1)***	$-22.6/-14.1$	-19.9 (2.3)***	$-24.5/-15.3$
	(ii) OSA severity at baseline			-0.5 (0.4)	$-1.3/0.3$
	(iii) Excessive daytime sleepiness at baseline			-1.2 (2.3)	$-5.8/3.4$
	(iv) Attitudes to CPAP treatment after 2 weeks			2.1 (3.1)	$-4.1/8.4$
	(v) Side effects of CPAP treatment after 6 months			1.6 (1.6)	$-1.6/4.8$
	Model statistics	$F(1, 50) = 76.44, P < 0.001, R^2 = 0.60$		$F(5, 46) = 16.60, P < 0.001, R^2 = 0.64$	

*** $P < 0.001$.

6 months was strongly predictive of CPAP use at 12 months. Findings suggest that habit is relevant to CPAP adherence and that the CHI-5 is sensitive to habit.

4.1. Validity of the CHI-5. The CHI-5 was adapted from the SRHI by a multiprofessional expert panel supported by established CPAP users. Our intention was to develop a parsimonious and conceptually clear tool to capture CPAP adherence habits in clinical practice. Researchers and clinicians have proposed that the effects of habit on behaviour can be attributed to automaticity [19, 30]: while habits arise from and are expressed in repeated performance, the reason that habits prompt behaviour is because they are automated. Commentators have thus reasoned that indicators of frequency are conceptually redundant within a habit index, as the contribution of past behaviour to habit should be adequately reflected by items pertaining to the automaticity with which action proceeds [29]. However, we chose to include behavioural frequency items within the CHI-5 scale, to help distinguish habit from other types of automatic actions which do not develop through repeated performance [30]. Our item selection strategy seems to have been successful, as the five items showed favourable face validity (i.e., comprehensibility, readability, clarity, and layout) among 20 patients with CPAP treated OSAS, and strong item-total and interitem correlations were observed. The composite five-item scale was also found to have a single-factor structure that explained 76% of variation in item scores, indicating unidimensionality. These results suggest that the CHI-5 is a psychometrically sound measurement instrument.

4.2. Clinical Applications of the CHI-5. Adherence to CPAP-treatment is a multifaceted problem [11] and low adherence to long-term treatment is well-documented. Theory and empirical evidence suggest that habit strength predicts the frequency with which behaviour is enacted [27], and our data suggested that habit strength predicts long-term adherence to CPAP treatment in patients with OSA. We could explain two-thirds of the variance in total CPAP use in hours after 12 months by using the CHI-5 score after 6 months, though explained variance was slightly lower when using a cut-off for adherence of >4 h/night. Furthermore, the strong impact of habit strength on objective adherence after 12 months was not altered when controlling for objective or self-assessed covariates that have previously been identified as predictors of adherence (i.e., OSA severity at baseline, excessive daytime sleepiness at baseline, improvement of ESS score after 6 months, attitude to CPAP treatment after two weeks, and side effects to CPAP treatment after 6 months).

An increased number of patients with severe OSA will need CPAP over the following years [1]. It is therefore of great importance to identify those patients where habit development might become a problem. Factors that might influence adherence include disease and patient characteristics, treatment titration procedures, technological device factors, and side effects, as well as psychological and social factors [18, 36]. Markers for the severity of OSA, such as the AHI, are of importance for the choice of a suitable treatment but are only weakly correlated with self-reported symptom severity and quality of life [5]. In the present study, although a high degree of dropout was observed, the baseline AHI, daytime sleepiness, and attitude towards treatment did not have any significant association to objective CPAP use after 12 months. As argued by Weaver and Grunstein [5], the patients' perceptions of their life situation may not automatically reveal the objective severity of the illness or the need for treatment and may therefore not be of importance for the development of habits. However, patients describe desires to avoid symptoms, knowledge about risks, fears of negative social consequences, and positive attitudes to CPAP treatment as facilitators for adherence [11]. In the present study attitude to CPAP treatment after 2 weeks did not have a significant association to CPAP use after 12 months. Cognitive interventions (i.e., CBT) have proved to be of importance for adherence [18].

OSA can cause severe impairments of the whole life situation for both the patient and partner before, as well as during the first period of CPAP treatment [5]. Developing a desirable habit (i.e., to start using the CPAP as a routine every night during the first month) or breaking an undesirable habit (i.e., to take up or increase the CPAP use after a period of nonadherence) can be difficult [11] but may be pertinent to promoting adherence. Low habit strength might, according to our findings, have a detrimental impact on long-term CPAP adherence. Verplanken [37] stresses that habit formation takes time and is facilitated by stability and repetition. Habits form in an asymptotic manner, with early repetitions leading to greatest gains in habit, which then reduce over time as a habit strength plateau is reached [38]. The degree of dedication to routine CPAP use during the early stages of formation may influence the sustainability of the behaviour and as long as the patient retains the CPAP device during the early initiation period, habit development will remain possible. The effects of different types of spousal support [39] have been studied in relation to adherence to CPAP and could be of importance for habit formation. We did not measure spousal support, but a supporting spouse might help to create a stable psychosocial environment, as well as positive cues that can be triggered for repetition and habit development. The interaction between healthcare personnel and patient can also be of importance but has not been studied in a habitual perspective. Olsen et al. [40], however, showed that motivational interviewing can improve adherence. Furthermore, communication patterns and shared decision making [41] have proved important for adherence in other patient groups and may be of importance in targeted interventions to develop a habitual CPAP use.

While we sought to validate the CHI-5 partly via exploration of its utility as a predictor of long-term CPAP adherence, the index has other clinically relevant applications. The scale could be administered repeatedly during the initiation process, for example, before each scheduled follow-up visit, to identify which CPAP users who are likely to require extra educational and emotional support. It can together with other instruments, such as SECI and ACTI, add important information regarding the patient perspective especially in the beginning of the initiation procedure (i.e., the early habit formation). CHI-5 is likely to be sensitive to the habit formation process. Although often conceived as a dichotomous variable (habit versus no habit), habit strength is better portrayed on a continuum [42]. A study in which participants were asked to repeat a behaviour daily and to self-report the automaticity of the behaviour found that an abbreviated version of the SRHI was sensitive to increases in habit strength with repetition [38]. The CHI-5 is likely to be useful for offering a potential explanation for low adherence among CPAP patients with low habit strength. Given the strong association observed between self-reported CPAP use habit and CPAP adherence rates, habit formation represents an important goal for CPAP users. While our data illustrate the power of habit to predict behaviour, our design, whereby habit was measured only at 6 months after initiation of CPAP treatment, precluded examination of the processes and duration of CPAP habit formation. Further work is needed to document the processes, as well as factors of importance for habit formation in CPAP.

4.3. Limitations. This is, to our knowledge, the first study that examines habits in CPAP treated patients. No other suitable instrument for measuring habits in this context is available. The drop-out rate was fairly high during the study. A larger sample might have led to a greater variation in the response pattern. According to general recommendations for 10 observations per item, the sample size was adequate for the validation analyses of the CHI-5 [34], but the sample was relatively small for regression analyses limiting the possibilities to include other potential predictors (e.g., age, gender, and educational level). Yet, despite this, habit was identified as a significant predictor for long-term CPAP adherence, even where controlling for four covariates, testifying to the unique and strong contribution of habit to CPAP use.

5. Conclusion

This is the first study investigating the reliability and predictive validity of a questionnaire measuring habits in relation to CPAP treatment. Acceptable measurement properties indicate that the CHI-5 can be used to measure habits to CPAP treatment in patients with OSA when intervening to improve adherence. Compared to other constructs, habits seem to hold great importance for CPAP adherence. Although more research is needed to show it conclusively, the present study indicates that focusing on habit-strengthening interventions in the education of patients, as well as in the education of healthcare personnel in charge of the CPAP initiation, offers a new and potentially important component for increasing CPAP adherence.

Conflict of Interests

The authors declare that there is no conflict of interests regarding the publication of this paper.

References

[1] A. I. Pack and T. Gislason, "Obstructive sleep apnea and cardiovascular disease. A perspective and future directions," *Progress in Cardiovascular Diseases*, vol. 51, no. 5, pp. 434–451, 2009.

[2] M. A. Martínez-García, F. Campos-Rodríguez, P. Catalán-Serra et al., "Cardiovascular mortality in obstructive sleep apnea in the elderly: role of long-term continuous positive airway pressure treatment: a prospective observational study," *American Journal of Respiratory and Critical Care Medicine*, vol. 186, pp. 909–916, 2012.

[3] J. M. Marin, S. J. Carrizo, E. Vicente, and A. G. N. Agusti, "Long-term cardiovascular outcomes in men with obstructive sleep apnoea-hypopnoea with or without treatment with continuous positive airway pressure: an observational study," *The Lancet*, vol. 365, no. 9464, pp. 1046–1053, 2005.

[4] L. J. Epstein, D. Kristo, P. J. Strollo Jr. et al., "Clinical guideline for the evaluation, management and long-term care of obstructive sleep apnea in adults," *Journal of Clinical Sleep Medicine*, vol. 5, no. 3, pp. 263–276, 2009.

[5] T. E. Weaver and R. R. Grunstein, "Adherence to continuous positive airway pressure therapy: the challenge to effective treatment," *Proceedings of the American Thoracic Society*, vol. 5, no. 2, pp. 173–178, 2008.

[6] S. Olsen, S. Smith, and T. P. S. Oei, "Adherence to continuous positive airway pressure therapy in obstructive sleep apnoea sufferers: a theoretical approach to treatment adherence and intervention," *Clinical Psychology Review*, vol. 28, no. 8, pp. 1355–1371, 2008.

[7] A. M. Sawyer, N. S. Gooneratne, C. L. Marcus, D. Ofer, K. C. Richards, and T. E. Weaver, "A systematic review of CPAP adherence across age groups: clinical and empiric insights for developing CPAP adherence interventions," *Sleep Medicine Reviews*, vol. 15, no. 6, pp. 343–356, 2011.

[8] N. B. Kribbs, A. I. Pack, L. R. Kline et al., "Objective measurement of patterns of nasal CPAP use by patients with obstructive sleep apnea," *American Review of Respiratory Disease*, vol. 147, no. 4, pp. 887–895, 1993.

[9] A. Brostrom, A. Strömberg, J. Mårtensson, M. Ulander, L. Harder, and E. Svanborg, "Association of Type D personality to perceived side effects and adherence in CPAP-treated patients with OSAS," *Journal of Sleep Research*, vol. 16, no. 4, pp. 439–447, 2007.

[10] A. Brostrom, A. Strömberg, M. Ulander, B. Fridlund, J. Mårtensson, and E. Svanborg, "Perceived informational needs, side-effects and their consequences on adherence—a comparison between CPAP treated patients with OSAS and healthcare personnel," *Patient Education and Counseling*, vol. 74, no. 2, pp. 228–235, 2009.

[11] A. Brostrom, P. Nilsen, P. Johansson et al., "Putative facilitators and barriers for adherence to CPAP treatment in patients with obstructive sleep apnea syndrome: a qualitative content analysis," *Sleep Medicine*, vol. 11, no. 2, pp. 126–130, 2010.

[12] A. Brostrom, K. F. Årestedt, P. Nilsen, A. Strömberg, M. Ulander, and E. Svanborg, "The side-effects to CPAP treatment inventory: the development and initial validation of a new tool for the measurement of side-effects to CPAP treatment," *Journal of Sleep Research*, vol. 19, no. 4, pp. 603–611, 2010.

[13] I. Smith, V. Nadig, and T. J. Lasserson, "Educational, supportive and behavioural interventions to improve usage of continuous positive airway pressure machines for adults with obstructive sleep apnoea," *Cochrane Database of Systematic Reviews*, no. 2, Article ID CD007736, 2009.

[14] A. M. Moran, D. E. Everhart, C. E. Davis, K. L. Wuensch, D. O. Lee, and H. A. Demaree, "Personality correlates of adherence with continuous positive airway pressure (CPAP)," *Sleep and Breathing*, vol. 15, no. 4, pp. 687–694, 2011.

[15] S. Olsen, S. Smith, T. Oei, and J. Douglas, "Health belief model predicts adherence to CPAP before experience with CPAP," *European Respiratory Journal*, vol. 32, no. 3, pp. 710–717, 2008.

[16] C. Poulet, D. Veale, N. Arnol, P. Lévy, J. L. Pepin, and J. Tyrrell, "Psychological variables as predictors of adherence to treatment by continuous positive airway pressure," *Sleep Medicine*, vol. 10, no. 9, pp. 993–999, 2009.

[17] A. Brostrom, M. Ulander, P. Nilsen, E. Svanborg, and K. F. Årestedt, "The attitudes to CPAP treatment inventory: development and initial validation of a new tool for measuring attitudes to CPAP treatment," *Journal of Sleep Research*, vol. 20, no. 3, pp. 460–471, 2011.

[18] A. M. Sawyer, A. Canamucio, H. Moriarty, T. E. Weaver, K. C. Richards, and S. T. Kuna, "Do cognitive perceptions influence CPAP use?" *Patient Education and Counseling*, vol. 85, no. 1, pp. 85–91, 2011.

[19] P. Nilsen, B. Gardner, and A. Brostrom, "Accounting for the role of habit in lifestyle intervention research," *European Journal of Cardiovascular Nursing*, vol. 12, pp. 5–6, 2013.

[20] T. L. Webb and P. Sheeran, "Does changing behavioral intentions engender behavior change? A meta-analysis of the experimental evidence," *Psychological Bulletin*, vol. 132, no. 2, pp. 249–268, 2006.

[21] C. J. Armitage, "Can the theory of planned behavior predict the maintenance of physical activity?" *Health Psychology*, vol. 24, no. 3, pp. 235–245, 2005.

[22] B. Gardner, "A review and analysis of the use of "habit" in understanding, predicting and influencing health-related behaviour," *Health Psychology Review*, 2014.

[23] B. Verplanken and W. Wood, "Interventions to break and create consumer habits," *Journal of Public Policy and Marketing*, vol. 25, no. 1, pp. 90–103, 2006.

[24] B. Verplanken, "Habits and implementation intentions," in *ABC of Behavior Change*, J. Kerr, R. Weitkunat, and M. Moretti, Eds., pp. 99–111, Elsevier, London, UK, 2005.

[25] P. Lally, J. Wardle, and B. Gardner, "Experiences of habit formation: a qualitative study," *Psychology, Health and Medicine*, vol. 16, no. 4, pp. 484–489, 2011.

[26] H. Triandis, *Interpersonal Behavior*, Brooks-Cole, Monterey, Calif, USA, 1977.

[27] P. Lally and B. Gardner, "Promoting habit formation," *Health Psychology Review*, vol. 7, supplement 1, pp. S137–S158, 2013.

[28] B. Gardner, G.-J. de Bruijn, and P. Lally, "A systematic review and meta-analysis of applications of the self-report habit index to nutrition and physical activity behaviours," *Annals of Behavioral Medicine*, vol. 42, no. 2, pp. 174–187, 2011.

[29] B. Verplanken and S. Orbell, "Reflections on past behavior: a self-report index of habit strength," *Journal of Applied Social Psychology*, vol. 33, no. 6, pp. 1313–1330, 2003.

[30] B. Gardner, C. Abraham, P. Lally, and G. J. de Bruijn, "Towards parsimony in habit measurement: testing the convergent and predictive validity of an automaticity subscale of the Self-Report Habit Index," *International Journal of Behavioral Nutrition and Physical Activity*, vol. 10, article 102, 2012.

[31] P. S. Jones, J. W. Lee, L. R. Phillips, X. E. Zhang, and K. B. Jaceldo, "An adaptation of Brislin's translation model for cross-cultural research," *Nursing Research*, vol. 50, no. 5, pp. 300–304, 2001.

[32] M. W. Johns, "A new method for measuring daytime sleepiness: the Epworth sleepiness scale," *Sleep*, vol. 14, no. 6, pp. 540–545, 1991.

[33] J. C. Nunnally and I. H. Bernstein, *Psychometric Theory*, McGraw-Hill, New York, NY, USA, 1994.

[34] M. A. Pett, N. R. Lackey, and J. J. Sullivan, *Making Sense of Factor Analysis: the Use of Factor Analysis for Instrument Development in Health Care Research*, SAGE, Thousand Oaks, Calif, USA, 2003.

[35] G. Norman and D. Streiner, *Biostatistics: the Bare Essentials*, B.C. Decker, London, UK, 3rd edition, 2008.

[36] M. Diaz-Abad, W. Chatila, M. R. Lammi, I. Swift, G. E. D'Alonzo, and S. L. Krachman, "Determinants of CPAP adherence in Hispanics with obstructive sleep apnea," *Sleep Disorders*, vol. 2014, Article ID 878213, 6 pages, 2014.

[37] B. Verplanken, "Beyond frequency: habit as mental construct," *British Journal of Social Psychology*, vol. 45, no. 3, pp. 639–656, 2006.

[38] P. Lally, C. H. M. van Jaarsveld, H. W. W. Potts, and J. Wardle, "How are habits formed: modelling habit formation in the real world," *European Journal of Social Psychology*, vol. 40, no. 6, pp. 998–1009, 2010.

[39] M. Elfström, S. Karlsson, P. Nilsen, B. Fridlund, E. Svanborg, and A. Broström, "Decisive situations affecting partners' support to continuous positive airway pressure-treated patients with obstructive sleep apnea syndrome: a critical incident technique analysis of the initial treatment phase," *Journal of Cardiovascular Nursing*, vol. 27, no. 3, pp. 228–239, 2012.

[40] S. Olsen, S. S. Smith, T. P. Oei, and J. Douglas, "Motivational interviewing (MINT) improves continuous positive airway pressure (CPAP) acceptance and adherence: a randomized controlled trial," *Journal of Consulting and Clinical Psychology*, vol. 80, pp. 151–163.

[41] C. Charles, A. Gafni, and T. Whelan, "Shared decision-making in the medical encounter: what does it mean? (Or it takes, at least two to tango)," *Social Science and Medicine*, vol. 44, no. 5, pp. 681–692, 1997.

[42] A. Moors and J. de Houwer, "Automaticity: a theoretical and conceptual analysis," *Psychological Bulletin*, vol. 132, no. 2, pp. 297–326, 2006.

16

Melatonin Supplementation in Patients with Complete Tetraplegia and Poor Sleep

Jo Spong,[1] Gerard A. Kennedy,[1,2] Douglas J. Brown,[3]
Stuart M. Armstrong,[4,5] and David J. Berlowitz[1]

[1] Institute for Breathing and Sleep, Austin Hospital, Heidelberg, VIC 3084, Australia
[2] School of Social Sciences & Psychology, Victoria University, St. Albans, VIC 3021, Australia
[3] Victorian Spinal Cord Service, Austin Hospital, Heidelberg, VIC 3084, Australia
[4] Brain Sciences Institute, Swinburne University, Hawthorn, VIC 3122, Australia
[5] The Bronowski Institute of Behavioural Neuroscience, Kyneton, VIC 3444, Australia

Correspondence should be addressed to David J. Berlowitz; david.berlowitz@austin.org.au

Academic Editor: Liborio Parrino

People with complete tetraplegia have interrupted melatonin production and commonly report poor sleep. Whether the two are related is unclear. This pilot study investigated whether nightly supplementation of 3 mg melatonin would improve objective and subjective sleep in tetraplegia. Five participants with motor and sensory complete tetraplegia ingested 3 mg melatonin (capsule) two hours prior to usual sleep time for two weeks. Full portable sleep studies were conducted in participants' homes on the night before commencing melatonin supplementation (baseline) and on the last night of the supplementation period. Endogenous melatonin levels were determined by assaying saliva samples collected the night of (just prior to sleep) and morning after (upon awakening) each sleep study. Prior to each sleep study measures of state sleepiness and sleep behaviour were collected. The results showed that 3 mg of melatonin increased salivary melatonin from near zero levels at baseline in all but one participant. A delay in time to Rapid Eye Movement sleep, and an increase in stage 2 sleep were observed along with improved subjective sleep experience with a reduction in time to fall asleep, improved quality of sleep and fewer awakenings during the night reported. Daytime sleepiness increased however. A randomised, placebo controlled trial with a larger sample is required to further explore and confirm these findings.

1. Introduction

For people living with tetraplegia, excessive daytime sleepiness, disturbed and poor quality sleep are a common problem [1]. A number of factors contribute to disturbed sleep in people with tetraplegia with the absence of increase in evening endogenous melatonin production after a complete cervical spinal cord injury (SCI) [2, 3] potentially being one. Melatonin is secreted nocturnally by the pineal gland and is believed to play a major modulatory role in the timing of circadian rhythms including the sleep-wake cycle [4]. The daily rhythm of melatonin secretion is regulated by an endogenous pacemaker, the suprachiasmatic nucleus (SCN, "circadian clock") which signals the pineal gland via a circuitous route involving other hypothalamic nuclei, brain stem nuclei,

the spinal cord, and peripheral sympathetic neurons from the superior cervical ganglion (SCG) [4]. Melatonin levels typically begin to increase two to three hours before sleep with peak levels between 02:00 and 04:00 and trough levels during the day [4].

Melatonin secretion following a SCI is low or abolished in those with complete tetraplegia, but relatively normal in those with complete paraplegia [2, 3, 5–7]. This suggests that the neural pathway controlling melatonin secretion passes through the cervical spinal cord and is interrupted between the SCN and the SCG. The fibres to the SCG are routed along with those of the autonomic nervous system and thus are disrupted in a manner analogous to the disruption that causes autonomic dysfunction [8]. Only one study has investigated the effect of abolished melatonin secretion on sleep in tetraplegia [9]. The study showed that total sleep time (TST) and sleep efficiency were significantly reduced, and rapid eye movement (REM) latency significantly delayed in complete tetraplegia compared with paraplegia. It was suggested that melatonin supplementation might assist in the restoration of normal sleep in people with tetraplegia [9].

Timed daily doses of melatonin in able-bodied people have been shown to reduce sleep onset time, improve sleep maintenance, increase REM sleep, and correct circadian based insomnias [10–15]. Timed daily administration of exogenous melatonin is also the current treatment of choice for "non-24-hour sleep/wake disorder" (free-running circadian rhythms) in people who are functionally blind and have complete or partial attenuation of ocular light transmission from the retina to the circadian clock [16, 17]. Despite such evidence that melatonin supplementation can improve sleep in able-bodied and blind people, there have been no studies investigating whether melatonin supplementation can improve sleep in people with complete tetraplegia. This pilot study is the first to investigate whether timed, nightly supplementation of 3 mg melatonin affects sleep in tetraplegia.

2. Methods

2.1. Participants. Five people (four male) with complete tetraplegia who had been treated by the Victorian Spinal Cord Service, Australia, were recruited. Patients diagnosed as having "complete" tetraplegia (American Spinal Injuries Association Impairment Scale (AIS) level A) have no motor or sensory function below the lesion level [18]. Two able-bodied participants were recruited to provide melatonin positive controls. Exclusion criteria were a history of major psychological/psychiatric disturbances, neurological damage (other than SCI), and significant comorbidity. Participants did not undertake transmeridian flight prior to or during the study. The project was approved by the Austin Health Human Research Ethics Committee, and all participants provided informed consent before the study began. The study is registered at http://www.anzctr.org.au/ (083167).

2.2. Procedure. Participants completed a 7-day sleep diary recording their intake of medication, caffeine, and alcohol, the type and duration of exercise performed, their bedtime, sleep onset and awakening times, the number of nocturnal awakenings, and the duration of any daytime naps. At the completion of the 7-day sleep diary, participants underwent a baseline sleep study (polysomnography) recorded in their home using a portable sleep monitoring device (Compumedics Somte, Abbottsford, VIC, Australia). Sleep study measures included central electroencephalography (C4/A1, C3/A2), bilateral electrooculography, electromyography (chin and diaphragmatic), electrocardiography, blood oxygen saturation, nasal pressure (airflow), leg movements, body position, and respiratory movements of the chest and abdomen. The portable sleep monitoring device does not contain a light sensor and as such, sleep efficiency and sleep onset latency could not be measured.

Beginning on the evening following the baseline sleep study, participants ingested one 3 mg melatonin capsule every night for two weeks, approximately two hours before their usual sleep time; the typical, natural onset time of endogenous melatonin [19]. The dose of 3 mg of melatonin for supplementation reflected the typical dose of melatonin prescribed in Australia. Participants had standard home lighting which would not have interfered with their melatonin production. On the last night of the two-week melatonin supplementation period, participants underwent a second home sleep study. Sleep was staged in 30-second epochs, arousals marked, respiratory events scored, and summary indices calculated according to international standard criteria [20, 21] by an independent, experienced sleep scientist blinded to treatment phase and participant.

Prior to each sleep study participants completed two questionnaires, the Karolinska Sleepiness Scale (KSS) [22] and the Basic Nordic Sleepiness Questionnaire (BNSQ) [23]. The KSS measures state sleepiness on a 9-point scale where 1 indicates feeling extremely alert and 9 indicates extreme sleepiness. Participants were asked to rate their level of sleepiness at mid-day of the day of each sleep study. The KSS is a more appropriate measure of state sleepiness for this population compared to others which ask questions that are often not applicable to people with this level of disability. The KSS has also been used in previous research investigating sleep in people with tetraplegia [24, 25]. The BNSQ is a general sleep questionnaire that has been validated in the spinal patient population [26]. It assesses sleep behaviour and symptoms of sleep disturbances during the past three months [1, 26] via 14 five-point scale questions (high score indicates a poorer condition or greater frequency) and six quantitative questions. In this study, BNSQ questions 1, 2, and 7 were used to assess sleep initiation, questions 3, 4, and 5 to examine waking behavior during sleep and early morning, questions 8, 9, and 15 to assess sleepiness (typical trait morning and daytime sleepiness), questions 10 and 11 to assess daytime functioning (inability to maintain wakefulness), questions 6, 12, 13, 14, and 20 to assess sleep quality, and questions 16, 17, and 18 to assess the presence of Obstructive Sleep Apnoea (OSA). The BNSQ that was administered on the last night of melatonin supplementation assessed participants' sleep/wake behavior and symptoms of sleep disturbances across the previous two weeks (melatonin supplementation period).

Saliva samples (2–4 mL) were collected just prior to sleep onset on the night of each sleep study and the following morning upon awakening to measure the participants' endogenous melatonin levels. Saliva collected from the two able-bodied participants (melatonin controls) provided an assay reference level. The control participants did not perform any other task in this study.

2.3. Data Analysis. Results from the sleep diary, sleep studies, and questionnaires are summarized as medians (range) and Wilcoxon Signed Rank Test used to compare baseline and melatonin supplementation data. For the 7-day sleep diary, medians for each variable were calculated for each participant and then group medians generated from these values. Missing values on the questionnaire items were generated by calculating the sample average for the specific item. BNSQ items relating to work days were analysed for those known to be in the work force (n = 2). Similarly, BNSQ items relating to OSA were only analysed for those not being treated for OSA. The error range associated with the saliva assay of melatonin is 10.2% (E. Sorich, ARL Pathology, Personal Communication). The reportable concentration levels of the saliva assay ranged between 0.5 and 50 pg/mL. 50 pg/mL was the maximum dilution level for this saliva assay (J. Evans, Healthscope Pathology, Personal Communication).

3. Results

The median (range) age of the tetraplegia participants was 42 years (26–68 yrs), Body Mass Index (kg/m^2) was 20.8 (18.5–32.9), and number of years living with complete tetraplegia was 17.1 years (4.1–23.9 yrs). At the time of the study, three participants had a diagnosis of OSA, two of whom were treated with Continuous Positive Airway Pressure (CPAP) therapy and one with a mandibular advancement splint. All participants continued their usual medications throughout the trial period. The individual characteristics of each participant are presented in Table 1.

3.1. Sleep Diary. Median (range) analyses from the 7-day sleep diary showed that the usual bedtime of the sample was 22:00 h (21:00 h–00:00 h) and time to fall asleep was 15 minutes (1.5–180 mins). The median number of awakenings was one (0–3) where the group would be awake for approximately 15 mins (0 sec–120 mins) before falling back to sleep. Morning wake time was 06:30 h (06:00 h–06:30 h) with a rising out of bed at 07:15 h (06:00 h–08:30 h). The number of naps taken during the day ranged between zero and one. Four participants reported doing exercise (stretches, weights) during the week for between 30 and 120 minutes. Intake of alcohol, drugs, or caffeine during the week was reported by four participants.

3.2. Saliva Samples: Endogenous Melatonin Concentration Levels. Melatonin levels measured at baseline for the tetraplegia sample were essentially zero (Figure 1) in all but participant 3. Supplementation of 3 mg melatonin two hours prior to sleep increased melatonin concentration to levels comparable with those of the positive controls in all but participant 4 (Figure 1).

3.3. Sleep Studies: Objective Sleep. The sleep parameters showing a noticeable change following melatonin supplementation were the proportion of stage two sleep and REM latency. Administration of 3 mg melatonin resulted in a 15.4% increase in the proportion of time spent in stage 2 sleep and a one-hour delay in REM latency (Table 2). Examination of REM latency for each participant (Figure 2) shows that the delay was pronounced for three of the five participants. Conversely, REM latency shortened for participant 5. No statistically significant differences were observed in these trends.

3.4. Questionnaires: Subjective Sleep. Subjective sleep improved following melatonin supplementation (Table 3), specifically for the BNSQ questions regarding sleep initiation (questions 1 and 2(b)), awakenings during the night and early morning (questions 4 and 5), quality of sleep (question 6), and daytime functioning (question 11); however, feeling sleepy during the day increased following melatonin supplementation (questions 8 and 9), as did sleep apnoea symptoms (questions 16 and 18). There was no change in state sleepiness (KSS, Table 3). Individual responses to the sleep-related scaled BNSQ questions showed that those with an increase in salivary melatonin generally reported improved sleep (Figure 3). Conversely, participant 4 who showed no change in salivary melatonin trended towards reporting similar or poorer rather than improved sleep. Only the change in BNSQ 4 following melatonin supplementation reached statistical significance.

4. Discussion

This study replicates earlier reports of reduced melatonin production in people with complete tetraplegia [2, 3]. It also shows that it is possible to increase circulating melatonin concentration levels in people with chronic complete tetraplegia by administering exogenous melatonin and that the increase in melatonin is generally associated with an improved subjective sleep experience.

Although the melatonin concentration levels of the tetraplegia sample were generally low at baseline there was a degree of intersubject variability in our findings. The higher baseline melatonin reading in the morning for participant 3 was unexpected. Possible explanations include preservation of the melatonin pathway and assay variability. The increase in melatonin concentration following supplementation was also variable, with participant 4 showing no observable rise in melatonin at all and the increase in melatonin level for participant 5 only evident in the morning sample. This variability may possibly be due to differences in hepatic catabolism or other changes in metabolism in participants deprived of endogenous melatonin for many years. The results of participants 4 and 5 suggest poor or delayed absorption of melatonin.

Benzodiazepine medication has been found to suppress the nocturnal rise in plasma melatonin or shift its day-night rhythmicity [27]. This drug interaction may also explain why participant 4, who was taking diazepam at the time of this study, had no observable rise in salivary melatonin; however, melatonin concentration increased for participant 3 who was also taking diazepam, suggesting that any drug interaction may have a variable consequence across individuals.

This study has shown that it is possible to increase circulating melatonin levels in people with chronic tetraplegia; however whether such levels are equivalent to or exceed normal nocturnal values is impossible to determine with the limited reportable concentration levels of this saliva assay (i.e., 0.5 to 50 pg/mL).

Despite the increase in saliva melatonin concentration levels, melatonin supplementation did not improve TST or reduce REM latency, the sleep parameters identified in earlier research [9] as being significantly altered for people with

TABLE 1: Individual characteristics of each participant.

Participant code	Sex	Age (yrs)	BMI (kg/m^2)	Injury level and AIS score	Years since SCI	Medications	Treatment
1	M	46	32.9	C5A	23.3	Baclofen, Temazepam	CPAP
2	M	68	27.7	C4A	23.9	Baclofen	CPAP
3	F	28	20.3	C5A	4.10	Baclofen, Diazepam	—
4	M	42	20.8	C6A	17.10	Baclofen, Diazepam	Oral Splint
5	M	26	18.5	C6A	10.10	Baclofen	—
Positive control							
1	M	43	24.8	—	—	—	—
2	F	31	20.7	—	—	—	—

BMI: Body Mass Index, AIS: American Spinal Injury Association Impairment Scale, SCI: Spinal Cord Injury, CPAP: Continuous Positive Airway Pressure.

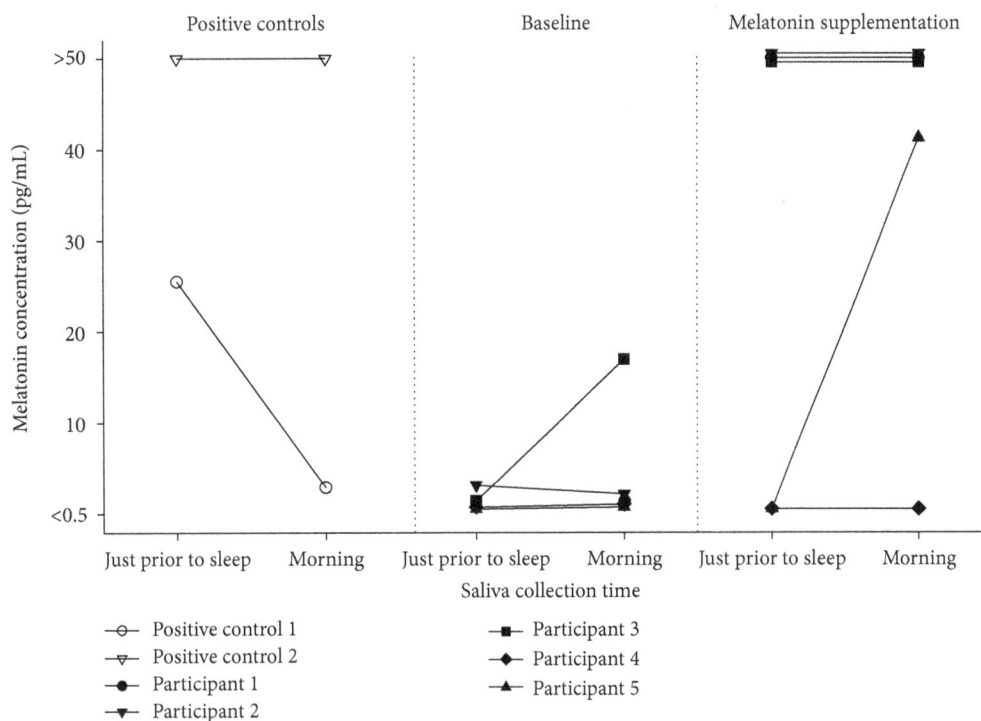

FIGURE 1: Melatonin concentrations (pg/mL) from saliva sampled just prior to sleep and after awakening for the positive controls and for the participants with complete tetraplegia at baseline and two weeks after melatonin supplementation. Note: reportable pg/mL range for this saliva assay was 0.5 to 50. Melatonin concentration values for three participants with a ceiling pg/ml were slightly altered on graph to show visually that three participants obtained this maximum reportable value.

complete tetraplegia. We observed that the TST remained relatively stable and REM latency was increased by a further 60 minutes. Previous authors have found similar prolongation of REM following the administration of one and five mg of melatonin to people with insomnia and healthy participants 15 minutes or two hours prior to bedtime [28, 29]. In both the previous research and the current study, the importance of and the mechanism underlying the delay in REM latency after melatonin supplementation is not clear.

Benzodiazepine medications have been known to delay or suppress REM sleep [30]. Two participants in our trial were taking Diazepam and one taking Temazepam; however any affect on REM latency would be expected to be similar between these participant's baseline and melatonin supplementation sleep studies. Furthermore, an effect of medication does not account for the pronounced delay in REM latency for the participants who were not using benzodiazepines.

The improvement in subjective sleep experience following melatonin supplementation appeared specific to sleep initiation, sleep quality, daytime functioning, and awakenings. There is no evidence to suggest that the improved subjective sleep was due to the chronobiotic (phase shifting) properties of melatonin [31]. Rather, participants may have experienced the hypnotic properties associated with melatonin. Exogenous melatonin may act as a hypnotic by attenuating wake-promoting signals from the SCN [32, 33] and/or as a

TABLE 2: Sleep study findings recorded at baseline (the night before commencing melatonin supplementation) and on last night of two-week melatonin supplementation period.

	Baseline	Melatonin Supplementation
AI	6.2 (3.8–22.5)	5.8 (3.3–33.5)
AHI	7.6 (3.6–57.7)	3.5 (1.2–48.6)
Stage 1%	1.3 (0–4.4)	2.2 (1.7–2.9)
Stage 2%	45.9 (32.7–68.7)	61.3 (40–68.5)
Stage 3%	15.8 (4.1–35.1)	19 (3.4–32.3)
Stage 4%	14.6 (0–30)	10.9 (0–13.4)
Stage REM%	13.1 (7.8–36.1)	14.2 (10.8–25.2)
REM latency	92 (63.5–169.5)	152.5 (66.5–213.5)
TST	332.5 (90–353.5)	338.5 (292–365)
SpO2 < 90%	0.6 (0–37.6)	0.8 (0.4–21.1)
# Awake times	7 (4–24)	7 (4–40)
Time spent awake	16 (6–149)	20 (5–136.5)

Note: values are median (range). AI (Arousal Index) = number of arousals per hour of sleep; AHI (Apnoea/Hypopnoea Index) = number of apnoeas/hypopnoeas per hour of sleep; TST (Total Sleep Time) = minutes sleep; Time spent awake = minutes spent awake during night after first falling asleep. No statistically significant differences were observed between the baseline and melatonin supplementation sleep study parameters.

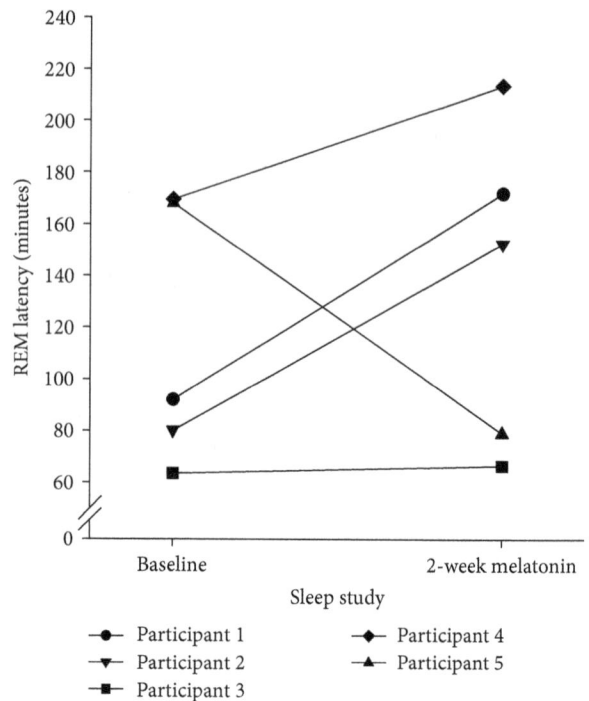

FIGURE 2: Individual REM latencies recorded for each participant at baseline (the night prior to commencing melatonin supplementation) and on last night of two-week melatonin supplementation period.

hypothermic, decreasing body temperature to promote sleep [34, 35]. It is generally accepted that melatonin administered during the day, when endogenous levels are absent, has a sleep-promoting effect [13, 33, 36, 37]. Past research that has administered melatonin closer to the time of habitual sleep in able-bodied subjects, however, has produced less consistent findings [32, 38–40]. In the current study we added exogenous melatonin to a system with no endogenous melatonin, a situation more analogous to daytime administration in the able-bodied and as such, the novel finding of a sedative effect in this situation is perhaps not surprising.

An increase in morning and daytime sleepiness was reported by participants 1 and 4. This observation raises the possibility that chronic tetraplegia may be associated with an alteration in melatonin absorption, metabolism, and/or excretion. Such alteration may have resulted in higher circulating melatonin in these participants during the day and subsequently increased sleepiness. Further understanding and characterizing of the time course of melatonin concentration in people with tetraplegia is required. The determination of Cmax and the half-life of melatonin would help distinguish the delivery time of melatonin for this population.

4.1. Limitations. The use of benzodiazepines, muscle relaxants, or breathing aids is often avoided in sleep research to limit any confounding effects they have on sleep architecture and quality. Unlike the able-bodied population, the prevalence of OSA and other symptoms resulting from the cervical spinal cord injury such as pain and spasm is extremely high [25]. Subsequently the prescription of these medications is very common. The continued use of these medications by participants in this pilot study was allowed in attempt to minimize the effect that these confounding symptoms have on sleep. Further, to not include people who had a diagnosis

of OSA and to exclude those on treatment would severely limit the portion of the tetraplegia population which these results could be generalised to.

The scope of this study did give rise to limitations which future research should consider. This pilot study is limited by the number of saliva samples collected and sleep studies performed. An increase in sampling would not only provide additional, more complete information about the circadian rhythm of melatonin production in people with tetraplegia but would also control for possible night-to-night variability between baseline and postsupplementation testing sessions. Measures of other circadian markers, such as core body temperature, would assist in understanding the effect that melatonin supplementation has on circadian phase in this population.

The nature of the home based setting in this study also gives rise to external variables which could not be controlled. The home based studies were selected for this study due to the logistic difficulties experienced in performing laboratory based studies in this population. Although the study presents data collected in the participants' natural living environment where sleep characteristics are not controlled by laboratory assessment and settings, it is difficult to monitor confounding variables such as diet and temperature. More obviously, this study is also limited by its sample size, which should be increased to validate the trends observed in this study.

This study showed that supplementation of 3 mg melatonin had an effect on both objective and subjective sleep for a person with complete tetraplegia. The improvement in

TABLE 3: Subjective sleep reports the night prior to (baseline) and last night of the two-week melatonin supplementation phase.

	Baseline	Supplementation
KSS	2 (2–4)	2 (1–4)
BNSQ1. Have you had any difficulties in falling asleep?	2 (1–5)	1 (1–3)
BNSQ2. For how long (how many minutes on average) do you stay awake in bed before you fall asleep (after lights out)?		
(a) Working days	5.8 (1.5–10)	5.5 (1–10)
(b) During free time	20 (1.5–60)	15 (1–30)
BNSQ3. How often do you wake up during the night?	5 (4-5)	5 (3–5)
BNSQ4. How many times do you usually wake up in one night?[b]	3 (3-4)	2 (2-3)*
BNSQ5. How often have you awakened very early in the morning without being able to fall back to sleep?	2 (1–3)	1 (1–4)
BNSQ6. How well have you been sleeping?[c]	3 (2–4)	2 (1–3)
BNSQ7. Have you used sleeping pills (by prescription)?	1 (1–5)	1 (1–5)
BNSQ8. Do you feel excessively sleepy in the morning?	1 (1–3)	3 (1–4)
BNSQ9. Do you feel excessively sleepy in the daytime?	1 (1–4)	2 (1–3)
BNSQ10. Have you suffered from an irresistible tendency to fall asleep while at work?	2 (1–3)	2 (1–2)
BNSQ11. Have you suffered from an irresistible tendency to fall asleep during free time?	2 (1–3)	1 (1-2)
BNSQ12. How many hours do you usually sleep per night?	6 (6-7)	6.5 (6-7)
BNSQ13. At what time do you usually go to bed (in order to sleep)?		
(a) During a working week	10:15 pm (9 pm–11:30 pm)	10:50 pm (9:40 pm–12 am)
(b) During free days	11 pm (9 pm–1:30 am)	12 am (9:40 pm–12 am)
BNSQ14. At what time do you usually wake up?		
(a) During a working week	6:30 am	6:30 am
(b) During free days	6:30 am (6:15 am–8 am)	6:30 am (2:30 am–9:30 am)
BNSQ15a. How often do you have a nap during daytime?	1 (1–4)	1 (1–3)
BNSQ15b. If you take a nap, how long does it usually last (minutes)?	40 (20–60)	32.5 (20–45)
BNSQ16. Do you snore while sleeping (ask other people)?	2 (1–3)	3 (1–5)
BNSQ17. In what way do you snore (ask other people about the quality of your snoring)?[d]	3 (1–5)	3 (1–5)
BNSQ18. Have you had breathing pauses (sleep apnoea) during sleep (have other people noticed that you have pauses in respiration when you sleep)?	1	3 (1–5)
BNSQ20. How many hours of sleep do you need per night (how many hours would you sleep if you had the possibility to sleep as long as you need to)?	7 (6–10)	7 (6–10)

*$P < 0.05$. Note: values are medians (range). The basic scale for answer alternatives is as follows: 1 = never or less than once a month; 2 = less than once per week; 3 = on 1-2 days per week; 4 = on 3–5 days per week; 5 = daily or almost daily.[b] Answer alternatives: 1 = usually I don't wake up at night; 2 = once per night; 3 = two times; 4 = 3-4 times; 5 = at least five times per night[c]. Answer alternatives: 1 = well; 2 = rather well; 3 = neither well nor badly; 4 = rather badly; 5 = badly[d]. Answer alternatives: 1 = i don't snore; 2 = my snoring sounds regular and it is of low voice; 3 = it sounds regular but rather loud; 4 = it sounds regular but it is very loud (other people hear my snoring in the next room); 5 = i snore very loud and intermittently (there are silent breathing pauses when snoring is not heard and at times very loud snorts with gasping).

subjective sleep experience suggests that melatonin supplementation may have a therapeutic role in tetraplegia. Due to the recruited sample size, however, only trends could be observed in this study with many changes following supplementation not reaching statistical significance likely due to a lack of statistical power. Therefore a larger, placebo-controlled, randomised trial is required to validate these findings. It would be of benefit to further explore melatonin absorption, the changes in sleep architecture, the apparent hypnotic effects, and the relationships between symptoms

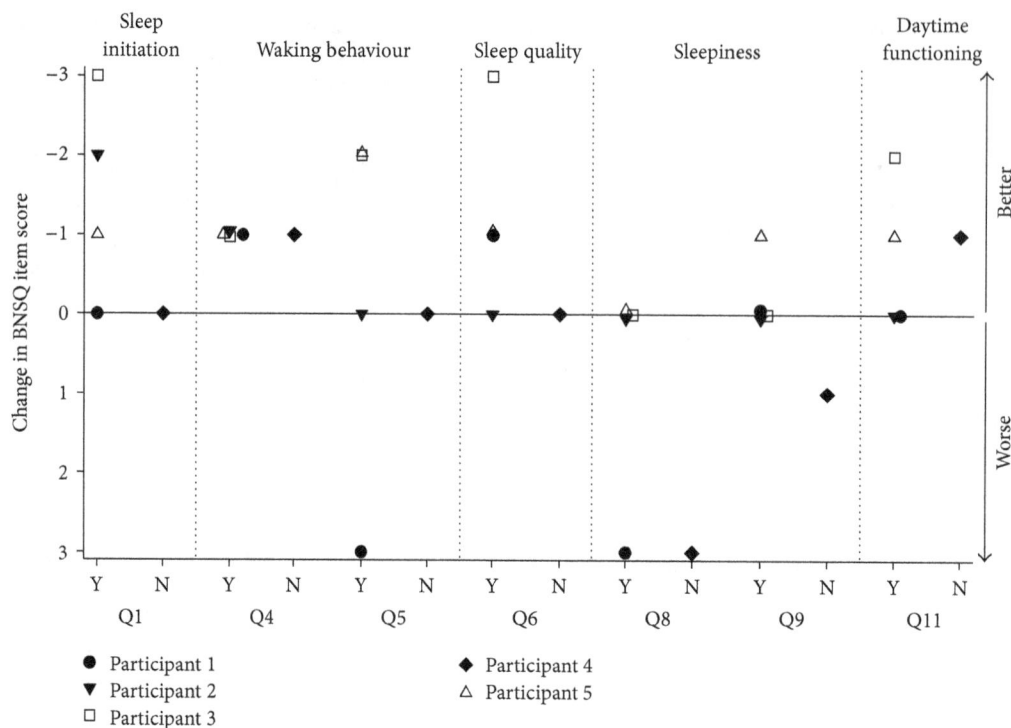

FIGURE 3: Change in individual participant responses to BNSQ scaled questions after two weeks of melatonin supplementation. Y = participants who showed an increase in melatonin concentration levels, N = the participant with no change in melatonin concentration level. Negative scores indicate improvement on the BNSQ item; positive scores indicate poorer sleep experience or functioning, 0 represents no change.

and sleep architecture that 3 mg melatonin supplementation has on people with SCI.

Conflict of Interests

Professor S. M. Armstrong is a member of the advisory board to Lundbeck (Australia). Dr. J. Spong, Dr. G. A. Kennedy, Associate Professor D. J. Brown and Dr. D. J. Berlowitz declare no potential conflict of interests.

Acknowledgments

The authors acknowledge the generous support of the participants and the assistance of Tom Churchward from the Austin Health sleep laboratory.

References

[1] F. Biering-Sørensen and M. Biering-Sørensen, "Sleep disturbances in the spinal cord injured: an epidemiological questionnaire investigation, including a normal population," Spinal Cord, vol. 39, no. 10, pp. 505–513, 2001.

[2] R. J. H. M. Verheggen, H. Jones, J. Nyakayiru et al., "Complete absence of evening melatonin increase in tetraplegics," The FASEB Journal, vol. 26, no. 7, pp. 1–6, 2012.

[3] J. M. Zeitzer, N. T. Ayas, S. A. Shea, R. Brown, and C. A. Czeisler, "Absence of detectable melatonin and preservation of cortisol and thyrotropin rhythms in tetraplegia," Journal of Clinical Endocrinology and Metabolism, vol. 85, no. 6, pp. 2189–2196, 2000.

[4] A. Brzezinski, "Melatonin in humans," The New England Journal of Medicine, vol. 336, no. 3, pp. 186–195, 1997.

[5] A. R. Gezici, A. Karakaş, R. Ergün, and B. Gündüz, "Rhythms of serum melatonin in rats with acute spinal cord injury at the cervical and thoracic regions," Spinal Cord, vol. 48, no. 1, pp. 10–14, 2010.

[6] L. W. Kneisley, M. A. Moskowitz, and H. G. Lynch, "Cervical spinal cord lesions disrupt the rhythm in human melatonin excretion," Journal of Neural Transmission, Supplement, no. 13, pp. 311–323, 1978.

[7] Y. Li, D. H. Jiang, M. L. Wang, D. R. Jiao, and S. F. Pang, "Rhythms of serum melatonin in patients with spinal lesions at the cervical, thoracic or lumbar region," Clinical Endocrinology, vol. 30, no. 1, pp. 47–56, 1989.

[8] C. J. Mathias and H. L. Frankel, "Autonomic disturbances in spinal cord lesions," in Autonomic Failure: A Textbook of clinical Disorders of the Autonomic Nervous System, C. J. Mathias and R. Bannister, Eds., pp. 494–513, Oxford Medical Publications, Oxford, UK, 1999.

[9] F. A. J. L. Scheer, J. M. Zeitzer, N. T. Ayas, R. Brown, C. A. Czeisler, and S. A. Shea, "Reduced sleep efficiency in cervical spinal cord injury; association with abolished night time melatonin secretion," Spinal Cord, vol. 44, no. 2, pp. 78–81, 2006.

[10] M. Dahlitz, B. Alvarez, J. Vignau, J. English, J. Arendt, and J. D. Parkes, "Delayed sleep phase syndrome response to melatonin," The Lancet, vol. 337, no. 8750, pp. 1121–1124, 1991.

[11] I. Haimov, P. Lavie, M. Laudon, P. Herer, C. Vigder, and N. Zisapel, "Melatonin replacement therapy of elderly insomniacs," Sleep, vol. 18, no. 7, pp. 598–603, 1995.

[12] D. Kunz, R. Mahlberg, C. Müller, A. Tilmann, and F. Bes, "Melatonin in patients with reduced REM sleep duration: two randomized controlled trials," *Journal of Clinical Endocrinology and Metabolism*, vol. 89, no. 1, pp. 128–134, 2004.

[13] M. L. N. Pires, A. A. Benedito-Silva, L. Pinto, L. Souza, L. Vismari, and H. M. Calil, "Acute effects of low doses of melatonin on the sleep of young healthy subjects," *Journal of Pineal Research*, vol. 31, no. 4, pp. 326–332, 2001.

[14] R. J. Wurtman and I. Zhdanova, "Improvement of sleep quality by melatonin," *The Lancet*, vol. 346, no. 8988, p. 1491, 1995.

[15] I. V. Zhdanova, R. J. Wurtman, C. Morabito, V. R. Piotrovska, and H. J. Lynch, "Effects of low oral doses of melatonin, given 2–4 hours before habitual bedtime, on sleep in normal young humans," *Sleep*, vol. 19, no. 5, pp. 423–431, 1996.

[16] R. L. Sack, A. J. Lewy, M. L. Blood, J. Stevenson, and L. D. Keith, "Melatonin administration to blind people: phase advances and entrainment," *Journal of Biological Rhythms*, vol. 6, no. 3, pp. 249–261, 1991.

[17] D. J. Skene and J. Arendt, "Circadian rhythm sleep disorders in the blind and their treatment with melatonin," *Sleep Medicine*, vol. 8, no. 6, pp. 651–655, 2007.

[18] M. E. Cohen, J. F. Ditunno, W. H. Donovan, and F. M. Maynard, "A test of the 1992 international standards for neurological and functional classification of spinal cord injury," *Spinal Cord*, vol. 36, no. 8, pp. 554–560, 1998.

[19] H. J. Burgess and L. F. Fogg, "Individual differences in the amount and timing of salivary melatonin secretion," *PLoS ONE*, vol. 3, no. 8, Article ID e3055, 2008.

[20] American Association of Sleep Medicine, "Sleep-related breathing disorders in adults: recommendations for syndrome definition and measurement techniques in clinical research. The Report of an American Academy of Sleep Medicine Task Force," *Sleep*, vol. 22, no. 5, pp. 667–689, 1999.

[21] A. Rechtschaffen and A. Kales, *A Manual of Standardized Terminology, Techniques and Scoring System for Sleep Stages in Human Subjects*, Brain Information Service, Brain Information Institute, University of California, Los Angeles, Calif, USA, 1968.

[22] M. Gillberg, G. Kecklund, and T. Akerstedt, "Relations between performance and subjective ratings of sleepiness during a night awake," *Sleep*, vol. 17, no. 3, pp. 236–241, 1994.

[23] M. Partinen and T. Gislason, "Basic nordic sleep questionnaire (BNSQ): a quantitated measure of subjective sleep complaints," *Journal of Sleep Research, Supplement*, vol. 4, supplement 1, pp. 150–155, 1995.

[24] J. Spong, D. Riley, J. Ross, R. J. Pierce, D. J. Brown, and D. J. Berlowitz, "Sleep health in tetraplegia—a Victorian population survey," *Respirology*, vol. 13, article A73, 2008.

[25] D. J. Berlowitz, J. Spong, I. Gordon, M. E. Howard, and D. J. Brown, "Relationships between objective sleep indices and symptoms in a community sample of people with tetraplegia," *Archives of Physical Medicine and Rehabilitation*, vol. 93, no. 7, pp. 1246–1252, 2012.

[26] F. Biering-Sorensen, M. Biering-Sorensen, and J. Hilden, "Reproducibility of Nordic sleep questionnaire in spinal cord injured," *Paraplegia*, vol. 32, no. 11, pp. 780–786, 1994.

[27] M. Kabuto, I. Namura, and Y. Saitoh, "Nocturnal enhancement of plasma melatonin could be suppressed by benzodiazepines in humans," *Endocrinologia Japonica*, vol. 33, no. 3, pp. 405–414, 1986.

[28] S. P. James, W. B. Mendelson, D. A. Sack, N. E. Rosenthal, and T. A. Wehr, "The effect of melatonin on normal sleep," *Neuropsychopharmacology*, vol. 1, no. 1, pp. 41–44, 1987.

[29] S. P. James, D. A. Sack, N. E. Rosenthal, and W. B. Mendelson, "Melatonin administration in insomnia," *Neuropsychopharmacology*, vol. 3, no. 1, pp. 19–23, 1990.

[30] S. Nishino, E. Mignot, and W. Dement, "Sedative-hypnotics," in *Essentials of Clinical Psychopharmacology*, A. Schatzberg and C. Nemeroff, Eds., pp. 283–301, American Psychiatric, Washington, DC, USA, 2001.

[31] D. Dawson and S. M. Armstrong, "Chronobiotics—drugs that shift rhythms," *Pharmacology and Therapeutics*, vol. 69, no. 1, pp. 15–36, 1996.

[32] R. L. Sack, R. J. Hughes, D. M. Edgar, and A. J. Lewy, "Sleep-promoting effects of melatonin: at what dose, in whom, under what conditions, and by what mechanisms?" *Sleep*, vol. 20, no. 10, pp. 908–915, 1997.

[33] F. A. J. L. Scheer and C. A. Czeisler, "Melatonin, sleep, and circadian rhythms," *Sleep Medicine Reviews*, vol. 9, no. 1, pp. 5–9, 2005.

[34] A. Cagnacci, J. A. Elliott, and S. S. C. Yen, "Melatonin: a major regulator of the circadian rhythm of core temperature in humans," *Journal of Clinical Endocrinology and Metabolism*, vol. 75, no. 2, pp. 447–452, 1992.

[35] K. Kräuchi, C. Cajochen, M. Pache, J. Flammer, and A. Wirz-Justice, "Thermoregulatory effects of melatonin in relation to sleepiness," *Chronobiology International*, vol. 23, no. 1-2, pp. 475–484, 2006.

[36] C. J. van den Heuvel, S. A. Ferguson, M. Mila MacChi, and D. Dawson, "Melatonin as a hypnotic: con," *Sleep Medicine Reviews*, vol. 9, no. 1, pp. 71–80, 2005.

[37] I. V. Zhdanova, "Melatonin as a hypnotic: pro," *Sleep Medicine Reviews*, vol. 9, no. 1, pp. 51–65, 2005.

[38] D. Dawson, N. L. Rogers, C. J. van den Heuvel, D. J. Kennaway, and K. Lushington, "Effect of sustained nocturnal transbuccal melatonin administration on sleep and temperature in elderly insomniacs," *Journal of Biological Rhythms*, vol. 13, no. 6, pp. 532–538, 1998.

[39] R. J. Hughes, R. L. Sack, and A. J. Lewy, "The role of melatonin and circadian phase in age-related sleep- maintenance insomnia: assessment in a clinical trial of melatonin replacement," *Sleep*, vol. 21, no. 1, pp. 52–68, 1998.

[40] I. V. Zhdanova, R. J. Wurtman, H. J. Lynch et al., "Sleep-inducing effects of low doses of melatonin ingested in the evening," *Clinical Pharmacology and Therapeutics*, vol. 57, no. 5, pp. 552–558, 1995.

17

Sleep and Military Members: Emerging Issues and Nonpharmacological Intervention

Cary A. Brown, Robyn Berry, and Ashley Schmidt

Department of Occupational Therapy, Faculty of Rehabilitation Medicine, University of Alberta, 2-64 Corbett Hall, Edmonton, AB, Canada T6G 2G4

Correspondence should be addressed to Cary A. Brown; cary.brown@ualberta.ca

Academic Editor: Marco Zucconi

Background. Many individuals who work in the military experience sleep deficiency which presents a significant problem given the nature of their work. The cause of their sleep problems is likely multifactorial, stemming from the interplay between their personal health, habits and lifestyle juxtaposed with the stress of their military work such as emotional and physical trauma experienced in service. *Objective.* To present an overview of sleep deficiency in military members (MMs) and review of nonpharmacological treatment options. *Discussion.* Although there are a number of promising nonpharmacological treatment options available for people working in the military who experience problems sleeping, testing interventions within the context of the military are still in the early stages. Further research utilizing rigorous design and standardized, context appropriate outcome measures is needed to help treat this burgeoning problem.

1. Introduction

The objective of this report is to present an overview of the significance of sleep deficiency (SD) in military members (MMs) and highlight the current state of the evidence for non-pharmacological, evidence-based sleep interventions (NPSIs) [1].

2. Background

Sleep deficiency is a growing problem for people of all ages and significantly impacts many aspects of an individual's life. It is now emerging that persons in the military experience even greater challenges with sleep deficiency than most members of the general public [2–4]. Sleep deficiency is defined by the National Centre on Sleep Disorders Research [5] as, "...too little sleep, poor quality sleep or sleep problems including diagnosed sleep disorders." Restorative sleep is needed for optimal brain function and overall health. Individuals with sleep deficiency have an increased risk of age-related illnesses such as diabetes, hypertension, obesity, and memory loss [6]. Emerging studies have also identified that SD is not simply a symptom of an existing illness but also acts as a risk factor, increasing the likelihood of developing health conditions such as diabetes, hypertension [7], impaired judgment and depression [8], and chronic pain [9].

2.1. Prevalence of Sleep Deficiency for Military Members. Sleep deficiency is common during and after deployment for MM [10, 11]. Research reports that over 75% of deployed military members rated their sleep quality as significantly worse than their sleep prior to deployment [4]. The literature suggests that the most common sleep disorders found in a MM are sleep breathing disorders and movement disorders [11, 12]. As well, insomnia is a common, unrelenting, and debilitating complaint for those returning from military deployment [10].

Military members have higher rates of life and job dissatisfaction, depression, and negative mental health when compared to the overall working population [2]. Sleep deficiency is a common feature of many of conditions that veterans live with as documented in a 2011 Canadian survey [3]. This survey found that 90% of veterans were diagnosed with at least one physical health condition, 50% reported at least one mental health condition, and almost 70% had between four to six physical and mental health conditions. Similar issues have been identified in American MM [4].

2.2. Etiology of Sleep Deficiency in MM. Sleep deficiency in MM is likely caused by the interaction of a number of factors. These factors include environmental and social influences, comorbid physical and mental health, individual habits, beliefs and lifestyle choices, preenlistment sleep quality as well as emotional and physical trauma experienced in service. For example, physical health could be changed by practices such as physical overtraining, dietary routines, and prolonged physiological arousal consequent to hyper-vigilance. Chronic pain, ruminations such as thinking about the traumatic event, general worries, and substance misuse [33–36] also contribute to the development of SD.

There are three main routes that MM can acquire sleep deficiency: presence of a preexisting sleep conditions such as sleep apnea, during their military service, or due to a traumatic event or injury during combat. New recruits may also bring poor sleep hygiene practices with them when they join the military. These practices may include alcohol use, smoking, irregular hours, substance misuse to self-medicate for sleep/wake cycle disruption, and extended electronic device use. Some military members are predisposed to SD due to physical inactivity, lifestyle choices, substance misuse, exposure to extreme environments (noise, heat, and light), beliefs about sleep and activity, comorbid conditions that contribute to SD (e.g., pain), and certain medications [33]. Weight, smoking, and alcohol use are all risk factors for sleep apnea. Sleep apnea is highly prevalent in MM with prevalence rates of 37.5% in active MM reported in 2005 [37, 38] and as high as 62.7% in a 2013 study of 110 MMs recently returned from combat [39].

Posttraumatic stress disorder (PTSD) is a growing concern for MM and a relationship between PTSD and SD problems (such as fragmented sleep, insomnia, nightmares, night terrors, and night time anxiety attacks) has been well documented [34–36]. Preexisting SD is believed to be a risk factor for a MM to develop PTSD and restorative sleep appears to serve a protective function [7]. Post-traumatic stress disorder appears to have a bidirectional relationship with SD. Chronic sleep deficiency may be a risk factor for developing PTSD and symptoms of PTSD lead to the development of SD [35, 40, 41]. This is congruent with the apparent bidirectional relationship demonstrated between a range of medical and psychiatric disorders and insomnia, as insomnia may reciprocally predispose patients to relapse or exacerbate a recurrence of the condition [41].

A final area to highlight is the relationship between mild traumatic brain injury (mTBI) and sleep [42, 43]. The number of reported mTBI incidents and concussions in youth is growing [44] and active, apparently fit, young people bring these pre-existing injuries with them into military service. There is also an increased incidence of head trauma, mTBI, and blast related concussion injuries in active MM [45]. Persons with TBI demonstrate significantly lower levels of evening melatonin production, reduced slow wave sleep, and elevated depression all of which disrupt circadian regulation and restorative sleep [46]. A study of 26 adults with mTBI found that light, nonrapid eye movement (NREM) sleep was significantly higher and REM stage sleep was lower than controls [42]. Because REM sleep is important for cognitive function, memory, and new learning, these findings are particularly of concern given the high cognitive demand of many military roles. This is an important new area to explore.

Once enlisted, existing SD is compounded and new sleep problems emerge as a consequence of the environmental, physical, and psychological challenges military service presents to restorative sleep [33]. These challenges include communal sleeping, training, and field action that is highly alerting and does not allow for a "wind-down" period prior to sleep and psychologically unsettling events. A study of British soldiers found that 19.5% snored and this behavior can have a serious negative impact on the sleep of others in communal settings [38]. Additionally, the appropriate timing of daylight exposure needed for circadian regulation may not be possible. The military can also promote a culture in which self-care activities like sleep are believed to have little standing value and demonstrate a personal shortcoming such that the individual is perceived to lack the stamina required for the demands of active service. As Bray [10] points out in this culture the acceptance of sleep deprivation and efforts to function in a sleep deprived state can be seen as indelibly heroic.

2.3. How Sleep Deficiency Impacts Military Members. There is strong evidence that SD significantly impacts cognitive, emotional, and physical functioning in MM [10]. Attention, alertness, memory, routine task performance, and physical performance are all negatively affected by SD [47]. For example, MMs who have an average of four to six hours of sleep per night or have not slept in over 16 hours show a noticeable decrease in performance [48]. After four days of sleep deprivation the MM participants in one study were no longer effective and demonstrated impaired decision making and reaction time [47]. Given that these individuals can face life threatening tactical decisions on a daily basis, impaired judgment or performance can have dangerous outcomes [48]. Military members with SD perform similarly on neurocognitive exams to those who had consumed three alcoholic beverages [10]. They also have poorer work effectiveness and subsequently increased accident rates [10]. Research reports that are between 12 and 25% of the most severe military accidents have been linked to fatigue [49].

3. Interventions for Sleep Deficiency

Current treatments for SD include both pharmacological and nonpharmacological approaches [8, 35, 50].

3.1. Pharmacological Treatments. Medications for SD in military members are the same as those used with civilians and can include antidepressants, sedatives/hypnotics, and adrenergic antagonists/anticonvulsants. To date, there is sparse research into the outcomes of these medications specific to MMs. This lack can be problematic given the quite unique range of biological, physiological, and emotional stressors MMs are exposed to as compared to the civilian population and more targeted research is indicated. As with the civilian population these interventions need to be used with caution because of side effects and potential to suppress the Rapid

TABLE 1: Categories of NPSI methodological quality as scored with EPHPP.

(a) Imagery rehearsal therapy alone or in combination

Imagery rehearsal therapy (i) Strong [13] (ii) Moderate [14–16]	Imagery rehearsal therapy + education (i) Strong [17] (ii) Moderate [18] (iii) Weak [19]	Imagery rehearsal therapy + cognitive behavioral approaches (i) Moderate [20–22] (ii) Weak [23]	

(b) Other

Multicomponent (i) Moderate [24] (ii) Weak [25]	Biofeedback (i) Moderate [26] (ii) Weak [12]	Cognitive behavioral approaches (i) Strong [27, 28]	Relaxation (i) Weak [29]
Mind body bridging (i) Moderate [30]	Flooding (i) Moderate [31]	Fitness (i) Weak [32]	

Eye Movement (REM) stage of sleep [49]. The benefit of drug therapies in the treatment of SD is controversial and there is limited evidence to support positive outcomes in long-term use [51] and particularly during deployment [52]. In addition, many side effects have been noted with the use of medications with resultant impaired cognition, insight, new learning, and other cortical functions [35]. Long-term use of medication for SD can reduce stages three and four of the sleep cycle which are necessary for physiological restoration and metabolism [51, 53, 54]. Recent guidelines [50] recommend short courses of corrective sleep medication and more long-term strategies of non-pharmacological sleep interventions (NPSIs) for SD.

The use of Modafinil (a psychostimulant available in the US since 2003) also warrants discussion in this overview. In some areas of the military this drug is used to suppress the normal circadian drive for sleep and foster prolonged states of cognitive arousal. Dongsoo's recent review of the Modafinil literature highlighted that the pharmacological mechanism of the drug is not yet clear and that some studies have identified concerns with potential abuse for recreational purposes, addiction, and the negative consequences of extended periods of sleeplessness on the immune system [55].

3.2. Nonpharmacological Interventions (NPSIs). Little is known about NPSI interventions for SD in the unique context of MM and veterans [9]. A number of psychological and behavioural treatments have been successful to treat insomnia in a range of populations [51]. These include stimulus control therapy, sleep restriction therapy, relaxation training, cognitive therapy, sleep hygiene education, and cognitive behavioural therapy [41, 51]. In the small body of research that exists which focuses on MM and veterans behavioral treatment for insomnia [4, 10], basic sleep hygiene principles [33], bright light therapy for MM experiencing combat-related PTSD [56], and biofeedback [57] have shown to be promising interventions.

A recent structured critical review of the methodological quality of NPSI research specific to MM [1] employed the Effective Public Health Practice Project (EPHPP) quality assessment tool [58, 59] and the Jadad quality of randomization scale [60]. The review yielded only 21 studies specific to military populations (see Table 1). Imagery Rehearsal Therapy (IRT) alone [13–16], in combination with sleep hygiene education [17–19], and combined with cognitive behavioral

approaches (CBAs) [20–23], was the most frequently studied NPSI and demonstrated the strongest overall methodological quality. Other NPSIs, such as multicomponent interventions [24, 25], Biofeedback [12, 26], relaxation [29], Mind Body Bridging [30], Flooding [31], and fitness programs [32] demonstrated only weak to moderate methodological quality and were studied less frequently. Two separate studies of cognitive behavioral approaches [27, 28] were also retrieved and rated as methodologically strong. An important positive finding was that 20 of the 21 studies were rated as strong in the domain of outcome measures. Encouragingly many of the outcome measures used in these studies are relevant and pragmatic for use in clinical settings. Overall research for NPSIs is in the preliminary stage and there is currently limited evidence of efficacy such that policy makers can strategically target service delivery. Further research is required for the effectiveness of NPSIs for military member's sleep disorders before the research can be deemed as being considered conclusive.

4. Discussion

There is a clear need for researchers to develop methodologically sound studies to address the unique context and complexity of factors that interact to precipitate and perpetuate SD in MM. An important consideration in any intervention is acceptability to the patient. Reassuringly, there is evidence to suggest MMs are not adverse to NPSIs. For example, Sloberg's [61] survey of 640 active-duty naval personnel found that 61.6% used complementary and alternative medicine (CAM) therapies within the last year. Sloberg also noted that this was comparable to CAM use in the general population. Part of this acceptability is of course the ability to apply an intervention in a simple to apply and nonstigmatizing fashion. However, many of the NPSIs we reviewed were not readily pragmatic, requiring additional training or equipment to implement either during active duty or in the home setting. This is a concern because pragmatic NPSIs that are incorporated into active duty can serve a health promotion and illness preventative function [4]. Additionally, the lack of NPSI outcome studies with a qualitative design is a concern. This is an important gap in the research because qualitative methods add the external validity and deeper insight needed to enhance our understanding of NPSIs as they apply to the complex context of sleep in MM. Finally, there is also a need for research involving both genders of young MM engaged in active duty. Much of the research involves predominantly older male veterans and is nonreflective of the current MM demographic of a younger, more gender-balanced population. For example in Canada, 46.7% of the military population are female and 52.6% of MM are below the age of 39 [2].

5. Conclusion

The evidence base for interventions for NPSI in MM is still under development and cannot be considered conclusive but can be viewed as promising. NPSIs are widely used, can be highly pragmatic, and are often congruent with principles of health self-management and personal control. Encouragingly, the literature has consistently demonstrated positive NPSI outcomes with no reported adverse effects. This literature highlights emerging and extensive opportunities for both research and clinical applications. It is important to note that while gaps in the extant research and methodological weakness in a study's design may result in a lack of evidence for the specific intervention, it does not follow that the intervention has no merit and should be discarded. Rather there is a clear need for more rigorous research within the unique context of military service. The unmet need to better assess and provide NPSI for SD in military members is of particular concern. The evidence is clear that SD impacts the physical, cognitive, and emotional functioning essential for military members to perform their jobs properly. The mission now is to bridge this research to practice gap so that clinicians and their MM patients can move forward with meaningful and effective sleep interventions.

References

[1] C. A. Brown, R. Berry, A. Schmidt, and M. Tan, "Rehabilitation and the military: working together for a good night's sleep," 2012, http://www.wix.com/carybrown/npsi-for-military.

[2] J. Park, "A profile of the Canadian forces. Statistics Canada, perspectives," Catalogue 75-001-X, 2008.

[3] Canada Veterans Affairs, "Survey on transition to civilian life: report on the health of regular force veterans," 2011, http://publications.gc.ca/collections/collection_2011/acc-vac/V32-231-1-2011-eng.pdf.

[4] A. L. Peterson, J. L. Goodie, W. A. Satterfield, and W. L. Brim, "Sleep disturbance during military deployment," Military Medicine, vol. 173, no. 3, pp. 230–235, 2008.

[5] National Center on Sleep Disorders Research, "National Institutes of Health Sleep Disorders Research Plan," 2011, National Institutes of Health, http://www.nhlbi.nih.gov/health/prof/sleep/201101011NationalSleepDisordersResearchPlanDHHSPublication11-7820.pdf.

[6] E. Van Cauter and K. Spiegel, "Sleep as a mediator of the relationship between socioeconomic status and health: a hypothesis," Annals of the New York Academy of Sciences, vol. 896, pp. 254–261, 1999.

[7] O. M. Buxton and E. Marcelli, "Short and long sleep are positively associated with obesity, diabetes, hypertension, and cardiovascular disease among adults in the United States," Social Science and Medicine, vol. 71, no. 5, pp. 1027–1036, 2010.

[8] A. D. Krystal, "Sleep and psychiatric disorders: future directions," Psychiatric Clinics of North America, vol. 29, no. 4, pp. 1115–1130, 2006.

[9] L. M. McCracken and G. L. Iverson, "Disrupted sleep patterns and daily functioning in patients with chronic pain," Pain Research and Management, vol. 7, no. 2, pp. 75–79, 2002.

[10] R. M. Bray, J. L. Spira, K. R. Olmsted, and J. J. Hout, "Behavioral and occupational fitness," Military Medicine, vol. 175, supplement 1, pp. 39–56, 2010.

[11] V. Mysliwiec, L. McGraw, R. Pierce, P. Smith, B. Trapp, and B. J. Roth, "Sleep disorders and associated medical comorbidities in active duty military personnel," Sleep, vol. 36, no. 2, pp. 167–174, 2013.

[12] R. N. McLay and J. L. Spira, "Use of a portable biofeedback device to improve insomnia in a combat zone, a case report," Applied Psychophysiology Biofeedback, vol. 34, no. 4, pp. 319–321, 2009.

[13] J. M. Cook, G. C. Harb, P. R. Gehrman et al., "Imagery rehearsal for posttraumatic nightmares: a randomized controlled trial," Journal of Traumatic Stress, vol. 23, no. 5, pp. 553–563, 2010.

[14] D. Forbes, A. J. Phelps, A. F. McHugh, P. Debenham, M. Hopwood, and M. Creamer, "Imagery rehearsal in the treatment of posttraumatic nightmares in Australian veterans with chronic combat-related PTSD: 12-month follow-up data," Journal of Traumatic Stress, vol. 16, no. 5, pp. 509–513, 2003.

[15] D. Forbes, A. Phelps, and T. McHugh, "Treatment of combat-related nightmares using imagery rehearsal: a pilot study," Journal of Traumatic Stress, vol. 14, no. 2, pp. 433–442, 2001.

[16] M. Lu, A. Wagner, L. Van Male, A. Whitehead, and J. Boehnlein, "Imagery rehearsal therapy for posttraumatic nightmares in U.S. Veterans," Journal of Traumatic Stress, vol. 22, no. 3, pp. 236–239, 2009.

[17] M. E. Long, M. E. Hammons, J. L. Davis et al., "Imagery rescripting and exposure group treatment of posttraumatic nightmares in Veterans with PTSD," Journal of Anxiety Disorders, vol. 25, no. 4, pp. 531–535, 2011.

[18] C. M. Nappi, S. P. A. Drummond, S. R. Thorp, and J. R. McQuaid, "Effectiveness of imagery rehearsal therapy for the treatment of combat-related nightmares in veterans," Behavior Therapy, vol. 41, no. 2, pp. 237–244, 2010.

[19] J. Wanner, M. E. Long, and E. J. Teng, "Multi-component treatment for posttraumatic nightmares in Vietnam veterans: two case studies," Journal of Psychiatric Practice, vol. 16, no. 4, pp. 243–249, 2010.

[20] G. C. Harb, J. M. Cook, P. R. Gehrman, G. M. Gamble, and R. J. Ross, "Post-traumatic stress disorder nightmares and sleep disturbance in Iraq war veterans: a feasible and promising treatment combination," Journal of Aggression, Maltreatment and Trauma, vol. 18, no. 5, pp. 516–531, 2009.

[21] L. M. Swanson, T. K. Favorite, E. Horin, and J. T. Arnedt, "A combined group treatment for nightmares and insomnia in combat veterans: a pilot study," Journal of Traumatic Stress, vol. 22, no. 6, pp. 639–642, 2009.

[22] C. S. Ulmer, J. D. Edinger, and P. S. Calhoun, "A multi-component cognitive-behavioral intervention for sleep disturbance in Veterans with PTSD: a pilot study," Journal of Clinical Sleep Medicine, vol. 7, no. 1, pp. 57–68, 2011.

[23] K. L. Berlin, M. K. Means, and J. D. Edinger, "Nightmare reduction in a Vietnam veteran using imagery rehearsal therapy," Journal of Clinical Sleep Medicine, vol. 6, no. 5, pp. 487–488, 2010.

[24] L. M. Perlman, J. L. Cohen, M. J. Altiere et al., "A multidimensional wellness group therapy program for veterans with comorbid psychiatric and medical conditions," *Professional Psychology*, vol. 41, no. 2, pp. 120–127, 2010.

[25] A. S. Hryshko-Mullen, L. S. Broeckl, C. K. Haddock, and A. L. Peterson, "Behavioral treatment of insomnia: the Wilford Hall Insomnia program," *Military Medicine*, vol. 165, no. 3, pp. 200–207, 2000.

[26] G. Tan, T. K. Dao, D. L. Smith, A. Robinson, and M. P. Jensen, "Incorporating Complementary and Alternative Medicine (CAM) therapies to expand psychological services to veterans suffering from chronic pain," *Psychological Services*, vol. 7, no. 3, pp. 148–161, 2010.

[27] J. D. Edinger and W. S. Sampson, "A primary care "friendly" cognitive behavioral insomnia therapy," *Sleep*, vol. 26, no. 2, pp. 177–182, 2003.

[28] J. D. Edinger, M. K. Olsen, K. M. Stechuchak et al., "Cognitive behavioral therapy for patients with primary insomnia or insomnia associated predominantly with mixed psychiatric disorders: a randomized clinical trial," *Sleep*, vol. 32, no. 4, pp. 499–510, 2009.

[29] C. G. Watson, J. R. Tuorila, K. S. Vickers, L. P. Gearhart, and C. M. Mendez, "The efficacies of three relaxation regimens in the treatment of PTSD in Vietnam War veterans," *Journal of Clinical Psychology*, vol. 53, no. 8, pp. 917–923, 1997.

[30] Y. Nakamura, D. L. Lipschitz, R. Landward, R. Kuhn, and G. West, "Two sessions of sleep-focused mind-body bridging improve self-reported symptoms of sleep and PTSD in veterans: a pilot randomized controlled trial," *Journal of Psychosomatic Research*, vol. 70, no. 4, pp. 335–345, 2011.

[31] N. A. Cooper and G. A. Clum, "Imaginal flooding as a supplementary treatment for PTSD in combat veterans: a controlled study," *Behavior Therapy*, vol. 20, no. 3, pp. 381–391, 1989.

[32] C. M. Shapiro, P. M. Warren, J. Trinder et al., "Fitness facilitates sleep," *European Journal of Applied Physiology*, vol. 53, no. 1, pp. 1–4, 1984.

[33] Z. Pouliot, M. Peters, H. Neufeld, K. Delaive, and M. H. Kryger, "Sleep disorders in a military population," *Military Medicine*, vol. 168, no. 1, pp. 7–10, 2003.

[34] P. Swales, "Sleep and posttraumatic stress disorder (PTSD)," 2011, http://www.veterans.gc.ca/eng/mental-health/support/factssho.

[35] L. J. Lamarche and J. De Koninck, "Sleep disturbance in adults with posttraumatic stress disorder: a review," *Journal of Clinical Psychiatry*, vol. 68, no. 8, pp. 1257–1270, 2007.

[36] T. A. Mellman, R. Kulick-Bell, L. E. Ashlock, and B. Nolan, "Sleep events among veterans with combat-related posttraumatic stress disorder," *American Journal of Psychiatry*, vol. 152, no. 1, pp. 110–115, 1995.

[37] C. J. Lettieri, A. H. Eliasson, T. Andrada, A. Khramtsov, M. Raphaelson, and D. A. Kristo, "Obstructive sleep apnea syndrome: are we missing an at-risk population?" *Journal of Clinical Sleep Medicine*, vol. 1, no. 4, pp. 381–385, 2005.

[38] N. Okpala, R. Walker, and A. Hosni, "Prevalence of snoring and sleep-disordered breathing among military personnel," *Military Medicine*, vol. 176, no. 5, pp. 561–564, 2011.

[39] V. Mysliwiec, J. Gill, H. Lee et al., "Sleep disorders in U.S. military personnel: a high rate of comorbid insomnia and obstructive sleep apnea," *Chest*, 2013.

[40] A. Germain, M. K. Shear, M. Hall, and D. J. Buysse, "Effects of a brief behavioral treatment for PTSD-related sleep disturbances:

a pilot study," *Behaviour Research and Therapy*, vol. 45, no. 3, pp. 627–632, 2007.

[41] M. T. Smith, M. I. Huang, and R. Manber, "Cognitive behavior therapy for chronic insomnia occurring within the context of medical and psychiatric disorders," *Clinical Psychology Review*, vol. 25, no. 5, pp. 559–592, 2005.

[42] S. Schreiber, G. Barkai, T. Gur-Hartman et al., "Long-lasting sleep patterns of adult patients with minor traumatic brain injury (mTBI) and non-mTBI subjects," *Sleep Medicine*, vol. 9, no. 5, pp. 481–487, 2008.

[43] R. J. Castriotta and J. M. Lai, "Sleep disorders associated with traumatic brain injury," *Archives of Physical Medicine and Rehabilitation*, vol. 82, no. 10, pp. 1403–1406, 2001.

[44] S. R. R. Buzzini and K. M. Guskiewicz, "Sport-related concussion in the young athlete," *Current Opinion in Pediatrics*, vol. 18, no. 4, pp. 376–382, 2006.

[45] R. W. Evans, "Posttraumatic headaches among United States soldiers injured in Afghanistan and Iraq," *Headache*, vol. 48, no. 8, pp. 1216–1225, 2008.

[46] J. A. Shekleton, D. L. Parcell, J. R. Redman, J. Phipps-Nelson, J. L. Ponsford, and S. M. W. Rajaratnam, "Sleep disturbance and melatonin levels following traumatic brain injury," *Neurology*, vol. 74, no. 21, pp. 1732–1738, 2010.

[47] T. O. Rognum, F. Vartdal, and K. Rodahl, "Physical and mental performance of soldiers on high- and low-energy diets during prolonged heavy exercise combined with sleep deprivation," *Ergonomics*, vol. 29, no. 7, pp. 859–867, 1986.

[48] J. Curry, "Sleep management and soldier readiness: a guide for leaders and soldiers," 2005, Infantry Magazine, http://www.thefreelibrary.com/Sleep+management+and+soldier+readiness%3A+a+guide+for+leaders+and...-a0141213094.

[49] J. A. Caldwell and J. L. Caldwell, "Fatigue in military aviation: an overview of U.S. military-approved pharmacological countermeasures," *Aviation Space and Environmental Medicine*, vol. 76, supplement 7, pp. C39–C51, 2005.

[50] S. L. Schutte-Rodin, L. Broch, D. Buysee, C. Dorsey, and M. Sateia, "Clinical guideline for the evaluation and management of chronic insomnia in adults," *Journal of Clinical Sleep Medicine*, vol. 4, no. 5, pp. 487–504, 2008.

[51] C. M. Morin, L. Bélanger, C. Bastien, and A. Vallières, "Long-term outcome after discontinuation of benzodiazepines for insomnia: a survival analysis of relapse," *Behaviour Research and Therapy*, vol. 43, no. 1, pp. 1–14, 2005.

[52] G. P. Krueger, "Sustained work, fatigue, sleep loss and performance: a review of the issues," *Work and Stress*, vol. 3, no. 2, pp. 129–141, 1989.

[53] D. X. Freedman, J. S. Derryberry, and D. D. Federman, "Drugs and insomnia. The use of medications to promote sleep," *Journal of the American Medical Association*, vol. 251, no. 18, pp. 2410–2414, 1984.

[54] National Institutes of Health Consensus Development Conference Statement, "The treatment of sleep disorders of older-people," *Sleep*, vol. 14, no. 2, pp. 169–177, 1991.

[55] K. Dongsoo, "Practical use and risk of Modafinil, a novel waking drug," *Environmental Health and Toxicology*, vol. 27, Article ID e2012007, 2012.

[56] K. McCann, "Sleep disturbances in soldiers with combat PTSD improved by bright light therapy," 2010, Science Daily, http://www.sciencedaily.com/releases/2010/06/100607065552.htm.

[57] R. D. Gevirtz and C. Dalenberg, "Heart rate variability biofeedback in the treatment of trauma symptoms," *Biofeedback*, vol. 36, no. 1, pp. 22–23, 2008.

[58] B. H. Thomas, D. Ciliska, M. Dobbins, and S. Micucci, "A process for systematically reviewing the literature: providing the research evidence for public health nursing interventions," *Worldviews on Evidence-Based Nursing*, vol. 1, no. 3, pp. 176–184, 2004.

[59] N. Jackson and E. Waters, "Criteria for the systematic review of health promotion and public health interventions," *Health Promotion International*, vol. 20, no. 4, pp. 367–374, 2005.

[60] A. R. Jadad, R. A. Moore, D. Carroll et al., "Assessing the quality of reports of randomized clinical trials: is blinding necessary?" *Controlled Clinical Trials*, vol. 17, no. 1, pp. 1–12, 1996.

[61] B. J. Sloberg, *Self-efficacy and the use of alternative medicine practices by active duty military stationed on board a United States naval warship [Ph.D. thesis]*, Touro University International, Cypress, Calif, USA, 2006.

18

No Difference in Sleep and RBD between Different Types of Patients with Multiple System Atrophy: A Pilot Video-Polysomnographical Study

Maria-Lucia Muntean,[1,2] **Friederike Sixel-Döring,**[1] **and Claudia Trenkwalder**[1,3]

[1] *Paracelsus Elena Klinik, Klinik Straße 16, 34128 Kassel, Germany*
[2] *Department of Neurosciences, University of Medicine and Pharmacy, Victor Babes Straße 43, 400012 Cluj-Napoca, Romania*
[3] *Department of Neurosurgery, University of Göttingen, Robert Koch Straße 40, 37075 Göttingen, Germany*

Correspondence should be addressed to Maria-Lucia Muntean; luciamuntean@yahoo.com

Academic Editor: Marco Zucconi

Background. Patients with multiple system atrophy (MSA), similarly to patients with alpha-synucleinopathies, can present with different sleep problems. We sought to analyze sleep problems in the two subtypes of the disease MSA cerebellar type (MSA-C) and MSA parkinsonian type (MSA-P), paying special attention to REM sleep disturbances and periodic limb movements (PLMs). *Methods.* In the study we included 11 MSA-C and 27 MSA-P patients who underwent one night polysomnography. For the analysis, there were 37 valid polysomnographic studies. *Results.* Sleep efficiency was decreased in both groups (MSA-C, 64.27% ± 12.04%; MSA-P, 60.64% ± 6.01%). The PLM indices using standard measures, in sleep (PLMS) and while awake (PLMW), were high in both groups (MSA-C patients: PLMS index 72 ± 65, PLMW index 38 ± 33; MSA-P patients: PLMS index 66 ± 63, PLMW index 48 ± 37). Almost one-third of the MSA patients of both groups presented features of RLS on video-polysomnography. RBD was described in 8/11 (73%) patients with MSA-C and 19/25 (76%) patients with MSA-P ($P = 0.849$). *Conclusion.* Our results showed very similar polysomnographic results for both MSA-P and MSA-C patients as a probable indicator for the similar pathologic mechanism of the disease and especially of its sleep problems.

1. Introduction

Nighttime sleep disturbances are a recognized problem in multiple system atrophy (MSA) patients. These disturbances have long been observed, but the studies published to date have only included small sample sizes. Nighttime sleep problems in patients with MSA include REM sleep behavior disorder (RBD) [1], periodic limb movements (PLMs) [2], restless legs syndrome (RLS) [2], or RLS like symptoms [3–6]. All of them lead to sleep fragmentation and decreased sleep efficiency [7, 8].

In MSA, as in other alpha-synucleinopathies, RBD can be present, with a prevalence of up to 90% [9], and sometimes can antedate the occurrence of motor symptoms [10, 11]. RBD and REM sleep without atonia (RWA) in MSA and PD patients may be related to lesions of brainstem nuclei and pontomedullary pathways, as suggested in previous studies [3, 12].

On the other hand, clinically defined RLS seems to be less frequent in MSA patients when compared to patients with other synucleinopathies [13]. However, most patients with RLS have PLMs during sleep, an unspecific sign of both RLS or other sleep disorders. The pathology of PLMs in patients with parkinsonism is not yet clarified, but a few theories have been put forward. One hypothesis concerns the involvement of the dopaminergic system of neurotransmission [14]. A second hypothesis is the suprasegmental disinhibition at the brainstem or spinal cord level [15].

There is only sparse data in the published literature comparing the polysomnographic (PSG) parameters in MSA patients and referring to the two different types of the disease according to Gilman et al.'s classification [16]. In this context,

TABLE 1: Description of the study population with valid PSGs.

Demographics	MSA-C ($n = 11$) (29.73%)	MSA-P ($n = 26$) (70.27%)	P value
Female (%)	5 (45.45)	14 (54.55)	NS
Male (%)	6 (53.85)	12 (46.15)	NS
Age, years	67.64 ± 5.55	66.19 ± 9.17	NS
Disease duration, years	4.27 ± 2.76	3.44 ± 2.28	NS
BMI	27.28 ± 3.07	27.61 ± 4.50	NS
MMSE	26.36 ± 4.82	28 ± 1.37	NS
Signs and symptoms, n (%)			
Cerebellar	11 (100)	3 (11.54)	0.000
Extrapyramidal	10 (90.91)	26 (100)	NS
Pyramidal	2 (18.18)	6 (23.08)	NS
Concomitant diseases, n (%)			
Cardiovascular*	4 (36.36)	12 (46.15)	NS
Psychiatric**	3 (27.27)	9 (34.61)	NS
Medication			
L-dopa, mg/day	391.67 ± 270.49	747.89 ± 439.50	0.017
n (%)	6 (55)	19 (73)	NS
Dopamine agonists, mg/day	0	319.67 ± 299.47	NA
n (%)	0	6 (23)	NA
Amantadine, mg/day	300	250 ± 100	NS
n (%)	1 (9.09)	4 (15.38)	NS
SSRIs, n (%)	3 (27.27)	11 (42.31)	NS
Opioids, n (%)	1 (9.09)	1 (3.85)	NS
Benzodiazepines, n (%)	2 (18.18)	6 (23.08)	NS
Other antipsychotics, n (%)	2 (18.18)	0	NA

Values are mean ± SD, Dopamine agonists dose = L-dopa equivalent dose according to Tomlinson et al., 2010 [17], MSA-C: multiple system atrophy cerebellar predominant, MSA-P: multiple system atrophy parkinsonian predominant, BMI: body mass index, MMSE: Mini Mental State Examination, L-dopa: levodopa, SSRIs: selective serotonin reuptake inhibitors, NS: not significant (P value > 0.05), NA: not applicable.
*Clinically relevant hypertension or any other form of heart disease. **Clinically relevant psychiatric conditions.

we aimed to analyze sleep problems in the two subtypes of MSA patients (MSA-C and MSA-P) and paid special attention to REM sleep disturbances and limb movements during the night.

2. Methods

The study was approved by the Ethics Committee of the Landesärztekammer Hessen in the context of Parkinson Syndromes in PSG studies. All subjects agreed to take part in the study and signed a written informed consent form that included the video-assessment.

We enrolled 38 patients with both MSA-P and MSA-C in this sleep laboratory study. The patients were referred for diagnosis or treatment of their disease and were investigated in our sleep lab because of subjective nighttime sleep problems, RLS like symptoms, probable RBD, or other nighttime disturbances including suspicious stridor. Three patients were evaluated as *de novo* Parkinson syndromes, who later proved to be MSA patients.

The demographical data, clinical findings, concomitant diseases, medication during the day, when the polysomnography was performed and Parkinson Disease Sleep Scale-version 2, (PDSS-2) scores [18], when available, were

obtained. We paid special attention to comorbidities such as cardiovascular and psychiatric conditions. The data were obtained from the admission charts of the patients who were previously diagnosed by cardiologists or psychiatrists.

2.1. Diagnosis. The diagnosis of MSA was established according to the 2008 Consensus Criteria established by Gilman et al. [16]. Patients were separated into two groups: MSA with predominant parkinsonism (MSA-P) and MSA with predominant cerebellar ataxia (MSA-C). Clinical symptoms of patients are described in Table 1.

2.2. Polysomnography. Nighttime sleep recordings started immediately after connecting the patient and calibration with lights off at 22:00 and ended at 6:00 the next morning. Cardiorespiratory PSG (Xltec: Excel Tech Ltd., Oakville, ON, Canada) was applied including bilateral monopolar central electroencephalography (EEG) with two channels, electrooculogram (EOG), chin and bilateral tibialis anterior surface electromyography (EMG), air flow registration, tracheal sound registration by microphone, thoracic and abdominal belts to measure respiratory movements, electrocardiography (EKG), and oximetry. All patients were documented with an infrared video recording synchronized to the PSG. A sleep laboratory technician monitored each recording. Sleep (including sleep stages), PLMs, and apneas were scored visually by a trained technician according to standard criteria [1, 19]. PLMs were scored in sleep and in wakefulness only if they occurred in a series of at least four consecutive movements lasting 0.5 to 5 seconds each with an intermovement interval of 4 to 90 seconds, in accordance with international scoring rules [2, 20]. The number of PLMs per hour of time in bed (PLM index), and the number of PLMs during wakefulness per hour of wake time (PLMW index), the number of PLMs during sleep per hour of total sleep time (PLMS index) were evaluated separately. All sleep evaluations were reviewed and supervised by board-certified sleep specialists. Sleep efficiency was defined as total sleep time (TST)/time in bed (TIB). Quantitative analysis of sleep stages was calculated as a percentage of TST. RBD was diagnosed by second per second review in time-synchronized video analysis of all REM episodes by experienced raters in accordance with EEG, EOG, and chin EMG. RBD was defined as the presence of REM sleep without atonia (RWA) together with complex movements or vocalizations during REM sleep apparently associated with dreaming or dream-enacting behaviors visible in time-synchronized video-PSG according to criteria established by Schenck et al. [21] and the International Classification of Sleep Disorders, second edition (ICSD-2) [1] with one modification as historical information was not included. Severity of RBD was quantified using the RBD severity scale (RBDSS). On the RBDSS, motor events in REM sleep were rated on a digital scale from 0–3 according to the localization and severity of movements. The scales rates the following: no visible movement but registration of RWA scored as 0, slight movements including facial movements, jerks or movements restricted to the distal extremities scored as 1, movements involving the proximal extremities, complex and/or violent behaviors scored as 2, and any axial involvement with a possibility of falling or observed falls scored as 3; vocalizations were rated as absent, indicated by "0", or present, indicated by "1", for any sound generated during REM sleep other than respiratory noises. Motor and vocalization scores were separated by a full stop [22].

We analysed RWA using chin EMG activity in REM sleep according to the criteria published by Frauscher et al. [23]. We evaluated the mentalis muscle. For scoring phasic or tonic EMG activity, the recording was divided into 3 sec mini-epochs. Each 3 sec mini-epoch was scored as having or not having "any" EMG activity, irrespective of whether it contained tonic, phasic, or a combination of both EMG activities. Finally, we also calculated the percentage of 3 sec mini-epochs with "any" chin EMG activity.

RLS-like symptoms were defined according to the video-polysomnographic assessment and clinical interview after the sleep study in those subjects, when PLMS and restlessness were obvious, since there is no structured targeted interview for RLS patients with Parkinson syndromes available. If not all 4 diagnostic features were fulfilled or could be obtained, we called it RLS-like syndrome.

Sleep apneas were defined as an apnea-hypnea index (AHI) of 5 or more in accordance with Ruehland et al. [24].

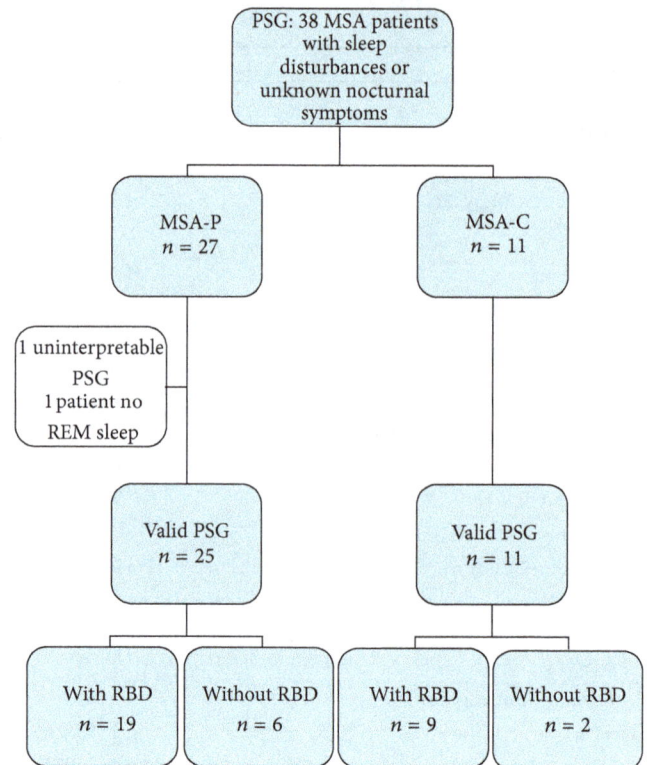

FIGURE 1: Study tree of the MSA patients. RBD = REM sleep behavior disorder, PSG = polysomnography.

2.3. Analysis. The statistical analysis was made in an environment for statistical computing and graphics, ("R", version 1.15.1) [25]. The association between two qualitative variables was assessed using the Fisher exact test. The strength of the association was assessed with odds ratio along with the 95% confidence intervals. To check for differences between two independent groups of quantitative data, Mann Whitney U test was used.

3. Results

3.1. Patient Population. Thirty-eight patients with MSA were referred to the sleep laboratory within approximately 2 years, out of a total of 50 MSA patients who were hospitalized in the Paracelsus Elena-Klinik at that time. One patient with MSA-P had a sleep efficiency of only 4% in the PSG, thus providing insufficient sleep to allow further analysis. This patient was excluded from the study. Therefore the study group consisted of 37 MSA patients with interpretable PGSs. There were 19 females and 18 males with an average age of 66.62 ± 8.21 years. The study tree of patients is presented in Figure 1. The MSA-C group consisted of 11 patients (5 females and 6 males, average age 67.64 ± 5.55) and the MSA-P group consisted of 26 patients (14 females and 10 males, average age 66.19 ± 9.17). One patient from the MSA-P group failed to enter REM sleep; therefore this patient was excluded from the REM sleep analysis. The demographics of the study population, together with the concurrent medical conditions and medication, are presented in Table 1.

TABLE 2: Polysomnographic characteristics of MSA-C and MSA-P patients.

	MSA-C ($n = 11$)	MSA-P ($n = 26$)	Significance P value
Sleep efficiency, %	64.27 ± 12.04	60.64 ± 16.01	NS
Sleep latency, min	25.74 ± 17.33	29.76 ± 41.54	NS
Sleep stage 1, % of TST	23.47 ± 8.46	26.63 ± 9.84	NS
Sleep stage 2, % of TST	52.15 ± 8.67	47.55 ±14.61	NS
Sleep stage 3, % of TST	4.70 ± 6.70	8.58 ± 11.55	NS
Sleep REM, % of TST	19.68 ± 9.84	17.24 ± 11.08	NS
REM latency, min	123.09 ± 81.62	141.72 ± 103.93	NS
Awakenings, total	18.09 ± 9.27	23.69 ± 8.24	NS
Awakenings index/h	4.01 ± 1.96	5.83 ± 3.75	NS
PLM index	64 ± 55	61 ± 48	NS
PLMS index	72 ± 65	66 ± 63	NS
PLMW index	38 ± 33	48 ± 37	NS
RLS-like, n (%)	3 (30.77)	8 (27.27)	NS

TST: total sleep time. Sleep efficiency was calculated as % of sleep during time in bed; sleep stages were calculated as % of TST; index of periodic leg movements (PLM) was calculated per hour of time in bed (PLM index), per hour of sleep (PLMS index), and per hour of wakefulness (PLMW index), awakening index = total number of awakenings in TST, RLS-like: restless legs symptoms, MSA-C: multiple system atrophy cerebellar predominant, MSA-P: multiple system atrophy parkinsonian predominant, NS: nonsignificant (P value > 0.05).

TABLE 3: The percentage of "any" EMG activity in MSA patients with RBD.

	"Any" EMG activity Mean ± SD (%)	
MSA-C patients	With RBD	Without RBD
	46.79 ± 21.17	7.35 ± 7.94
MSA-P patients	With RBD	Without RBD
	51 ± 36.96	17.72 ± 31.51

SD: standard deviation, RBD: REM Sleep Behavior Disorder, MSA-C: multiple system atrophy cerebellar predominant, MSA-P: multiple system atrophy parkinsonian predominant.

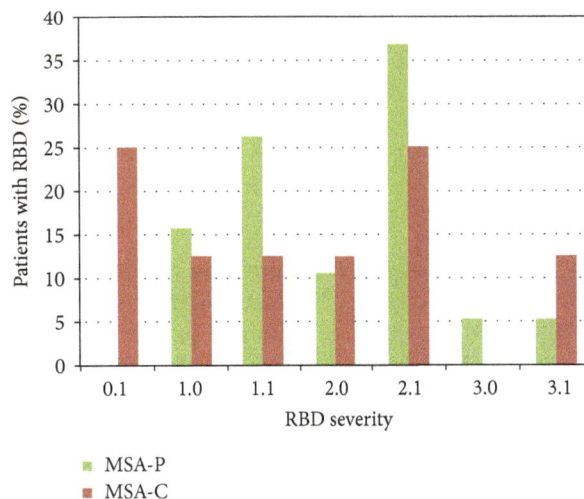

FIGURE 2: Representation of MSA patients according to RBD severity evaluated with RBDSS. RBSS = REM sleep behavior disorder severity scale, MSA-C = multiple system atrophy cerebellar predominant, MSA-P = multiple system atrophy parkinsonian predominant.

3.2. Medical Conditions.

The body mass index (BMI) did not differ significantly between the two groups. The incidences of cardiovascular and psychiatric comorbidities in MSA-C and MSA-P patients were not significantly different.

Daily levodopa dose was higher in patients with MSA-P compared to MSA-C patients ($P = 0.017$). No difference was observed in the dosage and number of patients using dopamine agonists, amantadine, selective serotonin reuptake inhibitors (SSRIs), and opioids in the two MSA patient groups.

3.3. Subjective Sleep Evaluation.

The overall subjective quality of nighttime sleep (item 1 score on PDSS-2) was 1.55 ± 1.08 for MSA-C patients and 1.59 ± 1.23 for MSA-P patients, with no statistically significant difference. The total PDSS-2 scores were as follows: 17.91 ± 4.41 in the MSA-C group and 19.64 ± 6.90 in the MSA-P group (no statistically significant difference).

3.4. Sleep Parameters.

The results of the PSG studies of the two subtypes of MSA patients are shown in Table 2 and results of RWA in both subtypes are shown in Table 3. RBD (according to the modified ICSD-2 criteria [1]) was described in 8/11 (73%) patients with MSA-C and 19/25 (76%) patients with MSA-P. There was no difference in the incidence as well as in the severity of clinical RBD between the two groups ($P = 0.849$). Violent manifestations were noted in only two of the MSA-P and one of the MSA-C patients. Details of RBD severity are represented in Figure 2.

The results of the EMG analysis of the mentalis muscle in relation to RBD are presented in Table 3. These show that MSA-C patients with RBD presented an average percentage of EMG activity in REM sleep of 46.79% ± 21.17% < compared to an average percentage of only 7.35% ± 7.94% for patients without RBD. In the MSA-P group the average percentage of EMG activity for patients with RBD was 51% ± 36.96% compared to only 17.72% ± 31.51% for the patients without RBD. The comparison between the RWA in both groups with RBD was not significantly different.

TABLE 4: Respiratory parameters at PSG in MSA patients.

	MSA-C (n = 11)	MSA-P (n = 26)	Significance P value
Sleep apnea, n (%)	7 (64)	11 (42)	NS
Min SaO2, %	82.22 ± 13.24	81.69 ± 10.99	NS
Average SaO2, %	94.68 ± 1.69	93.79 ± 2.80	NS

NS: not significant (P value > 0.05), SaO2: oxygen saturation, MSA-C: multiple system atrophy cerebellar predominant, MSA-P: multiple system atrophy parkinsonian predominant, PSG: polysomnography.

In the MSA-C group, 3 patients with RBD were using SSRIs, and none from the patients without RBD. In the MSA-P group, 8 patients with RBD were using SSRIs, compared to 3 patients without RBD. No statistical analysis was performed, due to the small number of patients in each group.

Respiratory events of MSA patients are represented in Table 4.

4. Discussion

Our study population consisted of MSA patients who were referred for sleep studies due to different or unclear nighttime sleep disturbances. The PSG results of the two groups of MSA patients (MSA-C and MSA-C) could be compared due to similarities in patient demographics and in clinical features.

We noted a high frequency of sleep problems in MSA patients both MSA-C and MSA-P, consistent with the results of Wetter et al. and Tison et al. [3, 11]. Taking into account the localization of the pathologic processes in the two MSA subtypes we expected to find different nighttime sleep problems in the two groups. The results of the study, however, which showed very similar nighttime problems and PSG results for both MSA-P and MSA-C patients, are a probable indicator for the similar pathologic mechanism of the disease and especially of its sleep problems. This is mainly a pilot study with a descriptive analysis and due to the small number of participants in each subgroup statistically significant differences cannot be expected. It could be considered a preliminary study, and more patients should be investigated to confirm that there is no difference in sleep parameters of these two subgroups of MSA patients.

The subjective sleep evaluation was undertaken using the PDSS-2 scale. Overall quality of sleep assessed by the first question of the scale showed a moderate quality of sleep. No difference was observed between the two MSA subtype patient groups concerning subjective nighttime sleep problems.

Sleep efficiency was decreased in both MSA groups (64.27% ± 12.04%, resp. 60.64% ± 16.01%) compared to the values of elderly normals available in the literature (76.5% ± 2.2%) [26]. MSA patients also presented fragmentation of sleep during the night either due to limb movements or to sleep apnea.

The assessment of motor activity in sleep for the patients included in the study was performed using the standard criteria for routine practice in our sleep laboratory at that time. Some authors use more quantitative data to analyze motor parameters in sleep, for example, using the periodicity

index [27]. We consider it an important new method, but it is, until now, not the gold standard for analysing PLMs in neurodegeneration.

An important finding of our study is the fact that MSA patients in the sleep laboratory featured a high number of PLMs. The PLM indices, both PLM during sleep and PLM while awake, were much higher (MSA-C patients: PLM index 64 ± 55; MSA-P patients: PLM index 61 ± 48) than those reported in PD patients in the same PSG laboratory (PLM index 36 ± 40) [28]. Iranzo et al. found a similarly high index of PLMs in MSA patients, also using standard PLM assessments, which could suggest a dysfunction in the structures that modulate sleep [29]. One explanation for the difference between PLM indices between MSA and PD patients could be that the spinal-cerebellar pathways involved in PLM generation are probably more affected in MSA than in PD patients. It would therefore be of interest to use more elaborated assessments for measuring PLMS, such as the periodicity index [27] to see, if the difference between PD, RLS, and MSA is related to movements with periodicity or just to single movements while motor activity is increased during sleep. The overall dosages of dopamine agonists in MSA patients were in general lower compared to PD patients, which could also contribute to an increased number of limb movements in MSA patients.

Almost a third of the MSA patients presented RLS features on the video-PSG with obvious restlessness at night in the PSG-video. Spontaneous reporting of these symptoms, however, is rare. This implies that a more thorough questioning of MSA patients about RLS is needed in order to detect these symptoms before referring patients to sleep studies. We classified these patients as "RLS-like" syndrome as used by others [5] when not all diagnostic features were met or obtained.

We assumed that due to the more specific involvement of pontine and cerebellar structures including the olivoponto-cerebellar structures in the pathology of MSA-P [30], these patients should have a higher prevalence of RLS than MSA-C patients. The results of the study, however, did not support this hypothesis.

The presence of RWA was high in both MSA patient groups. We analysed the chin EMG activity in sleep with the method described by Frauscher et al. [23] although the method has not been validated for MSA patients. Thus we noted a high percentage of EMG activity in MSA patients with RBD compared to MSA patients without RBD in both MSA subtypes (for MSA-C patients 46,79% versus 7,35% and for MSA-P patients 51% versus 17,72%). There was an interindividual variability of chin EMG activity, but the mean values fall within the range given by Frauscher et al.. The cut-off value for 100% specificity for RBD in PD patients was 18,2% in the group of Frauscher et al. [23]. This comparison deserves attention, as it is the first study that uses the Frauscher method in MSA patients.

Our results are supported by the work of Nomura et al. who revealed RWA in 68.8% of patients with MSA [31].

The relationship between SSRIs and the presence of polysomnographically-diagnosed RBD could not be statistically analysed due to the small number of patients in each group. In the literature, Frauscher et al. showed a significant association between RBD and SSRI use in a population with different sleep disorders, but not in neurodegenerative patients [32].

SSRIs were used in therapeutic doses either for depressive symptoms or with the aim of improving MSA symptoms. It is assumed that a serotonergic depletion occurs in the brainstem nuclei of MSA-patients [33]. A first small randomized trial of our group could show improvement of motor symptoms and speech with paroxetine in MSA patients [34]. In our current study, more MSA-P patients than MSA-C patients have been treated with SSRIs, although the difference between the two groups did not reach the significance threshold. The neurodegenerative changes of the brain or neuropharmacological alterations leading to RBD may therefore be more important than any pharmacological imbalance that is caused by serotonergic treatment in patients, who are not or not yet diagnosed with neurodegeneration.

A number of MSA patients in both groups presented with sleep apnea that could be explained either by the pathologic process of the disease or by an increase in BMI. The average values in both groups were situated above the normal weight limit. The upper normal weight limit according to the World Health Organization is $24.99 \, kg/m^2$. This shows that many of the MSA patients were overweight, which could be a contributing factor to their nighttime sleep disturbances, especially their respiratory problems [35]. However, PD patients have similar BMIs, and it is still unclear if neurodegeneration leads to preponderance because of immobility or if those who are overweight have a higher risk of parkinsonism [36].

This study showed once more that sleep problems in MSA patients represent a frequent and serious problem. Patients are referred to the sleep laboratory for various nocturnal complaints, which were difficult to diagnose from history only. After PSG analysis their subjective sleep disturbances proved to be sleep fragmentation, RBD, PLMS, RLS, or several phenomena combined. One of the limitations of this study is represented by the fact that we included only MSA patients who had subjective complaints of sleep, and not the entire group of MSA patients.

Even though the pathology of the two subtypes of MSA is somewhat different we did not notice any significant difference in the occurrence of sleep disturbances in MSA-C and MSA-P patients thus possibly arguing for a common disease entity. This could be considered as a preliminary study. More patients are expected to be included in this type of analysis in order to better clarify the results.

Conflict of Interests

The authors of this paper have no conflict of interests to declare.

Disclosure

Maria-Lucia Muntean has received travel expenses from Abbott, Boehringer Ingelheim, and Lundbeck. Friederike Sixel-Döring has received educational lecture fees and honoraria from Boehringer Ingelheim, Cephalon, Medtronic, Orion Pharma, Roche Pharma, and Schwarz Pharma. She serves on an advisory board for Orion Pharma. Claudia Trenkwalder has received honoraria for consultancy from Boehringer Ingelheim, UCB, Novartis, Orion Pharma, Mundipharma, Britannia, and Solvay. She has received lecture honoraria from Boehringer Ingelheim, GlaxoSmithKline, UCB Schwarz Pharma, and Mundipharma. This study was not supported by the industry.

Acknowledgments

Dr. Muntean has received a grant from EFNS through the Department to Department Cooperation Program, which made the research for this study possible.

References

[1] American Academy of Sleep Medicine, *REM Sleep Behavior Disorder*, American Academy of Sleep Medicine, Westchester, Ill, USA, 2nd edition, 2005.

[2] American Academy of Sleep Medicine, *International Classification of Sleep Disorders, Revised: Diagnostic and Coding Manual*, American Academy of Sleep Medicine, Chicago, Ill, USA, 2001.

[3] T. C. Wetter, V. Collado-Seidel, T. Pollmächer, A. Yassouridis, and C. Trenkwalder, "Sleep and periodic leg movement patterns in drug-free patients with Parkinson's disease and multiple system atrophy," *Sleep*, vol. 23, no. 3, pp. 361–367, 2000.

[4] I. Aricò, R. Condurso, F. Granata, L. Nobili, O. Bruni, and R. Silvestri, "Nocturnal frontal lobe epilepsy presenting with restless leg syndrome-like symptoms," *Neurological Sciences*, vol. 32, no. 2, pp. 313–315, 2011.

[5] L. Ferini-Strambi, "RLS-like symptoms: differential diagnosis by history and clinical assessment," *Sleep Medicine*, vol. 8, supplement 2, pp. S3–S6, 2007.

[6] C. R. Baumann, I. Marti, and C. L. Bassetti, "Restless legs symptoms without periodic limb movements in sleep and without response to dopaminergic agents: a restless legs-like syndrome?" *European Journal of Neurology*, vol. 14, no. 12, pp. 1369–1372, 2007.

[7] R. Manni, R. Morini, E. Martignoni, C. Pacchetti, G. Micieli, and A. Tartara, "Nocturnal sleep in multisystem atrophy with autonomic failure: polygraphic findings in ten patients," *Journal of Neurology*, vol. 240, no. 4, pp. 247–250, 1993.

[8] J. R. Neil, B. C. Holzer, and D. G. Spiker, "EEG sleep alterations in olivopontocerebellar degeneration," *Neurology*, vol. 30, no. 6, pp. 660–662, 1980.

[9] G. Plazzi, R. Corsini, F. Provini et al., "REM sleep behavior disorders in multiple system atrophy," *Neurology*, vol. 48, no. 4, pp. 1094–1097, 1997.

[10] B. F. Boeve, M. H. Silber, C. B. Saper et al., "Pathophysiology of REM sleep behaviour disorder and relevance to neurodegenerative disease," *Brain*, vol. 130, no. 11, pp. 2770–2788, 2007.

[11] F. Tison, G. K. Wenning, and N. P. Quinn, "REM sleep behaviour disorder as the presenting symptom of multiple system atrophy," *Journal of Neurology Neurosurgery and Psychiatry*, vol. 58, no. 3, pp. 379–385, 1995.

[12] T. Shimizu, Y. Inami, Y. Sugita et al., "REM sleep without muscle atonia (stage 1-REM) and its relation to delirious behavior

during sleep in patients with degenerative diseases involving the brain stem," *Japanese Journal of Psychiatry and Neurology*, vol. 44, no. 4, pp. 681–692, 1990.

[13] R. L. Gama, D. G. Távora, R. C. Bomfim, C. E. Silva, V. M. de Bruin, and P. F. C. de Bruin, "Sleep disturbances and brain MRI morphometry in Parkinson's disease, multiple system atrophy and progressive supranuclear palsy: a comparative study," *Parkinsonism and Related Disorders*, vol. 16, no. 4, pp. 275–279, 2010.

[14] T. C. Wetter, K. Stiasny, J. Winkelmann et al., "A randomized controlled study of pergolide in patients with restless legs syndrome," *Neurology*, vol. 52, no. 5, pp. 944–950, 1999.

[15] S. F. Bucher, K. C. Seelos, W. H. Oertel, M. Reiser, and C. Trenkwalder, "Cerebral generators involved in the pathogenesis of the restless legs syndrome," *Annals of Neurology*, vol. 41, no. 5, pp. 639–645, 1997.

[16] S. Gilman, G. K. Wenning, P. A. Low et al., "Second consensus statement on the diagnosis of multiple system atrophy," *Neurology*, vol. 71, no. 9, pp. 670–676, 2008.

[17] C. L. Tomlinson, R. Stowe, S. Patel, C. Rick, R. Gray, and C. E. Clarke, "Systematic review of levodopa dose equivalency reporting in Parkinson's disease," *Movement Disorders*, vol. 25, no. 15, pp. 2649–2653, 2010.

[18] C. Trenkwalder, R. Kohnen, B. Högl et al., "Parkinson's disease sleep scale-validation of the revised version PDSS-2," *Movement Disorders*, vol. 26, no. 4, pp. 644–652, 2011.

[19] A. Kales, A. Rechtschaffen, and University of California LABIS, Network NNI, "A manual of standardized terminology, techniques and scoring system for sleep stages of human subjects," A. Rechtschaffen and A. Kales, Eds., U.S. National Institute of Neurological Diseases and Blindness, Neurological Information Network, Bethesda, Md, USA, 1968.

[20] Atlas Task Force of the American Sleep Disorders Association, C. Guilleminault, and C. Chairman, "Recording and scoring leg movements," *Sleep*, vol. 16, pp. 748–759, 1993.

[21] C. H. Schenck, S. R. Bundlie, M. G. Ettinger, and M. W. Mahowald, "Chronic behavioral disorders of human REM sleep: a new category of parasomnia," *Sleep*, vol. 9, no. 2, pp. 293–308, 1986.

[22] F. Sixel-Döring, M. Schweitzer, B. Mollenhauer, and C. Trenkwalder, "Intraindividual variability of REM sleep behavior disorder in Parkinson's disease: a comparative assessment using a new REM sleep behavior disorder severity scale (RBDSS) for clinical routine," *Journal of Clinical Sleep Medicine*, vol. 7, no. 1, pp. 75–80, 2011.

[23] B. Frauscher, A. Iranzo, C. Gaig et al., "Normative EMG values during REM sleep for the diagnosis of REM sleep behavior disorder," *Sleep*, vol. 35, no. 6, pp. 835–847, 2012.

[24] W. R. Ruehland, P. D. Rochford, F. J. O'Donoghue, R. J. Pierce, P. Singh, and A. T. Thornton, "The new AASM criteria for scoring hypopneas: impact on the apnea hypopnea index," *Sleep*, vol. 32, no. 2, pp. 150–157, 2009.

[25] R Development Core Team, "a language and environment for statistical computing," Vienna: R Foundation for Statistical Computing, 2010, http://www.R-project.org.

[26] A. N. Vgontzas, M. Zoumakis, E. O. Bixler et al., "Impaired nighttime sleep in healthy old versus young adults is associated with elevated plasma interleukin-6 and cortisol levels: physiologic and therapeutic implications," *Journal of Clinical Endocrinology and Metabolism*, vol. 88, no. 5, pp. 2087–2095, 2003.

[27] R. Ferri, S. Fulda, F. I. Cosentino, F. Pizza, and G. Plazzi, "A preliminary quantitative analysis of REM sleep chin EMG

in Parkinson's disease with or without REM sleep behavior disorder," *Sleep Medicine*, vol. 13, no. 6, pp. 707–713, 2012.

[28] F. Sixel-Döring, E. Trautmann, B. Mollenhauer, and C. Trenkwalder, "Associated factors for REM sleep behavior disorder in Parkinson disease," *Neurology*, vol. 77, pp. 1048–1054, 2011.

[29] A. Iranzo, J. Santamaría, D. B. Rye et al., "Characteristics of idiopathic REM sleep behavior disorder and that associated with MSA and PD," *Neurology*, vol. 65, no. 2, pp. 247–252, 2005.

[30] C. Trenkwalder and W. Paulus, "Restless legs syndrome: pathophysiology, clinical presentation and management," *Nature Reviews Neurology*, vol. 6, no. 6, pp. 337–346, 2010.

[31] T. Nomura, Y. Inoue, B. Högl et al., "Comparison of the clinical features of rapid eye movement sleep behavior disorder in patients with Parkinson's disease and multiple system atrophy," *Psychiatry and Clinical Neurosciences*, vol. 65, no. 3, pp. 264–271, 2011.

[32] B. Frauscher, V. Gschliesser, E. Brandauer et al., "REM sleep behavior disorder in 703 sleep-disorder patients: the importance of eliciting a comprehensive sleep history," *Sleep Medicine*, vol. 11, no. 2, pp. 167–171, 2010.

[33] O. Flabeau, W. G. Meissner, and F. Tison, "Multiple system atrophy: current and future approaches to management," *Therapeutic Advances in Neurological Disorders*, vol. 3, no. 4, pp. 249–263, 2010.

[34] E. Friess, T. Kuempfel, S. Modell et al., "Paroxetine treatment improves motor symptoms in patients with multiple system atrophy," *Parkinsonism and Related Disorders*, vol. 12, no. 7, pp. 432–437, 2006.

[35] 2012, http://apps.who.int/bmi/index.jsp?introPage=intro_3.html.

[36] C. G. Bachmann and C. Trenkwalder, "Body weight in patients with Parkinson's disease," *Movement Disorders*, vol. 21, no. 11, pp. 1824–1830, 2006.

19

Oximetry Signal Processing Identifies REM Sleep-Related Vulnerability Trait in Asthmatic Children

Geovanny F. Perez,[1] **Maria J. Gutierrez,**[2] **Shehlanoor Huseni,**[1] **Khrisna Pancham,**[1] **Carlos E. Rodriguez-Martinez,**[3,4,5] **Cesar L. Nino,**[6] **and Gustavo Nino**[1,7]

[1] *Division of Pulmonary and Sleep Medicine, Children's National Medical Center, Washington, DC 20010, USA*
[2] *Division of Pediatric Rheumatology, Allergy & Immunology, Pennsylvania State University College of Medicine, Hershey, PA 17033, USA*
[3] *Department of Pediatrics, School of Medicine, Universidad Nacional de Colombia, Bogota, Colombia*
[4] *Department of Pediatric Pulmonology and Pediatric Critical Care Medicine, School of Medicine, Universidad El Bosque, Bogota, Colombia*
[5] *Research Unit, Military Hospital of Colombia, Bogota, Colombia*
[6] *Department of Electronics Engineering, Javeriana University, Bogota, Colombia*
[7] *Department of Integrative Systems Biology and Center for Genetic Medicine Research, Children's National Medical Center, George Washington University, Washington, DC 20010, USA*

Correspondence should be addressed to Gustavo Nino; nino.gustavo@gmail.com

Academic Editor: Giora Pillar

Rationale. The sleep-related factors that modulate the nocturnal worsening of asthma in children are poorly understood. This study addressed the hypothesis that asthmatic children have a REM sleep-related vulnerability trait that is independent of OSA. *Methods.* We conducted a retrospective cross-sectional analysis of pulse-oximetry signals obtained during REM and NREM sleep in control and asthmatic children ($n = 134$). Asthma classification was based on preestablished clinical criteria. Multivariate linear regression model was built to control for potential confounders (significance level $P \leq 0.05$). *Results.* Our data demonstrated that (1) baseline nocturnal respiratory parameters were not significantly different in asthmatic versus control children, (2) the maximal % of SaO_2 desaturation during REM, but not during NREM, was significantly higher in asthmatic children, and (3) multivariate analysis revealed that the association between asthma and REM-related maximal % SaO_2 desaturation was independent of demographic variables. *Conclusion.* These results demonstrate that children with asthma have a REM-related vulnerability trait that impacts oxygenation independently of OSA. Further research is needed to delineate the REM sleep neurobiological mechanisms that modulate the phenotypical expression of nocturnal asthma in children.

1. Introduction

Asthma is a chronic inflammatory disease characterized by worsening of symptoms during sleep [1, 2]. This nocturnal vulnerability of asthmatic individuals has been previously attributed to increased vagal tone, decreased sympathetic activity, reduced functional residual capacity of the lungs (affecting the small airways), endogenous circadian system changes during the night, and a higher risk for obstructive sleep apnea (OSA) in the asthmatic population [2–4].

Interestingly, several studies have reported that asthmatic patients deteriorate more during the morning hours with the majority of respiratory arrests and sudden deaths occurring from midnight to 8 am [5, 6]. The latter phenomenon suggests a greater influence of the rapid eye movement (REM) sleep in the asthmatic condition since this sleep stage predominates during the second part of the night [7].

REM sleep is considered particularly important in the pathogenesis of OSA and other sleep-related breathing abnormalities [8–12]. It has also been suggested that REM sleep is characterized by nocturnal bronchoconstriction [13]. In the context of pediatric asthma, we have recently identified that asthmatic children with OSA have more REM sleep-related breathing abnormalities relative to children with OSA alone [14]. These findings suggested that asthmatic patients have a REM sleep vulnerability trait that predisposes them to have more respiratory abnormalities during this sleep stage. In support of this notion, Catterall et al. have previously demonstrated that stable adult asthmatics have irregular breathing and hypoxemia clustered during REM sleep [15]. Importantly, OSA worsens during REM sleep as well [8–12], thus REM-related breathing abnormalities in asthmatic individuals may be just a reflection of the well-known association between asthma and OSA [4]. Accordingly, to better delineate the link between asthma and REM sleep in children, our current study investigated whether asthmatic children have more REM sleep-related hypoxemia independently of the presence of OSA. To this end, we conducted stage specific (REM versus NREM sleep) signal processing of the pulse-oximetry channel recorded during overnight polysomnography (PSG) in asthmatic children without OSA as previously described [14]. Our main hypothesis was that asthmatic children without OSA would have more REM-related hypoxemia, expressed as the maximal percentage of SaO_2 desaturation during REM sleep, relative to control children without asthma. Secondary analysis evaluated the influence of modulatory factors of REM-related breathing abnormalities, such as gender, age, and ethnicity [16], in the association between REM-related hypoxemia and asthma in children.

2. Materials and Methods

2.1. Subjects. A database of all children that underwent routine overnight polysomnogram (PSG) at the Penn State Sleep Research and Treatment Center (SRTC) between January 2010 and June 2011 was reviewed. Patients were eligible for the study if their PSG ruled out the diagnosis of obstructive sleep apnea (OSA). Almost all patients were referred to PSG to rule out OSA. OSA was defined as an obstructive apnea-hypopnea index (OAHI) ≥ 1.5 events per hour [17–20]. Only the patient's initial PSG was included in the study. Infants, school age children, and young adolescents were included (2–13 years). Patients were excluded if they had need for supplemental oxygen or positive airway pressure, central hypoventilation syndromes, congenital heart disease, severe developmental delay, cerebral palsy, genetic syndromes, craniofacial abnormalities, or neuromuscular disorders. Patients without complete clinical and PSG data available were also excluded from the study. Asthma status was determined based on electronic medical records reviewed in Penn State Children's Hospital and Penn State SRTC. This study was approved by the Institutional Review Board of Penn State College of Medicine.

2.2. PSG Protocol, Scoring, and Analysis. Standard pediatric overnight PSG was performed on all patients. During 9-10 hours, the child's sleep was continuously recorded to a computerized system (Twin PSG software; Grass Technologies. Inc., West Warwick, RI, USA) and scored manually in 30-second epochs according to the American Academy of Sleep Medicine (AASM) standardized criteria [17]. PSG measurements included electroencephalograms (EEG), electrooculograms (EOG), electrocardiogram (ECG), mental-submental electromyogram (EMG), thoracic and abdominal wall motion (respiratory inductance plethysmography), pulse oximetry (with 2 s averaging time), end-tidal carbon dioxide monitoring, combined nasal/oral thermistor, and nasal pressure. Sleep stages and respiratory events were scored according to the AASM pediatric scoring criteria [17]. Five AASM sleep stages were identified (wake stage = W, stage 1 = N1, stage 2 = N2, stage 3 = N3, and stage REM = R). For the purpose of this investigation, we used OAHI and respiratory data calculated for W stage (beginning of PSG), non-REM stage (represented by N1, N2, and N3), and REM sleep. The OAHI was calculated separately during REM, NREM sleep, and total sleep time (TST). Pulse-oximetry signal was examined separately and carefully cleaned from artifacts. "Maximal percentage of SaO_2 desaturation" was calculated with the formula (SaO_2 baseline − SaO_2 nadir)/SaO_2 baseline, and it was individually measured during NREM and REM sleep stages as previously described [14]. Additional respiratory analyses were conducted to obtain baseline SaO_2 during TST, wake, NREM, and REM sleep.

2.3. Asthma Status and Other Covariables. Clinical and demographic variables were obtained reviewing electronic medical records in Penn State Children's Hospital and Penn State Sleep Research and Treatment Center. "Asthma" was defined in this pediatric population using a definition that required the presence of at least one of the following criteria: (1) ever being diagnosed with asthma by a physician on the basis of criteria recommended for children 0–4 and 5–11 years of age in the National Institute Of Health (NIH) National Asthma Education and Prevention Program (NAEPP) Guidelines [1] and (2) use of asthma therapy and/or presence of asthma symptoms in the past 12 months. Other covariables investigated included age, race, sex, body mass index (BMI), percent of REM sleep, total sleep time (TST), and TST in supine position.

2.4. Statistical Analysis. Data were analyzed using the software SAS version 9.3 or later (SAS Institute Inc., Cary, NC, USA). Exploratory data analysis on main variables were performed for the entire study population and stratified according to asthma status. SaO_2 parameters were calculated separately for REM and NREM sleep. For pair-wise relationships, two-sample t-test was used to compare the mean value of the continuous outcome measures such as SaO_2-derived measurements, and chi-square test was used to compare the proportion of positive signals for binary outcomes. Multivariate linear regression model was built to study the joint effect of asthma and maximal percentage of SaO_2 desaturation during REM with control of possible confounders such as gender, age, and ethnicity. Significance was taken at the $P < 0.05$ level.

3. Results

3.1. Study Population. 134 children and young adolescents (2–13 years) were included in this study. The total study population was subdivided into one group with asthma ($n = 46$) and another group without the disease ($n = 88$). Comparison of demographic, anthropometric, and baseline PSG variables between these two groups revealed no significant differences (Tables 1 and 2).

3.2. Children with Asthma Are Susceptible to Nocturnal Hypoxemia during REM Sleep. We first examined pulse-oximetry signals at baseline and during sleep stages (REM versus NREM) in children with asthma and contrasted them with those seen in children without this condition (control). As shown in Table 2, the mean SaO_2 parameters obtained during wake, REM, and NREM sleep were not significantly different in asthmatic children compared to those in the control group (Table 2). In the same way, the maximal percentage of SaO_2 during REM and NREM was not significantly different in those children without asthma (REM 4.4% ± SD 2.4 versus NREM 4.2% ± SD 2.5, $P = 0.38$) (Figure 1). The mean SaO_2 nadir in the asthma group was slightly lower (93.49 ± SD 2.2) relative to the control group (94.14 ± SD 1.5), but this difference did not reach statistically significance ($P = 0.08$) probably because this nadir included REM and NREM sleep values. In contrast, children with asthma had a maximal percentage of SaO_2 desaturation that was significantly higher during REM relative to that seen in NREM (REM 6.2% ± SD 2.9 versus NREM 4.4 ± SD 2.0, $P = 0.001$).

3.3. The Association between Asthma and REM-Related Hypoxemia Is Independent of Gender, Age, and Ethnicity. REM-related breathing abnormalities have been linked to younger age and female gender [16]. Accordingly, we built a multivariate linear regression model to assess the confounder effect of age, gender, and ethnicity in the relationship between asthma and maximal percentage of SaO_2 desaturation during REM sleep (Table 3). After adjusting for these covariables, we found that the effect of asthma in REM-related hypoxemia (maximal % REM SaO_2 desaturation) is independent of age, gender, and ethnicity (adjusted $P = 0.04$, Table 3).

4. Discussion

The most important finding of the current study is that the maximal percentage of SaO_2 desaturation during REM, but not during NREM, is significantly greater in asthmatic children without OSA. Accordingly, our data suggest that children with asthma have a REM-related vulnerability trait that impacts oxygenation independently of OSA according to PSG criteria.

There is clear evidence supporting the worsening of asthma during sleep. The largest study of the prevalence of nocturnal asthma symptoms was reported by Turner-Warwick [21]. This survey of 7729 patients with asthma revealed that 74% awoke at least once per week with asthma symptoms [21]. Several asthma studies have also shown decreased pulmonary function and increased inflammatory

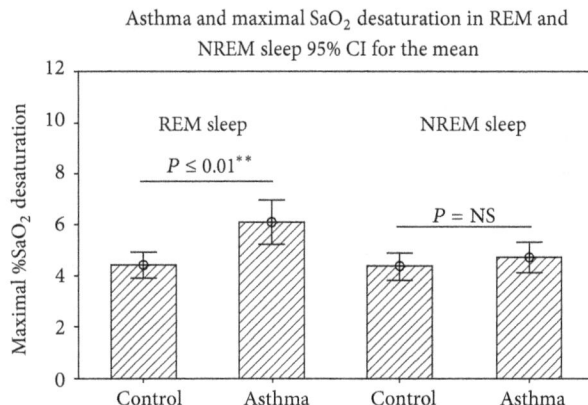

FIGURE 1: Maximal SaO_2 desaturation in REM and NREM sleep by asthma status in children. Data are presented as mean and 95% confidence interval (CI). REM: rapid eye movement; NREM: nonrapid eye movement; SaO_2: Oxygen saturation; P values are obtained by two-sample student t-test.

markers at nighttime. Kelly et al. [22] demonstrated that the forced expiratory volume in the first second (FEV1) of patients with asthma is significantly worse at 4:00 A.M. compared to 4 P.M. [22]. Bonnet et al. performed inhalation challenges every 4 h for 13 consecutive times in asthmatic patients and found 24 hour oscillations in the pulmonary sensitivity to histamine and methacholine, with at least doubling concentrations required for the same effect at certain times of day [23]. Additionally, Kraft et al. [24] reported that patients with nocturnal asthma exhibit higher concentrations of inflammatory markers in the distal airways (leukocyte, neutrophil, and eosinophil counts) at nighttime [24]. Collectively, these data support the prevailing notion that the asthmatic condition is highly influenced by the nocturnal phase of circadian rhythms.

In concert with circadian changes at night, specific sleep stages appear to modulate the phenotypical expression of asthma. Shapiro et al. reported that nocturnal bronchoconstriction may be associated with REM sleep [13]. Catterall et al. also identified that individuals with chronic stable asthma have irregular breathing and greater fluctuations in SaO_2 during REM sleep relative to controls [15]. In children, we have recently reported that asthmatic subjects with OSA have clustering of obstructive events and hypoxemia during REM sleep compared to children with OSA alone [14]. Based on these observations, our current study postulated that asthmatic children without OSA also have nocturnal respiratory abnormalities during REM sleep. To test this hypothesis, we conducted signal processing of the pulse-oximetry channel used during PSG to calculate stage specific (REM versus NREM) means and maximal SaO_2 desaturations as previously described [14]. Our data demonstrated that children with asthma have greater REM-related maximal SaO_2 desaturation relative to those children without asthma.

There are several neurobiological mechanisms that might underlie the potential modulatory role of REM in asthma. REM sleep is characterized by increased cholinergic outflow and ablated noradrenergic signals in the brainstem [25–27], which are in turn critical modulators of the caliber and

TABLE 1: Demographic profile of subjects.

Factors/variables	Total ($n = 134$)	Control ($n = 88$, 66%)	Asthma ($n = 46$, 34%)	P value
Demographic variables				
Gender				0.28
Female	58 (43%)	41 (46%)	17 (37%)	
Male	76 (57%)	47 (54%)	29 (63%)	
Age: mean (SD)	6.32 (2.9)	6.1 (2.9)	6.8 (2.9)	0.18
Ethnicity				0.95
White	96 (62%)	55 (67%)	41 (65%)	
Others	49 (37%)	27 (33%)	22 (35%)	
BMI: mean (SD)	18.5 (5.3)	17.8 (4.3)	19.6 (5.9)	0.08

For quantitative variables, data are presented as mean ± standard deviation (SD). BMI: body mass index; for categorical variables, data are presented as count number (column percentage). *P* values are obtained by either two-sample *t*-test or chi-square test, depending on the type of variables.

TABLE 2: Polysomnographic parameters of subjects.

Factors/variables	Control ($n = 88$, 66%)	Asthma ($n = 46$, 34%)	P value
Sleep study parameters			
OAHI			
Events/hr; mean (SD)	0.35 (0.4)	0.39 (0.4)	0.65
Total sleep time (TST)			
Min; mean (SD)	535 (61)	526 (41)	0.28
TST supine %			
Mean (SD)	43.3 (27.2)	46.3 (22)	0.67
REM (%)			
Mean (SD)	18.8 (5.1)	21.3 (4.9)	0.35
Max % REM SAO$_2$ desaturation			
Mean (SD)	**4.4 (2.5)**	**6.2 (2.8)**	**0.001**[**]
Max % NREM SAO$_2$ desaturation			
Mean (SD)	4. 4 (2.5)	4.7 (2.0)	0.38
SAO$_2$ (wake)			
Mean (SD)	97.3 (1.4)	97.2 (0.9)	0.54
SAO$_2$ (REM, average)			
Mean (SD)	97 (1.0)	97 (1.2)	0.85
SAO$_2$ (NREM, average)			
Mean (SD)	96.8 (1.0)	96.6 (1.2)	0.28

For quantitative variables, data are presented as mean ± standard deviation (SD). SAO$_2$: saturation of oxygen; REM: rapid eye movement; OAHI: obstructive apnea-hypopnea index. For categorical variables, data are presented as count number (column percentage). *P* values are obtained by either two-sample *t*-test or chi-square test, depending on the type of variables. Statistically significant results are shown in bold font.

TABLE 3: Multivariate regression analysis results for the association between rhinitis and REM-OAHI adjusted by co-variables.

Predictors	Parameter estimate	SE	P-value
Multivariate regression analysis for max % REM SAO$_2$ desaturation			
Asthma	**1.26**	**0.62**	**0.04**[*]
Age yrs	−0.08	0.10	0.41
Gender	−0.90	0.59	0.13
Ethnicity	−0.18	0.27	0.50

Data are presented as parameter estimate, standard error (SE). REM: rapid eye movement; OAHI: obstructive apnea-hypopnea index. Adjusted *P*-values are obtained by multiple linear regression.
Statistically significant results are shown in bold font.

reactivity of the lower airways in mice [25–27]. In addition, animal models of allergic asthma have illustrated that allergic lung inflammation may affect central noradrenergic control of cholinergic outflow to the airways, thereby augmenting bronchoconstrictive reflex responses in the asthmatic state [28]. The tone of the accessory respiratory muscles is also markedly decreased during REM sleep, which may reduce pulmonary reserve and lead to hypoventilation-hypoxemia in many respiratory conditions including asthma [29]. The latter

information, together with our current findings, support the notion that REM sleep neurobiology plays a key role in the normal functioning of the lower airways and so it might modulate the nocturnal manifestations of asthma children.

In evaluating the implications of the present observations, it is important to mention that our investigation used a cross-sectional design with a retrospective cohort of children. Thus, this study has the potential limitations of any retrospective analysis such as selection bias and misclassification of disease (information bias) resulting from inaccurate documentation in medical records. In terms of potential confounders, our design and statistical analysis accounted for several important covariables for the association between REM-related hypoxemia and asthma. For instance, our study excluded children with chronic lung disease, neuromuscular disorders, cerebral palsy, craniofacial abnormalities, and dysmorphic genetic syndromes, as they have a higher risk for nocturnal hypoxemia. Nonetheless, snoring was not evaluated and was likely present in a large number of children included in the study, so they cannot be necessarily regarded as otherwise healthy children with asthma. On the other hand, the strengths of our study included the relatively large sample size and the use of objective data to evaluate the influence of REM in asthma (PSG scoring and sleep-stage signal processing).

In summary, we feel that enough evidence is presented to support the concept that children with asthma have a REM-related vulnerability trait that impacts oxygenation independently of OSA. Further research is needed to delineate the biological link between REM-sleep and the physiology of the lower airways during health and disease. New knowledge in this area may allow the discovery of mechanistic pathways that connect airway inflammation and function with sleep biology, which in turn may result in novel strategies for the treatment of nocturnal symptoms of asthma.

Conflict of Interests

The authors declare that they have no conflict of interests.

Acknowledgment

This work was supported in part by the National Institute of Health (NIH), Career Development Award 1K12HL090020/NHLBI, Bethesda, MD, USA. Gustavo Nino (GN).

References

[1] "National Asthma Education and Prevention Program Expert Panel Report 3," US Department of Health and Human Services, National Institute of Health, NIH publication number 08-5406, 2007.

[2] H. Greenberg and R. I. Cohen, "Nocturnal asthma," *Current Opinion in Pulmonary Medicine*, vol. 18, no. 1, pp. 57–62, 2012.

[3] M. Litinski, F. A. J. L. Scheer, and S. A. Shea, "Influence of the circadian system on disease severity," *Sleep Medicine Clinics*, vol. 4, no. 2, pp. 143–163, 2009.

[4] M. Alkhalil, E. Schulman, and J. Getsy, "Obstructive sleep apnea syndrome and asthma: what are the links?" *Journal of Clinical Sleep Medicine*, vol. 5, no. 1, pp. 71–78, 2009.

[5] M. R. Hetzel, T. J. H. Clark, and M. A. Branthwaite, "Asthma: analysis of sudden deaths and ventilatory arrests in hospital," *The British Medical Journal*, vol. 1, no. 6064, pp. 808–811, 1977.

[6] G. M. Cochrane and T. J. H. Clark, "A survey of asthma mortality in patients between ages 35 and 64 in the Greater London hospitals in 1971," *Thorax*, vol. 30, no. 3, pp. 300–305, 1975.

[7] R. A. España and T. E. Scammell, "Sleep neurobiology for the clinician," *Sleep*, vol. 27, no. 4, pp. 811–820, 2004.

[8] A. I. Pack, L. R. Kline, J. C. Hendricks, N. B. Kribbs, and J. B. Neilly, "Neural mechanisms in the genesis of sleep apnea," *Progress in Clinical and Biological Research*, vol. 345, pp. 177–188, 1990.

[9] L. Kubin, R. O. Davies, and A. I. Pack, "Control of upper airway motoneurons during REM sleep," *News in Physiological Sciences*, vol. 13, no. 2, pp. 91–97, 1998.

[10] V. B. Fenik, R. O. Davies, and L. Kubin, "REM sleep-like atonia of hypoglossal (XII) motoneurons is caused by loss of noradrenergic and serotonergic inputs," *The American Journal of Respiratory and Critical Care Medicine*, vol. 172, no. 10, pp. 1322–1330, 2005.

[11] A. Oksenberg, E. Arons, K. Nasser, T. Vander, and H. Radwan, "REM-related obstructive sleep apnea: the effect of body position," *Journal of Clinical Sleep Medicine*, vol. 6, no. 4, pp. 343–348, 2010.

[12] B. Mokhlesi and N. M. Punjabi, "'REM-related' obstructive sleep apnea: an epiphenomenon or a clinically important entity?" *Sleep*, vol. 35, no. 1, pp. 5–7, 2012.

[13] C. M. Shapiro, J. R. Catterall, I. Montgomery, G. M. Raab, and N. J. Douglas, "Do asthmatics suffer bronchoconstriction during rapid eye movement sleep?" *The British Medical Journal*, vol. 292, no. 6529, pp. 1161–1164, 1986.

[14] M. J. Gutierrez, J. Zhu, C. E. Rodriguez-Martinez, C. L. Nino, and G. Nino, "Nocturnal phenotypical features of obstructive sleep apnea (OSA) in asthmatic children," *Pediatric Pulmonology*, vol. 48, no. 6, pp. 592–600, 2013.

[15] J. R. Catterall, N. J. Douglas, P. M. A. Calverley et al., "Irregular breathing and hypoxaemia during sleep in chronic stable asthma," *The Lancet*, vol. 1, no. 8267, pp. 301–304, 1982.

[16] B. B. Koo, S. R. Patel, K. Strohl, and V. Hoffstein, "Rapid eye movement-related sleep-disordered breathing: influence of age and gender," *Chest*, vol. 134, no. 6, pp. 1156–1161, 2008.

[17] C. Iber, S. Ancoli-Israel, A. L. Chesson Jr., and S. F. Quan, *The AASM Manual for the Scoring of Sleep and Associated Events: Rules, Terminology and Technical Specifications*, American Academy of Sleep Medicine, Westchester, Ill, USA, 2007.

[18] N. Traeger, B. Schultz, A. N. Pollock, T. Mason, C. L. Marcus, and R. Arens, "Polysomnographic values in children 2–9 years old: additional data and review of the literature," *Pediatric Pulmonology*, vol. 40, no. 1, pp. 22–30, 2005.

[19] H. E. Montgomery-Downs, L. M. O'Brien, T. E. Gulliver, and D. Gozal, "Polysomnographic characteristics in normal preschool and early school-aged children," *Pediatrics*, vol. 117, no. 3, pp. 741–753, 2006.

[20] M. B. Witmans, T. G. Keens, S. L. D. Ward, and C. L. Marcus, "Obstructive hypopneas in children and adolescents: normal values," *The American Journal of Respiratory and Critical Care Medicine*, vol. 168, no. 12, p. 1540, 2003.

[21] M. Turner-Warwick, "Epidemiology of nocturnal asthma," *The American Journal of Medicine*, vol. 85, no. 1, pp. 6–8, 1988.

[22] E. A. B. Kelly, J. J. Houtman, and N. N. Jarjour, "Inflammatory changes associated with circadian variation in pulmonary function in subjects with mild asthma," *Clinical and Experimental Allergy*, vol. 34, no. 2, pp. 227–233, 2004.

[23] R. Bonnet, R. Jorres, U. Heitmann, and H. Magnussen, "Circadian rhythm in airway responsiveness and airway tone in patients with mild asthma," *Journal of Applied Physiology*, vol. 71, no. 4, pp. 1598–1605, 1991.

[24] M. Kraft, R. Djukanovic, S. Wilson, S. T. Holgate, and R. J. Martin, "Alveolar tissue inflammation in asthma," *The American Journal of Respiratory and Critical Care Medicine*, vol. 154, no. 5, pp. 1505–1510, 1996.

[25] M. A. Haxhiu, P. Kc, K. V. Balan, C. G. Wilson, and R. J. Martin, "Modeling of sleep-induced changes in airway function: implication for nocturnal worsening of bronchial asthma," *Advances in Experimental Medicine and Biology*, vol. 605, pp. 469–474, 2008.

[26] M. A. Haxhiu, S. O. Mack, C. G. Wilson, P. Feng, and K. P. Strohl, "Sleep networks and the anatomic and physiologic connections with respiratory control," *Frontiers in Bioscience*, vol. 8, pp. d946–d962, 2003.

[27] M. A. Haxhiu, P. Kc, C. T. Moore et al., "Brain stem excitatory and inhibitory signaling pathways regulating bronchoconstrictive responses," *Journal of Applied Physiology*, vol. 98, no. 6, pp. 1961–1982, 2005.

[28] C. G. Wilson, S. Akhter, C. A. Mayer et al., "Allergic lung inflammation affects central noradrenergic control of cholinergic

outflow to the airways in ferrets," *Journal of Applied Physiology*, vol. 103, no. 6, pp. 2095–2104, 2007.

[29] J. R. Catterall, P. M. A. Calverley, W. MacNee et al., "Mechanism of transient nocturnal hypoxemia in hypoxic chronic bronchitis and emphysema," *Journal of Applied Physiology*, vol. 59, no. 6, pp. 1698–1703, 1985.

20

Asthma Control and Its Relationship with Obstructive Sleep Apnea (OSA) in Older Adults

Mihaela Teodorescu,[1,2,3] **David A. Polomis,**[2] **Ronald E. Gangnon,**[4] **Jessica E. Fedie,**[1,2]
Flavia B. Consens,[5] **Ronald D. Chervin,**[5] **and Mihai C. Teodorescu**[1,3,6]

[1] *James B. Skatrud Pulmonary/Sleep Research Laboratory, Medical Service, William S. Middleton Memorial Veterans Hospital, Madison, WI, USA*
[2] *Section of Allergy, Pulmonary and Critical Care Medicine, USA*
[3] *Center for Sleep Medicine and Sleep Research/Wisconsin Sleep, University of Wisconsin School of Medicine and Public Health, Madison, WI, USA*
[4] *Department of Biostatistics and Medical Informatics and Population Health Sciences, University of Wisconsin School of Medicine and Public Health, Madison, WI, USA*
[5] *Department of Neurology and Sleep Disorders Center, University of Michigan Health System, Ann Arbor, MI, USA*
[6] *Section of Geriatrics and Gerontology, University of Wisconsin School of Medicine and Public Health, Madison, WI, USA*

Correspondence should be addressed to Mihai C. Teodorescu; mct@medicine.wisc.edu

Academic Editor: Giora Pillar

Background/Objectives. Asthma in older individuals is poorly understood. We aimed to characterize the older asthma phenotype and test its association with obstructive sleep apnea (OSA). *Design*. Cross-sectional. *Setting*. Pulmonary and Asthma/Allergy clinics. *Participants*. 659 asthma subjects aged 18–59 years (younger) and 154 aged 60–75 (older). *Measurements*. Sleep Apnea scale of Sleep Disorders Questionnaire (SA-SDQ), asthma severity step (1–4, severe if step 3 or 4), established OSA diagnosis, continuous positive airway pressure (CPAP) use, and comorbidities. *Results*. Older versus younger had worse control, as assessed by asthma step, lung function, and inhaled corticosteroid use. Among older subjects, after controlling for known asthma aggravators, OSA diagnosis was the only factor robustly associated with severe asthma: on average, OSA was associated with nearly 7 times greater likelihood of severe asthma in an older individual (OR = 6.67). This relationship was of greater magnitude than in younger subjects (OR = 2.16). CPAP use attenuated the likelihood of severe asthma in older subjects by 91% ($P = 0.005$), much more than in the younger asthmatics. *Conclusion*. Diagnosed OSA increases the risk for worse asthma control in older patients, while CPAP therapy may have greater impact on asthma outcomes. Unrecognized OSA may be a reason for poor asthma control, particularly among older patients.

1. Introduction

Asthma is a major health problem in the general population. As many patients develop asthma in childhood or adolescence, large community studies have focused on asthma in early years. While the prevalence is estimated to be 6.5–17% [1] and may be similar to that seen in younger adults, asthma is frequently underrecognized as a geriatric respiratory disorder and often remains undiagnosed [2]. This may be due to the fact that older adults tend to underreport symptoms, have limited subjective awareness, lack perception or attribution to pulmonary pathology [2], or lack access to lung function testing such as spirometry and peak flow [3].

Asthma-associated morbidity and mortality increase with older age [4]. The number of unscheduled ambulatory visits, emergency visits, and hospitalizations is high in elderly asthmatics [5]. Elderly individuals with asthma in comparison to young adults have 14-fold higher asthma-related death rates and are twice as likely to be hospitalized in a given year [6]. Death rates attributable to asthma increase exponentially after age of 65 [7], with women and particularly black women being the most affected [8]. Nonetheless, suboptimal therapeutic management has often been the norm [4], perhaps as a result of the poor recognition and understanding of this phenotype. Inhaled corticosteroids were historically underutilized, with deviation from recommended clinical guidelines. In addition, therapeutic decisions may have been hampered by the fact that many randomized treatment trials excluded patients older than 65 years, or those with substantial comorbidity [9].

Quality of sleep in older patients with asthma is poorer compared to those with chronic obstructive pulmonary disease (COPD) or chronic bronchitis [10]. Whereas some comorbid conditions, such as rhinitis and gastroesophageal reflux disease (GERD), are well recognized to aggravate asthma, little is known about the potential role of obstructive sleep apnea (OSA), another condition with high prevalence in the elderly [11]. Accumulating data in younger samples suggests a role of OSA in asthma control. Treatment of OSA with continuous positive airway pressure (CPAP) improves asthma symptoms, peak flow rates, and quality of life [12, 13]. The sleep disorder is also an important risk factor for frequent exacerbations in difficult-to-control asthma patients [14].

We therefore used data from a sizeable, ongoing survey [15] to examine whether clinically-diagnosed and untreated OSA predicts asthma control among older patients and to assess whether the magnitude of such associations resembles those found among younger patients. Our hypothesis was that OSA predicts worse asthma control in older patients, as it does in the young. Preliminary results of this work have been published in abstract form [16]. Subsets of these data have been analyzed on other aspects of the relationships between OSA and asthma, which were included in our prior reports [15–17].

2. Methods

2.1. Study Participants. The sample included asthma patients returning for routine follow-up visits at the University of Michigan Pulmonary Clinics and Asthma-Airways Center and at the University of Wisconsin Allergy and Pulmonary Clinics. Subjects were enrolled as part of a larger ongoing study on the relationship between OSA and asthma, including use of informed consent and approval from each Institutional Review Board. Data were collected between May 2004 and April 2006 (at the University of Michigan) and July 2007 and December 2009 (at the University of Wisconsin). As required by the design of the parent study, patients 18–75 years old who were able and willing to provide informed consent and complete our survey were invited to participate. All subjects had specialist-diagnosed and managed asthma [18]. Patients underwent history, physical examination, asthma control assessments, and spirometry with each clinic visit. Those at urgent asthma-related visits or pregnant women were not enrolled.

2.2. Survey Content. The self-administered survey package, distributed by study assistants, is comprised of two questionnaires and additional questions on demographics. The first instrument, the Sleep Apnea scale of the Sleep Disorders Questionnaire (SA-SDQ) assesses OSA symptoms and summarizes its risk [19]. This scale consists of eight symptom items inquiring about loud snoring disruptive to the bed partner, cessation of breathing in sleep, sudden gasping arousals, worsening of snoring while supine or after alcohol, nocturnal sweating and nasal congestion, and history of hypertension. Responses are recorded on a 5-point Likert scale ("never" to "always"). Demographic data on weight, age, smoking, and body mass index (BMI) are rated on a 1 to 5 scale, with the overall SA-SDQ score ranging between 12 and 60. This scale was validated in a large sample of sleep patients [19].

The second survey instrument asked about frequency of daytime and nighttime asthma symptoms (as below) following the National Asthma Education and Prevention Program classification of asthma severity based on clinical features [20], as we previously reported [15]; two additional items asked about duration of asthma symptoms and physician-established diagnosis.

2.3. Medical Records Review. Reviews were conducted by study physicians to extract information on established diagnoses of lung disease (such as allergic bronchopulmonary aspergillosis, chronic obstructive pulmonary disease, and interstitial lung diseases), on OSA diagnosis (which had been established by clinical polysomnography (PSG)), and whether or not CPAP was being used as documented in the clinic visit notes at the time of the survey. PSG indices or objective CPAP use were not collected in this study. Also, information was extracted on other comorbidities (e.g., GERD, rhinitis, chronic sinusitis, nasal polyps, and psychiatric diseases such as depression, anxiety, panic, or bipolar disorders) and current asthma medications, and from spirometry to help assess asthma step.

The asthma step was assigned, according to NAEPP guidelines [20], as we previously reported [15], in order of increasing severity: (i) step 1 (mild-intermittent asthma), patients with daytime symptoms ≤ 2 days/week, nighttime symptoms ≤ 2 nights/month, Forced Expiratory Volume in first second (FEV$_1$) $\geq$ 80% predicted and peak expiratory flow rates (PEFR) variability <20%; (ii) step 2 (mild-persistent asthma), patients with daytime symptoms 3–6 days/week, nighttime symptoms more than 2 nights/month (3-4 nights/month), FEV$_1$ $\geq$ 80% and PEFR variability 20–30%; (iii) step 3 (moderate-persistent asthma), patients with daily asthma symptoms, nocturnal symptoms $\geq$5/month (or >once/week), FEV$_1$ between >60%–<80% or PEFR variability >30%; (iv) step 4 (severe-persistent asthma), patients with continuous daytime symptoms, frequent nighttime symptoms, FEV$_1$ $\leq$ 60% or PEFR variability >30%. The PEFR variability was calculated by dividing the difference between the highest and the lowest daily PEF value by the daily mean PEF and multiplying the result by 100 [21]. Attempts were made to obtain current peak flow diaries from patients or their medical records; due to their limited availability, for uniformity, the peak flow variability could not be used in asthma step assessment. The asthma step was determined by the most severe remaining qualifying features.

2.4. Data Analysis. Subjects were categorized into an older (60–75 years) or younger group (18–59 years). Baseline characteristics were summarized as mean ± standard deviation (SD) for continuous variables and percentages for categorical variables. The BMI was stratified per CDC criteria (<25, 25–29.9 and ≥30 kg/m^2) and used as an ordinal variable. Occurrence of OSA symptoms "usually" or "always" (responses of 4 or 5 on the SA-SDQ) defined "habitual" symptoms. The validated cutoffs of SA-SDQ ≥36 for men and ≥32 for women defined high OSA risk [19]. Age at asthma onset was computed based on current age and duration of asthma symptoms, and age at physician-established diagnosis was recorded. Asthma step 3 or 4 defined severe asthma. To assess for any differential expression of relationships between daytime or nighttime asthma symptoms with OSA, daytime asthma symptoms occurring >2 days/week defined persistent daytime symptoms, and nighttime symptoms occurring >2 nights/month defined persistent nighttime symptoms.

The initial analysis was conducted on data from subjects without OSA and those with diagnosed OSA but not on CPAP treatment at the time of survey. Two-sample *t*-test, *chi*-squared, or Fisher exact test were used, as appropriate, to test for group differences in baseline variables. Ordinal logistic or logistic regression were used to test for univariate relationships of asthma step or severe asthma as the dependent variables with OSA diagnosis, BMI and traditional contributors to asthma control (demographics [age, gender and African-American race], rhinitis, chronic sinusitis, nasal polyps, GERD, and psychiatric disease) [14, 22]. The same techniques were employed to fit multivariate models with asthma step, severe asthma or persistent asthma symptoms as the outcomes, and OSA diagnosis as the predictor, while controlling for the above covariates, regardless of their univariate associations with these asthma outcomes.

Secondly, data from subjects with diagnosed OSA were separately tested among each group, for associations of CPAP use with asthma step or severe asthma as the dependent variables. These multivariate logistic regression models were adjusted only for obesity, due to the small sample size of CPAP users, particularly in the older.

Statistical computations were conducted using SAS software Version 9.2 (SAS Institute, Cary, NC). A two-sided *P*-value < 0.05 was required for statistical significance. Trends were noted when *P*-values ranged 0.05–0.10.

3. Results

Among 1,026 subjects invited to participate, 952 (93%) agreed and completed the survey. Of these, 64 subjects had comorbid lung disease and were excluded from the analyses.

For the initial analysis, among 140 (36 older and 104 younger) subjects with previously diagnosed OSA, those 75 (16 older and 59 younger subjects) on treatment at the time of survey were excluded from analyses, as beneficial effects of CPAP treatment for OSA on asthma have been reported

[12, 13]. Among the remaining 813 subjects, 154 (19%) were elderly and 659 (81%) young, among whom the main results are reported. The subsequent analysis encompassed solely the 140 subjects with diagnosed OSA, regardless of their treatment status at the time of survey.

3.1. Phenotypic Characteristics of Older and Younger Asthma Subjects. Table 1 presents the demographic, physiologic, and clinical characteristics of the two groups. As compared to the young, older individuals had later onset of asthma symptoms and longer duration of physician-established diagnosis. They exhibited several indices of worse disease control, including physiologic measures and more frequent use of inhaled corticosteroid (ICS) at the time of survey. Older asthmatics had a higher prevalence of nasal polyps and GERD and a lower prevalence of psychiatric diseases. No statistically significant differences emerged in the other clinical variables presented (all $P > 0.10$). Table 2 depicts the distribution of asthma severity step and severe asthma (step 3 or 4) among the older and young groups. As before, when accounting for symptoms, a tendency towards higher step category was seen in the older group, and a significantly larger proportion of older subjects (49% versus 39%, $\chi^2 = 5.53$, $P = 0.02$) were in the severe asthma category. When evaluating the pattern of asthma symptoms, in comparison to the young, older subjects had similar frequencies of persistent daytime symptoms (31% versus 35%, $\chi^2 = 0.77$, $P = 0.38$), but they less often had nighttime symptoms (29% versus 39%, $\chi^2 = 5.50$, $P = 0.02$).

3.2. OSA Diagnosis and Symptoms in the Older and Younger Asthma Subjects. Table 3 presents the OSA diagnosis (clinically-diagnosed and untreated), SA-SDQ scores, and responses on its symptom-items. A larger proportion of older as opposed to younger subjects had OSA (13% versus 7%, $P = 0.01$); likewise, the mean SA-SDQ scores were higher in the older than in the young, and a higher proportion of older subjects (34% versus 25%, $P = 0.03$) achieved scores placing them at high risk for OSA, as defined by previously validated cutoffs [19]. Among individual SA-SDQ symptom items, witnessed apneas tended to be more prevalent in older patients who also had a significantly increased prevalence of current/history of hypertension; there was a lower prevalence of gasping arousals in the older relative to the younger patients.

3.3. Associations of Clinically-Diagnosed and Untreated OSA with Asthma Severity in the Older and Younger Asthma Subjects. Among older patients, in univariate ordinal logistic regression analyses (Table 4), statistically significant associations of asthma step with OSA and a history of GERD were noted, and trends were observed with BMI and rhinitis. In contrast, age, gender, African-American race, chronic sinusitis, nasal polyps, and a psychiatric history were not significantly associated with asthma step. Associations with OSA were of similar magnitude in the older and younger subjects. When examining severe asthma (Table 5), significant associations were also noted with OSA and GERD, and the

TABLE 1: Demographic and physiologic characteristics, medical history, and medication use for older and younger asthma subjects.

Characteristic	Mean ± SD, or Number (%) of Subjects		P value
	Older (n = 154)	Younger (n = 659)	
Age (y)	66 ± 4	42 ± 11	<0.0001
Gender (female)	95 (62%)	448 (68%)	0.14
BMI (kg × m^{-2})	29 ± 6	29 ± 7	0.36
<25	38 (25%)	214 (32%)	
25–29.9	52 (34%)	204 (31%)	0.17
≥30	64 (42%)	241 (37%)	
Race			0.65
African-American	7 (5%)	35 (5%)	
White	145 (94%)	598 (91%)	
Others*	2 (1%)	26 (4%)	
Current smokers	4 (3%)	33 (5%)	0.28
Age of asthma onset (y)	39 ± 21	22 ± 15	<0.0001
Age at physician-established asthma diagnosis (y)	41 ± 20	23 ± 16	<0.0001
FEV$_1$% predicted	87 ± 19	94 ± 19	0.0002
FVC% predicted	84 ± 16	93 ± 16	<0.0001
FEV$_1$/FVC	73 ± 9	77 ± 9	<0.0001
FEF$_{25-75}$% predicted	56 ± 27	71 ± 31	<0.0001
History of rhinitis	137 (89%)	598 (91%)	0.50
History of chronic sinusitis	54 (35%)	192 (29%)	0.15
History of nasal polyps	32 (21%)	88 (13%)	0.02
History of GERD	84 (55%)	285 (43%)	0.01
History of psychiatric disease	29 (19%)	190 (29%)	0.01
Using inhaled corticosteroid (ICS)	132 (86%)	500 (76%)	0.008
Using oral corticosteroid	16 (10%)	54 (8%)	0.38
Using inhaled long-acting bronchodilator	97 (63%)	379 (58%)	0.22
Using antileukotriene agents	32 (21%)	182 (28%)	0.08
Using inhaled anticholinergic	10 (6%)	49 (7%)	0.69
Using theophylline	4 (3%)	13 (2%)	0.54

Definition of abbreviations: SD: standard deviation; BMI: body mass index; FEV$_1$%: forced expiratory volume in first second; FVC%: forced vital capacity; FEF$_{25-75}$%: forced expiratory flow between 25% and 75% of vital capacity (all of these physiologic variables are expressed as percentages of predicted values); GERD: gastroesophageal reflux disease.
* Included Asians, Hawaiian/Pacific Islander, and American Indians/Alaskans.

TABLE 2: Distribution of asthma severity step and severe asthma (step 3 or 4) among older and younger asthma subjects.

	Older (n = 154) number (%)	Younger (n = 659) number (%)	P value
Asthma step			
1	64 (42%)	312 (47%)	0.08
2	14 (9%)	90 (14%)	
3	44 (29%)	138 (21%)	
4	32 (21%)	119 (18%)	
Severe asthma	76 (49%)	257 (39%)	0.02

relationship with OSA was of greater magnitude in the older than in the young.

In a multivariate model (Table 6) that included all the above variables as covariates, only OSA was significantly associated with asthma severity step: having an OSA diagnosis increased the odds of a worse asthma severity step on average by 191% (OR = 2.91, 95% confidence interval [1.15–7.36]), independent of the other characteristics. Associations of OSA with asthma step in older subjects seemed of greater magnitude than in the younger subjects. In a reiteration of this model using severe asthma as the dependent variable (Table 7), much more robust associations with OSA were observed in the older than in the younger subjects: independent of covariates, an OSA diagnosis raised the likelihood of severe asthma on average by 567% (OR = 6.67, 95% confidence interval [1.74–25.56]) in the older subjects versus 161% (2.61 [1.28–5.33]) in the younger subjects.

3.4. Pattern of Asthma Symptoms and Their Associations with Clinically-Diagnosed and Untreated OSA in Older and Younger Asthma Subjects. A differential expression of the relationships between daytime or nighttime asthma symptoms with OSA was noted (Table 8): in the older subjects, nighttime asthma symptoms were primarily related to OSA (4.56 [1.55–13.43]), whereas in the younger subjects daytime

TABLE 3: OSA (clinically-diagnosed and untreated), SA-SDQ scores, and frequencies of individual symptoms (when present with any frequency), in older and younger asthma subjects.

	Mean ± SD or number (%) of subjects		P value
	Older ($n = 154$)	Younger ($n = 659$)	
OSA	20 (13%)	45 (7%)	0.01
SA-SDQ score	30.2 ± 6.4	27.7 ± 7.6	<0.0001
Snoring	126 (82%)	511 (78%)	0.25
Habitual snoring*	37 (24%)	172 (26%)	0.60
Witnessed apneas	50 (32%)	167 (25%)	0.07
Sudden gasping arousals	48 (31%)	276 (42%)	0.01
Excessive sweating at night	109 (71%)	481 (73%)	0.58
Current or history of hypertension	87 (56%)	182 (28%)	<0.0001
Nasal congestion during sleep	118 (77%)	485 (74%)	0.44
Snoring worse when supine	103 (67%)	433 (66%)	0.78
Snoring worse after alcohol	51 (33%)	236 (36%)	0.53

Definition of abbreviations: OSA: obstructive sleep apnea; SA-SDQ: Sleep Apnea scale of the Sleep Disorders Questionnaire (range 12–60); *Habitual snoring: snoring occurring "usually" or "always" (responses of 4 or 5 on the SA-SDQ).

TABLE 4: Univariate associations of asthma severity step with OSA (clinically-diagnosed and untreated) and other traditional factors of asthma control, in the older and younger asthma subjects.

	Older ($n = 154$)		Younger ($n = 659$)	
	Odds ratio [95% confidence interval]	P value	Odds ratio [95% confidence interval]	P value
OSA	3.44 [1.43–8.27]	<0.0001	3.61 [2.07–6.31]	<0.0001
Age	1.04 [0.97–1.11]	0.30	1.01 [1.00–1.02]	0.12
Gender (female versus male)	0.97 [0.54–1.77]	0.93	1.35 [1.00–1.83]	0.05
BMI (categorized)	1.37 [0.95–1.98]	0.09	1.84 [1.54–2.20]	<0.0001
African-American (versus all others)	1.90 [0.48–7.55]	0.36	4.04 [2.14–7.60]	<0.0001
Rhinitis	0.43 [0.17–1.09]	0.08	0.27 [0.17–0.44]	<0.0001
Chronic sinusitis	0.67 [0.36–1.23]	0.20	0.93 [0.68–1.28]	0.67
Nasal polyps	0.92 [0.45–1.88]	0.82	1.35 [0.90–2.04]	0.15
GERD	1.94 [1.08–3.51]	0.03	1.64 [1.23–2.18]	0.0007
Psychiatric disease	1.26 [0.60–2.62]	0.54	1.50 [1.10–2.04]	0.01

Definition of abbreviations: OSA: obstructive sleep apnea; BMI: body mass index (kg/m^2); GERD: gastroesophageal reflux disease.

TABLE 5: Univariate associations of severe asthma (step 3 or 4) with OSA (clinically-diagnosed and untreated) and other traditional factors of asthma control, in the older and younger asthma subjects.

	Older ($n = 154$)		Younger ($n = 659$)	
	Odds ratio [95% confidence interval]	P value	Odds ratio [95% confidence interval]	P value
OSA	7.20 [2.02–25.74]	0.002	4.26 [2.19–8.28]	<0.0001
Age	1.04 [0.97–1.11]	0.30	1.01 [1.00–1.02]	0.12
Gender (female versus male)	0.97 [0.54–1.77]	0.93	1.35 [1.00–1.83]	0.05
BMI (categorized)	1.37 [0.95–1.98]	0.09	1.84 [1.54–2.20]	<0.0001
African-American (versus all others)	1.90 [0.48–7.55]	0.36	4.04 [2.14–7.60]	<0.0001
Rhinitis	0.43 [0.17–1.09]	0.08	0.27 [0.17–0.44]	<0.0001
Chronic sinusitis	0.67 [0.36–1.23]	0.20	0.93 [0.68–1.28]	0.67
Nasal polyps	0.92 [0.45–1.88]	0.82	1.35 [0.90–2.04]	0.15
GERD	1.94 [1.08–3.51]	0.03	1.64 [1.23–2.18]	0.0007
Psychiatric disease	1.26 [0.60–2.62]	0.54	1.50 [1.10–2.04]	0.01

Definition of abbreviations: OSA: obstructive sleep apnea; BMI: body mass index (kg/m^2); GERD: gastroesophageal reflux disease.

TABLE 6: Multivariate associations of asthma severity step with OSA (clinically-diagnosed and untreated) and other traditional factors of asthma control, in the older and younger asthma subjects.

	Older ($n = 154$)		Younger ($n = 659$)	
	Odds ratio [95% confidence interval]	P value	Odds ratio [95% confidence interval]	P value
OSA	2.91 [1.15–7.36]	0.02	2.07 [1.14–3.75]	0.02
Age	1.03 [0.96–1.10]	0.48	1.00 [0.99–1.02]	0.89
Gender (female versus male)	0.89 [0.46–1.74]	0.74	1.45 [1.06–1.99]	0.02
BMI (categorized)	1.22 [0.82–1.81]	0.32	1.60 [1.32–1.93]	<0.0001
African-American (versus all others)	0.76 [0.17–3.43]	0.72	3.08 [1.60–5.93]	0.0008
Rhinitis	0.48 [0.19–1.25]	0.14	0.36 [0.22–0.59]	<0.0001
Chronic Sinusitis	0.60 [0.29–1.24]	0.17	0.88 [0.62–1.26]	0.49
Nasal Polyps	1.34 [0.55–3.26]	0.52	1.26 [0.79–1.95]	0.33
GERD	1.58 [0.86–2.92]	0.14	1.22 [0.89–1.67]	0.22
Psychiatric disease	1.33 [0.60–2.97]	0.48	1.31 [0.94–1.82]	0.11

Definition of abbreviations: OSA: obstructive sleep apnea; BMI: body mass index (kg/m^2); GERD: gastroesophageal reflux disease.

TABLE 7: Multivariate associations of severe asthma (step 3 or 4) with OSA (clinically-diagnosed and untreated) and other traditional factors of asthma control, in the older and younger asthma subjects.

	Older ($n = 154$)		Younger ($n = 659$)	
	Odds ratio [95% confidence interval]	P value	Odds ratio [95% confidence interval]	P value
OSA	6.67 [1.74–25.56]	0.006	2.61 [1.28–5.33]	0.008
Age	1.06 [0.98–1.14]	0.17	1.01 [0.99–1.02]	0.45
Gender (female versus male)	1.32 [0.61–2.86]	0.49	1.48 [1.03–2.11]	0.04
BMI (categorized)	1.06 [0.68–1.65]	0.81	1.49 [1.20–1.84]	0.0003
African-American (versus all others)	1.89 [0.27–13.24]	0.52	4.26 [1.89–9.59]	0.0005
Rhinitis	0.40 [0.12–1.28]	0.12	0.45 [0.25–0.81]	0.007
Chronic sinusitis	0.38 [0.16–0.91]	0.03	0.81 [0.54–1.22]	0.31
Nasal polyps	1.73 [0.60–4.96]	0.31	1.32 [0.78–2.23]	0.30
GERD	1.35 [0.67–2.71]	0.41	1.30 [0.91–1.85]	0.16
Psychiatric disease	1.68 [0.65–4.33]	0.28	1.05 [0.72–1.54]	0.81

Definition of abbreviations: OSA: obstructive sleep apnea; BMI: body mass index (kg/m^2); GERD: gastroesophageal reflux disease.

TABLE 8: Multivariate associations of persistent daytime and nighttime asthma symptoms with OSA (clinically-diagnosed and untreated) with adjustment for age, gender, race (African-American versus. all others), rhinitis, chronic sinusitis, nasal polyps, gastroesophageal reflux disease, and psychiatric disease, in the older and younger asthma subjects.

	Older ($n = 154$)		Younger ($n = 659$)	
	Odds ratio [95% confidence interval]	P value	Odds ratio [95% confidence interval]	P value
Persistent daytime symptoms	2.00 [0.71–5.65]	0.19	2.66 [1.32–5.35]	0.006
Persistent nighttime symptoms	4.56 [1.55–13.43]	0.006	1.35 [0.70–2.63]	0.37

asthma symptoms were associated with OSA (2.66 [1.32–5.32]), both after adjustment for the same variables shown in Tables 6 and 7.

3.5. Relationships of Asthma Severity with CPAP Use among Older and Younger Subjects with Clinically-Diagnosed OSA. Among clinically-diagnosed OSA subjects ($n = 140$), the frequency of CPAP use was not significantly different between the older and younger groups (21% versus 31%, $\chi^2 = 1.62$, $P = 0.20$). In older subjects, with adjustment for BMI, CPAP use was associated with a reduced likelihood of worse asthma step by 86% (0.14 [0.04–0.56], $P = 0.005$) and of severe asthma by 91% (0.09 [0.02–0.49], $P = 0.005$); these

relationships were of greater magnitude in older subjects than in younger subjects, where CPAP use attenuated the likelihood of worse asthma step by 58% (0.42 [0.20–0.88], $P = 0.02$) and that of severe asthma by 57% (0.43 [0.18–1.03], $P = 0.06$).

4. Discussion

This analysis of a large clinic-based sample of patients with asthma shows for the first time that older as compared to younger asthmatics have worse asthma control and that poor control in older subjects may depend on comorbid OSA more than it does in younger subjects. Moreover,

CPAP use attenuated the likelihood of worse asthma control, statistically, more robustly in older than in younger subjects. In marked contrast to OSA symptoms, traditionally recognized risk factors for asthma such as BMI, female gender, African-American race, rhinitis, and GERD showed little or no independent predictive value for asthma control among older persons. Collectively, these data suggest that underlying OSA may contribute to worse asthma control, particularly in the older patients, independent of other known asthma aggravators.

This clinic-based asthma sample is likely representative of older asthma patients, including those with unrecognized OSA, who are managed in specialty clinic settings. There was a high participation rate in our survey study (95%). Obesity rates were consistent with current estimates of obesity in this age group [23]. Mean duration of asthma was comparable with that reported in other studies [24]. Subjects demonstrated a higher FEV_1/FVC ratio and much higher use of inhaled corticosteroids than what has been reported previously [2, 4], indicating appropriate use of treatment guidelines for asthma control in our sample. The high prevalence of patients with rhinitis (88%) reflects that this sample was recruited in good part from Allergy clinics. Rhinitis was not associated with asthma step in our population, likely due to its rigorous management by expert providers, which counteracted its detrimental influence on asthma control. Smoking was remarkably infrequent in our sample as compared to others [25], which may reflect a historical trend toward lower smoking rates or more effective education and interventions in two university clinic settings. Nonetheless, this finding supports the absence of confounding by comorbid chronic obstructive lung disease.

Despite vigorous management, nearly half (49%) of our older subjects had worse asthma control (severe asthma: steps 3 and 4) as compared with 39% in the younger group, consistent with other reports [26]. This finding suggests that other factors for poor control of asthma, besides those usually recognized, may be at play. One explanation may be that older patients have worse physiological changes compared with younger asthmatics; however, no age effect was found in intraluminal obstruction and subepithelial collagen in a study of individuals who died from asthma [27]. Our data suggest an alternate explanation for this relationship.

We found a significant association of diagnosed OSA with worse asthma control (asthma step) among older patients. Associations of potential clinical significance have been identified between asthma and OSA, such that treatment for comorbid OSA improved asthma symptoms [12, 13, 28], use of rescue bronchodilator, peak expiratory flow rates [12], and disease-specific quality of life [29]. However, these data came from younger subjects, and to our knowledge, our study is the first to extend identification of OSA as a potential adverse contributor to asthma control to the aged. While asthma is an important cause of morbidity and mortality in older individuals, in regard to sleep and respiratory diseases in older persons, little data are available, pertaining mainly to disrupted sleep. Older patients with chronic airway obstruction, relative to controls, have a higher prevalence and greater severity of sleep difficulties and morning tiredness

[10]. Furthermore, among older individuals with obstructive lung disease, sleep quality is worse in asthmatics than in individuals with COPD and chronic bronchitis [10].

For the first time, we report that the association of OSA with worse asthma control was of greater magnitude in older than in younger individuals (Tables 6 and 7) and, likewise, that CPAP use more robustly in the older than in the young attenuated the likelihood of worse asthma control. It is known that older adults are at increased risk for OSA and for more severe disease, which may be an explanation for our observation. Prevalence estimates for OSA among persons over 65 years of age, compared to those for the middle aged, are approximately 2-3 times higher [30]. In a large cohort of healthy older persons, the prevalence of OSA as defined by apnea hypopnea index (AHI) > 15 respiratory events/hr was 53%, and 37% had severe OSA (AHI > 30) [31]. Our sample demonstrates similar rates of snoring with a sample of 134 older subjects of similar age (mean 64.1 ± 9.1 years) and BMI (29.3 ± 5.3 kg/m^2) [32]. Furthermore, in the most recent Wisconsin Sleep Cohort data, regardless of gender and BMI strata, the oldest group (50–70 years old) consistently demonstrated higher OSA (AHI ≥ 5 events/h) prevalence including that of clinically-significant (AHI ≥ 5 and daytime sleepiness) and of more severe (AHI ≥ 15 and daytime sleepiness) disease [33]. Age-related changes in the upper airway anatomy have been shown, including an increase in the soft palate length and parapharyngeal fat pads independent of BMI, as well as a decrease in the upper airway size [34, 35]. Aging also affects upper airway function by decreasing the genioglossus's response to negative pressure, a greater reduction in genioglossus and tensor palatini activity at sleep onset, and an increase in pharyngeal collapsibility and resistance independent of BMI and gender [34, 36, 37]. These effects may be compounded in older asthmatics by the effects of sleep on their lung properties—important determinants of upper airway patency during sleep [38]. There is an augmented decline in functional residual capacity (FRC) during sleep in patients with asthma: as compared to normal controls, among asthmatics, the FRC is significantly reduced while sleeping supine than during supine wakefulness. Loss of lung elastic recoil may reduce the effectiveness of lung volume stabilizing the upper airway during sleep [38]. Furthermore, in elderly asthmatics, an association between FRC (estimating degree of hyperinflation) and duration of asthma, as well as an inverse relationship of FEV_1% predicted with duration of asthma has been shown; however, the former was independent of the degree of airflow limitation, suggesting that the duration of asthma is associated with both the degree of airflow limitation and hyperinflation [39]. This study suggested that with longer asthma duration, in time these abnormalities may become irreversible, as a reflection of distal airway and/or parenchymal changes as well as proximal airway remodeling [39]. Conversely, in regards to CPAP use, one predictor of beneficial effects of CPAP is the severity of disease. In one large study, the oxygen desaturation index (ODI) showed the strongest association with long-term adherence to CPAP; age was not a detrimental factor [40].

PSG in young asthma individuals of different severities and controls did find lower mean nocturnal SaO_2 and higher AHIs with more severe asthma, compared with controls [41]. Therefore, a higher severity of disease, particularly its degree of hypoxemia in elderly asthma patients, could be a factor in their more reported benefit with CPAP.

Another interesting and intriguing observation from this study is the differential pattern of associations of OSA observed with asthma symptoms: more with nighttime in older and more with daytime in younger individuals (Table 8). This has to be better understood in future studies, but one possibility remains that sleep in older patients with chronic airway obstruction being marked by more disruptions and awakenings [10] may render them more aware of their nighttime asthma symptoms than the young.

How OSA can worsen asthma in general remains unknown, but there are several plausible pathways. The concept of a relationship between upper and lower airways called the *integrated airway* [42] is used to describe an inflammatory process within a continuous airway as opposed to distinct pathologies [43] and may also underlie the interaction of OSA with asthma. Repetitive upper airway obstruction results in intrathoracic pressure swings, frequent arousals, and intermittent hypoxemia that contribute to an inflammatory milieu, as demonstrated through associations with cardiovascular and cerebrovascular diseases [44, 45]. Other putative mechanisms include SDB-induced resistive loading [46] of an already challenged lower airways system during sleep [47], enhanced vagal tone during obstructive events [28], increased nonspecific bronchial reactivity [48, 49], altered chemical arousal thresholds [50], and upper airway occlusion [51], all of which may promote bronchoconstriction. Although experimental human studies of intermittent hypoxia are lacking, exposure to sustained hypoxia led to cough suppression [52] and impaired symptom perception in individuals with asthma [53]. OSA could also promote GERD [54], which is a well-recognized trigger of asthma [55].

Our data suggest a potential role of OSA in asthma control independent of other factors known to worsen this disease, such as obesity, particularly in the elderly [56, 57]. Studies of the relationship between obesity and asthma in older persons are scarce and do not account for OSA as a potential mediator, though obesity is an important risk factor for OSA [30]. In a population-based longitudinal study of older Norwegians, a U-shaped association between asthma and BMI was found [58]. However, our study adds new evidence to suggest that much of the association between obesity and asthma may in fact be explained by OSA. In our older subjects, accounting for OSA completely attenuated (Tables 6 and 7) the trends of BMI with asthma initially noted in univariate analyses (Tables 4 and 5). One other study that systematically assessed OSA syndrome in difficult-to-control asthmatics did report an increased risk for OSA (3.1 (1.1–9.0)), less severe airway obstruction, and eosinophilic inflammation and concluded that other factors, rather than airway inflammation alone, explain the relationship between obesity and asthma [59].

Among limitations to our study, we relied on the use of a questionnaire-based approach (SA-SDQ) to evaluate OSA symptoms prospectively and of previously clinically-documented diagnosis of OSA. Additionally, owing to lack of availability and heterogeneity of testing we did not have meaningful PSG data available. Costs of prospective PSG would have been prohibitive for an early-stage investigation of this size, and selection bias might well have been more prominent, as far fewer than 93% of approached patients would have agreed to participate. The SA-SDQ has been validated in a large sample of sleep patients with high internal validity, good sensitivity, and specificity [19]. Although lower threshold scores than those used herein have been validated in patients with epilepsy [60], application of those lower thresholds to patients with pulmonary fibrosis reduced the performance of the survey instrument, despite retention of a good correlation between SA-SDQ and OSA severity [61]. These data suggest that the original cutoffs [19], which we used in our study, may be more suitable for patients with chronic lung diseases.

The cross-sectional design of this study limits conclusions about causality. Although asthma may be a risk factor for the development of OSA [62], our data fit with those from interventional studies [12, 13, 28, 29] and plausible mechanisms, as reviewed above, to suggest a detrimental effect of OSA on asthma control. Lastly, our sample included subjects aged up to 75 years, a restriction imposed by the design of the parent study. Our anecdotal observation conducting this survey is that there were quite small numbers of patients over 75 years of age attending our tertiary Allergy and Pulmonary clinics; therefore, we do not feel that this age restriction is likely to have had substantial impact on our findings. These patients may have unique comorbidity and cognitive profiles making them suitable for inclusion in future studies, specifically targeted to the older asthma patient population.

In conclusion, this first study of asthma and its relationship with OSA among well-characterized patients finds in older individuals worse indices of disease control than in the young. It also shows associations of OSA diagnosis with worse asthma control indices that were independent of obesity and other recognized asthma aggravators and in great part attenuated by CPAP use. These associations were of greater magnitude in the older than in the younger subjects, suggesting that the former may draw greater benefit from treating OSA. These data are correlative and cannot prove causation, but they raise the possibility that in many cases, OSA may be an unrecognized contributor to asthma control in older persons. If so, identification and treatment of OSA may improve asthma control particularly in these patients.

Authors' Contribution

Mihaela Teodorescu, Mihai C. Teodorescu, and Ronald D. Chervin were responsible for the conception and design of the paper. Mihaela Teodorescu, David A. Polomis, Jessica E. Fedie, and Mihai C. Teodorescu were responsible for the acquisition of subjects and/or data. Mihaela Teodorescu and Ronald E. Gangnon were responsible for data analysis. Mihaela Teodorescu, Ronald E. Gangnon, Flavia B. Consens,

Ronald D. Chervin, and Mihai C. Teodorescu were responsible for the interpretation of the data. Mihaela Teodorescu and Mihai C. Teodorescu were responsible for the drafting of the paper. Ronald E. Gangnon, Jessica E. Fedie, Flavia B. Consens, and Ronald D. Chervin were responsible for the critical review of the paper.

Acknowledgments

This work was conducted at the University of Michigan Health System, Ann Arbor, MI and the University of Wisconsin, Madison, WI. The authors are grateful to all patients for their participation in the survey, as well as to all providers in clinics at the two institutions for assisting with patient recruitment. This study was funded by the University of Michigan General Clinical Research Center (MO1 RR00042); University of Michigan, Department of Neurology Training Grant (T32 NS007222); University of Wisconsin School of Medicine and Public Health, Department of Medicine; the Medical Education and Research Committee-New Investigator Award, University of Wisconsin School of Medicine and Public Health, Madison, WI; 1UL1RR025011 from the Clinical and Translational Science Award (CTSA) program of the National Center for Research Resources, National Institutes of Health for asthma-sleep apnea research; and with additional resources from the William S. Middleton Memorial Veterans Hospital, Madison, WI (to Dr. Mihaela Teodorescu).

References

[1] P. Barua and M. S. O'Mahony, "Overcoming gaps in the management of asthma in older patients: new insights," *Drugs and Aging*, vol. 22, no. 12, pp. 1029–1059, 2005.

[2] K. Parameswaran, A. J. Hildreth, D. Chadha, N. P. Keaney, I. K. Taylor, and S. K. Bansal, "Asthma in the elderly: underperceived, underdiagnosed and undertreated; a community survey," *Respiratory Medicine*, vol. 92, no. 3, pp. 573–577, 1998.

[3] P. L. Enright, "The diagnosis and management of asthma is much tougher in older patients," *Current Opinion in Allergy and Clinical Immunology*, vol. 2, no. 3, pp. 175–181, 2002.

[4] P. L. Enright, R. A. Kronmal, M. W. Higgins, M. B. Schenker, and E. F. Haponik, "Prevalence and correlates of respiratory symptoms and disease in the elderly," *Chest*, vol. 106, no. 3, pp. 827–834, 1994.

[5] S. S. Braman, "Asthma in the elderly," *Clinics in Geriatric Medicine*, vol. 19, no. 1, pp. 57–75, 2003.

[6] G. B. Diette, J. A. Krishnan, F. Dominici et al., "Asthma in older patients: factors associated with hospitalization," *Archives of Internal Medicine*, vol. 162, no. 10, pp. 1123–1132, 2002.

[7] Center for Disease Control and Prevention, Asthma Surveillance Data, http://www.cdc.gov/asthma/asthmadata.htm.

[8] J. Moorman and D. Mannino, "Increasing U.S. asthma mortality rates: who is really dying?" *Journal of Asthma*, vol. 38, no. 1, pp. 65–71, 2001.

[9] P. G. Gibson, V. M. McDonald, and G. B. Marks, "Asthma in older adults," *The Lancet*, vol. 376, no. 9743, pp. 803–813, 2010.

[10] R. Antonelli Incalzi, R. Pistelli, C. Imperiale et al., "Effects of chronic airway disease on health status of geriatric patients,"

Aging Clinical and Experimental Research, vol. 16, no. 1, pp. 26–33, 2004.

[11] S. Ancoli-Israel, D. F. Kripke, M. R. Klauber, W. J. Mason, R. Fell, and O. Kaplan, "Sleep-disordered breathing in community-dwelling elderly," *Sleep*, vol. 14, no. 6, pp. 486–495, 1991.

[12] C. Shu Chan, A. J. Woolcock, and C. E. Sullivan, "Nocturnal asthma: role of snoring and obstructive sleep apnea," *American Review of Respiratory Disease*, vol. 137, no. 6, pp. 1502–1504, 1988.

[13] T. U. Ciftci, B. Ciftci, S. Firat Guven, O. Kokturk, and H. Turktas, "Effect of nasal continuous positive airway pressure in uncontrolled nocturnal asthmatic patients with obstructive sleep apnea syndrome," *Respiratory Medicine*, vol. 99, no. 5, pp. 529–534, 2005.

[14] A. ten Brinke, P. J. Sterk, A. A. M. Masclee et al., "Risk factors of frequent exacerbations in difficult-to-treat asthma," *European Respiratory Journal*, vol. 26, no. 5, pp. 812–818, 2005.

[15] M. Teodorescu, F. B. Consens, W. F. Bria et al., "Correlates of daytime sleepiness in patients with asthma," *Sleep Medicine*, vol. 7, no. 8, pp. 607–613, 2006.

[16] M. Teodorescu, F. B. Consens, W. F. Bria et al., "Predictors of habitual snoring and obstructive sleep apnea risk in patients with asthma," *Chest*, vol. 135, no. 5, pp. 1125–1132, 2009.

[17] M. Teodorescu, D. A. Polomis, S. V. Hall et al., "Association of obstructive sleep apnea risk with asthma control in adults," *Chest*, vol. 138, no. 3, pp. 543–550, 2010.

[18] Standards for the diagnosis and care of patients with chronic obstructive pulmonary disease (COPD) and asthma, "This official statement of the American Thoracic Society was adopted by the ATS Board of Directors," *The American Review of Respiratory Disease*, vol. 136, no. 1, pp. 225–244, 1987.

[19] A. B. Douglass, R. Bornstein, G. Nino-Murcia et al., "The Sleep Disorders Questionnaire I: creation and multivariate structure of SDQ," *Sleep*, vol. 17, no. 2, pp. 160–167, 1994.

[20] US Department of Health and Human Services, National Institute of Health, National asthma education and prevention program: practical guide for the diagnosis and management of asthma, expert panel report 2, http://www.nhlbi.nih.gov.ezproxy.library.wisc.edu/guidelines/archives/epr-2/index.htm.

[21] C. Janson, W. De Backer, T. Gislason et al., "Increased prevalence of sleep disturbances and daytime sleepiness in subjects with bronchial asthma: a population study of young adults in three European countries," *European Respiratory Journal*, vol. 9, no. 10, pp. 2132–2138, 1996.

[22] "Expert panel report 3 (EPR-3): guidelines for the diagnosis and management of asthma," Full Report, US Department of Health and Human Services. National Institute of Health, National Heart, Lung and Blood Institute. National Asthma Education and Prevention Program, 2007, http://www.nhlbi.nih.gov/guidelines/asthma/asthgdln.pdf.

[23] D. E. Arterburn, P. K. Crane, and S. D. Sullivan, "The coming epidemic of obesity in elderly Americans," *Journal of the American Geriatrics Society*, vol. 52, no. 11, pp. 1907–1912, 2004.

[24] L. Rogers, C. Cassino, K. I. Berger et al., "Asthma in the elderly: cockroach sensitization and severity of airway obstruction in elderly nonsmokers," *Chest*, vol. 122, no. 5, pp. 1580–1586, 2002.

[25] W. C. Bailey, J. M. Richards Jr., C. M. Brooks, S.-J. Soong, and A. L. Brannen, "Features of asthma in older adults," *Journal of Asthma*, vol. 29, no. 1, pp. 21–28, 1992.

[26] K. Huss, P. L. Naumann, P. J. Mason et al., "Asthma severity, atopic status, allergen exposure, and quality of life in elderly

persons," *Annals of Allergy, Asthma and Immunology*, vol. 86, no. 5, pp. 524–530, 2001.

[27] T. R. Bai, J. Cooper, T. Koelmeyer, P. D. Pare, and T. D. Weir, "The effect of age and duration of disease on airway structure in fatal asthma," *American Journal of Respiratory and Critical Care Medicine*, vol. 162, no. 2 I, pp. 663–669, 2000.

[28] C. Guilleminault, M. A. Quera-Salva, N. Powell et al., "Nocturnal asthma: snoring, small pharynx and nasal CPAP," *European Respiratory Journal*, vol. 1, no. 10, pp. 902–907, 1988.

[29] C. Lafond, F. Sériès, and C. Lemière, "Impact of CPAP on asthmatic patients with obstructive sleep apnoea," *European Respiratory Journal*, vol. 29, no. 2, pp. 307–311, 2007.

[30] T. Young, P. E. Peppard, and D. J. Gottlieb, "Epidemiology of obstructive sleep apnea: a population health perspective," *American Journal of Respiratory and Critical Care Medicine*, vol. 165, no. 9, pp. 1217–1239, 2002.

[31] E. Sforza, F. Roche, C. Thomas-Anterion et al., "Cognitive function and sleep related breathing disorders in a healthy elderly population: the synapse study," *Sleep*, vol. 33, no. 4, pp. 515–521, 2010.

[32] R. A. Stoohs, H.-C. Blum, M. Haselhorst, H. W. Duchna, C. Guilleminault, and W. C. Dement, "Normative data on snoring: a comparison between younger and older adults," *European Respiratory Journal*, vol. 11, no. 2, pp. 451–457, 1998.

[33] P. E. Peppard, T. Young, J. H. Barnet et al., "Increasedprevalence of sleep-disordered breathing in adults," *American Journal of Epidemiology*. In press.

[34] A. Malhotra, Y. Huang, R. Fogel et al., "Aging influences on pharyngeal anatomy and physiology: the predisposition to pharyngeal collapse," *American Journal of Medicine*, vol. 119, no. 1, pp. 72–e9, 2006.

[35] S. E. Martin, R. Mathur, I. Marshall, and N. J. Douglas, "The effect of age, sex, obesity and posture on upper airway size," *European Respiratory Journal*, vol. 10, no. 9, pp. 2087–2090, 1997.

[36] M. Eikermann, A. S. Jordan, N. L. Chamberlin et al., "The influence of aging on pharyngeal collapsibility during sleep," *Chest*, vol. 131, no. 6, pp. 1702–1709, 2007.

[37] C. Worsnop, A. Kay, Y. Kim, J. Trinder, and R. Pierce, "Effect of age on sleep onset-related changes in respiratory pump and upper airway muscle function," *Journal of Applied Physiology*, vol. 88, no. 5, pp. 1831–1839, 2000.

[38] D. P. White, "The pathogenesis of obstructive sleep apnea: advances in the past 100 years," *American Journal of Respiratory Cell and Molecular Biology*, vol. 34, no. 1, pp. 1–6, 2006.

[39] C. Cassino, K. I. Berger, R. M. Goldring et al., "Duration of asthma and physiologic outcomes in elderly nonsmokers," *American Journal of Respiratory and Critical Care Medicine*, vol. 162, no. 4 I, pp. 1423–1428, 2000.

[40] M. Kohler, D. Smith, V. Tippett, and J. R. Stradling, "Predictors of long-term compliance with continuous positive airway pressure," *Thorax*, vol. 65, no. 9, pp. 829–832, 2010.

[41] J. Y. Julien, J. G. Martin, P. Ernst et al., "Prevalence of obstructive sleep apnea-hypopnea in severe versus moderate asthma," *Journal of Allergy and Clinical Immunology*, vol. 124, no. 2, pp. 371–376, 2009.

[42] E. O. Meltzer, J. Szwarcberg, and M. W. Pill, "Allergic rhinitis, asthma, and rhinosinusitis: diseases of the integrated airway," *Journal of Managed Care Pharmacy*, vol. 10, no. 4, pp. 310–317, 2004.

[43] L. Bjermer, "Time for a paradigm shift in asthma treatment: from relieving bronchospasm to controlling systemic inflammation," *Journal of Allergy and Clinical Immunology*, vol. 120, no. 6, pp. 1269–1275, 2007.

[44] A. S. M. Shamsuzzaman, B. J. Gersh, and V. K. Somers, "Obstructive sleep apnea: implications for cardiac and vascular disease," *Journal of the American Medical Association*, vol. 290, no. 14, pp. 1906–1914, 2003.

[45] H. K. Yaggi, J. Concato, W. N. Kernan, J. H. Lichtman, L. M. Brass, and V. Mohsenin, "Obstructive sleep apnea as a risk factor for stroke and death," *The New England Journal of Medicine*, vol. 353, no. 19, pp. 2034–2041, 2005.

[46] E. L. Bijaoui, V. Champagne, P. F. Baconnier, R. John Kimoff, and J. H. T. Bates, "Mechanical properties of the lung and upper airways in patients with sleep-disordered breathing," *American Journal of Respiratory and Critical Care Medicine*, vol. 165, no. 8, pp. 1055–1061, 2002.

[47] R. D. Ballard, "Sleep, respiratory physiology, and nocturnal asthma," *Chronobiology International*, vol. 16, no. 5, pp. 565–580, 1999.

[48] C.-C. Lin and C.-Y. Lin, "Obstructive sleep apnea syndrome and bronchial hyperreactivity," *Lung*, vol. 173, no. 2, pp. 117–126, 1995.

[49] N. Nandwani, R. Caranza, and C. D. Hanning, "Obstructive sleep apnoea and upper airway reactivity," *Journal of Sleep Research*, vol. 7, no. 2, pp. 115–118, 1998.

[50] S. M. Garay, D. Rapoport, and B. Sorkin, "Regulation of ventilation in the obstructive sleep apnea syndrome," *American Review of Respiratory Disease*, vol. 124, no. 4, pp. 451–457, 1981.

[51] R. B. Berry, K. G. Kouchi, D. E. Der, M. J. Dickel, and R. W. Light, "Sleep apnea impairs the arousal response to airway occlusion," *Chest*, vol. 109, no. 6, pp. 1490–1496, 1996.

[52] D. J. Eckert, P. G. Catcheside, D. L. Stadler, R. McDonald, M. C. Hlavac, and R. D. McEvoy, "Acute sustained hypoxia suppresses the cough reflex in healthy subjects," *American Journal of Respiratory and Critical Care Medicine*, vol. 173, no. 5, pp. 506–511, 2006.

[53] D. J. Eckert, P. G. Catcheside, J. H. Smith, P. A. Frith, and R. Doug McEvoy, "Hypoxia suppresses symptom perception in asthma," *American Journal of Respiratory and Critical Care Medicine*, vol. 169, no. 11, pp. 1224–1230, 2004.

[54] A. M. Zanation and B. A. Senior, "The relationship between extraesophageal reflux (EER) and obstructive sleep apnea (OSA)," *Sleep Medicine Reviews*, vol. 9, no. 6, pp. 453–458, 2005.

[55] S. M. Harding, "Gastroesophageal reflux: a potential asthma trigger," *Immunology and Allergy Clinics of North America*, vol. 25, no. 1, pp. 131–148, 2005.

[56] D. A. Beuther, S. T. Weiss, and E. R. Sutherland, "Obesity and asthma," *American Journal of Respiratory and Critical Care Medicine*, vol. 174, no. 2, pp. 112–119, 2006.

[57] L.-P. Boulet, Q. Hamid, S. L. Bacon et al., "Symposium on obesity and asthma—november 2, 2006," *Canadian Respiratory Journal*, vol. 14, no. 4, pp. 201–208, 2007.

[58] J.-M. Kvamme, T. Wilsgaard, J. Florholmen, and B. K. Jacobsen, "Body mass index and disease burden in elderly men and women: the tromso study," *European Journal of Epidemiology*, vol. 25, no. 3, pp. 183–193, 2010.

[59] I. H. Van Veen, A. Ten Brinke, P. J. Sterk, K. F. Rabe, and E. H. Bel, "Airway inflammation in obese and nonobese patients with difficult-to-treat asthma," *Allergy*, vol. 63, no. 5, pp. 570–574, 2008.

[60] K. J. Weatherwax, X. Lin, M. L. Marzec, and B. A. Malow, "Obstructive sleep apnea in epilepsy patients: the Sleep Apnea scale of the Sleep Disorders Questionnaire (SA-SDQ) is a useful screening instrument for obstructive sleep apnea in a disease-specific population," *Sleep Medicine*, vol. 4, no. 6, pp. 517–521, 2003.

[61] L. H. Lancaster, W. R. Mason, J. A. Parnell et al., "Obstructive sleep apnea is common in idiopathic pulmonary fibrosis," *Chest*, vol. 136, no. 3, pp. 772–778, 2009.

[62] M. Knuiman, A. James, M. Divitini, and H. Bartholomew, "Longitudinal study of risk factors for habitual snoring in a general adult population: the Busselton Health Study," *Chest*, vol. 130, no. 6, pp. 1779–1783, 2006.

21

Restless Leg Syndrome in Diabetics Compared with Normal Controls

Mehdi Zobeiri[1] and Azita Shokoohi[2]

[1] *Department of Internal Medicine, School of Medicine, Imam Reza Hospital, Kermanshah University of Medical Sciences, Kermanshah, Iran*
[2] *Kermanshah University of Medical Sciences, Kermanshah, Iran*

Correspondence should be addressed to Mehdi Zobeiri; mehdizobeiri@yahoo.com

Academic Editor: Michael R. Littner

Introduction. Restless leg syndrome (RLS) is a common sleep disorder which is characterized by urge to move the legs accompanied by disturbing and uncomfortable leg sensation during night and rest. This common condition affects 7–10% of general population and is frequently unrecognized, misdiagnosed, and poorly managed. Several clinical conditions like diabetes have been associated with secondary form of RLS. This study analyzed the frequency and possible risk factor for RLS development in diabetic patient. *Material and Methods.* This descriptive case-control study was done on 140 consecutive outpatient diabetics and age, sex, and body mass index matched control group. RLS was diagnosed by criteria of the International RLS Study Group. *Results.* Prevalence of RLS was 28.6% in diabetes and 7.1% in control group ($P = 0.001$). Sex difference was not significant and with rising duration of diabetes prevalence of RLS was not increased. *Discussion.* With regarding significant association between RLS and diabetes and its negative impact on quality of life/health outcome/sleep/daytime activity/cognitive function/ and mental state of diabetic patient/higher awareness of RLS among physicians and related health worker suggested.

1. Introduction

Restless legs syndrome (RLS) is a common sleep disorder characterized by unpleasant night sensations (tingling, creeping) in the legs and rarely arms that are temporarily relieved by movement and leads to a severe difficulty in initiating and maintaining sleep [1–3].

RLS typically worse during periods of rest, relaxation, or inactivity and may be accompanied with major impact on daytime function and quality of life [2, 3]. RLS is a common disease that occurs in 7–10% of general population, increasing with age and affecting women more often than men and parity is a major factor in explaining the sex difference [1, 4–6].

RLS is often familial or idiopathic, recognized as primary but may be associated with, renal failure, iron deficiency, rheumatoid arthritis, polyneuropathy, cryoglobulinemia, and infection [6]. Primary RLS is familial in up to two-thirds of patients believed to be an autosomal dominant disorder and

secondary form is most common in those presenting for the first time in later life [7, 8].

This neurological problem despite trials for better recognition remains an undiagnosed clinical condition [4, 9]. Diagnosis of RLS is purely clinical and there is no specific test [2, 7].

The essential clinical diagnostic criteria for restless legs syndrome were developed and approved by workshop participants and the executive committee of the International Restless Legs Syndrome Study Group as specified by the National Institutes of Health, and all four essential criteria must be met for a positive diagnosis in more than five times per month [2, 10]. Diabetic patients have 4–4.4-time more risk of developing RLS than in the general population although in one study no relation detected [2, 6, 11]. Significant association between RLS and diabetes is not wonderful because of etiologic role of diabetes in producing polyneuropathy and renal failure [10]. The aims of this investigation were to look for an association between RLS and diabetes in a case-control study and to identify possible risk factors for the development of RLS in diabetic patients.

2. Material and Methods

This is a case-control study between 140 consecutive patients with diabetes attending the diabetes center of the Kermanshah University Hospital, which were recruited from March 2007 to July 2007 and the control group consists of 140 patients without diabetes who were admitted in the ENT department. Data collection was done by physician from check list which includes demographic information, variables related to diabetes, and diagnostic criteria of RLS which were assessed with standardized, validated questions addressing the 4 minimal criteria for RLS as defined by International Restless legs Syndrome Study Group. Both groups were matched based on age, sex, and body mass index (BMI). Exclusion criteria were renal disease, iron deficiency anemia, rheumatoid arthritis, and pregnancy. In diabetic patient, disease duration and type of diabetes determined but polyneuropathy were not assessed. Data were analyzed by use of two dimensional frequency tables and calculation of tchouprov qualitative correlation coefficient for relation of risk factors and diabetes type. For summarizing quantitative variables, data are displayed in tables as means and standard deviations and Z test was used for comparison of RLS prevalence between two groups. In order to matching between two groups independent chi-square and as needed Fisher's exact test and Mann-Whitney U test were used.

3. Results

Mean age in diabetic was 46.3±13.93 and in control group was 44.02 ± 19.1 ($P = 0.252$). Mean BMI in diabetic was 25.19 ± 3.73 and in control group was 24.61±3.11 ($P = 0.159$). In each group, 80 (57.1%) were female and 60 (42.9%) were male. As a whole RLS prevalence was 17.9% which is 28.6% in diabetic and 7.1% in control group ($P = 0.001$).

General characteristics of RLS frequency in the diabetic patients and of the nondiabetic controls are reported in Table 1 (more than 5 times per month regarded as positive RLS symptom).

Between related variables in diabetic and control, only hypertension was significantly higher in diabetic groups (Table 2).

Characteristics of variables in both diabetic and control groups with and without RLS are depicted in Table 3.

The only difference was hypertension, which was significantly higher among RLS groups.

4. Discussion

The prevalence of RLS in our diabetic patients (28.6%) was significantly higher than nondiabetic controls (7.1%), whereas it was higher with respect to previous studies carried out in subjects with type 2 diabetes [10]. The studies are consistent with the idea that RLS is a common condition, at least in populations derived from Western Europe and USA

TABLE 1: RLS frequency in diabetic patients and of the nondiabetic controls.

RLS symptom	Study groups		
	Diabetic	Control	Total
Never	52 (37.1%)	84 (60%)	136 (48.6%)
Seldom (one time per month)	19 (13.6%)	23 (16.4%)	42 (15%)
Sometimes (2–4 times per month)	29 (20.7%)	23 (16.4%)	52 (18.6%)
Often (5-6 times per month)	25 (17.9%)	7 (5%)	32 (11.4%)
Always (≥16 times per month)	15 (10.7%)	3 (2.1%)	18 (6.4%)
Total	140 (100%)	140 (100%)	280 (100%)

TABLE 2: Frequency of related variables in diabetic patients and of the nondiabetic controls.

Variables	Groups		
	Diabetic	Control	P
Smoking	22	9	0.013
Alcohol consumption	2	1	0.562
Hypertension	40	18	0.001
Exercise	82	28	0.001
(24.9) BMI mean	3.73 ± 25.19	3.11 ± 24.61	0.159
Mean age	13.93 ± 46.31	19.10 ± 44.02	0.252

TABLE 3: Comparison of related variable in groups with and without RLS.

variables	Groups		
	Without RLS (%)	With RLS (%)	P
Smoking	23 (10)	8 (16)	0.22
Alcohol consumption	2 (0.86)	1 (2)	0.428
Hypertension	40 (1.73)	18 (36)	0.003
Exercise	86 (37.3)	24 (48)	0.164
(24.9) BMI mean	(24.6 ± 3.3)	(25.9 ± 3.6)	0.18
Total	230	50	

RLS was not significantly more common in female than male (20% versus 15%) ($P = 0.280$). 27% of diabetic patients with ≤10 years and 34% with ≥10 years diabetic duration had RLS ($P = 0.429$).

with prevalence between 5.8 and 11.4% [12]. A number of epidemiological studies of RLS prevalence from Asia found lower prevalence in Japanese (2–4%) and Singapore (0.1%) populations [13, 14].

IRAN and its western parts like Kermanshah city have peoples belonging to Caucasian race [15].

More than four times higher prevalence of RLS in diabetic than nondiabetic control suggests strong association between RLS and diabetes. Because of some association between neuropathy and RLS, increased risk for RLS in diabetic may reflect partial consequences of diabetic neuropathy rather than diabetes per se [16].

Cho et al. show more than two time higher confirmed RLS prevalence in diabetics than control with osteoarthritis through face-to-face interviews using the 18-item Hopkins Diagnostic Questionnaire, which removes RLS mimics [16].

Polyneuropathy is a risk factor for RLS in diabetic patients but after adjusting for the presence of polyneuropathy diabetes remains an independent risk factor for RLS [8].

In this study, polyneuropathy was not evaluated and RLS symptoms were assessed as a whole. Studies have documented the relative iron stores depletion and impaired dopaminergic neurotransmission of brain which is a probable pain control system in RLS patients [12, 17]. Iron is needed for dopamine synthesis and, at least in animal models, iron deficiency during early life can result in lifetime abnormalities of the dopamine system [6, 12].

In the diabetic population, RLS seems to be independent from the iron status of patients [8, 10]. Hypertension was higher in diabetic and control group with RLS which seems to be partially related to RLS.

Mean age of study groups suggest secondary form of RLS which is most common in those presenting for the first time in later life [6]. Women were not significantly affected than men although in two studies significant higher prevalence of women was found and parity defined as a major factor in explaining the sex difference [1, 6]. Prevalence of RLS was not increased with rising duration of diabetes, while there was witnessed increases with age [6].

RLS as a sleep disorder may have impact on diabetes management and health outcome [17, 18].

It is associated with impairs sleep quality, drug consumption at night, daytime activity, cognitive function, and depressive and anxious symptoms and may be a risk factor for hypertension and cardiovascular disease [17, 19, 20].

RLS as a one of the most intriguing chronic sensory-motor disorders is frequently unrecognized, misdiagnosed, and poorly managed [8, 21]. Awareness about RLS is poor among medical professionals and diagnosis of RLS was missed not only by general physicians, but also by specialists like neurologists and psychiatrists [22–24]. RLS symptoms are not reported by patients to their health care providers. So, identification and suitable management of RLS, especially in diabetic populations, are recommended [8, 21].

Conflict of Interests

The authors declare that there is no conflict of interests regarding the publication of this paper.

References

[1] K. Berger, J. Luedemann, C. Trenkwalder, U. John, and C. Kessler, "Sex and the risk of restless legs syndrome in the general population," *Archives of Internal Medicine*, vol. 164, no. 2, pp. 196–202, 2004.

[2] R. P. Allen, D. Picchietti, W. A. Hening et al., "Restless legs syndrome: diagnostic criteria, special considerations, and epidemiology. A report from the restless legs syndrome diagnosis and epidemiology workshop at the National Institutes of Health," *Sleep Medicine*, vol. 4, no. 2, pp. 101–119, 2003.

[3] G. J. Lavigne and J. Y. Montplaisir, "Restless legs syndrome and sleep bruxism: prevalence and association among Canadians," *Sleep*, vol. 17, no. 8, pp. 739–743, 1994.

[4] B. Phillips, T. Young, L. Finn, K. Asher, W. A. Hening, and C. Purvis, "Epidemiology of restless legs symptoms in adults," *Archives of Internal Medicine*, vol. 160, no. 14, pp. 2137–2141, 2000.

[5] S. Happe, N. Treptau, R. Ziegler, and E. Harms, "Restless legs syndrome and sleep problems in children and adolescents with insulin-dependent diabetes mellitus type 1," *Neuropediatrics*, vol. 36, no. 2, pp. 98–103, 2005.

[6] G. Merlino, L. Fratticci, M. Valente et al., "Association of restless leqs syndrome in type 2 diabetes: a case-control study," *Sleep*, vol. 30, no. 7, pp. 866–871, 2007.

[7] M. Maheswaran and C. A. Kushida, "Restless legs syndrome in children," *Medscape General Medicine*, vol. 8, no. 2, article 79, 2006.

[8] P. E. Cotter and S. T. O'Keeffe, "Restless leg syndrome: is it a real problem?" *Therapeutics and Clinical Risk Management*, vol. 2, no. 4, pp. 465–475, 2006.

[9] C. Sitaru, V. Cristea, and S. M. Florea, "Restless legs syndrome—relevant aspects for internal medicine specialists," *Romanian Journal of Internal Medicine*, vol. 37, no. 3, pp. 275–286, 1999.

[10] R. P. Skomro, S. Ludwig, E. Salamon, and M. H. Kryger, "Sleep complaints and restless legs syndrome in adult type 2 diabetics," *Sleep Medicine*, vol. 2, no. 5, pp. 417–422, 2001.

[11] S.-C. Lai and R.-S. Chen, "Restless legs syndrome," *Acta Neurologica Taiwanica*, vol. 17, no. 1, pp. 54–65, 2008.

[12] W. A. Hening, R. P. Allen, C. J. Earley, D. L. Picchietti, and M. H. Silber, "An update on the dopaminergic treatment of restless legs syndrome and periodic limb movement disorder," *Sleep*, vol. 27, no. 3, pp. 560–583, 2004.

[13] T. Nomura, Y. Inoue, M. Kusumi, Y. Oka, and K. Nakashima, "Email-based epidemiological surveys on restless legs syndrome in Japan," *Sleep and Biological Rhythms*, vol. 6, no. 3, pp. 139–145, 2008.

[14] E. K. Tan, A. Seah, S. J. See, E. Lim, M. C. Wong, and K. K. Koh, "Restless legs syndrome in an Asian population: a study in Singapore," *Movement Disorders*, vol. 16, no. 3, pp. 577–579, 2001.

[15] "Irano-Afghan race," Wikipedia, the free Encyclopedia.

[16] Y. W. Cho, G. Y. Na, J. G. Lim et al., "Prevalence and clinical characteristics of restless legs syndrome in diabetic peripheral neuropathy: comparison with chronic osteoarthritis," *Sleep Medicine*, vol. 14, pp. 1387–1392, 2013.

[17] E. Karroum, E. Konofal, and I. Arnulf, "Restless-legs syndrome," *Revue Neurologique*, vol. 164, no. 8-9, pp. 701–721, 2008.

[18] N. G. Cuellar and S. J. Ratcliffe, "A comparison of glycemic control, sleep, fatigue, and depression in type 2 diabetes with and without restless legs syndrome," *Journal of Clinical Sleep Medicine*, vol. 4, no. 1, pp. 50–56, 2008.

[19] A. S. Walters and D. B. Rye, "Review of the relationship of restless legs syndrome and periodic limb movements in sleep to hypertension, heart disease, and stroke," *Sleep*, vol. 32, no. 5, pp. 589–597, 2009.

[20] A. S. Walters and D. B. Rye, "Evidence continues to mount on the relationship of restless legs syndrome/periodic limb movements in sleep to hypertension, cardiovascular disease, and stroke," *Sleep*, vol. 33, no. 3, p. 287, 2010.

[21] F. G. Dantas, J. L. Mederios, K. S. Farias, and C. D. Ribeiro, "Restless legs syndrome in institutional eldery," *Arquivos de Neuro-Psiquiatria*, vol. 66, no. 2b, pp. 328–330, 2008.

[22] C. Möller, T. C. Wetter, J. Köster, and K. Stiasny-Kolster, "Differential diagnosis of unpleasant sensations in the legs: prevalence of restless legs syndrome in a primary care population," *Sleep Medicine*, vol. 11, no. 2, pp. 161–166, 2010.

[23] R. P. Allen, P. Stillman, and A. J. Myers, "Physician-diagnosed restless legs syndrome in a large sample of primary medical care patients in western Europe: prevalence and characteristics," *Sleep Medicine*, vol. 11, no. 1, pp. 31–37, 2010.

[24] R. Gupta, V. Lahan, and D. Goel, "Restless legs syndrome: a common disorder, but rarely diagnosed and barely treated—an Indian experience," *Sleep Medicine*, vol. 13, pp. 838–841, 2012.

22

Insomnia in Sweden: A Population-Based Survey

Lena Mallon,[1] Jan-Erik Broman,[1] Torbjörn Åkerstedt,[2] and Jerker Hetta[3]

[1] *Department of Neuroscience, Psychiatry, Uppsala University, SE-75185 Uppsala, Sweden*
[2] *Stress Research Institute, Stockholm University, SE-10691 Stockholm, Sweden*
[3] *Department of Clinical Neuroscience, Psychiatry, Karolinska Institutet, SE-14186 Stockholm, Sweden*

Correspondence should be addressed to Lena Mallon; lena.mallon@ltdalarna.se

Academic Editor: Michel M. Billiard

Aims. Estimate the prevalence of insomnia and examine effects of sex, age, health problems, sleep duration, need for treatment, and usage of sleep medication. *Methods.* A sample of 1,550 subjects aged 18–84 years was selected for a telephone interview. The interview was completed by 1,128 subjects (72.8%). *Results.* 24.6% reported insomnia symptoms. Insomnia disorder, that is, insomnia symptoms and daytime consequences, was reported by 10.5%. The prevalence was similar among all age groups, with the exception of women aged 40–49 years who demonstrated a significantly higher prevalence, 21.6%. Having at least one physical or psychiatric disorder was reported by 82.8% of subjects with insomnia disorder. Mean sleep duration for subjects with insomnia disorder was 5.77 hours on weeknights and 7.03 hours on days off/weekends. The corresponding figures for subjects without insomnia disorder were 7.04 hours and 7.86 hours, respectively. Among those with insomnia disorder 62.5% expressed a need for treatment, and 20.0% used prescribed sleep medication regularly. *Conclusions.* Insomnia disorder is highly prevalent in the population. There are significant associations between insomnia disorder and physical and psychiatric disorders. A majority of subjects with insomnia disorder expressed a need for treatment, indicating a public health problem.

1. Introduction

Several epidemiological studies have been conducted in order to estimate the prevalence of insomnia in the general population. The reported prevalence rates vary considerably, and differences in how insomnia is defined contribute to this variation.

Also, some variability may be explained by differences in how information is obtained, that is, questionnaire or interview surveys.

Some studies report insomnia symptoms, that is, difficulties initiating and/or maintaining sleep, without restrictive criteria, while others include duration, frequency, or severity criteria. Studies without restrictive criteria produce prevalence estimates from 25% to 48% [1], while studies using some form of duration, frequency, or severity gradations report prevalence rates from 9% to 34% [1, 2]. The diagnosis of insomnia disorder according to classification systems, such as the DSM-IV [3], ICD-10 [4], or ICSD-2 [5] also requires daytime impairment, and with this definition the prevalence

rates of insomnia decrease to about 6% to 12% [6, 7]. A consistent finding is that women are more likely to have insomnia [8]. Almost all studies report an increase in insomnia symptoms with age [9, 10], while there are mixed results concerning insomnia disorder [6, 7].

Subjects with insomnia generally report shorter sleep duration compared to normal sleepers [6], and high levels of comorbidity between insomnia and medical disorders have been demonstrated in epidemiological surveys [11, 12]. Among physical disorders heart disease, hypertension, breathing problems, urinary problems, and pain conditions are more common in subjects with insomnia. Moreover, a survey reported that about half of subjects with insomnia also met criteria for a psychiatric disorder [13]. Although effective behavioural and pharmacological therapies exist for insomnia, many insomnia sufferers do not seek help [14] or use sleep medication [6, 14].

It is important to have accurate estimates of the sex- and age-related prevalence of insomnia and its correlates in the general population in order to understand the public health effect of the disorder. Given the differences in the definition of insomnia in epidemiological research it is difficult to draw conclusions about the true prevalence of the disorder.

This study aims to evaluate the prevalence of insomnia and to identify factors associated with insomnia in the general adult population in Sweden. We used a definition of insomnia disorder that includes insomnia symptoms and detrimental effects on daytime functioning, and our definition of insomnia disorder is thereby close to the DSM-IV insomnia disorder diagnosis [3].

2. Methods

2.1. Procedure. The study was initiated by the Swedish Council on Health Technology Assessment (SBU). Data were collected by a telephone interview commissioned to the Central Bureau of Statistics (SCB), a governmental agency, in Sweden. Data collection was done with a software package designed specifically for this type of computer-assisted phone survey. After a brief description of the aims of the study and after obtaining verbal consent to proceed with the interview, data were collected.

2.2. Participants. A sample of 1,550 subjects living in Sweden, 18–84 years of age, representative for the population and proportionally stratified for age and sex was selected for a telephone interview. The interview was completed by 1128 subjects (72.8%). The characteristics of the sample are shown in Table 1. The sample consisted of 52.1% women and the mean age was 47.8 years (SD = 18.0).

2.3. Material. The interview consisted of 39 questions covering demographics, work conditions, sleep complaints, daytime impairment due to sleep complaints, sleep duration, physical and psychiatric disorders, need for treatment, and usage of prescriptive sleep medication.

Sleep initiation problems were assessed by asking "How often have you had difficulties falling asleep during the last month?" to be answered on a five-point scale (1 = never or less than once a month; 2 = less than once a week; 3 = 1-2 times per week; 4 = 3–5 times per week; 5 = daily or almost daily). Sleep maintenance problems were assessed by asking "How many times do you wake up during the night?" to be answered on a five-point scale (1 = never; 2 = once; 3 = twice; 4 = 3-4 times; 5 = at least 5 times). Insomnia symptoms were defined as sleep initiation problems at least 3 times per week (scores 4 and 5) and/or sleep maintenance problems at least 3 times per night (scores 4 and 5).

Daytime consequences were assessed by asking "Have your sleep complaints interfered with your daily life during the last month?" (1 = no interference, 2 = minor interference; 3 = moderate interference; 4 = severe interference; 5 = very severe interference).

Insomnia disorder was defined as having insomnia symptoms and at least moderate interference with daytime functioning (scores 3 to 5).

Sleep duration was assessed by asking subjects to estimate sleep duration on weeknights and on days off/weekends.

TABLE 1: Characteristics of the sample ($N = 1128$).

	Men		Women	
	N	%	N	%
Age groups (years)				
18–29	117	21.7	106	18.0
30–39	102	18.9	89	15.1
40–49	87	16.1	111	18.9
50–59	78	14.4	90	15.3
60–69	95	17.6	101	17.2
70–84	61	11.3	91	15.5
Physical and psychiatric disorders				
Hypertension	68	12.6	107	18.2
Asthma	68	12.6	73	12.4
Heart disease	37	6.9	39	6.6
Diabetes	35	6.5	27	4.6
Gastrointestinal disorder	86	15.9	134	22.8
Urogenital disorder	37	6.9	36	6.1
Cancer	17	3.1	14	2.4
Joint pain	98	18.1	172	29.3
Fibromyalgia	2	0.4	20	3.4
Other physical disorders	45	8.3	90	15.3
Psychiatric disorder	26	4.8	41	7.0
Burnout	19	3.5	35	6.0
Depression	42	7.8	70	11.9
Sleep duration (hours)				
Weeknights (mean ± SD)	6.87 ± 1.12		6.93 ± 1.24	
Weekends/days off (mean ± SD)	7.85 ± 1.51		7.70 ± 1.55	

The answer was expressed as a continuous variable. Physical and psychiatric disorders were ascertained by asking (in a yes/no question) if respondents had hypertension, asthma, heart disease, diabetes, gastrointestinal disorder, urogenital disorder, cancer, joint pain, fibromyalgia, psychiatric disorder, burnout, depression, or any other disorder.

Subjects were asked (in a yes/no question) "Do you think you need treatment for your sleep problems?" Usage of prescriptive sleep medication was ascertained by the question "How often during the last month have you used prescriptive sleep medication?" (1 = never or less than once per month, 2 = less than once per week, 3 = 1-2 times per week, 4 = 3–5 times per week, and 5 = daily or almost daily). Usage at least 3 times per week (scores 4 and 5) was considered regular usage. Unfortunately we do not have any information about the nature of sleep medication. The type of sleep medication asked about was "on prescription," that is, not sold over the counter. In Sweden the dominating drugs in this class are zopiclone, zolpidem, and propiomazine.

2.4. Data Analyses. All analyses were carried out using IBM SPSS Statistics, version 20.0. Standard methods were used to calculate mean values and standard deviations (SDs).

TABLE 2: Prevalence (%) and odds ratios (95% confidence interval) of insomnia symptoms and insomnia disorder by age groups in men (*n* = 537) and women (*n* = 587).

	Insomnia symptoms		Insomnia disorder	
	Men	Women	Men	Women
Age groups (yrs)				
18–29	16.2 [10.6–24.0]	23.6 [16.5–32.5]	6.8 [3.5–12.9]	9.4 [5.2–16.5]
30–39	17.6 [11.5–26.2]	32.6 [23.7–42.9]	6.9 [3.5–12.9]	13.5 [7.9–22.1]
40–49	18.4 [11.6–27.8]	26.1 [18.8–35.0]	11.5 [6.4–19.9]	21.6 [15.0–30.2]
50–59	15.4 [9.0–25.0]	27.8 [19.6–37.8]	5.1 [2.0–12.5]	13.3 [7.8–21.9]
60–69	21.1 [14.1–30.3]	30.7 [22.5–40.3]	4.2 [1.6–10.3]	12.9 [7.7–20.8]
70–84	31.1 [20.9–43.6]	36.3 [27.1–46.5]	8.2 [3.5–17.8]	9.9 [5.3–17.7]
Total	19.4 [16.2–22.9]	29.3 [25.8–33.1]	7.1 [5.2–9.6]	13.6 [11.1–16.6]

TABLE 3: Sleep duration on week nights and on weekends/days off in subjects with insomnia disorder (*n* = 118) and in subjects without insomnia disorder (*n* = 1005).

	Sleep duration on week nights (hrs)		Sleep duration on weekends/days off (hrs)	
	Mean	SD	Mean	SD
Subjects with insomnia disorder	5.77	1.64	7.04[***]	2.41
Subjects without insomnia disorder	7.03	1.05	7.86[***]	1.37

SD: standard deviation: [***] $P < .001$.

When the comparison involved continuous variables the Mann-Whitney U test was used, and the chi-square test was used for differences between proportions.

Ninety-five percent confidence intervals were calculated for prevalence rates and odds ratios. Linear regression models were used to calculate correlations between continuous variables. To identify associations between insomnia disorder and physical and mental disorders age-adjusted and multivariate logistic regression analyses were conducted. Results are presented as odds ratios (OR) with 95% confidence intervals.

3. Results

3.1. Prevalence of Insomnia Symptoms. The prevalence of having difficulties initiating sleep only was 10.7%, and the prevalence of having sleep maintenance problems only was also 10.7%. The prevalence of insomnia symptoms, that is, sleep initiation problems and/or sleep maintenance problems, was 24.6%. Women reported insomnia symptoms more often than men, 29.3% versus 19.4% (χ^2 = 14.9; $P < .001$). In all age groups insomnia symptoms were more frequent in women (Table 2). Insomnia symptoms were significantly predicted by sex (OR, 1.69; 95% CI, 1.28–2.23; $P < .001$). The highest prevalence of insomnia symptoms was in the oldest age group, 70 to 84 years, in which 31.1% of men and 36.3% of women reported insomnia symptoms. With the youngest age group as a reference we found that insomnia symptoms remained comparable between age groups with the exception of men aged 70 to 84 years who had a significant higher prevalence rate (OR, 2.33 95% CI, 1.12–4.85; $P < .05$).

3.2. Prevalence of Insomnia Disorder. Of those with insomnia symptoms 42.9% reported concomitant impairment of daytime functioning and were classified as having insomnia disorder. The prevalence of insomnia disorder was 10.5%, and more women than men reported insomnia disorder, 13.6% versus 7.1% (χ^2 = 12.7; $P < .001$). In all age groups insomnia disorder was more frequent in women (Table 2). Thus, insomnia disorder was significantly predicted by sex (OR, 2.08; 95% CI, 1.38–3.12; $P < .001$). The prevalence of insomnia disorder remained comparable between age groups with the exception of women aged 40 to 49 years who demonstrated a significant higher prevalence rate, 21.6% (OR, 2.65; 95% CI, 1.20–5.85; $P < .05$).

3.3. Sleep Duration. Subjects with insomnia disorder reported shorter sleep duration on weeknights compared to subjects without insomnia disorder, 5.77 ± 1.64 hours versus 7.03 ± 1.05 hours (t = 11.2; $P < .0001$). They also reported shorter sleep duration on days off/weekends, 7.04 ± 2.41 hours, compared to subjects without insomnia disorder, 7.86 ± 1.37 hours (t = 15.9; $P < .0001$) (Table 3). Both groups extended their sleep on days off/weekends. On days off/weekends 42.4% of subjects with insomnia disorder and 43.4% of subjects without insomnia disorder extended their sleep with at least one hour.

3.4. Comorbid Disorders. Having at least one physical or psychiatric disorder was reported by 82.8% of subjects with insomnia disorder compared to 54.2% of subjects without insomnia disorder (OR, 1.78; 95% CI, 1.58–1.98; $P < .001$). In subjects with insomnia disorder there was no sex difference in the prevalence of comorbid disorders (OR, 0.74; 95% CI, 0.24–2.24; n.s.), but there was a difference between age groups (OR, 1.72; 95% CI, 1.20–2.48; $P < .01$). The prevalence of comorbid disorders increased with advancing age, and all of the insomniacs aged 60 and above reported at least

TABLE 4: Prevalence (%) and odds ratios (95% confidence interval) of physical and psychiatric disorders in subjects without insomnia disorder ($n = 1005$) and in subjects with insomnia disorder ($n = 118$).

	Subjects without insomnia disorder	Subjects with insomnia disorder	Subjects with insomnia; univariate analyses[a]	Subjects with insomnia; multivariate analyses[b]
	%	%	OR (95% CI)	OR (95% CI)
Hypertension	14.8	22.4	1.67 (1.04–2.67)	0.98 (0.53–1.83)
Asthma	10.9	25.6	2.81 (1.77–4.44)	1.96 (1.11–3.44)
Heart disease	5.9	14.4	2.69 (1.51–4.80)	1.13 (0.50–2.54)
Diabetes	5.1	8.5	1.75 (0.86–3.54)	1.53 (0.67–3.51)
Gastrointestinal disorder	16.3	45.8	4.32 (2.90–6.44)	2.36 (1.46–3.82)
Urogenital disorder	5.8	12.7	2.38 (1.30–4.34)	1.72 (0.80–3.66)
Cancer	2.8	2.5	0.91 (0.27–3.04)	0.30 (0.07–1.24)
Joint pain	21.3	46.6	3.22 (2.18–4.76)	1.91 (1.16–3.15)
Fibromyalgia	1.1	9.5	9.41 (3.98–22.23)	5.04 (1.88–13.53)
Other physical disorder	11.2	18.6	1.83 (1.10–3.02)	1.16 (0.63–2.13)
Psychiatric disorder	3.7	24.1	8.32 (4.86–14.23)	2.00 (0.91–4.37)
Burnout	2.5	23.7	12.17 (6.81–21.76)	2.19 (0.99–4.85)
Depression	6.2	40.5	10.40 (6.64–16.28)	4.91 (2.63–9.17)

OR: odds ratio; CI: confidence interval findings are significant when CIs do not include 1.00.
[a] Adjusted for age in 5-year strata.
[b] Multivariate analyses adjusted for age in 5-year strata, all physical and psychiatric disorders.

one physical or psychiatric disorder. All disorders, with the exception of diabetes and cancer, were more common in subjects with insomnia disorder (Table 4). In unadjusted logistic regression analyses significant associations were found between insomnia disorder and several of the disorders. In multivariate logistic regression analysis including all disorders, the association between insomnia disorder and many of the disorders were reduced to a nonsignificant level. Significant associations remained between insomnia disorder and asthma, gastrointestinal disorders, joint pain, fibromyalgia, and depression. The strongest association found was with depression (OR, 4.91; 95% CI, 2.63–9.17; $P < .001$). In subjects with insomnia disorder there was no sex difference (OR, 0.78; 95% CI, 0.36–1.71; n.s.), or difference between age groups (OR, 0.97; 95% CI, 0.77–1.21; n.s.) in the prevalence of depression.

3.5. Need for Treatment and Usage of Prescriptive Sleep Medication. Among those with insomnia disorder 62.5% expressed a need for treatment, and 22.0% used prescriptive sleep medication regularly. There was no age or sex difference in expressed need for treatment or usage of sleep medication. Subjects with insomnia disorder who were depressed used sleep medication more often than insomniacs without depression, 33.3% versus 17.1% (OR, 3.00; 95% CI, 1.22–7.37; $P < .05$).

4. Discussion

The main finding of the present study is that the prevalence of insomnia disorder is 10.5%, and women are 2.08 more likely to report insomnia disorder. Insomnia disorder did not increase with advancing age since being older decreased the probability of daytime impairment due to insomnia symptoms. There was, however, a significant rise in reports of insomnia disorder in women aged 40–49 years. Subjects with insomnia disorder slept less than 6 hours on weeknights, but 42.4% were able to extend sleep with more than 1 hour on days off/weekends. There was a strong overlap between insomnia disorder and physical and psychiatric disorders, most often with depression. A majority of subjects with insomnia disorder expressed a need for treatment, indicating that they are troubled and worried about their sleep, while 20.0% used sleep medication.

Advantages of the present study include the nationally representative sample, the high response rate, the broad age range, the comprehensive definition of insomnia disorder, and the wide range physical and psychiatric disorders included. Data were collected by telephone interview, and telephone interviews assessing DSM-IV psychiatric disorders have been shown to yield results comparable to other strategies [15].

One limitation is that sleep maintenance problems were assessed by the number of awakenings, and an additional question about duration of wake time would have been good. However, we think that 3 or more awakenings will include most individuals with sleep maintenance problems. This categorization has been shown to be related to daytime symptoms [16]. Individuals with 1 or 2 long awakenings should of course be regarded as having problems, but when we examined sleep duration in this group there were only few subjects with sleep duration less than 6 hours.

The measure of physical and psychiatric health according to number of disorders reported is relatively coarse but common in epidemiologic studies. The reliability of some self-reported diagnoses, for example, diabetes, is good [16], but others have shown poor reliability [17]. In the present study occurrence of depression was based on subjects' response to a single question about having depression. Previously the value of single-item depression screening has been established [18]. A limitation is that certain physical and psychiatric disorders, life style factors such as excessive drinking, and other concomitant medication than sleep-promoting medication which we did not deal with in this study could influence the results. Another restraint is that the question about sleep medication usage focused on prescribed medications.

This study demonstrates that subjects with insomnia disorder had a higher prevalence of several physical and psychiatric disorders compared to subjects without insomnia disorder. The cross-sectional nature of the study does not permit us to disentangle cause and effect; we can only demonstrate associations. Insomnia disorder and other health problems are either causally related to each other or other factors may influence this relationship. As such, we cannot say that insomnia disorder is a result of a physical or psychiatric disorder or that insomnia caused or exacerbated the disorder. However, from longitudinal studies we know that insomnia disorder actually plays a role in disorder development [19–22].

One aim of the present study was to provide valid estimates of the prevalence of insomnia disorder. Our definition of insomnia disorder is based on insomnia symptoms with frequency criteria, accompanying daytime consequences and a duration criterion of four weeks, and is thereby close to the DSM-IV insomnia disorder diagnosis [3]. The prevalence of insomnia disorder in our study was 10.5% and is similar to that of other studies [7, 14, 23].

In this study insomnia disorder was more common in women, but we found no association with advancing age. There was, however, a significant rise in insomnia disorder in women aged 40 to 49 years. Other surveys have also demonstrated a rise in insomnia disorder frequency in middle rather than old age [12, 24].

It has been shown that women more easily express emotional distress and somatic symptoms, like sleep complaints, compared to men [25]. It has also been shown that there are gender differences in coping styles [26] and exposure to stressful life events [27]. Menopause has been suggested as an explanation for the discrepancy between men and women in the prevalence of insomnia in mid-life. A recent study showed that postmenopausal women (53–58 yrs) had more nocturnal awakenings compared to premenopausal women (44–48 yrs), but the frequency of difficulty falling asleep, snoring, and use of sleep medication did not differ between the groups [28].

Although the elderly have difficulties initiating and maintaining sleep many do not report daytime impairment. With advancing age sleep becomes more fragmented and "lighter" due to increased percentage of stage one sleep and decreased percentage of slow wave sleep [29]. It has been shown that there is an age-related reduction in sleep duration and depth required to maintain daytime alertness [30] and that reduced night-time sleep quality in older people does not cause increased daytime sleep propensity [31]. These changes appear to be, at least in part, related to an age-related reduction in the homeostatic drive for sleep and a reduced strength

of the circadian signal [32]. Furthermore, a study showed that age was not predictive of insomnia when social satisfaction and activity status were controlled [33], suggesting that life style changes and inactivity accompanying old age can contribute to the lack of reports of daytime impairment.

Generally epidemiological surveys only assess sleep duration without comparing sleep on weeknights to sleep on days off/weekends. In agreement with previous studies subjects with insomnia disorder reported shorter sleep duration than subjects without insomnia disorder [6]. Surprisingly, we found that 42.4% of subjects with insomnia disorder increased their sleep duration with at least one hour on days off/weekends. This may partly be explained by a reduced stress experienced during weekends. Still it casts some doubts about these subjects having true insomnia disorder. This aspect has not been studied extensively earlier but should indeed be investigated in future studies. Our findings run counter to a survey from Spain demonstrating that subjects with insomnia did not to extend their time in bed on weekends [6] but is in agreement with a study from South Korea where subjects with difficulties initiating sleep slept at least three extra hours on days off and weekends [34].

Our study confirms that insomnia disorder rarely occurs alone. It is by far more common as a comorbid condition than as a single sleep problem. We found that 82.8% of subjects with insomnia disorder reported one or more disorders which is similar to findings from a survey where 86.1% of subjects with insomnia reported medical health problems [11]. Depression was reported by 40.5% of subjects with insomnia disorder, and subjects with insomnia disorder were 4.91 times as likely to have depression compared to subjects without insomnia disorder. We found no variation in association between insomnia disorder and depression between age groups, indicating that depression and insomnia disorder are related to each other with similar strength across life. In addition, we found that fibromyalgia, gastrointestinal disorder, and asthma were associated with insomnia disorder. These findings are in line with a survey that demonstrated that insomnia disorder was most strongly associated with psychiatric conditions, conditions characterised by psychological properties, and pain conditions [9]. Also, an association between gastroesophageal reflux disease and sleep problems has previously been reported [35].

In the present study a majority of subjects with insomnia disorder expressed a need for treatment, while 20.0% used prescribed sleep medication regularly. Other surveys from different countries report that a majority of subjects with insomnia do not use sleep medication. Rates of sleep medication usage in subjects with insomnia range from 21.5% to 33.2% [6, 14]. Variation in usage may be due to different definitions of sleep medication usage, but also cultural, social, or economic dissimilarities as well as differences in attitudes to sleep complaints and sleep medication.

5. Conclusions

This study provides important information about several aspects of the epidemiology of insomnia disorder, and the results have public health implications. The prevalence of insomnia disorder was 10.5%, and it did not increase with advancing age. This may suggest that many elderly adapt their life stylein such a way that potential daytime consequences of disturbed sleep are not manifested. Insomnia disorder was strongly related to physical and psychiatric disorders, most notably depression, underlining the importance of investigating and treating insomnia in subjects with physical and psychiatric disorders. The cause-effect relationship is difficult to establish, but there is evidence that treatment of insomnia disorder should be considered separately and independent of other cooccurring disorders [36]. A majority of subjects with insomnia disorder expressed a need for treatment, but only one-fifth used prescribed sleep medication. This study confirms that insomnia disorder is a public health issue, and improved recognition and adequate treatment strategies are required.

Conflict of Interests

The authors declare that there is no conflict of interests regarding the publication of this paper.

Acknowledgments

Research grants were provided by the Swedish Research Council, Stockholm Council Research Foundation, and SBU (the Swedish Council on Health Technology Assessment).

References

[1] M. M. Ohayon, "Epidemiology of insomnia: what we know and what we still need to learn," *Sleep Medicine Reviews*, vol. 6, no. 2, pp. 97–111, 2002.

[2] M. M. Ohayon and G. Bader, "Prevalence and correlates of insomnia in the Swedish population aged 19–75 years," *Sleep Medicine*, vol. 11, no. 10, pp. 980–986, 2010.

[3] American Psychiatric Association, *Diagnostic and Statistical Manual of Mental Disorders (DSM-IV-R)*, American Psychiatric Association, Washington, DC, USA, 4th edition, 2000.

[4] World Health Organisation, *International Statistical Classification of Diseases and Related Health Problems (ICD)*, 10th revision, World Health Organisation, Geneva, Switzerland, 2nd edition, 1994.

[5] American Academy of Sleep Medicine, *International Classification of Sleep Disorders: Diagnostic and Coding Manual (ICSD)*, American Sleep Disorders Association, Rochester, Minn, USA, 2nd edition, 2005.

[6] M. M. Ohayon and T. Sagales, "Prevalence of insomnia and sleep characteristics in the general population of Spain," *Sleep Medicine*, vol. 11, no. 10, pp. 1010–1018, 2010.

[7] S. Pallesen, I. H. Nordhus, G. H. Nielsen et al., "Prevalence of insomnia in the adult Norwegian population," *Sleep*, vol. 24, no. 7, pp. 771–779, 2001.

[8] B. Zhang and Y. K. Wing, "Sex differences in insomnia: a meta-analysis," *Sleep*, vol. 29, no. 1, pp. 85–93, 2006.

[9] B. Sivertsen, S. Krokstad, S. Øverland, and A. Mykletun, "The epidemiology of insomnia: associations with physical and mental health. The HUNT-2 study," *Journal of Psychosomatic Research*, vol. 67, no. 2, pp. 109–116, 2009.

[10] M. M. Ohayon and C. F. Reynolds III, "Epidemiological and clinical relevance of insomnia diagnosis algorithms according to the DSM-IV and the International Classification of Sleep Disorders (ICSD)," *Sleep Medicine*, vol. 10, no. 9, pp. 952–960, 2009.

[11] D. J. Taylor, L. Mallory, K. L. Lichstein, H. H. Durrence, B. W. Riedel, and A. J. Bush, "Comorbidity of chronic insomnia with medical problems," *Sleep*, vol. 30, pp. 213–218, 2007.

[12] R. Stewart, A. Besset, P. Bebbington et al., "Insomnia comorbidity and impact and hypnotic use by age group in a national survey population aged 16 to 74 years," *Sleep*, vol. 29, no. 11, pp. 1391–1397, 2006.

[13] M. M. Ohayon, M. Caulet, and P. Lemoine, "Comorbidity of mental and insomnia disorders in the general population," *Comprehensive Psychiatry*, vol. 39, no. 4, pp. 185–197, 1998.

[14] C. M. Morin, M. LeBlanc, M. Daley, J. P. Gregoire, and C. Mérette, "Epidemiology of insomnia: prevalence, self-help treatments, consultations, and determinants of help-seeking behaviors," *Sleep Medicine*, vol. 7, no. 2, pp. 123–130, 2006.

[15] P. Rhode, P. M. Lewinsohn, and J. R. Seeley, "Comparability of telephone and face to face interviews in assessing axis I and axis II disorders," *The American Journal of Psychiatry*, vol. 154, no. 11, pp. 1593–1598, 1997.

[16] M. M. Ohayon, "Nocturnal awakenings and difficulty resuming sleep: their burden in the European general population," *Journal of Psychosomatic Research*, vol. 69, no. 6, pp. 565–571, 2010.

[17] C. Nord, A. Mykletun, and S. D. Fosså, "Cancer patients' awareness about their diagnosis: a population-based study," *Journal of Public Health Medicine*, vol. 25, no. 4, pp. 313–317, 2003.

[18] L. Mallon and J. Hetta, "Detecting depression in questionnaire studies: comparison of a single question and interview data in community sample of older adults," *European Journal of Psychiatry*, vol. 16, no. 3, pp. 135–144, 2002.

[19] L. Mallon, J. E. Broman, and J. Hetta, "Relationship between insomnia, depression, and mortality: a 12-year follow-up of older adults in the community," *International Psychogeriatrics*, vol. 12, no. 3, pp. 295–306, 2000.

[20] L. Mallon, J. E. Broman, and J. Hetta, "Sleep complaints predict coronary artery disease mortality in males: a 12-year follow-up study of a middle-aged Swedish population," *Journal of Internal Medicine*, vol. 251, no. 3, pp. 207–216, 2002.

[21] L. Mallon, J. E. Broman, and J. Hetta, "High incidence ofdiabetes in men with sleep complaints or short sleep duration: a 12-year follow-up study of a middle-aged population," *Diabetes Care*, vol. 28, no. 11, pp. 2762–2767, 2005.

[22] E. O. Bixler, A. Kales, C. R. Soldatos, J. D. Kales, and S. Healey, "Prevalence of sleep disorders in the Los Angeles metropolitan ares," *The American Journal of Psychiatry*, vol. 136, no. 10, pp. 1257–1262, 1979.

[23] M. M. Ohayon and M. Partinen, "Insomnia and global sleep dissatisfaction in Finland," *Journal of Sleep Research*, vol. 11, no. 4, pp. 339–346, 2002.

[24] M. A. Grandner, J. L. Martin, N. P. Patel et al., "Age and sleep disturbances among American men and women: data from the U.S. Behavioral Risk Factor Surveillance System," *Sleep*, vol. 35, no. 3, pp. 395–406, 2012.

[25] A. J. Barsky, H. M. Peekna, and J. F. Borus, "Somatic symptom reporting in women and men," *Journal of General Internal Medicine*, vol. 16, no. 4, pp. 266–275, 2001.

[26] S. Nolen-Hoeksema, "Sex differences in unipolar depression: evidence and theory," *Psychological Bulletin*, vol. 101, no. 2, pp. 259–282, 1987.

[27] E. McGrath, G. P. Keita, B. R. Strickland, and N. F. Russo, "Women and depression: risk factors and treatment issues," Final Report, The American psychological Association's National Task Force on Women and Depression, 1990.

[28] L. Lampio, P. Polo-Kantola, O. Polo, T. Kauko, J. Aittokallio, and T. Saaresranta, "Sleep in midlife women: effects of menopause, vasomotor symptoms, and depressive symptoms," *Menopause*. In press.

[29] D. L. Bliwise, "Sleep in normal aging and dementia," *Sleep*, vol. 16, no. 1, pp. 40–81, 1993.

[30] D. J. Dijk, J. A. Groeger, N. Stanley, and S. Deacon, "Age-related reduction in daytime sleep propensity and nocturnal slow wave sleep," *Sleep*, vol. 33, no. 2, pp. 211–223, 2010.

[31] E. B. Klerman and D. J. Dijk, "Age-Related Reduction in the Maximal Capacity for Sleep-Implications for Insomnia," *Current Biology*, vol. 18, no. 15, pp. 1118–1123, 2008.

[32] D. J. Dijk, J. F. Duffy, E. Kiel, T. L. Shanahan, and C. A. Czeisler, "Ageing and the circadian and homeostatic regulation of human sleep during forced desynchrony of rest, melatonin and temperature rhythms," *Journal of Physiology*, vol. 516, no. 2, pp. 611–627, 1999.

[33] M. M. Ohayon, J. Zulley, C. Guilleminault, S. Smirne, and R. G. Priest, "How age and daytime activities are related to insomnia in the general population: consequences for older people," *Journal of the American Geriatrics Society*, vol. 49, no. 4, pp. 360–366, 2001.

[34] M. M. Ohayon and S. C. Hong, "Prevalence of insomnia and associated factors in South Korea," *Journal of Psychosomatic Research*, vol. 53, no. 1, pp. 593–600, 2002.

[35] C. Jansson, H. Nordenstedt, M. A. Wallander et al., "A population-based study showing an association between gastroesophageal reflux disease and sleep problems," *Clinical Gastroenterology and Hepatology*, vol. 7, no. 9, pp. 960–965, 2009.

[36] L. Culpepper, "Secondary insomnia in the primary care setting: review of diagnosis, treatment, and management," *Current Medical Research and Opinion*, vol. 22, no. 7, pp. 1257–1268, 2006.

23

Association between Sleep Disturbances and Leisure Activities in the Elderly: A Comparison between Men and Women

Amanda Hellström,[1,2] **Patrik Hellström,**[1] **Ania Willman,**[1,3] **and Cecilia Fagerström**[1,4]

[1] School of Health Science, Blekinge Institute of Technology, 371 79 Karlskrona, Sweden
[2] Department of Health Sciences, Lund University, 221 00 Lund, Sweden
[3] Department of Care Science, Malmö University, 205 06 Malmö, Sweden
[4] Blekinge Centre of Competence, 371 81 Karlskrona, Sweden

Correspondence should be addressed to Amanda Hellström; amanda.hellstrom@bth.se

Academic Editor: Giora Pillar

It has been suggested that physical or social activity is associated with fewer sleep disturbances among elderly people. Women report more sleep disturbances than men, which could indicate a variation in activity patterns between the genders. The aim of this study was to investigate associations between sleep disturbances and leisure activities in men and women ($n = 945$) aged ≥ 60 years in a Swedish population. Sleep disturbances were measured using eight dichotomous questions and seventeen variables, covering a wide range of leisure activities. Few leisure activities were found to be associated with sleep disturbances and their importance decreased when the models were adjusted for confounders and gender interactions. After clustering the leisure activities and investigating individual activities, sociointellectual activities were shown to be significant for sleep. However, following adjustment for confounders and gender interactions, home maintenance was the only activity significant for sleep. Being a female increased the effect of home maintenance. Besides those leisure activities, poor/fair self-rated health (OR 7.50, CI: 4.27–11.81) and being female (OR 4.86, CI: 2.75–8.61) were found to have the highest association with poor sleep. Leisure activities pursued by elderly people should focus on activities of a sociointellectual nature, especially among women, to promote sleep.

1. Introduction

It is suggested that leisure activities, such as physical and social activities and spending time outdoors, influence the timing of sleep and the robustness of the sleep-wake rhythm [1, 2]. Physical and social activities have also been found to improve sleep quality, efficiency, and duration [3, 4]. However, extremely short/long sleep duration has been associated with higher morbidity among elderly people (≥ 60 years) [5]. Fewer daytime activities and frequent naps during the day contribute to changes in the sleep-wake rhythm, which might lead to poor sleep quality [6]. This implies that elderly people need stimulating activities during the day if they are to sleep well at night.

Sleep changes throughout life. Elderly people usually go to sleep and rise earlier (i.e., phase-advanced sleep) [1], especially elderly women [7]. There is a decrease in sleep efficiency

and deep sleep (N3) [6]. The most common sleep disturbances in elderly people are nocturnal awakening, difficulty falling asleep, and early awakening [8]. Some of the changes in sleep can be attributed to normal ageing and others to medical conditions [1]. Most of the insomnia that occurs in old age is chronic, and long-term use of sleep medication is known to lead to impaired memory and daytime functioning [8]. There is thus a need for nonpharmacological management of sleep disturbances among elderly people.

Several randomised controlled trials (RCTs) [3, 9–11] have demonstrated sleep benefits when performing activities in people aged ≥ 55 years. Low-intensity physical activities, such as tai-chi, as well as high-intensity physical activities and social activities, all improve sleep quality, duration, and efficiency [3, 9, 10]. However, instead of investigating a set of predetermined activities, an alternative approach could be to investigate the activities that elderly people pursue in their leisure time. Leisure activities can be defined as activities that are enjoyable for the individual, are chosen freely, and derive from the interests and skills of the individual [12]. Leisure activities can include physical, social as well as cultural, or creative components.

Activity has been defined with considerable variation. It cannot be concluded therefore that all activities influence a common physiological mechanism, or that activities affecting sleep depend on energy expenditure. Morgan [13] investigated different levels of customary physical activity (CPA) and sleep quality. Included in CPA were outdoor productive activities (e.g., gardening), indoor productive activities (e.g., housework), outdoor walking, shopping, and leisure activities. The results showed that CPA was related significantly to insomnia whereas social engagement and daily walks were not [13]. Associations between physical and/or social activities and sleep have been investigated previously in several studies although the findings are inconclusive regarding the establishment of statistically significant improvements in sleep. Another difficulty is the definition of "physical and social activity". The inconclusive findings could possibly be explained by the nature of the activities that were included or that they are sorted into physical or social. Not investigating activities solely on the group level but also as individual activities could lead to greater understanding of which activities might be beneficial to sleep.

In elderly people, the association between leisure activities and sleep disturbances cannot be investigated without taking into account confounding variables. A confounder can be described as a variable that blurs or distorts the real effect of exposure [14]. Possible confounders of the association between sleep disturbances and leisure activity are gender, cognition, health, functional ability, and mood. Sleep disturbances in elderly people are found to be associated with female gender, depression, impaired cognitive function, and perceived poor health [15–18]. The association between poor health and sleep disturbances in people aged ≥60 years is well known [5, 19, 20] although sleep may also be affected by the functional status of the person [7]. In order to be active, a person needs functional ability and a willingness to engage in activities. Sleep disturbances have also been linked to mood disorders and other psychiatric illnesses among elderly people [21, 22]. Furthermore, mood disorders, such as depression or rumination and neuroticism, are more frequent in women [23].

Women report sleep disturbances to a greater extent [24], and sleep disturbances seem to increase with old age [25] as does the use of sleep medication [26]. Investigation of active ageing in the elderly showed that women are more often widowed, have a lower level of education, and are homemakers. Women also report more diseases and poorer self-rated health compared to men [27]. The different prerequisites of men and women could imply that men and women also have deviating activity patterns. Previous research highlights the seriousness of sleep disturbances and the importance of investigating sleep-promoting interventions in men and women separately. The aim of this study was to investigate associations between sleep disturbances and leisure activities

in elderly (≥60 years) men and women in a Swedish population.

2. Methods

2.1. Design and Sample. This cross-sectional study included participants ($n = 945$) enrolled in the longitudinal "Swedish National Study on Aging and Care-Blekinge" (SNAC-B). Data were provided by the survey, which was carried out in 2007–2009. Participants lived in a municipal area in south-east Sweden with a population of approximately 64,000. Ten age clusters, ranging from 60 to 96+ years, were included in the SNAC-B sample. There was randomised selection of the four younger age clusters (60, 66, 72, and 78 years) and total inclusion of the clusters of people aged 81, 84, 87, 90, 93, and 96+ years [28]. The SNAC-B sample is intended to be representative of the Swedish population. However, in the present study there was a slight overrepresentation of the oldest age (90+). Data within the SNAC-B study were collected through medical examinations, interviews, and self-administered questionnaires [28]. Demographic data, as well as data on sleep, leisure activities, functional status, and general health, were collected from the SNAC-B self-administered questionnaire.

2.2. Measurements. Sleep disturbances were measured by means of eight questions developed for the Comprehensive Assessment and Referral Evaluation interview schedule [29] and which were applied previously in a three-year followup study of elderly people [30]. The questions are dichotomous (yes/no) and based on self-reports. Examples of questions are as follows. *Is your sleep interrupted during the night?*, *Do you have difficulty falling asleep?*, and *Do you wake up early?* A cut-off figure of ≥4 sleep disturbances at the third quartile of the total sample was considered to be the demarcation point between those who sleep well (0–3 sleep disturbances) and those who sleep poorly (≥4 sleep disturbances). The cut-off point is based on the assumption that 10–25% of the general population suffer from persistent insomnia and with a higher prevalence among people aged >65 years [31, 32]. For the descriptive analyses, questions about use of sleep medication and sleep duration were added.

Leisure activities were measured using 17 dichotomous items, covering a wide range of activities (Table 1). In order to obtain a picture of the participants' exercise habits, two questions concerning light and intensive physical activity were amalgamated into one variable and dichotomised question, revealing whether or not the person performed regular exercise. The new variable comprised activities such as jogging, walking, cycling, gardening, exercising, swimming, skiing, skating, and ball games. The highest frequency was registered, irrespective of intensity. All people who participated in physical activity at least once a week were considered to exercise. Leisure activities were investigated as clusters of activities and as individual activities (Table 1).

Functional status was measured using the Instrumental Activities of Daily Living (IADL) items: shopping, cooking, cleaning, washing, and transportation. Each item had

TABLE 1: The leisure activities presented as clusters and individual activities and their association with sleep disturbances.

Cluster of leisure activities	Individual leisure activities	Correlation with sleep disturbances		P value	
		Group level	Individual level	Group level	Individual level
Physical outdoor activities	Exercise	−0.223	−0.095	<0.001	0.007
	Gardening		−0.167		<0.001
	Strolling in the country		−0.174		<0.001
	Picking berries		−0.140		<0.001
	Hunting and fishing		−0.121		0.001
Sociointellectual activities	Home maintenance	−0.248	−0.215	<0.001	<0.001
	Repairing cars/machines		−0.193		<0.001
	Playing chess/cards		−0.108		0.002
	Using/surfing the Internet/playing computer games		−0.129		<0.001
Creative activities	Knitting, weaving, or sewing	0.047	−0.090	0.165	0.010
	Playing an instrument		−0.040		0.286
	Painting, drawing, or pottery		−0.012		0.832
Cultural activities	Reading a daily paper	−0.005	−0.060	0.888	0.125
	Reading magazines/journals		−0.023		0.560
	Reading books		−0.014		0.751
	Watching TV		−0.026		0.578
	Listening to music		−0.024		0.562

Note: correlations between clusters and individual leisure activities were calculated using Spearman's RHO and Pearson's Chi-squared test.

the following response alternatives: dependent, partly dependent, or independent. The people who were dependent and partly dependent were classified as dependent, thus creating five dichotomous IADL items. The five items were then amalgamated into a dichotomous variable (dependent on one or more activity/independent).

Mood was measured by using a subscale of the Life Satisfaction Index [33]. In a factor analysis by Liang [34], three factors were found: mood, zest, and congruence. These factors have been validated in a sample of elderly people [35]. The mood factor comprises three items: *I am just as happy as when I was younger, My life could be happier than it is now,* and *These are the best years of my life.* All questions are answered with agree, uncertain, or disagree. The item *My life could be happier than it is now* was reversed before the total score was computed. The response alternatives "uncertain" and "disagree" were amalgamated for items 1 and 3, and "agree" and "uncertain" were amalgamated for *My life could be happier than it is now.* Mood scores are shown as being above or below the median value of the measurement (Md 1, range 0–3).

General health was measured using an item from the Short Form 12 questionnaire (SF12) with five response alternatives, ranging from poor to excellent [36]. The five original responses were then transformed into three responses: poor/fair health, good health, and very good/excellent health.

This was done in order to fit the variable's variation in the sample.

Cognition was measured using the *Mini Mental State Examination* (MMSE), which measures various cognitive processes. It can be used as a screening device for cognitive impairment, and three levels of cognition are defined. The score range is 0–30, where a score of 0–17 indicates severe cognitive impairment, 18–23 indicates mild cognitive impairment, and 24–30 indicates no cognitive impairment [37]. For this study, a cut-off at ≥24 of the MMSE has been made, separating those with cognitive impairment, regardless of severity, from those without impairment.

2.3. Statistical Analysis. Data were analysed using PASW Statistics 21.0 (SPSS Inc. Chicago, IL, USA). Descriptive analyses and group comparisons were made using the χ^2 test and the Mann-Whitney U-test on continuous variables. Yates' continuity correction was used in four field tables [38]. The ten age clusters used in SNAC-B were reduced to three clusters: 60 and 66 years (retirement age); 72- and 78-year-olds; and 81 years and above, in order to increase the number of people in each cluster.

Associations between variables were calculated using Spearman's RHO and multiple logistic regressions. Correlations using Spearman's RHO between sleep disturbances, confounding variables, and leisure activities were investigated. Only variables found to be significant ($P < 0.05$) through crosstabulation and associated with sleep disturbances in Spearman's RHO (Table 1) were entered into the multiple logistic regressions. The modelling was performed in three steps. Firstly, associations between sleep disturbances and clustered activities were investigated. Secondly, associations between sleep disturbances and individual leisure activities were investigated. Thirdly, associations between sleep disturbances and individual leisure activities and interactions between gender and the main effects found in the second model (2a) were investigated. All the crude models were adjusted for the confounder variables: gender, age, general health, functional ability, and mood. All multiple logistic regressions were performed using a backward, stepwise likelihood ratio (LR) method and were presented as odds ratios (ORs) with 95% confidence intervals (CIs). Goodness of fit of the regression models was performed using the Hosmer-Lemeshow test [39]. Collinearity diagnostics (VIF) was used to check for multicollinearity between the independent variables and was shown to be acceptable. Response alternatives that were considered to have the lowest association with ≥4 sleep disturbances were chosen as references for each variable. Subjects with an internal dropout in one or several variables were excluded from the models. The level of significance was set at $P < 0.05$.

2.4. Ethical Considerations. Written and verbal consent was obtained from participants. The study was approved by the Regional Ethical Review Board in Lund (LU 605-00, LU 744-00).

3. Results

3.1. Sample Description. Of the 945 people included in the study, 55.4% were women. The mean age of the women was 74.3 years (SD 10.3), while the mean age of the men was 72.8 years (SD 10.1) (Table 2). Women reported greater use of sleep, medication, greater dependence on medication for sleep, and more coexisting sleep disturbances than men (Table 2). Sleep disturbances due to pain and itching tended to be more common in women. The mean sleep duration was 6.7 hours for women and 6.9 hours for men. Sleep duration in the sample ranged from two to 12 hours, representing extreme sleep durations. Although there was a significant difference between the genders, both men and women reported interrupted sleep during the night, waking up early, and difficulty falling asleep as the three most common sleep disturbances. There were no significant differences between the genders with regard to early waking and daytime napping (Table 2).

There were significant differences in sleep disturbances between age cohorts and with regard to general health, functional status, and mood. Among the poor sleepers, 59.8% perceived their general health as poor or fair compared to 27.4% of the good sleepers. People with poor sleep were frequently more dependent when performing daily activities than those who slept well (34.5% versus 16.6%). Of those who slept poorly, 70.6% reported low mood (Table 3).

3.2. Sleep Disturbances and Leisure Activities. The most common leisure activities among both poor and good sleepers were reading the daily paper (95.5% versus 97.7%), reading journals or magazines (84.5% versus 86.4%), watching television (95.9% versus 97%), and listening to music (87.7% versus 89.4%) (Table 3). Significant differences existed between poor and good sleepers with regard to performance of regular exercise, gardening, strolling in the country, picking berries, home maintenance, repairing cars/machinery, playing chess/cards, and using the Internet/playing computer games.

Logistic regressions were performed to assess the associations between leisure activities and reports of ≥4 sleep disturbances. The first model contained the two clusters of leisure activities found to be associated significantly with sleep disturbance using univariate analyses (Table 1). Performing no sociointellectual activities increased the odds ratio of sleep disturbances (OR 3.75, CI: 1.49–9.43) as did performing only one sociointellectual activity (OR 3.15, CI: 1.26–7.88) compared to performing four sociointellectual activities. Physical outdoor activities did not contribute to Model 1a (Table 4). After adding the confounding variables gender, age cohorts, functional ability, general health, and mood (Model 1b, Table 4), none of the clusters of leisure activities mattered. Instead, being a woman (OR 3.12, CI: 2.16–4.52), aged 81 or older (OR 1.68, CI: 1.09–2.58), and perceiving one's health as good (OR 3.36, CI: 2.00–5.62) or poor/fair (OR 6.97, CI: 4.24–11.45) increased the odds ratio (OR) of having poor sleep.

A second model was then performed: investigating associations between sleep disturbances, individual leisure activities, and confounding variables (Table 5). Five leisure activities were found to be the main effects. Gardening (OR 1.45, CI: 1.00–2.08), strolling in the country (OR 1.47, CI: 1.01–2.14), home maintenance (OR 1.60, CI: 1.08–2.39), repairing cars/machines (OR 2.20, CI: 1.28–3.77), and playing chess/cards (OR 1.69, CI: 1.13–2.52) were all found to be significant for poor sleep (Model 2a). However, after adjusting for health, functional ability, gender, mood, and age, the highest odds ratio of sleep disturbances were among those reporting poor/fair health (OR 6.82, CI: 4.14–11.22), followed by those with good health (OR 3.33, CI: 1.99–5.58). Being a woman compared to being a man yielded three times the odds of poor sleep (OR 3.06, CI: 2.11–4.43). People aged 81 or older were 1.60 times likely to report poor sleep compared to those of retirement age. No significant difference was found between those of retiring age and those aged 72 or 78 years (OR 0.91, CI: 0.59–1.41). Of the leisure activities, only playing chess/cards, which is a sociointellectual activity, remained significant, with an odds ratio of 1.54 (CI: 1.01–2.35) (Table 5).

The second part of the aim was to investigate differences between men and women with regard to leisure activities associated with sleep disturbances and interactions between gender and activities. A third model was created containing the main effects found in Model 2a (gardening, strolling in the country, home maintenance, repairing cars/machines, and playing chess/cards). "Gender" was also added to the equation, as well as interactions between gender and each of the activities. Performing home maintenance (OR 2.26,

TABLE 2: Sleep disturbances, sleep duration, sleep medication, general health, functional status, cognition, and mood among men and women in the total sample. Percentages in brackets, significant values in bold.

	Men $n = 421$	Women $n = 524$	χ^2 value	df	P value	Missing data (n)
Mean age (SD)	72.8 (SD 10.1)	74.3 (SD 10.3)			**0.035**[2]	0
Difficulty falling asleep	74 (17.9)	188 (36.5)	38.2	1	**<0.001**[1]	17
Taking or being dependent on medication for sleep	51 (12.3)	103 (19.9)	9.3	1	**0.002**[1]	12
Sleep interrupted during the night	325 (77.9)	446 (86.4)	11.0	1	**0.001**[1]	12
Difficulty sleeping (falling/staying asleep) due to moods or tension	71 (17.3)	165 (32.7)	27.5	1	**<0.001**[1]	30
Difficulty sleeping due to pain or itching	54 (13.0)	111 (21.8)	11.5	1	**0.001**[1]	21
Inability to return to sleep after waking at night	45 (10.9)	112 (21.8)	18.7	1	**<0.001**[1]	17
Waking up early	236 (57.0)	308 (60.2)	0.8	1	0.367[1]	19
Feeling tired and sleeping for more than two hours during the day	33 (8.0)	39 (7.6)	0.0	1	0.910[1]	17
Sleep disturbances 0–8			45.9	1	**<0.001**[1]	61
Poor sleep ≥4	55 (13.9)	165 (33.9)				
Good sleep 0–3	342 (86.1)	322 (66.1)				
Sleep duration in hours	6.9 (SD 1.2)	6.7 (SD 1.3)			**0.048**[2]	119
Mean, (SD), (min–max)	(3–12)	(2–11)				
			7.56		**0.023**[3]	119
Short sleep ≤5 h	39 (10.9)	83 (17.7)				
Normal sleep 6–9 h	312 (87.2)	376 (80.3)				
Long sleep ≥10 h	7 (2.0)	9 (1.9)				
Prescribed sleep medication			20.9	4	**<0.001**[3]	10
Never	339 (81.5)	367 (70.7)				
Sometimes per month	35 (8.4)	48 (9.2)				
Several times per month	3 (0.7)	9 (1.7)				
Sometimes per week	8 (1.9)	34 (6.6)				
Every night	31 (7.5)	61 (11.8)				
General health			7.91	2	**0.019**[3]	15
Poor/fair	131 (31.6)	207 (40.1)				
Good	129 (31.2)	152 (29.5)				
Very good/excellent	134 (37.2)	157 (30.4)				
Functional status			5.997	1	**0.014**[1]	3
Independent	342 (81.4)	389 (74.5)				
Dependent on 1–5 activities	78 (18.6)	133 (25.5)				
Cognition			0.091	1	**0.763**[1]	5
<24 MMSE	32 (7.6)	36 (6.9)				
≥24 MMSE	387 (92.4)	485 (93.1)				
Mood (below/over median = 1)			5.485	1	**0.019**[1]	34
Low	209 (51.4)	299 (59.3)				
High	198 (48.6)	205 (40.7)				

Note: [1]Yates' continuity correction, [2]Mann-Whitney's U-test, and [3]Pearson's χ^2 test.

CI: 1.17–4.35), playing chess/cards (OR 1.61, CI: 1.09–2.39), strolling in the country (OR 1.56, CI: 1.07–2.29), and gardening (OR 1.50, CI: 1.04–2.16) were the leisure activities linked to sleep disturbances (Table 6). Examination of the interactions between gender and activities showed that the interaction between gender and home maintenance had an OR 0.44 (CI: 0.20–0.94). The interpretation is that being a man and being active did not increase the effect on sleep disturbances. After adjusting the model with confounder variables (Table 6, Model 3b), the home maintenance activity

TABLE 3: Leisure activities, age, gender, general health, functional status, mood, cognition, sleep duration, and sleep medication among good and poor sleepers in the total sample. Percentages are in brackets, significant values in bold.

	Good sleepers 0–3 sleep disturbances $n = 664$	Poor sleepers ≥4 sleep disturbances $n = 220$	χ^2 value	df	P value	Missing data (n)
Leisure activities						
Exercise	498 (76.9)	144 (67.3)	7.2	1	**0.007**[2]	83
Gardening	491 (74.5)	125 (56.8)	23.8	1	**<0.001**[2]	5
Strolling in the country	515 (78.1)	133 (60.5)	25.7	1	**<0.001**[2]	5
Picking berries	373 (56.6)	89 (40.5)	16.6	1	**<0.001**[2]	5
Hunting and fishing	117 (17.8)	17 (7.7)	12.1	1	**0.001**[2]	5
Knitting, weaving, or sewing	202 (30.7)	89 (40.5)	6.7	1	**0.010**[2]	5
Playing an instrument	93 (14.0)	24 (10.9)	1.1	1	0.286[2]	1
Painting, drawing, or pottery	59 (9.0)	18 (8.2)	0.0	1	0.125[2]	5
Home maintenance	376 (57.1)	71 (32.3)	39.5	1	**<0.001**[2]	5
Repairing cars/machines	200 (30.3)	24 (10.9)	31.8	1	**<0.001**[2]	5
Playing chess/cards	197 (29.7)	41 (18.6)	9.7	1	**0.002**[2]	1
Using/surfing the Internet/playing computer games	290 (43.7)	64 (29.1)	14.2	1	**<0.001**[2]	1
Reading a daily paper	648 (97.7)	210 (95.5)	2.4	1	0.648[2]	1
Reading magazines/journals	573 (86.4)	186 (84.5)	0.3	1	0.56[2]	1
Reading books	485 (73.2)	164 (74.5)	0.1	1	0.751[2]	1
Watching TV	643 (97.0)	211 (95.9)	0.3	1	0.578[2]	1
Listening to music	593 (89.4)	193 (87.7)	0.3	1	0.562[2]	1
Age cohorts			29.5	2	**<0.001**[1]	61
Retirement age (60- and 66-year-olds)	289 (43.5)	61 (27.7)				
72- and 78-year-olds	212 (31.9)	65 (29.5)				
≥81-year-olds	163 (24.5)	94 (42.7)				
Gender			45.9	1	**<0.001**[2]	61
Women	322 (48.5)	165 (75.0)				
Men	342 (51.5)	55 (25.0)				
General health			91.9	2	**<0.001**[1]	69
Poor/fair	180 (27.4)	131 (59.8)				
Good	202 (30.7)	62 (28.3)				
Very good/excellent	275 (41.9)	26 (11.9)				
Functional status			31.8	1	**<0.001**[2]	64
Independent	551 (83.4)	144 (65.5)				
Dependent on 1–5 activities	110 (16.6)	76 (34.5)				
Mood (below/over median = 1)			31.0	1	**<0.001**[2]	83
Low	315 (48.9)	154 (70.6)				
High	329 (51.1)	64 (29.4)				
Cognition			0.230	1	0.631[2]	66
<24 MMSE	43 (6.5)	17 (7.8)				
≥24 MMSE	617 (93.5)	202 (92.2)				
Sleep duration (hours)			114.8	2	**<0.001**[1]	163
Short sleep ≤5 h	36 (6.2)	75 (36.6)				
Normal sleep 6–9 h	530 (91.9)	126 (61.5)				
Long sleep ≥10 h	11 (1.9)	4 (2.0)				

TABLE 3: Continued.

	Good sleepers 0–3 sleep disturbances $n = 664$	Poor sleepers ≥4 sleep disturbances $n = 220$	χ^2 value	df	P value	Missing data (n)
Prescribed sleep medication			217.6	4	**<0.001**[1]	63
Never	578 (87.3)	93 (42.3)				
Sometimes per month	47 (7.1)	29 (13.2)				
Several times per month	4 (0.6)	7 (3.2)				
Sometimes per week	7 (1.1)	32 (14.5)				
Every night	26 (3.9)	59 (26.8)				

Note: [1]Pearson's χ^2 test, [2]Yates' continuity correction.

TABLE 4: The two clusters of activities associated with sleep disturbances, with and without adjustment for confounders.

	Model 1a			Model 1b		
	OR	95% CI	P value	OR	95% CI	P value
Physical outdoor activities			**0.007**			
None	2.15	0.92–5.01	0.077			
One	1.80	0.81–3.96	0.148			
Two	1.70	0.80–3.61	0.168			
Three	1.06	0.51–2.20	0.881			
Four	0.80	0.39–1.65	0.546			
Sociointellectual activities			**<0.001**			
None	3.75	1.49–9.43	**0.005**			
One	3.15	1.26–7.88	**0.014**			
Two	1.92	0.76–4.88	0.170			
Three	0.69	0.24–2.02	0.497			
Gender (women)				3.12	2.16–4.52	**<0.001**
Age cohorts						**0.011**
72- and 78-year-olds				0.93	0.60–1.44	0.742
81 years or older				1.68	1.09–2.58	**0.018**
General health						**<0.001**
Good				3.36	2.00–5.62	**<0.001**
Poor/fair				6.97	4.24–11.45	**<0.001**

Notes: in model 1a physical outdoor activities and sociointellectual activities were entered. The model explained between 8.9% (Cox and Snell R^2) and 13.2% (Nagelkerke R^2), Hosmer and Lemeshow 0.662, chi-square 5.870 (df 8), missing $n = 85$. Model 1b included physical outdoor activities and sociointellectual activities and was adjusted for gender, age, functional ability, mood, and general health. The model explained between 16.1% (Cox and Snell R^2) and 23.8% (Nagelkerke R^2), Hosmer and Lemeshow 0.497, chi-square 7.377 (df 8), missing $n = 111$. Significant factors are presented in bold. Only the last step of the regression analyses is shown in the table.

decreased in significance (OR 2.09, CI: 1.07–4.07), as did the interaction between gender and home maintenance (OR 0.33, CI: 0.15–0.75). Other explanatory variables for sleep were poor/fair health, good health, and being a woman, while the age clusters did not reach statistical significance (Table 6). People who reported poor/fair health were almost seven times more likely to report having ≥4 sleep disturbances, allowing for all the factors in the model.

4. Discussion

The associations between leisure activities and sleep disturbances were investigated as well as comparisons between men and women in an elderly Swedish population. The number of activities performed was of less importance than performing specific activities. Physical outdoor and sociointellectual activities were those that were found to be of significance, both as clustered and individual activities. Individual activities presented as being associated significantly with fewer sleep disturbances were gardening, strolling in the country, playing chess/cards, repairing cars/machines, and home maintenance. Following modelling and the inclusion of confounders and gender interactions, it became clear that it is mainly sociointellectual activities that were of importance. Interactions between leisure activities and gender showed that home maintenance was significant in relation to sleep disturbances, especially in women. This remained after the model was adjusted.

TABLE 5: Individual leisure activities associated with sleep disturbances, with and without adjusting for confounders.

	Model 2a			Model 2b		
	OR	95% CI	P value	OR	95% CI	P value
Gardening	1.45	1.00–2.08	**0.048**			
Strolling in the country	1.47	1.01–2.14	**0.046**			
Home maintenance	1.60	1.08–2.39	**0.020**			
Repairing cars/machines	2.20	1.28–3.77	**0.004**			
Playing chess/cards	1.69	1.13–2.52	**0.011**	1.54	1.01–2.35	**0.046**
Gender (women)				3.06	2.11–4.43	**<0.001**
Age cohorts						**0.019**
72- and 78-year-olds				0.91	0.59–1.41	0.666
81 years or older				1.60	1.04–2.47	**0.034**
General health						**<0.001**
Good				3.33	1.99–5.58	**<0.001**
Poor/fair				6.82	4.14–11.22	**<0.001**

Note: in Model 2a exercise, gardening, strolling in the country, picking berries, hunting/fishing, home maintenance, repairing cars/machines, knitting/weaving/sewing, playing chess/cards, and using/surfing the Internet/playing computer games were entered. The model explained 8.2% (Cox and Snell R^2) to 12.1% (Nagelkerke R^2) of the variance, Hosmer and Lemeshow 0.563, chi-square 6.670 (df 8), missing $n = 85$. Model 2b included exercise, gardening, strolling in the country, picking berries, hunting/fishing, home maintenance, repairing cars/machines, knitting/weaving/sewing, playing chess/cards, and using/surfing the Internet/playing computer games and was adjusted for gender, functional ability, mood, general health, and age. The model explained between 16.5% (Cox and Snell R^2) and 24.4% (Nagelkerke R^2) of the variance, Hosmer and Lemeshow 0.260, chi-square 10.078 (df 8), missing $n = 111$. Only the last step of the regression analyses is shown in the table.

TABLE 6: Individual leisure activities and gender interactions associated with sleep disturbances, with and without adjusting for confounders.

	Model 3a			Model 3b		
	OR	95% CI	P value	OR	95% CI	P value
Gardening	1.50	1.04–2.16	**0.032**			
Strolling in the country	1.56	1.07–2.29	**0.022**			
Playing chess/cards	1.61	1.09–2.39	**0.017**	1.43	0.95–2.17	0.090
Home maintenance	2.26	1.17–4.35	**0.015**	2.09	1.07–4.07	**0.031**
Home maintenance × gender	0.44	0.20–0.94	**0.033**	0.33	0.15–0.75	**0.008**
Gender (women)	3.63	2.15–6.15	**<0.001**	4.86	2.75–8.61	**<0.001**
Age cohorts						**0.043**
72- and 78-year-olds				0.95	0.61–1.49	0.832
81 years or older				1.56	0.99–2.46	0.056
General health						**<0.001**
Good				3.40	2.02–5.73	**<0.001**
Poor/fair				7.50	4.27–11.81	**<0.001**

Note: in Model 3a gardening, strolling in the country, home maintenance, repair cars/machines, and playing chess/cards were entered together with gender and the interactions gardening × gender, strolling in the country × gender, playing chess/cards × gender, repairing cars/machines × gender, and home maintenance × gender. The model explained between 9.2% (Cox and Snell R^2) and 13.7% (Nagelkerke R^2) of the variance, Hosmer and Lemeshow 0.887, chi-square 2.973, (df 7), missing $n = 66$. Model 3b included gardening, strolling in the country, home maintenance, repair cars/machines, and playing chess/cards, gender, gardening × gender, strolling in the country × gender, playing chess/cards × gender, repairing cars/machines × gender, and home maintenance × gender and was adjusted for age, functional ability, mood, and general health. The model explained between 16.9% (Cox and Snell R^2) and 24.9% (Nagelkerke R^2) of the variance, Hosmer and Lemeshow 0.716, chi-square 5.386, (df 8), missing = 93. Only the last step of the regression analyses is shown in the table.

Gardening and strolling are outdoor activities, implying spending time in daylight/sunlight, which is known to be beneficial for sleep. Bennett [40] found that women preferred to perform indoor leisure activities, such as housework, whereas men frequently did more gardening and car maintenance. Armstrong and Morgan [41] also found that women performed outdoor activities to a lesser degree than men. If women are less likely to be involved in outdoor activities, this could be a possible explanation for the higher prevalence of sleep disturbances among women. Environmental and

social factors, such as being widowed or being a homemaker, are also associated with poorer sleep [24, 42]. These are circumstances that could have contributed to the observed gender differences but they were not investigated here and cannot be verified or refuted by the present study.

Playing chess/cards was defined as a sociointellectual activity that exercises the memory and mental activity and maintains social contacts and communication [43]. Playing games might have a possible effect on brain plasticity, which refers to physical changes in the neurons in response to stimuli. Motivating or challenging stimuli enhance connections between neurons in the brain, thus improving or maintaining cognitive ability [44]. Findings from human and animal studies show that the need for sleep is adjusted by the amount of brain plasticity during prior waking [45]. Exposure to challenging and novel experiences could possibly trigger homeostatic increases in sleep requirements and thus also in deep sleep [44, 45]. Chess in particular is said to stimulate memory, attention, concentration, creativity, and reasoning, which underlines the value of this activity in the elderly. Playing games requires rigorous thinking combined with agility [46]. Social interactions have also been found to protect against depression [47], which often occurs in conjunction with sleep disturbances [21].

Home maintenance was the only significant individual activity for sleep when the model was adjusted for confounding variables and gender interactions. Unfortunately, it is not feasible to verify the upcoming finding since the same association has not been described previously. However, home maintenance could provide intellectual stimulation and physical activity and be a marker of autonomy, depending on the task. In an Australian study, having your own home was considered to be a sign of being free and not having to answer to anyone. The house was seen as a symbol of independence and autonomy [48]. This is also supported by a study of remote communities in Scotland. Even if tasks in the home might take longer for an elderly person to perform, it was important to remain independent [49]. In both studies it was emphasised that staying in the house also meant keeping your social contacts [48, 49]. It is possible that home maintenance represents more than just the physical performance of maintenance.

It was interesting to note in our study that the interaction showed that being both male and active did not have a synergetic effect with regard to home maintenance. The addition of confounding variables to the model did not erase the effect of the interaction between home maintenance and gender. It remained significant but the odds were lower, that is, decreasing the effect of not being an active man. The gender difference could be explained by the high odds for gender (OR 3.63, CI: 2.15–6.15) and home maintenance itself (OR 2.26, CI: 1.17–4.35). The finding also implies that home maintenance is of greater importance to women than men with regard to sleep disturbances. Even if the findings cannot be validated by previous research, it is possible that the ability to maintain one's own household independently could be a marker that distinguishes poor sleepers from those with fewer sleep disturbances. Nevertheless, this needs to be investigated further.

Another factor affecting sleep was health. Perceiving one's general health as fair/poor stood out as the strongest variable associated with sleep disturbances, followed by gender and good general health in the final model (3b). Physical and mental factors, such as medical illnesses, low mood, physical disabilities, and poor perceived health, are known to be associated with sleep disturbances [42]. Women reported poor sleep to a greater degree than men (33.9% versus 13.9%). This is concordant with previous research, where women tend to have more difficulty sleeping than men [24], although studies

that included objective measurements indicate the opposite [7]. Use of sleep medication was higher for women than for men (18.4% versus 9.4%), which confirms the findings of Ineke Neutel and Patten [26]. A possible interpretation of the results could be that women have difficulty sleeping despite the use of sleep medication. Prolonged use of sleep medication in women has been associated with perceived poor health and negative health outcomes [19]. It could be assumed that the higher prevalence of sleep disturbances in women was related to poor health. Another explanation could be that women did not sleep quite as long as men, and in the present study shorter sleep was found to be associated significantly with sleep disturbances. Women reported poor/fair health, low mood, and impaired physical ability to a greater extent than men. Tanaka and Shirakawa [50] suggest that sleep could be the key to improving or maintaining mental and physical health among the elderly, underlining the importance of sleep promotion, especially in women. There are obvious differences between the sleep of men and women, and tailored interventions for sleep promotion that take into account gender should be considered.

An advantage of the study was that an investigation was made of a broad spectrum of leisure activities that varied in intensity and orientation. Previous research emphasises that nonpharmacological interventions aimed at sleep hygiene factors may improve nocturnal sleep and maintain cognitive functioning and quality of life [32, 51]. Consequently, management of sleep disturbances by encouraging active living may result in several health benefits. No causalities can be inferred from the findings although it is known that sleep deprivation has a detrimental effect on brain function. Sleep loss could also result in a decrease in the restorative functions of the body as well as immune functions, which implies reduced resistance to infections [50].

The sample in this study is representative of the ageing population in Sweden, which is an advantage when investigating factors that affect sleep disturbances. The downside of the data collection procedure is that the most fragile elderly people do not have the strength or willingness to participate. This is mirrored in part by the large number (77.4%) of physically independent people with very good/excellent health and mood who were included in the study. The sample resided in what is mostly a sparsely populated area with small towns, which may have affected the leisure activities that were pursued. Geographical differences in the selection of leisure activities have been shown previously [52]. Other activities that were crucial to sleep could possibly have been found if the investigation was in a city area or in another part of Sweden. The study sample was taken from a single geographical area of Sweden, which implies a need for further studies. Interestingly, commonly performed activities, such as exercise or reading, did not explain the variation in sleep disturbances.

The decision to make a cutoff at the third quartile of the sample with regard to good and poor sleep was based on previous studies. Approximately 30–60% of the general population in developed countries suffer from insomnia symptoms [21, 53, 54], 10–20% of whom have persistent insomnia [31]. Among elderly people, 12–25% of those aged

≥65 years have persistent insomnia [32]. The prevalence varies depending on whether it is symptoms of insomnia or persistent insomnia that are measured. The use of eight single items with dichotomous answers when measuring sleep disturbances meant that only the number of difficulties could be measured, not the frequency, which is a common measurement in sleep studies. However, the questions picked up features of insomnia well, insomnia being one of the most common sleep disturbances. The questions were thus considered relevant.

5. Conclusions

Our findings show that sociointellectual activities are beneficial for sleep. Physical activities, such as strolling in the country or gardening, were significant in the crude models although they became nonsignificant when the models were adjusted. Including gender interactions, home maintenance was the only activity found to be significant for sleep, particularly in women. Furthermore, it was emphasised that people who perceived their health as poor/fair ran a greater risk of sleep disturbances. Self-rated health and the ability to manage your own home could be important markers for sleep disturbances. However, the significance of doing home maintenance cannot be validated by previous research and needs to be investigated further.

Conflict of Interests

The authors declare that there is no conflict of interests regarding the publication of this paper.

Acknowledgments

The outhors would like to thank the participants, the participating counties, and the municipal authority. The Swedish National Study on Aging and Care (SNAC) receives financial support from the Swedish Ministry of Health and Social Affairs and the participating county councils, local authorities, and university departments. Special thanks are due to Claes Jogreus for his statistical expertise when performing the analyses. Finally, The authors would like to thank Lund University and Blekinge Institute of Technology for supporting the study.

References

[1] L. Ayalon and S. Ancoli-Israel, "Normal sleep in aging," in *Sleep: A Comprehensive Handbook*, T. L. Lee-Chiong, Ed., pp. 599–603, John Wiley & Sons, Hoboken, NJ, USA, 2005.

[2] V. P. J. Zarcone, "Sleep hygiene," in *Principles and Practice of Sleep Medicine*, M. H. Kryger, T. Roth, and W. C. Dement, Eds., pp. 657–661, WB Saunders, Philadelphia, Pa, USA, 3rd edition, 2000.

[3] K. C. Richards, C. Lambert, C. K. Beck et al., "Strength training, walking, and social activity improve sleep in nursing home and assisted living residents: randomized controlled trial," *Journal of the American Geriatrics Society*, vol. 59, no. 2, pp. 214–223, 2011.

[4] M. Soltani, M. R. Haytabakhsh, J. M. Najman et al., "Sleepless nights: the effect of socioeconomic status, physical activity, and lifestyle factors on sleep quality in a large cohort of Australian women," *Archives of Womens Mental Health*, vol. 15, no. 4, pp. 237–247, 2012.

[5] R. Faubel, E. Lopez-Garcia, P. Guallar-Castillón et al., "Sleep duration and health-related quality of life among older adults: a population-based cohort in Spain," *Sleep*, vol. 32, no. 8, pp. 1059–1068, 2009.

[6] D. L. Bliwise, "Sleep in normal aging and dementia," *Sleep*, vol. 16, no. 1, pp. 40–81, 1993.

[7] A. Fetveit, "Late-life insomnia: a review," *Geriatrics and Gerontology International*, vol. 9, no. 3, pp. 220–234, 2009.

[8] E. J. W. van Someren, "Circadian and sleep disturbances in the elderly," *Experimental Gerontology*, vol. 35, no. 9-10, pp. 1229–1237, 2000.

[9] M. R. Irwin, R. Olmstead, and S. J. Motivala, "Improving sleep quality in older adults with moderate sleep complaints: a randomized controlled trial of Tai Chi Chih," *Sleep*, vol. 31, no. 7, pp. 1001–1008, 2008.

[10] F. Li, K. J. Fisher, P. Harmer, D. Irbe, R. G. Tearse, and C. Weimer, "Tai chi and self-rated quality of sleep and daytime sleepiness in older adults: a randomized controlled trial," *Journal of the American Geriatrics Society*, vol. 52, no. 6, pp. 892–900, 2004.

[11] E. Naylor, P. D. Penev, L. Orbeta et al., "Daily social and physical activity increases slow-wave sleep and daytime neuropsychological performance in the elderly," *Sleep*, vol. 23, no. 1, pp. 87–95, 2000.

[12] G. Häggblom-Kronlöf and U. Sonn, "Interests that occupy 86-year-old persons living at home: associations with functional ability, self-rated health and sociodemographic characteristics," *Australian Occupational Therapy Journal*, vol. 53, no. 3, pp. 196–204, 2005.

[13] K. Morgan, "Daytime activity and risk factors for late-life insomnia," *Journal of Sleep Research*, vol. 12, no. 3, pp. 231–238, 2003.

[14] K. J. Jager, C. Zoccali, A. MacLeod, and F. W. Dekker, "Confounding: what it is and how to deal with it," *Kidney International*, vol. 73, no. 3, pp. 256–260, 2008.

[15] Y. S. Bin, N. S. Marshall, and N. Glozier, "The burden of insomnia on individual function and healthcare consumption in Australia," *Australian and New Zealand Journal of Public Health*, vol. 36, no. 5, pp. 462–468, 2012.

[16] R. Furihata, M. Uchiyama, S. Takahashi et al., "The association between sleep problems and perceived health status: a Japanese nationwide general population survey," *Sleep Medicine*, vol. 13, no. 7, pp. 831–837, 2012.

[17] I. Haimov, E. Hanuka, and Y. Horowitz, "Chronic insomnia and cognitive functioning among older adults," *Behavioral Sleep Medicine*, vol. 6, no. 1, pp. 32–54, 2008.

[18] I. Jaussent, Y. Dauvilliers, M.-L. Ancelin et al., "Insomnia symptoms in older adults: associated factors and gender differences," *American Journal of Geriatric Psychiatry*, vol. 19, no. 1, pp. 88–97, 2011.

[19] J. E. Byles, G. D. Mishra, M. A. Harris, and K. Nair, "The problems of sleep for older women: changes in health outcomes," *Age and Ageing*, vol. 32, no. 2, pp. 154–163, 2003.

[20] C. Fagerström and A. Hellström, "Sleep complaints and their association with comorbidity and health-related quality of life in an older population in Sweden," *Aging and Mental Health*, vol. 15, no. 2, pp. 204–213, 2011.

[21] N. S. Kamel and J. K. Gammack, "Insomnia in the elderly: cause, approach, and treatment," *American Journal of Medicine*, vol. 119, no. 6, pp. 463–469, 2006.

[22] M. M. Ohayon and T. Roth, "Place of chronic insomnia in the course of depressive and anxiety disorders," *Journal of Psychiatric Research*, vol. 37, no. 1, pp. 9–15, 2003.

[23] L. S. Leach, H. Christensen, A. J. Mackinnon, T. D. Windsor, and P. Butterworth, "Gender differences in depression and anxiety across the adult lifespan: the role of psychosocial mediators," *Social Psychiatry and Psychiatric Epidemiology*, vol. 43, no. 12, pp. 983–998, 2008.

[24] C. N. Soares, "Insomnia in women: an overlooked epidemic?" *Archives of Women's Mental Health*, vol. 8, no. 4, pp. 205–213, 2005.

[25] M. S. T. Giron, Y. Forsell, C. Bernsten, M. Thorslund, B. Winblad, and J. Fastbom, "Sleep problems in a very old population: drug use and clinical correlates," *Journals of Gerontology A*, vol. 57, no. 4, pp. M236–M240, 2002.

[26] C. Ineke Neutel and S. B. Patten, "Sleep medication use in Canadian seniors," *Canadian Journal of Clinical Pharmacology*, vol. 16, no. 3, pp. e443–e452, 2009.

[27] P. M. López, R. Fernández-Ballesteros, M. D. Zamarrón, and S. R. López, "Anthropometric, body composition and health determinants of active ageing: a gender approach," *Journal of Biosocial Science*, vol. 43, no. 5, pp. 597–610, 2011.

[28] M. Lagergren, L. Fratiglioni, I. R. Hallberg et al., "A longitudinal study integrating population, care and social services data. The Swedish National study on Aging and Care (SNAC)," *Aging and Clinical Experimental Research*, vol. 16, no. 2, pp. 158–168, 2004.

[29] J. A. Teresi, R. R. Golden, and B. J. Gurland, "Construct validity of indicator-scales developed from the comprehensive assessment and referral evaluation interview schedule," *Journals of Gerontology*, vol. 39, no. 2, pp. 147–157, 1984.

[30] G. Livingston, B. Blizard, and A. Mann, "Does sleep disturbance predict depression in elderly people? A study in inner London," *British Journal of General Practice*, vol. 43, no. 376, pp. 445–448, 1993.

[31] S. Ancoli-Israel, "The impact and prevalence of chronic insomnia and other sleep disturbances associated with chronic illness," *American Journal of Managed Care*, vol. 12, no. 8, pp. S221–S229, 2006.

[32] C. M. Morin, V. Mimeault, and A. Gagné, "Nonpharmacological treatment of late-life insomnia," *Journal of Psychosomatic Research*, vol. 46, no. 2, pp. 103–116, 1999.

[33] B. L. Neugarten, R. J. Havighurst, and S. S. Tobin, "The measurement of life satisfaction," *Journal of Gerontology*, vol. 16, pp. 134–143, 1961.

[34] J. Liang, "Dimensions of the life satisfaction index A: a structural formulation," *Journals of Gerontology*, vol. 39, no. 5, pp. 613–622, 1984.

[35] C. Fagerström, M. Lindwall, A. I. Berg, and M. Rennemark, "Factorial validity and invariance of the Life Satisfaction Index in older people across groups and time: addressing the heterogeneity of age, functional ability, and depression," *Archives of Gerontology and Geriatrics*, vol. 55, pp. 349–356, 2012.

[36] J. E. Ware Jr., M. Kosinski, and S. D. Keller, "A 12-item short-form health survey: construction of scales and preliminary tests of reliability and validity," *Medical Care*, vol. 34, no. 3, pp. 220–233, 1996.

[37] T. N. Tombaugh and N. J. McIntyre, "The mini-mental state examination: a comprehensive review," *Journal of the American Geriatrics Society*, vol. 40, no. 9, pp. 922–935, 1992.

[38] D. Altman, *Practical Statistics For Medical Research*, Chapman & Hall, London, UK, 1st edition, 1999.

[39] V. Bewick, L. Cheek, and J. Ball, "Statistics review 14: logistic regression," *Critical Care*, vol. 9, no. 1, pp. 112–118, 2005.

[40] K. M. Bennett, "Gender and longitudinal changes in physical activities in later live," *Age and Ageing*, vol. 27, supplement 3, pp. 24–28, 1998.

[41] G. K. Armstrong and K. Morgan, "Stability and change in levels of habitual physical activity in later life," *Age and Ageing*, vol. 27, supplement 3, pp. 17–23, 1998.

[42] D. J. Foley, A. A. Monjan, G. Izmirlian, J. C. Hays, and D. G. Blazer, "Incidence and remission of insomnia among elderly adults in a biracial cohort," *Sleep*, vol. 22, supplement 2, pp. S373–S378, 1999.

[43] G. T.-Y. Leung, K. F. Leung, and L. C. W. Lam, "Classification of late-life leisure activities among elderly Chinese in Hong Kong," *East Asian Archives of Psychiatry*, vol. 21, no. 3, pp. 123–127, 2011.

[44] D. E. Vance, P. McNees, and K. Meneses, "Technology, cognitive remediation, and nursing: directions for successful cognitive aging," *Journal of Gerontological Nursing*, vol. 35, no. 2, pp. 50–56, 2009.

[45] C. Cirelli, "Brain plasticity, sleep and aging," *Gerontology*, vol. 58, no. 5, pp. 441–445, 2012.

[46] N. Krogius, *Psychology in Chess*, RHM Press, New York, NY, USA, 1972.

[47] V. Carayanni, C. Stylianopoulou, G. Koulierakis, F. Babatsikou, and C. Koutis, "Sex differences in depression among older adults: are older women more vulnerable than men in social risk factors? The case of open care centers for older people in Greece," *European Journal of Ageing*, vol. 9, no. 2, pp. 177–186, 2012.

[48] D. M. de Jonge, A. Jones, R. Phillips, and M. Chung, "Understanding the essence of home: older people's experience of home in Australia," *Occupational Therapy International*, vol. 18, no. 1, pp. 39–47, 2011.

[49] G. King and J. Farmer, "What older people want: evidence from a study of remote Scottish communities," *Rural and Remote Health*, vol. 9, no. 2, p. 1166, 2009.

[50] H. Tanaka and S. Shirakawa, "Sleep health, lifestyle and mental health in the Japanese elderly: ensuring sleep to promote a healthy brain and mind," *Journal of Psychosomatic Research*, vol. 56, no. 5, pp. 465–477, 2004.

[51] I. Haimov, "Association between memory impairment and insomnia among older adults," *European Journal of Ageing*, vol. 3, no. 2, pp. 107–115, 2006.

[52] I. Nilsson, B. Löfgren, A. G. Fisher, and B. Bernspång, "Focus on leisure repertoire in the oldest old: the Umeå 85+ study," *Journal of Applied Gerontology*, vol. 25, no. 5, pp. 391–405, 2006.

[53] C. M. Morin, M. LeBlanc, M. Daley, J. P. Gregoire, and C. Mérette, "Epidemiology of insomnia: prevalence, self-help treatments, consultations, and determinants of help-seeking behaviors," *Sleep Medicine*, vol. 7, no. 2, pp. 123–130, 2006.

[54] M. M. Ohayon and T. Paiva, "Global sleep dissatisfaction for the assessment of insomnia severity in the general population of Portugal," *Sleep Medicine*, vol. 6, no. 5, pp. 435–441, 2005.

24

Fast-Acting Sublingual Zolpidem for Middle-of-the-Night Wakefulness

Joseph V. Pergolizzi Jr.,[1,2,3] Robert Taylor Jr.,[4] Robert B. Raffa,[5] Srinivas Nalamachu,[6,7] and Maninder Chopra[8]

[1] *Department of Medicine, School of Medicine, Johns Hopkins University, Baltimore, MD 21205, USA*
[2] *Department of Anesthesiology, Georgetown University School of Medicine, Washington, DC 20057, USA*
[3] *Department of Pharmacology, School of Medicine in Philadelphia, Temple University, PA 19140, USA*
[4] *NEMA Research, Inc., Naples, FL 34108, USA*
[5] *School of Pharmacy, Temple University, Philadelphia, PA 19140, USA*
[6] *Kansas University Medical Center, Kansas City, KS 66160, USA*
[7] *International Clinical Research, Leawood, KS 66211, USA*
[8] *Kirax Pharmaceuticals, Bonita Springs, FL 34134, USA*

Correspondence should be addressed to Robert Taylor Jr.; robert.taylor.phd@gmail.com

Academic Editor: Giora Pillar

Sleep disorders (somnipathies) are conditions characterized by disruptions of sleep quality or of sleep pattern. They can involve difficulty falling asleep (prolonged sleep onset latency), difficulty staying asleep (disturbance of sleep maintenance), sleep of poor quality (unrefreshing), or combinations of these and can lead to poor health and quality of life problems. A subtype of sleep-maintenance insomnia is middle-of-the-night wakefulness, a relatively common occurrence. Zolpidem, a nonbenzodiazepine benzodiazepine receptor agonist, allosterically modulates an ion channel and increases the influx of Cl^-, thereby dampening the effect of excitatory (sleep disrupting) input. Recently, product label changes to some zolpidem containing products have been implemented by the FDA in order to reduce the risk associated with their morning after residual side effects. A new formulation of zolpidem tartrate (Intermezzo) sublingual tablet, an approved product indicated exclusively for the treatment of middle-of-the-night wakefulness and difficulty returning to sleep, did not have its label changed. We present a short summary of its basic science and clinical attributes in light of the recent regulatory changes for zolpidem products.

1. Introduction

Middle-of-the-night wakefulness (sleep-maintenance insomnia), a core symptom of insomnia, is a somnipathy that affects about 30.0% of those with incident chronic insomnia at baseline and 18.0% of the general population [1] and may contribute to another core symptom of insomnia, unrefreshed sleep [2]. See Figure 1. Certain populations may be more severely impacted: 78.3% of chronic pain patients have difficulty staying asleep [3] and women between the ages of 40 and 59 years rate "awakening during the night" as their most frequent symptom of insomnia [4]. Although there are many pharmacological and nonpharmacological

options to treat sleep disorders, there had previously been no sleep aid indicated specifically for middle-of-the-night wakefulness. In fact, previous products were unsuited for this use because they are long acting and, if taken in the middle of the night, would require the patient to sleep for several hours past their normal wake time. It is known that relatively few insomniacs seek medical care [5] and those that do may still have symptoms a year later [6]. The reasons for this are unclear but may owe, at least in part, to the fact that patients suffering from middle-of-the-night wakefulness had no pharmacological options. This narrative review discusses a new formulation of the established pharmacological sleep aid zolpidem (Intermezzo, Transcept/Purdue Pharma cleared for

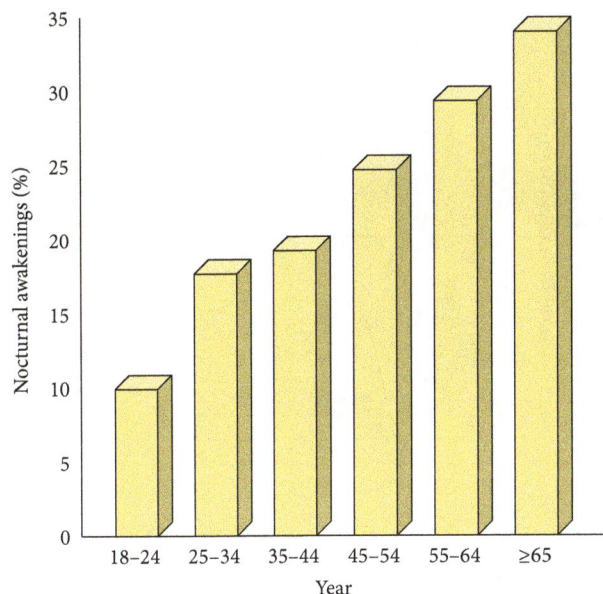

FIGURE 1: The prevalence of nightly nocturnal awakenings by age group (based on data from Ohayon) [64].

market by the Food and Drug Administration in November 2012), the first sleep aid indicated exclusively for the treatment of middle-of-the-night wakefulness and difficulty returning to sleep.

2. Sleep and GABAergic Transmission

In coordination with other neurotransmitters and neuromodulators, the inhibitory amino acid GABA (γ-aminobutyric acid), acting through the $GABA_A$ receptor, plays an important role in sleep/wake cycles [7–9]. The $GABA_A$ receptor is a ligand-gated ionotropic type receptor. Binding of the endogenous neurotransmitter GABA or an exogenous agonist analog increases Cl^- ion influx down its concentration difference from the extracellular side to the intracellular side of neurons. Since the transmembrane resting potential is already negative, the influx of Cl^- hyperpolarizes the neuron, that is, increases the transmembrane potential difference, producing a postsynaptic inhibitory potential (IPSP). The hyperpolarization means that the neuron is less likely to fire in response to an excitatory input. See Figure 2.

3. Benzodiazepines

Benzodiazepines have been the go to choice for short term treatment of insomnia. Benzodiazepines work by binding to the GABA receptors causing inhibition of neuronal excitation and result in increased total sleep time and shortened sleep latency [10, 11]. There are a number of FDA approved benzodiazepines for insomnia and they are generally considered safe and effective when used at recommended doses and for short term. However, their mechanism of action and long half life have been linked with a number of adverse effects. Common reported adverse effects include changes in sleep

architecture, daytime hangover, psychomotor impairment, rebound insomnia, withdrawal, drowsiness, dizziness, and headache [10, 11]. Daytime hangover has received much attention due to the increased association with impairing some daytime activities such as driving, resulting in many motor vehicle accidents [12]. To provide a safer treatment option for patients, recently nonbenzodiazpines (also known as z-hypnotics) have entered the market.

4. Zolpidem Pharmacodynamics

Chemically, zolpidem is an imidazopyridine not a benzodiazepine, but zolpidem acts as a benzodiazepine receptor agonist. It has a high binding affinity for the benzodiazepine receptor, which acts as a positive allosteric modulator of the $GABA_A$ receptor. Benzodiazepine receptor agonists, such as zolpidem, increase the neuronal transmembrane influx of Cl^- ions [13], which results in neuronal hyperpolarization and decreased neuronal excitability [14].

A large number of studies indicate that zolpidem has selective binding affinity and functional efficacy at the GABAA receptors containing $\alpha 1$ subunits [15]. Genetic studies of knock-in mice suggest the main target of zolpidem, GABAA receptors with $\alpha 1$ subunits, are involved in sedative action, while GABAA receptors with other subunits are associated with a variety of other activities, such as anxiety, myorelaxation, and cognitive function [16]. Similar genetic studies suggest that sleep continuity, as opposed to the motor sedative action, is mediated by subunits other than $\alpha 1$ [17]. Thus, the molecular mechanism underlying the clinical efficacy of zolpidem's hypnotic action is likely to be more complex, involving both $\alpha 1$ and other subunits.

Zolpidem is the active ingredient in several products commercially marketed to treat insomnia (see Table 1).

5. Pharmacokinetics of Sublingual Formulations

Two formulations of sublingual tablets are available: a higher-dose product (Edluar, 5 and 10 mg) indicated for difficulty with sleep onset and a fast-acting low-dose product (Intermezzo, 1.75 and 3.5 mg) indicated for middle-of-the-night wakefulness [18]. The low-dose product is available as a lozenge to be placed under the tongue and allowed to dissolve. A bicarbonate-carbonate buffer speeds absorption through the oral mucosa. Patients should be advised not to chew the lozenge or swallow it whole [18, 19]. Another formulation as an oral spray is available, which is considered bioequivalent to the fast-acting sublingual tablets [20]. Key pharmacokinetic properties of other zolpidem products appear in Table 2.

Doses of 1.75 and 3.5 mg produce a plasma concentration of >20 ng/mL within about 20 minutes, the level associated with sedation, and maintain it for about four hours [18]. Maximum serum concentration (C_{max}) is achieved in about 35–75 minutes with a half life of 2.5 hours. In normal healthy subjects (ages 21 to 45) the average C_{max} and AUC values for 3.5 mg Intermezzo were 77 ng/mL and 296 ng·h/mL, respectively, for women and 53 ng/mL and 198 ng·h/mL,

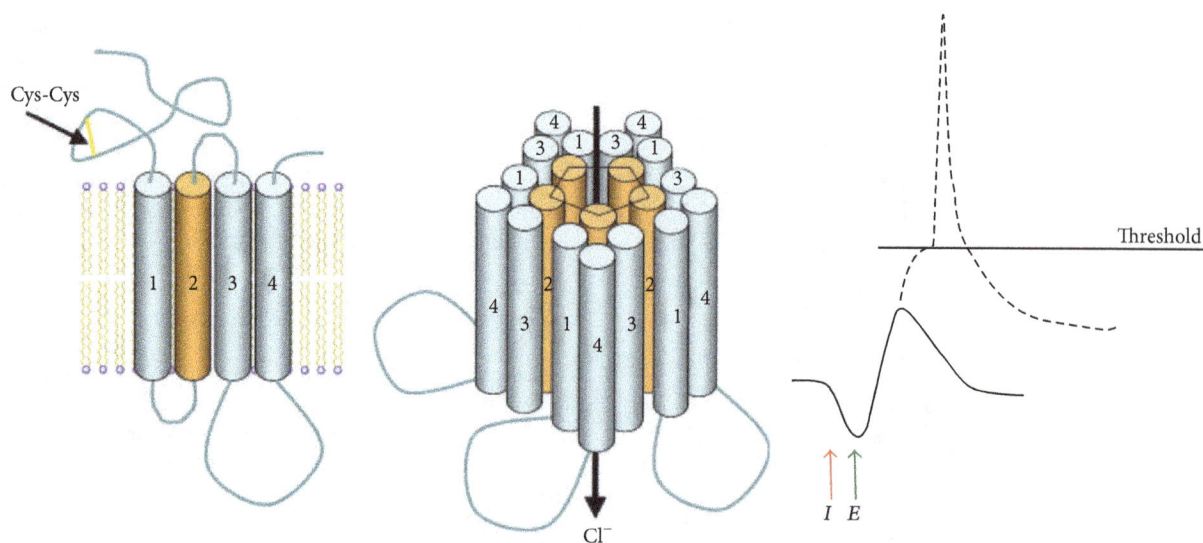

FIGURE 2: The pentameric structure of the GABA$_A$ receptor is composed of 4-transmembrane monomeric subunits (a disulfide bond in the *N*-terminal extracellular domain, characteristic of the family of cys-loop receptors which includes the GABA$_A$ receptor, is depicted). Zolpidem allosterically enhances Cl$^-$ influx, which hyperpolarizes the neuronal transmembrane potential (at I), thereby making it less likely to fire in response to excitatory input (at E).

TABLE 1: Zolpidem products currently marketed in the United States for treatment of insomnia. Zolpidem 10 mg tablets are marketed in Australia under the trade name Stilnox.

Brand Name	Manufacturer	Formulation	Indication	Strength(s)
Ambien [58]*	Sanofi	Immediate-release tablet	Difficulty with sleep initiation	5 and 10 mg
Ambien CR [59]	Sanofi	Controlled-release tablet (sometimes called extended-release or modified-release Ambien)	Difficulty with sleep onset and/or sleep maintenance	6.25 and 12.5 mg
Edluar [60]	Meda	Sublingual tablet	Difficulty falling asleep	5 and 10 mg
Intermezzo [19]	Transcept/Purdue Pharma	Fast-acting sublingual tablet	Middle-of-the-night wakefulness and difficulty returning to sleep	1.75 and 3.5 mg
Zolpimist [61]	NovaDel/ECR	Oral spray	Difficulty with sleep initiation (also being studied for middle-of-the-night wakefulness)	5 mg

All brand names are trademarks or registered trademarks of the manufacturer or drug owner.
*The patent on the Ambien immediate-release formulation has expired and generic products have been introduced into the market.

respectively, for men (C_{max} and AUC for 1.75 mg in women were 37 ng/mL and 151 ng·h/mL, resp.) [21]. At 12 hours, the drug is no longer detectable in plasma [22]. Thus, fast-acting low-dose zolpidem is associated with a rapid onset of short-term (four hours) sedation. This formulation does not appear to accumulate in the plasma, even after long-term administration [23].

The pharmacokinetic parameters, especially bioavailability, of sublingual zolpidem are variable depending on patient characteristics such as gender, age, or comorbidities. The pharmacokinetics of zolpidem differs by gender, resulting in gender-specific dosing [18, 24]. Gender differences in

the clearance of cytochrome-P (CYP) 3A4 substrates have been put forth as a possible explanation for different drug metabolism by gender of zolpidem and other agents [25]. A study of genetic polymorphisms of CYP3A4 and CYP2C19 among the Chinese Han people found that zolpidem is poorly metabolized by some individuals in this group [26], indicating that genetic factors may also play a role in zolpidem metabolism. In elderly patients taking 3.5 mg of sublingual zolpidem, C_{max} and $AUC_{0-4\,hr}$ were higher by 34% and 30%, respectively, than in nonelderly subjects. The C_{max} and AUC in elderly subjects were lower compared to elderly taking 3.5 mg, but higher than nonelderly taking 1.75 mg

TABLE 2: Pharmacokinetic parameters for zolpidem formulations.

Brand name	AUC(ng·h/mL)	C_{max} (ng/mL)	T_{max} (hours)	$T_{1/2}$ (hours)	Protein binding
Nonbenzodiazapines					
Ambien* 5 and 10 mg, respectively [58]		59 (range 29–113) and 121 (range 58–272)	1.6 for both	2.6 (range 1.4–4.5) and 2.5 (range 1.4–3.8)	92.5 ± 0.1%
Ambien CR 12.5 mg [59]	740 ng·hr/mL (range: 295 to 1359 ng·hr/mL)	134 (range 68.9–197)	1.5	Similar to above	92.5% ± 0.1%
Edluar 10 mg [60]		106 (range 52–205)	1.4	2.65 (range 1.75–3.77)	92.5% ± 0.1%
Intermezzo 3.5 mg [21]	Healthy Men: 198 Women: 296 *Elderly & hepatic impaired may vary	3.5 mg: men 53 and women 77. *Elderly & hepatic impaired may vary	0.6 to 1.25	2.5 (range 1.4 to 3.6)	93% ± 0.1%
Zolpimist 5 and 10 mg [61]		114 (range 19–197) and 210 (range 77–401), respectively	0.9 for both	2.7 (range 1.7–5.0) and 3.0 (range 1.7–8.4), respectively	92.5% ± 0.1%
Benzodiazapines					
Triazolam (Halcion) [62]		1–6	2	1.5–5.5	
Temazepam (Restoril) (30 mg) [63]		666 to 982 ng/mL (mean 865 ng/mL)	1.2 to 1.6 hours (mean 1.5 hours)	4–18	96

All brand names are trademarks or registered trademarks of the manufacturer or drug owner.
*The patent on the Ambien immediate-release formulation has expired and generic products have been introduced into the market.

[21]. In addition, patients who had hepatic impairment had mean C_{max} and AUC values two times and five times higher than patients with normal hepatic function when taking 20 mg oral zolpidem tartrate [21].

6. Efficacy

In a randomized, double-blind, placebo-controlled study, subjects with insomnia characterized by middle-of-the-night wakefulness were randomized into three groups [27]. Each group underwent a two-day treatment period followed by a five-to-12-day washout period. During treatment, subjects were awakened four hours after lights were turned off and administered one of the following: fast-acting zolpidem sublingual 3.5 mg or 1.75 mg or similar-looking placebo. Subjects were kept awake for 30 minutes and then allowed back to bed for another four hours. A total of 82 adults were enrolled and evaluated by both polysomnography and questionnaires about their sleep quality. All subjects crossed over into all three groups. Fast-acting low-dose sublingual zolpidem was found to confer a dose-related decrease in sleep latency to persistent sleep and total sleep time ($P < 0.001$) versus placebo and subjects taking the active agents did not exhibit impairment or sleepiness the following day. Fast-acting zolpidem sublingual 3.5 mg improved sleep quality ($P < 0.001$), ability to function, and level of refreshed sleep (both $P < 0.05$) versus placebo and zolpidem 1.75 mg also provided significantly higher levels of refreshed sleep versus placebo ($P < 0.05$).

7. Safety

In a randomized, three-arm, double-blind, placebo-controlled study conducted by Roth et al., adverse events were mild to moderate and reported by four, three, and seven subjects in the zolpidem 3.5 mg, zolpidem 1.75 mg, and placebo groups, respectively [27]. Events that were reported for active treatments included GI disorders, infections, urinary tract infection, glossodynia, increased blood pressure, nervous system disorders, headache, skin disorders, and contact dermatitis. Adverse events were not significantly greater in the active treatment arms.

In a double-blind, placebo-controlled study of 24 healthy volunteers, subjects were exposed to doses of 1.0, 1.75, and 3.5 mg of fast-acting sublingual zolpidem [22]. Subjects were randomized into each of the doses, separated by a washout period of 5–12 days. Medication was administered every morning at 8 AM and adverse events were assessed through length of study. A total of 48 adverse events (AEs) were reported, most of which occurred at higher doses. The most frequently reported AE was somnolence, reported by 12.5% of placebo subjects and 41.7% of subjects taking zolpidem 3.5 mg; fatigue was also reported at all doses. Dizziness and headache were reported by 4.2%, 12.5%, and 8.3% of the 1.75 mg, 3.5 mg, and placebo groups, respectively. Nausea was reported only at 3.5 mg doses (12.5%). One severe AE occurred and was deemed unrelated to treatment (epigastric pain; subject was in the 1.75 mg group). Two further AEs were considered unrelated to treatment (headache in the 1.75 mg group and dysmenorrheal in placebo) and were treated with acetaminophen and ibuprofen. All other AEs resolved without the need for treatment. Time of occurrence for AEs was not reported and statistical difference between placebo and active treatments was not conducted.

8. Morning Effects

Sleepdriving and other complex behaviors have been reported in the literature and popular media for other formulations of zolpidem [28–30], including reports of sleepdriving by prominent individuals [31]. Sleep-related complex behaviors associated with zolpidem have included sleep cooking, sleep eating, sleep shopping, and sleep conversations, usually associated with anterograde amnesia for the episode [32]. It is unclear why such behaviors occur. Enhancing GABA activity at the GABA$_A$ receptors might trigger hypnosedative behaviors and amnesia, the latter possibly the result of consolidating short-term to long-term memory, but this explanation is inadequate. Dosing may play a role; in the 15 cases involving zolpidem in a study of complex sleep-related behaviors, 10 involved taking ≥10 mg at bedtime; however, complex behaviors often occur with therapeutic-range doses. Drug-drug interactions may be involved; for example, a pharmacokinetic drug-drug interaction that inhibits cytochrome P450 metabolism could potentiate zolpidem. A pharmacodynamic drug-drug interaction could also occur for example, taking a drug which depresses the central nervous system (CNS) or enhances GABAergic activity could produce additive effects [32]. While several plausible, if incomplete, explanations have been set forth to explain complex behaviors, no single explanation or agent can elucidate all of the cases. In a study of traffic stops and arrests for sleepdriving or other forms of impaired driving while taking the so-called "z-hypnotics," including but not limited to zolpidem, it was found that impaired drives exhibited one or more of the following traits: they had higher-than-therapeutic serum concentrations of the drug while driving, they had failed to take the drug according to manufacturer's directions, or they had combined the sleeping agent with a CNS depressant or alcohol or both [33]. It should be noted that those taking z-drugs and detained for impaired driving are often unable to stand unassisted, and while they can speak, they have extremely poor motor control, in contrast to sleep walkers who can ambulate and maintain their balance.

In the case of sleepwalking, it has been suggested that such behavior is more common than generally believed, occurring in 1% to 15% of the general population and associated with sleep deficit—a common condition of insomniacs [34]. In a review of specific cases of sleep-related complex behaviors associated with zolpidem, these actions appear to be dose-dependent [30]. It may be that lower doses of zolpidem are associated with different rates of complex behaviors. For example, the literature reports a case of a patient who suffered from sleep eating with an extended-release formulation of zolpidem that resolved when changed to an immediate-release formulation [35]. Further studies are needed.

Recently the FDA has issued a change in product label for all zolpidem marketed products [36]. Reports have indicated that patient blood concentration levels may still be too high the morning after dose administration, resulting in residual somnolence and impairing activities that require alertness. These morning after effects have been shown to increase risk of car accidents and falls [37, 38]. Driving simulation and laboratory studies indicate that zolpidem blood concentration levels above 50 ng/mL are capable of impairing driving. Pharmacokinetic trials of zolpidem products reported a significant number of patients above this threshold the morning after administration. By lowering the recommended dose for these products, potential risk for these morning after effects may be reduced. It should be noted that Intermezzo's product label was not required to be changed due to it already being a lower dose formulation.

9. Abuse Potential

Zolpidem is a Schedule IV controlled substance in the United States according to the Controlled Substances Act. A retrospective study found that zolpidem had the potential for abuse and dependence in certain patients, particularly those with a history of substance abuse and those actively consuming multiple types of drugs [39], but it should be noted that low-dose, fast-acting zolpidem is a new product and was not included in this study. It is not clear if a low-dose, short-acting product would have less appeal to a potential abuser than higher-dose formulations. Zolpidem dependence with withdrawal symptoms has been reported in the literature, which was effectively managed with pregabalin [40].

Mechanistic animal studies on physical dependence and abuse liability of GABAA-α1-preferring drugs, such as zolpidem, have been equivocal. Some primate studies suggest that the GABAA-α1-subunit is involved in physical dependence, suggesting that the hypnotic and abuse liability activity of zolpidem might not be separated [41]. Other studies on genetic mice models suggest that subunits other than α1 (such as α3) are involved in reward-enhancing activity of various GABA agonists, including zolpidem [42].

Zolpidem does not appear to induce tolerance in insomniac patients, even with long-term use [43, 44]. The use of sublingual zolpidem 10 mg at bedtime over the course of one year did not induce tolerance in primary insomniacs [45], but it is uncertain whether a fast-acting sublingual formulation would exhibit a different tolerance profile.

10. Cancer

A retrospective health insurance database study ($n = 14{,}950$) in Taiwan found that zolpidem users had a greater risk than nonusers for developing any of several types of cancer (overall hazard ratio 1.68, 95% confidence interval, 1.57 to 3.56), with men at higher risk than women [46]. This risk increased with dose with greater use of zolpidem (defined here as ≥300 mg/year). Since this is a single retrospective study in a highly homogeneous population, it requires confirmation, particularly in light of such unusual findings. This study did not gather data from patients on smoking, alcohol consumption, or obesity, all of which may have contributed to higher cancer rates.

11. Zolpidem Use in Special Populations

11.1. Geriatric Patients. Zolpidem pharmacokinetics in general differs in younger and older patients; the elderly have an increased maximum serum concentration (C_{max}) and lower oral clearance rates, meaning that lower doses are recommended in individuals over the age of 60 [47]. A population-based cohort study found that ambulatory seniors were often prescribed supratherapeutic doses of zolpidem [48]. The recommended dose of zolpidem for geriatric patients is 5 mg/day (for long-acting formulations) and 1.75 mg/day for men and women of the fast-acting sublingual formulation [19].

11.2. Women. Insomnia is more common in women and may affect women differently than men [49]. Attempts have been made to correlate higher insomnia rates in women with greater rates of depression, mental health disorders, and hormonal disruptions, but, even taking those into account, women are more likely to experience insomnia than men [50]. Insomnia has been more closely correlated to pain and somatic symptoms in women than men [51]. Furthermore, insomnia prevalence in women increases with advancing age [50]. The apparent female predisposition to insomnia causes more elderly women than elderly men to take hypnotics and sedatives to facilitate sleep [52]. A Danish registry study ($n = 10,000$) found that female gender and advanced age were risk factors for the long-term use of zolpidem and other z-hypnotics [53]. Gender-specific dosing should be followed with zolpidem as drug clearance rates are slower in women than men. Women have a significantly higher serum concentration of zolpidem than men, as much as 40% greater, a factor that should be considered when making prescribing decisions [54]. In January of 2013, the FDA recommended that dosages be reduced for women of certain immediate-release zolpidem products (Ambien, Edluar, and Zolpimist) from 10 mg to 5 mg and extended-release zolpidem (Ambien CR) be dropped from 12.5 mg to 6.25 mg. The dosage of the lower-dose middle-of-the-night product (Intermezzo) remains unchanged as it was released to market with a lower dosage for women than men.

In a systematic review of the literature of driving studies involving a variety of sleeping agents ($n = 14$ studies), differences in driving ability by gender were noted the morning after taking a sleeping agent for flurazepam 30 mg and zolpidem 10 mg administered in the middle of the night, but not for ramelteon 8 mg, lormetazepam 1 and 2 mg, zaleplon 10 and 20 mg, and zopiclone 7.5 mg [55]. Women seem to be affected more by these drugs in terms of driving than men. It must be noted that these authors compared a variety of studies using different drugs, different study methodologies, and different patient populations; for instance, some studies enrolled only men or only women.

Zolpidem is classified as a category C drug for use during pregnancy, meaning that the risk of its use in this population cannot be ruled out. Zolpidem has been associated with adverse pregnancy outcomes in a population-based study in Taiwan [56].

12. Clinical Perspective

Since many sleeping products are available on the market, including several zolpidem formulations, the arrival of a new product may seem unnecessary. Fast-acting, low-dose sublingual zolpidem is important because it is indicated specifically for middle-of-the-night wakefulness, a need not previously addressed by the current products. Middle-of-the-night wakefulness is a core symptom of insomnia and not a rare one; it is one of the most common ways that insomnia presents. Prior zolpidem formulations were long-acting products that required patients to have at least eight hours reserved for sleep upon taking the medication. Patients taking a long-acting formulation and then arising while the drug was still in effect are thought to be at greater risk for unexpected and complex behaviors, such as sleepdriving [19].

Though there are treatment options being researched for the morning after effects such as sublingual Flumazenil, a $GABA_A$ receptor antagonist, these may not be suitable for all patients and additional medications may not be feasible [57]. Therefore, a fast-acting, low-dose product that is effective only for a four-hour time period meets a need not served by any of the other formulations.

When treating insomnia, clinicians should first rule out any underlying conditions that might be causing sleeplessness. Many patients with mild or occasional insomnia may benefit from nonpharmacological treatment options, such as lifestyle modifications or changes in sleep hygiene. There remain many patients who will require pharmacological therapy to manage the distressing symptoms of primary insomnia. Sleep aids are powerful agents and should be prescribed with patient education so that patients understand their potential risks as well as benefits. Considerable direct-to-consumer advertising of sleeping pills may encourage in some consumers a false notion that sleep aids are harmless drugs that can be consumed casually. Thus, clinicians must instill in patients the important concept that drugs to fight insomnia are powerful agents to be taken only as directed, when needed, and under medical supervision.

Since this is a new indication for zolpidem, clinicians should counsel patients about this agent and how to take it. In particular, a gender-specific (and age-specific) dosing regimen should be emphasized. The gender-specific dosing for fast-acting low-dose zolpidem also appears to recognize a previously overlooked consideration, namely, that women metabolize zolpidem differently than men. Since more women than men suffer from insomnia and more women take sleep aids, this is not a trivial consideration.

As with all drugs in this class and use in this application, adequate caution is required regarding possibly allergy to the drug substance, adverse effects, drug-drug interactions, and other potential problems that should be adequately reviewed before prescribing or taking.

13. Conclusion

Fast-acting sublingual zolpidem tartrate (Intermezzo) is a new low-dose formulation designed to specifically address the somnipathy of middle-of-the-night wakefulness. It is the first FDA-approved drug exclusively for this use. Since middle-of-the-night wakefulness is a frequent core symptom of primary insomnia, this new agent addresses an important need. The fast-acting low-dose sublingual formulation offers an interesting new option for the right patients.

Conflict of Interests

Joseph V. Pergolizzi Jr. is a consultant for Purdue Pharma, Grünenthal, Endo, Pfizer, INSYS Therapeutics, Baxter, and is a consultant and on the speakers bureau for Lilly USA. Srinivas Nalamachu has received consultancy honoraria or research grants from the following companies: Grünenthal, GmbH, Johnson & Johnson, Endo Pharmaceuticals, Cephalon, Teva, AlphPharma, King Pharmaceuticals, Allergan, Ipsen, Archmiedes, Insys, Zogenix, ProStakan, and Covidien. Robert B. Raffa is a speaker, consultant, and/or basic science investigator for several pharmaceutical companies involved in analgesic research, but he receives no royalty (cash or otherwise) from the sale of any product. Joseph V. Pergolizzi Jr., Srinivas Nalamachu, Robert Taylor Jr., Robert B. Raffa, and Maninder Chopra have no direct financial relation with the commercial identities mentioned in this paper that might lead to a conflict of interest. This paper was prepared with medical writing and editing services from Jo Ann LeQuang of LeQ Medical, Angleton, Texas, whose services were paid by the authors.

References

[1] R. Singareddy, A. N. Vgontzas, J. Fernandez-Mendoza et al., "Risk factors for incident chronic insomnia: a general population prospective study," *Sleep Medicine*, vol. 13, no. 4, pp. 346–353, 2012.

[2] K. Sarsour, D. L. Van Brunt, J. A. Johnston, K. A. Foley, C. M. Morin, and J. K. Walsh, "Associations of nonrestorative sleep with insomnia, depression, and daytime function," *Sleep Medicine*, vol. 11, no. 10, pp. 965–972, 2010.

[3] C. R. Green, S. K. Ndao-Brumblay, and T. Hart-Johnson, "Sleep problems in a racially diverse chronic pain population," *Clinical Journal of Pain*, vol. 25, no. 5, pp. 423–430, 2009.

[4] J. E. Blümel, A. Cano, E. Mezones-Holguín et al., "A multinational study of sleep disorders during female mid-life," *Maturitas*, vol. 72, no. 4, pp. 359–366, 2012.

[5] S. Sullivan, "Update on emerging drugs for insomnia," *Expert Opin Emerg Drugs*, vol. 17, no. 3, pp. 295–298, 2012.

[6] D. J. Buysse, "Chronic insomnia," *American Journal of Psychiatry*, vol. 165, no. 6, pp. 676–686, 2008.

[7] H. Möhler, "GABAA receptors in central nervous system disease: anxiety, epilepsy, and insomnia," *Journal of Receptors and Signal Transduction*, vol. 26, no. 5-6, pp. 731–740, 2006.

[8] D. Gerashchenko, J. P. Wisor, D. Burns et al., "Identification of a population of sleep-active cerebral cortex neurons," *Proceedings of the National Academy of Sciences of the United States of America*, vol. 105, no. 29, pp. 10227–10232, 2008.

[9] R. Winsky-Sommerer, "Role of GABAA receptors in the physiology and pharmacology of sleep," *European Journal of Neuroscience*, vol. 29, no. 9, pp. 1779–1794, 2009.

[10] A. K. Morin, C. I. Jarvis, and A. M. Lynch, "Therapeutic options for sleep-maintenance and sleep-onset insomnia," *Pharmacotherapy*, vol. 27, no. 1, pp. 89–110, 2007.

[11] S. Passarella and M.-T. Duong, "Diagnosis and treatment of insomnia," *American Journal of Health*, vol. 65, no. 10, pp. 927–934, 2008.

[12] T. Dassanayake, P. Michie, G. Carter, and A. Jones, "Effects of benzodiazepines, antidepressants and opioids on driving: a systematic review and meta-analysis of epidemiological and experimental evidence," *Drug Safety*, vol. 34, no. 2, pp. 125–156, 2011.

[13] A. Dang, A. Garg, and P. V. Rataboli, "Role of zolpidem in the management of insomnia," *CNS Neuroscience and Therapeutics*, vol. 17, no. 5, pp. 387–397, 2011.

[14] J. Costentin, "Treatment of insomnia. Pharmacological approaches and their limitations," *Bulletin of the National Academy of Medicine*, vol. 195, no. 7, pp. 1583–1595, 2011.

[15] D. J. Nutt and S. M. Stahl, "Searching for perfect sleep: the continuing evolution of GABAA receptor modulators as hypnotics," *Journal of Psychopharmacology*, vol. 24, no. 11, pp. 1601–1612, 2010.

[16] U. Rudolph and F. Knoflach, "Beyond classical benzodiazepines: novel therapeutic potential of GABA A receptor subtypes," *Nature Reviews Drug Discovery*, vol. 10, no. 9, pp. 685–697, 2011.

[17] I. Tobler, C. Kopp, T. Deboer, and U. Rudolph, "Diazepam-induced changes in sleep: role of the alpha 1 GABA(A) receptor subtype," *Proceedings of the National Academy of Sciences of the United States of America*, vol. 98, no. 11, pp. 6464–6469, 2001.

[18] "Low-dose sublingual zolpidem (intermezzo) for insomnia due to middle-of-the-night awakening," *The Medical Letter on Drugs and Therapeutics*, vol. 54, no. 1387, pp. 25–26, 2012.

[19] "Intermezzo (zoplidem tartrate) sublingual tablets," Highlights of prescribing information, 2012, http://app.purduepharma.com/xmlpublishing/pi.aspx?id=i.

[20] "Zolpidem oral spray (zolpimist) for insomnia," *The Medical Letter on Drugs and Therapeutics*, vol. 54, no. 1384, pp. 14–15, 2012.

[21] G. S. De Oliveira Jr., D. Agarwal, and H. T. Benzon, "Perioperative single dose ketorolac to prevent postoperative pain: a meta-analysis of randomized trials," *Anesthesia and Analgesia*, vol. 114, no. 2, pp. 424–433, 2012.

[22] T. Roth, D. Mayleben, B. C. Corser, and N. N. Singh, "Daytime pharmacodynamic and pharmacokinetic evaluation of low-dose sublingual transmucosal zolpidem hemitartrate," *Human Psychopharmacology*, vol. 23, no. 1, pp. 13–20, 2008.

[23] L. Staner, P. Danjou, and R. Luthringer, "A new sublingual formulation of zolpidem for the treatment of sleep-onset insomnia," *Expert Review of Neurotherapeutics*, vol. 12, no. 2, pp. 141–153, 2012.

[24] "Intermezzo-zolpidem tartrate tablet," Highlights of prescribing information, 2012, http://app.purduepharma.com/xmlpublishing/pi.aspx?id=i.

[25] M. Chetty, D. Mattison, and A. Rostami-Hodjegan, "Sex differences in the clearance of CYP3A4 substrates: exploring possible

reasons for the substrate dependency and lack of consensus," *Current Drug Metabolism*, vol. 13, no. 6, pp. 778–786, 2012.

[26] M. Shen, Y. Shi, and P. Xiang, "CYP3A4 and CYP2C19 genetic polymorphisms and zolpidem metabolism in the Chinese Han population: a pilot study," *Forensic Science International*, vol. 227, no. 1–3, pp. 77–81, 2012.

[27] T. Roth, S. G. Hull, D. A. Lankford et al., "Low-dose sublingual zolpidem tartrate is associated with dose-related improvement in sleep onset and duration in insomnia characterized by middle-of-the-night (MOTN) awakenings," *Sleep*, vol. 31, no. 9, pp. 1277–1284, 2008.

[28] R. Hoque and A. L. Chesson Jr., "Zolpidem-induced sleepwalking, sleep related eating disorder, and sleepdriving: fluorine-18-flourodeoxyglucose positron emission tomography analysis, and a literature review of other unexpected clinical effects of zolpidem," *Journal of Clinical Sleep Medicine*, vol. 5, no. 5, pp. 471–476, 2009.

[29] M. Najjar, "Zolpidem and amnestic sleep related eating disorder," *Journal of Clinical Sleep Medicine*, vol. 3, no. 6, pp. 637–638, 2007.

[30] C. Daley, D. E. McNiel, and R. L. Binder, "'I did what?' Zolpidem and the courts," *Journal of the American Academy of Psychiatry and the Law*, vol. 39, no. 4, pp. 535–542, 2011.

[31] K. Falkenberg, "Kerry Kennedy DUI arrest likely caused by sleepdriving—just like cousin Patrick's Capitol Hill crash (updated)," 2012, http://www.forbes.com/sites/kaifalkenberg/2012/07/14/kerry-kennedy-was-likely-sleep-driving-just-like-her-cousin-patrick/.

[32] C. R. Dolder and M. H. Nelson, "Hypnosedative-induced complex behaviours: incidence, mechanisms and management," *CNS Drugs*, vol. 22, no. 12, pp. 1021–1036, 2008.

[33] M. R. Pressman, "Sleepdriving: sleepwalking variant or misuse of z-drugs?" *Sleep Medicine Reviews*, vol. 15, no. 5, pp. 285–292, 2011.

[34] "Sleepwalking," 2012, http://www.sleepfoundation.org/article/sleep-related-problems/sleepwalking.

[35] A. Chiang and A. Krystal, "Report of two cases where sleep related eating behavior occurred with the extended-release formulation but not the immediate-release formulation of a sedative-hypnotic agent," *Journal of Clinical Sleep Medicine*, vol. 4, no. 2, pp. 155–156, 2008.

[36] US Food and Drug Administration, "FDA drug safety communication: risk of next-morning impairment after use of insomnia drugs; FDA requires lower recommended doses for certain drugs containing zolpidem (Ambien, Ambien CR, Edluar, and Zolpimist)," 2013, http://www.fda.gov/drugs/drugsafety/ucm334033.htm.

[37] B. P. Kolla, J. K. Lovely, M. P. Mansukhani, and T. I. Morgenthaler, "Zolpidem is independently associated with increased risk of inpatient falls," *Journal of Hospital Medicine*, vol. 8, no. 1, pp. 1–6, 2013.

[38] R. H. Farkas, E. F. Unger, and R. Temple, "Zolpidem and driving impairment—identifying persons at risk," *The New England Journal of Medicine*, vol. 369, no. 8, pp. 689–691, 2013.

[39] C. Victorri-Vigneau, E. Dailly, G. Veyrac, and P. Jolliet, "Evidence of zolpidem abuse and dependence: results of the French centre for evaluation and information on pharmacodependence (CEIP) network survey," *British Journal of Clinical Pharmacology*, vol. 64, no. 2, pp. 198–209, 2007.

[40] P. Oulis, G. Nakkas, and V. G. Masdrakis, "Pregabalin in zolpidem dependence and withdrawal," *Clinical Neuropharmacology*, vol. 34, no. 2, pp. 90–91, 2011.

[41] B. D. Fischer, L. P. Teixeira, M. L. van Linn, O. A. Namjoshi, J. M. Cook, and J. K. Rowlett, "Role of gamma-aminobutyric acid type A (GABAA) receptor subtypes in acute benzodiazepine physical dependence-like effects: evidence from squirrel monkeys responding under a schedule of food presentation," *Psychopharmacology*, vol. 227, no. 2, pp. 347–354, 2013.

[42] L. M. Reynolds, E. Engin, G. Tantillo et al., "Differential roles of GABA(A) receptor subtypes in benzodiazepine-induced enhancement of brain-stimulation reward," *Neuropsychopharmacology*, vol. 37, no. 11, pp. 2531–2540, 2012.

[43] L. Maarek, P. Cramer, P. Attali, J. P. Coquelin, and P. L. Morselli, "The safety and efficacy of zolpidem in insomniac patients: a long-term open study in general practice," *Journal of International Medical Research*, vol. 20, no. 2, pp. 162–170, 1992.

[44] D. Schlich, C. L'Heritier, J. P. Coquelin, and P. Attali, "Long-term treatment of insomnia with zolpidem: a multicentre general practitioner study of 107 patients," *Journal of International Medical Research*, vol. 19, no. 3, pp. 271–279, 1991.

[45] T. A. Roehrs, S. Randall, E. Harris, R. Maan, and T. Roth, "Twelve months of nightly zolpidem does not lead to dose escalation: a prospective placebo-controlled study," *Sleep*, vol. 34, no. 2, pp. 207–212, 2011.

[46] C. H. Kao, L. M. Sun, J. A. Liang, S. N. Chang, F. C. Sung, and C. H. Muo, "Relationship of zolpidem and cancer risk: a Taiwanese population-based cohort study," *Mayo Clinic Proceedings*, vol. 87, no. 5, pp. 430–436, 2012.

[47] J. O. Olubodun, H. R. Ochs, L. L. Von Moltke et al., "Pharmacokinetic properties of zolpidem in elderly and young adults: possible modulation by testosterone in men," *British Journal of Clinical Pharmacology*, vol. 56, no. 3, pp. 297–304, 2003.

[48] C. S. van der Hooft, G. W. 'T Jong, J. P. Dieleman et al., "Inappropriate drug prescribing in older adults: the updated 2002 Beers criteria—a population-based cohort study," *British Journal of Clinical Pharmacology*, vol. 60, no. 2, pp. 137–144, 2005.

[49] V. Krishnan and N. Collop, "Gender differences in sleep disorders," *Current Opinion in Pulmonary Medicine*, vol. 12, no. 6, pp. 383–389, 2006.

[50] B. Zhang and Y.-K. Wing, "Sex differences in insomnia: a meta-analysis," *Sleep*, vol. 29, no. 1, pp. 85–93, 2006.

[51] J. Zhang, S.-P. Lam, S. X. Li et al., "Insomnia, sleep quality, pain, and somatic symptoms: sex differences and shared genetic components," *Pain*, vol. 153, no. 3, pp. 666–673, 2012.

[52] K. Johnell and J. Fastbom, "Gender and use of hypnotics or sedatives in old age: a nationwide register-based study," *International Journal of Clinical Pharmacy*, vol. 33, no. 5, pp. 788–793, 2011.

[53] A. B. Andersen and M. Frydenberg, "Long-term use of zopiclone, zolpidem and zaleplon among Danish elderly and the association with sociodemographic factors and use of other drugs," *Pharmacoepidemiology and Drug Safety*, vol. 20, no. 4, pp. 378–385, 2011.

[54] L. C. Toner, B. M. Tsambiras, G. Catalano, M. C. Catalano, and D. S. Cooper, "Central nervous system side effects associated with zolpidem treatment," *Clinical Neuropharmacology*, vol. 23, no. 1, pp. 54–58, 2000.

[55] J. C. Verster and T. Roth, "Gender differences in highway driving performance after administration of sleep medication: a review of the literature," *Traffic Injury Prevention*, vol. 13, no. 3, pp. 286–292, 2012.

[56] L.-H. Wang, H.-C. Lin, C.-C. Lin, Y.-H. Chen, and H.-C. Lin, "Increased risk of adverse pregnancy outcomes in women

receiving zolpidem during pregnancy," *Clinical Pharmacology and Therapeutics*, vol. 88, no. 3, pp. 369–374, 2010.

[57] N. Katz, G. Pillar, E. Peled, A. Segev, and N. Peled, "Sublingual flumazenil for the residual effects of hypnotics: zolpidem and brotizolam," *Clinical Pharmacology in Drug Development*, vol. 1, no. 2, pp. 45–51, 2012.

[58] "Ambien (zolpidem tartrate) tablets highlights of prescribing information," May 2012, http://products.sanofi.us/ambien/ambien.pdf.

[59] "*Ambien CR*, Highlights of prescribing information," May 2012, http://products.sanofi.us/ambien_cr/ambienCR.html.

[60] Edluar: zolpidem tartrate sublingual tablets, "Highlights of prescribing information," October 1992, http://www.edluar.com/EDLUAR-PI.pdf.

[61] Zolpimist (zoplidem tartrate) oral spray, "Highlights of prescribing information," December 2008, http://www.accessdata.fda.gov/drugsatfda_docs/label/2008/022196lbl.pdf.

[62] Phizer, "Halcion triazolam tablets," USP CIV—Prescribing Information, 2013.

[63] Mallinckrodt, "Restoril (temazepam) Capsules USP," Prescribing Information, 2013.

[64] M. M. Ohayon, "Nocturnal awakenings and comorbid disorders in the American general population," *Journal of Psychiatric Research*, vol. 43, no. 1, pp. 48–54, 2008.

25

Determinants of CPAP Adherence in Hispanics with Obstructive Sleep Apnea

Montserrat Diaz-Abad,[1] **Wissam Chatila,**[2] **Matthew R. Lammi,**[3] **Irene Swift,**[2] **Gilbert E. D'Alonzo,**[2] **and Samuel L. Krachman**[2]

[1] *Division of Pulmonary and Critical Care Medicine, Sleep Disorders Center, University of Maryland School of Medicine, 685 West Baltimore Street, MSTF 800, Baltimore, MD 21201-1192, USA*

[2] *Division of Pulmonary, Critical Care, and Sleep Medicine, Temple University School of Medicine, 3401 North Broad Street, Philadelphia, PA 19140, USA*

[3] *Section of Pulmonary and Critical Care Medicine, Louisiana State University Health Sciences Center, 433 Bolivar Street New Orleans, LA 70112, USA*

Correspondence should be addressed to Montserrat Diaz-Abad; montse@kunhardt.net

Academic Editor: Diego Garcia-Borreguero

Purpose. We hypothesized that socioeconomic factors and a language barrier would impact adherence with continuous positive airway pressure (CPAP) among Hispanics with obstructive sleep apnea (OSA). *Methods.* Patients with OSA who were prescribed CPAP for at least 1 year and completed a questionnaire evaluating demographic data, socioeconomic status, and CPAP knowledge and adherence participated in the study. *Results.* Seventy-nine patients (26 males; 53 ± 11 yrs; body mass index (BMI) = 45 ± 9 kg/m^2) with apnea-hypopnea index (AHI) 33 ± 30 events/hr completed the study. Included were 25 Hispanics, 39 African Americans, and 15 Caucasians, with no difference in age, AHI, CPAP use, or BMI between the groups. While there was a difference in educational level ($P = 0.006$), income level ($P < 0.001$), and employment status ($P = 0.03$) between the groups, these did not influence CPAP adherence. Instead, overall improvement in quality of life and health status and perceived benefit from CPAP influenced adherence, both for the group as a whole ($P = 0.03$, $P = 0.004$, and $P = 0.001$, resp.), as well as in Hispanics ($P = 0.02$, $P = 0.02$, $P = 0.03$, resp.). *Conclusion.* In Hispanic patients with OSA, perceived benefit with therapy, rather than socioeconomic status or a language barrier, appears to be the most important factor in determining CPAP adherence.

1. Introduction

Obstructive sleep apnea (OSA) syndrome is a common disorder with a reported prevalence of 2% of women and 4% of men between the ages of 30 and 60 years old [1]. Effective treatment is important due to the identification of OSA as an independent risk factor for cardiovascular disease [2–4]. While continuous positive airway pressure (CPAP) therapy is effective at correcting sleep disordered breathing [5, 6] and improving daytime sleepiness [6, 7], adherence is poor [8–10]. Although a number of factors are suggested to influence adherence, the importance of many of the determinants remains unclear [11, 12].

CPAP adherence among minorities in the United States is reported to be lower, especially among African Americans [13–15]. Factors such as the neighborhood of residence and associated socioeconomic status appear important [16–18] and are known to influence overall medical care and follow-up among minority populations [19–23]. While CPAP adherence has been examined in Caucasian and African American patients, no prior study has examined CPAP adherence in Hispanic patients with OSA. In addition to socioeconomic factors, a language barrier may play a role. We hypothesized that among Hispanics with OSA CPAP adherence would be influenced by socioeconomic factors and a language-related lack of understanding of how and why to use CPAP therapy.

2. Methods

2.1. Patient Selection. We recruited consecutive patients over a one-year period that had been previously studied in a University Hospital Sleep Laboratory. Included were patients referred from the University Sleep Clinic as well as patients referred from outside specialists with an interest in sleep medicine. Patients who were asked to participate had been newly diagnosed with OSA by an overnight polysomnogram study, had undergone a CPAP titration, and had not used CPAP before. OSA was defined as an apnea-hypopnea index (AHI) of ≥5 events/hr with symptoms of excessive daytime sleepiness or an AHI ≥15 events/hr. Patients reviewed the results of their sleep studies and discussed therapy with the referring physician, who then prescribed the patient's CPAP. Specific instructions about use and care of their CPAP device were given by the durable medical equipment company who delivered and set up the CPAP at home. Patients referred from the University Sleep Clinic and from the outside specialists are routinely seen in follow-up 6–8 weeks after CPAP initiation to evaluate adherence. Patients are then seen as often as needed to optimize adherence or to change therapy if they are unable to tolerate CPAP. Once the patients are considered stable, they are instructed to follow-up on a yearly basis. Patients who had been prescribed CPAP and had it set up at home for at least 1 year (12–15 months) prior to enrollment into the study were selected. Patients were excluded from participating in the study if they (1) had associated obesity-related alveolar hypoventilation or central sleep apnea, (2) had other conditions that might interfere with sleep (underlying chronic respiratory disorders, uncontrolled allergies, heart failure, narcolepsy, and periodic leg movements), (3) had known pregnancy, (4) were unable to be located or refused to complete or return the questionnaire, and (5) refused or were unable to sign informed consent. The study was approved by the Institutional Review Board for Human Research (Temple University School of Medicine, Philadelphia, PA, USA).

2.2. Questionnaire. All study materials including the questionnaire and informed consent were mailed both in English and in Spanish to each patient at their last known address. The patients were instructed to mail back both the completed questionnaire and the signed informed consent in a stamped envelope that was provided. If the patients had not returned the questionnaire after 2 weeks, they were called once using their last known telephone phone number as a reminder and asked to complete and return the questionnaire. The questionnaire consisted of 30 questions divided into 2 main sections. The first section contained questions related to demographic and socioeconomic data, including age, gender, racial/ethnic background, level of education, yearly income, country of birth, and language that was spoken. The second section contained questions related to the diagnosis of OSA and CPAP adherence. Included were questions related to symptoms, familiarity with CPAP therapy, perceived benefit from therapy, and CPAP adherence. Good adherence was defined as reported use of CPAP at least 4 hours per night, 70% of the nights of the week [8]. The section also included questions related to the level of support from medical and technical personnel related to the implementation of CPAP.

2.3. Polysomnogram. Polysomnograms were performed in-laboratory and consisted of a recording of rib cage and abdominal motion (Respitrace; Ambulatory Monitoring; White Plains, NY, USA), with air flow measured using a pressure transducer. Snoring was monitored using a snore microphone. Other recordings included pulse oximetry (Cephalo Pro, Viasys Healthcare, Yorba Linda, CA, USA), electrocardiogram, electrooculogram, digastric electromyogram, and electroencephalogram. All variables were continuously recorded and stored in a computerized system (Viasys Healthcare; Yorba Linda, CA, USA). Sleep was staged and arousal defined using established criteria [24]. Obstructive apnea was defined by the lack of airflow for ≥10 seconds, associated with the presence of rib cage and abdominal movement [24]. Obstructive hypopnea was defined by a 50% decrease in airflow associated with a ≥3% decrease in oxygen saturation or an arousal [24]. Apnea was defined as central if there was a lack of respiratory effort during the period of absent airflow [24]. The AHI was calculated as the number of apneic and hypopneic events per hour of sleep. An arousal was defined as an abrupt shift of EEG frequency including alpha, theta, and/or frequencies >16 Hz (but not spindles) that lasts at least 3 seconds, with at least 10 seconds of stable sleep preceding the change [24]. Other calculated variables included total sleep time, sleep efficiency (total sleep time divided by time in bed), arousal index, and the percent of total sleep time with an arterial oxygen saturation (SpO_2) <90%. All patients had a baseline polysomnogram followed by a full night CPAP titration study or had a split night study with the initial portion performed off CPAP and the remainder of the night consisting of a CPAP titration. CPAP titrations were performed using recommended guidelines [25] with the patient's prescribed CPAP pressures based on studies that were considered optimal, good, or adequate as described in the guidelines. All of the polysomnogram studies were initially scored by a single senior technologist. The same author (SK) reviewed each study.

2.4. Statistical Analysis. Continuous data are presented as the mean ± SD. Differences in continuous variables between the CPAP adherent and nonadherent groups were evaluated using unpaired *t*-tests. Categorical data are presented as frequencies with percentages; between-group differences were analyzed using Fisher's exact test. Differences between ethnic groups were analyzed using one-way ANOVA with follow-up pairwise comparisons using a Bonferroni adjustment. A *P* value ≤ 0.05 was considered statistically significant. All data were analyzed using SAS V9.2 software.

3. Results

3.1. Patient Characteristics. A total of 219 patients who were diagnosed with OSA and treated with CPAP therapy over a one-year period were selected to participate in the study. Of the 219 questionnaires that were mailed, 79 patients (26 males,

TABLE 1: Baseline characteristics[*].

Variable	Total group	Hispanic	African American	Caucasian	P value
Patients, n	79	25	39	15	
Age, yrs	53 ± 11	54 ± 12	54 ± 13	56 ± 12	$P = 0.8$
Male, n (%)	26 (33)	8 (32)	7 (18)	3 (20)	$P = 0.4$
BMI, kg/m^2	45 ± 9	44 ± 7	40 ± 9	46 ± 13	$P = 0.7$
Baseline AHI, events/hr	33 ± 30	32 ± 24	34 ± 31	32 ± 38	$P = 0.3$
Lowest SpO$_2$, %	82 ± 9	85 ± 5	81 ± 10	81 ± 7	$P = 0.3$
% TST SpO$_2$ < 90%	8 ± 13	11 ± 16	8 ± 12	5 ± 7	$P = 0.7$
TST, min	308 ± 77	330 ± 70	324 ± 76	279 ± 79	$P = 0.2$
Sleep efficiency, %	78 ± 17	82 ± 15	80 ± 15	74 ± 19	$P = 0.4$
Arousal index, events/hr	18 ± 14	17 ± 10	17 ± 15	24 ± 16	$P = 0.2$
Sleep architecture, %TST					
N1, %	16 ± 14	16 ± 14	15 ± 12	17 ± 18	$P = 0.9$
N2, %	53 ± 16	51 ± 19	53 ± 13	56 ± 13	$P = 0.7$
N3, %	13 ± 11	12 ± 10	14 ± 11	13 ± 10	$P = 0.8$
REM, %	16 ± 13	16 ± 15	17 ± 9	14 ± 12	$P = 0.7$
CPAP, cm H$_2$O	12 ± 4	12 ± 3	13 ± 4	12 ± 4	$P = 0.7$

[*]Data are presented as mean ± SD or the number of patients. BMI: body mass index; AHI: apnea-hypopnea index; TST: total sleep time; REM: rapid eye movement; CPAP: continuous positive airway pressure.

53 ± 11 yrs, and BMI = 45 ± 9 kg/m^2) responded (36%) and returned their questionnaires (Table 1) and included 25 Hispanics, 39 African Americans, and 15 Caucasians (Table 1). Twenty questionnaires (9%) were returned unopened (incorrect address). The respondents had evidence of severe OSA with an AHI of 33 ± 30 events/hr with a mean CPAP requirement of 12 ± 4 cm H$_2$O (Table 1). The three population groups were similar in regard to age, sex, BMI, AHI, sleep quality, and CPAP requirement (Table 1). There was no difference in AHI or racial/ethnic distribution between the responders and nonresponders ($P = 0.5$ and $P = 0.3$, resp.).

3.2. CPAP Adherence. Overall, 63 patients reported that they are still using CPAP therapy, an average of 5.9 ± 1.9 hours/night and 5.7 ± 1.7 nights/week. There was no difference in the AHI in the group that was adherent with CPAP (35 ± 30 events/hr) compared to the group that was not using CPAP (24 ± 21 events/hr) ($P = 0.12$). However, the prescribed CPAP pressure was higher in the adherent group (12.9 ± 3.5 cm H$_2$O) compared to the nonadherent group (10.2 ± 2.8 H$_2$O) ($P = 0.01$). CPAP adherence was similar between the groups, both in regard to the number of nights/week (Caucasian = 5.5 ± 1.4; African American = 5.4 ± 2.0; Hispanics = 5.6 ± 1.8; $P = 0.9$) and hours/night (Caucasian = 6.4 ± 1.5; African Americans = 5.5 ± 1.8; Hispanics = 5.8 ± 2.2; $P = 0.8$) CPAP was used. The percentage of patients considered to have good adherence to CPAP was also similar between the groups: 46.4% of Caucasians, 56.4% of African Americans, and 48% of Hispanics; $P = 0.73$.

3.3. Socioeconomic and Language Differences. Between the 3 racial/ethnic groups, there was a difference in the educational level ($P = 0.006$), with 36% of the Hispanics having less

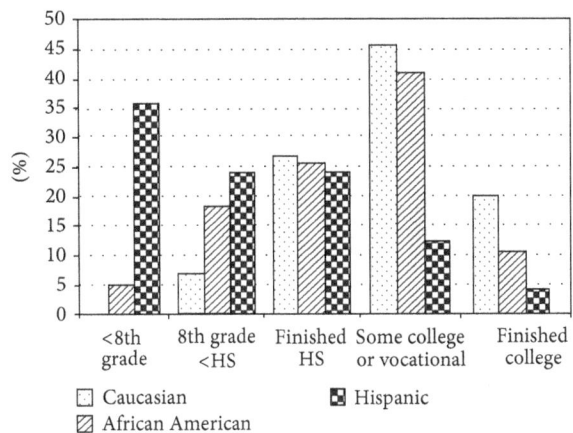

FIGURE 1: There was a significant difference in educational level between the 3 racial/ethnic groups ($P = 0.006$). Group by group comparison: Caucasian versus African American: $P = 0.7$; Caucasian versus Hispanic: $P = 0.04$; African American versus Hispanic: $P = 0.01$. HS = High school.

than an 8th grade education versus none in the Caucasian group and 5% in the African American group (Figure 1). In addition, there was a difference between groups in regard to income level ($P < 0.001$), with 79% of Hispanics earning less than \$15,000/yr versus 46% of African Americans and 27% of Caucasians (Figure 2). In relation to employment status, the Caucasian group was more often employed (Caucasian = 53%, African American = 33%, and Hispanics = 12%; $P = 0.03$) (Figure 3). In the Hispanic group, 80% were born outside the continental United States, having lived in the United States 29 ± 13 yrs, and 33% of Hispanics spoke only Spanish. Spoken language did not influence adherence, both in the combined patient group ($P = 0.35$) and within

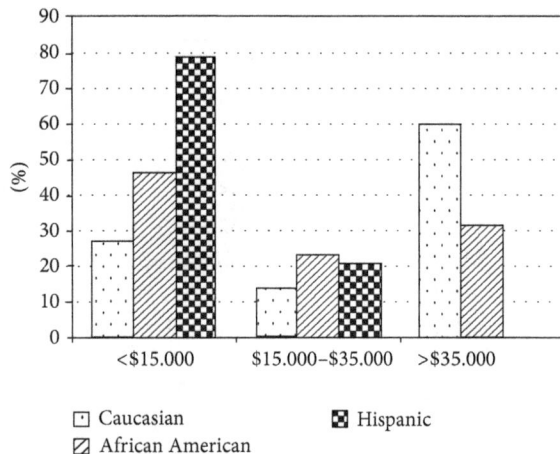

FIGURE 2: Between the 3 racial/ethnic groups there was a significant difference in income level ($P < 0.001$). Group by group comparison: Caucasian versus African American: $P = 0.2$; Caucasian versus Hispanic: $P < 0.001$; African American versus Hispanic: $P = 0.003$.

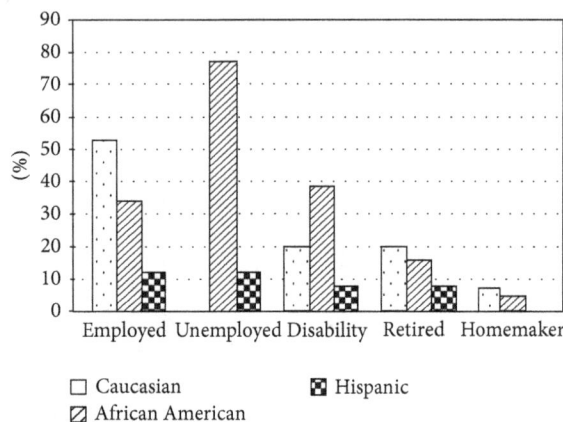

FIGURE 3: In regard to employment status, there was a significant difference between the 3 racial/ethnic groups ($P = 0.03$). Group by group comparison: Caucasian versus African American: $P = 0.47$; Caucasian versus Hispanic: $P = 0.02$; African American versus Hispanic: $P = 0.1$.

the Hispanic group ($P = 0.64$). Fifty-two percent of Hispanics reported that their physician made sure that the results of their sleep studies were explained in their language, 71% reported that the home company that set up their equipment had someone who spoke their language, and 91% stated that the home company adequately explained how to use their CPAP. However, on analysis, none of these variables appeared to influence CPAP adherence.

3.4. Determinants of CPAP Adherence. In regard to the determinants that were associated with CPAP adherence in the group as a whole, compared to the patients that were no longer using CPAP, those using CPAP more often reported an overall improvement in quality of life ($P = 0.03$) and health status ($P = 0.004$). In addition, those adherent with CPAP reported a greater perceived benefit from using CPAP

($P = 0.001$). Similar to the group as a whole, Hispanics who were adherent with CPAP more often noted an overall improvement in quality of life ($P = 0.02$) and health status ($P = 0.02$), compared to those that were no longer using CPAP. In addition, Hispanics who were adherent with CPAP therapy more often reported an initial improvement in symptoms ($P = 0.003$), as well as a greater perceived benefit from using CPAP ($P = 0.03$).

4. Discussion

While CPAP is an effective therapy in the treatment of OSA, the determinants that influence CPAP adherence are not completely defined [11, 12]. The influence that socioeconomic factors and a language barrier may have on CPAP adherence in Hispanic patients has not been fully investigated. There are 2 main findings in this study: (1) CPAP adherence in Hispanics is not related to noted differences in socioeconomic status or spoken language, and (2) the main factors associated with CPAP adherence in Hispanics are related to perceived benefit and improvement in quality of life and health status noted with treatment.

We had hypothesized that CPAP adherence would be influenced in Hispanics by socioeconomic status and a language barrier. However, these did not turn out to be determinants in regard to CPAP adherence. In the present study, for Hispanic patients and for the group as whole, CPAP adherence was associated with an overall improvement in quality of life and health status and a greater perceived benefit from using CPAP. In addition, Hispanic patients adherent with CPAP reported an initial improvement in their symptoms with the use of CPAP therapy.

Similar results have been reported by others. Kribbs et al. objectively examined CPAP usage in 35 patients with OSA [8]. At the initial 1-month follow-up, the 16 patients considered to be regular CPAP users (≥4 hrs/night on ≥70% of the days) reported more satisfaction with CPAP treatment and had a better level of energy during the day compared to the 19 patients who were irregular users of CPAP [8]. More recently, Wells et al. prospectively examined CPAP adherence at 30 days in 54 patients with OSA [26], noting that CPAP adherence was associated with an improvement in OSA symptoms.

In healthcare, racial differences have been reported when it comes to medication adherence [19, 20], with a known effect on diabetes and blood pressure control in minority populations [20–23]. In the treatment of OSA, racial differences in CPAP adherence have been noted by some [14, 15] but not all investigators [27]. Billings et al. examined the racial differences in CPAP adherence in 191 patients who were part of the HomePAP study [14]. At both 1 and 3 months, race was a predictor of CPAP use, with African American patients being less adherent based on the number of minutes of use per night as well as the percent of days that CPAP was used for ≥ 4 hrs/night. Means et al. found similar results in 499 veterans whose CPAP adherence data was reviewed from a clinical database at 30 and 90 days [15]. CPAP adherence was significantly higher in Caucasians versus African Americans at both time points based on the percentage of nights used as well the average hours per night. The presence of a mental health diagnosis had a negative impact on CPAP adherence in the African American patients but not in the Caucasian group [15].

Budhiraja et al. noted a lower daily CPAP usage in African Americans compared to Caucasians in 100 patients who were being studied to evaluate if CPAP adherence in the first few days of use predicted adherence at 30 days [13]. The study was limited by the lack of educational and socioeconomic data in assessing racial differences in adherence. Joo and Herdegen noted that African Americans were 5 times more likely to be nonadherent with CPAP therapy at 30 days as compared to Caucasians [18]. However, the results may have been biased by the much smaller number of Caucasians versus African Americans in the study. All of these studies are limited by the fact that they evaluated adherence for not more than 90 days and none of them evaluated adherence in Hispanic patients.

In contrast to the above studies, Scharf et al. evaluated self-reported CPAP adherence in 108 patients 3–9 months after they were diagnosed and treated with CPAP therapy [27]. There was no difference between African Americans and Caucasians both in regard to initial acceptance of CPAP therapy (48% versus 45%, resp.) and more long-term adherence (39% versus 35%, resp.). Age, Epworth Score, and respiratory disturbance index (RDI) were found to be associated with long-term CPAP adherence, but race was not. In the present study, CPAP adherence in Hispanics was similar to the other groups. In addition, unlike previous studies, we evaluated adherence after the patient had been prescribed CPAP for at least 1 year.

Socioeconomic factors have been suggested to influence CPAP adherence [14, 16, 17]. Simon-Tuval et al. evaluated CPAP acceptance in 162 patients with OSA who completed a 2-week adaptation period [17]. CPAP acceptance, as measured 4–6 weeks following completion of the adaptation period, was significantly greater in patients from a higher income level. Platt et al. retrospectively evaluated the importance of neighborhood-level socioeconomic status on CPAP adherence in 266 veterans with OSA [16]. After 1 week of use, CPAP adherence was found to be lower in patients from a low socioeconomic neighborhood (34%) compared to patients from a high socioeconomic neighborhood (62%). However, Billings et al. found that socioeconomic status by itself had no influence on CPAP adherence when evaluated at both 1 and 3 months [14]. In the present study, we also did not find socioeconomic status to influence CPAP adherence, despite significant differences in yearly income and educational levels, with 79% of Hispanics earning less than $15,000/yr and 36% having less than an 8th grade education.

There are a number of limitations within the study that need to be addressed. First, the study involved a relatively small number of patients. However, the number of patients evaluated is similar or higher than that of previous studies that have examined determinants of CPAP adherence [18, 26]. Second, CPAP adherence was self-assessed with the use of a questionnaire that was mailed to the patients, rather than being quantitatively monitored. Subjective assessment has been shown to overestimate actual CPAP usage by approximately 1 hour per night [28]. However, this would have affected all groups proportionally and be less likely to affect the main objective of the study, the evaluation of factors associated with CPAP adherence in Hispanics. Third, this was a cross-sectional survey of patients prescribed CPAP for at least 1 year and did not evaluate factors associated with early CPAP adherence. Finally, the results may not be representative of all Hispanics. Our urban Hispanic population consists mostly of immigrants from Puerto Rico. Whether similar findings apply to Hispanics in other demographic areas will have to be determined.

In conclusion, in Hispanics with OSA, there is no evidence that a language barrier is important in determining CPAP adherence. In addition, while the socioeconomic status was substantially lower in Hispanics patients, the perceived benefit and improvement in quality of life and health status obtained with CPAP therapy were the most important determinants for CPAP adherence. Larger, prospective studies are needed to confirm these findings.

Conflict of Interests

The authors declare that they have no conflict of interests.

Acknowledgment

This work was performed at Temple University Hospital Sleep Disorders Center, Temple University Health System, Philadelphia, PA

References

[1] T. Young, M. Palta, J. Dempsey, J. Skatrud, S. Weber, and S. Badr, "The occurrence of sleep-disordered breathing among middle-aged adults," *The New England Journal of Medicine*, vol. 328, no. 17, pp. 1230–1235, 1993.

[2] P. E. Peppard, T. Young, M. Palta, and J. Skatrud, "Prospective study of the association between sleep-disordered breathing and hypertension," *The New England Journal of Medicine*, vol. 342, no. 19, pp. 1378–1384, 2000.

[3] H. K. Yaggi, J. Concato, W. N. Kernan, J. H. Lichtman, L. M. Brass, and V. Mohsenin, "Obstructive sleep apnea as a risk factor for stroke and death," *The New England Journal of Medicine*, vol. 353, no. 19, pp. 2034–2041, 2005.

[4] E. Shahar, C. W. Whitney, S. Redline et al., "Sleep-disordered breathing and cardiovascular disease: cross-sectional results of the sleep heart health study," *American Journal of Respiratory and Critical Care Medicine*, vol. 163, no. 1, pp. 19–25, 2001.

[5] R. R. Grunstein, "Sleep-related breathing disorders: 5. Nasal continuous positive airway pressure treatment for obstructive sleep apnoea," *Thorax*, vol. 50, no. 10, pp. 1106–1113, 1995.

[6] P. Gay, T. Weaver, D. Loube, and C. Iber, "Evaluation of positive airway pressure treatment for sleep related breathing disorders in adults," *Sleep*, vol. 29, no. 3, pp. 381–401, 2006.

[7] J. P. McMahon, B. H. Foresman, and R. C. Chisholm, "The influence of CPAP on the neurobehavioral performance of patients with obstructive sleep apnea hypopnea syndrome: a systematic review," *Wisconsin Medical Journal*, vol. 102, no. 1, pp. 36–43, 2003.

[8] N. B. Kribbs, A. I. Pack, L. R. Kline et al., "Objective measurement of patterns of nasal CPAP use by patients with obstructive sleep apnea," *American Review of Respiratory Disease*, vol. 147, no. 4, pp. 887–895, 1993.

[9] H. M. Engleman, S. E. Martin, and N. J. Douglas, "Compliance with CPAP therapy in patients with the sleep apnoea/hypopnoea syndrome," *Thorax*, vol. 49, no. 3, pp. 263–266, 1994.

[10] M. K. Reeves-Hoche, R. Meck, and C. W. Zwillich, "Nasal CPAP: an objective evaluation of patient compliance," *American Journal of Respiratory and Critical Care Medicine*, vol. 149, no. 1, pp. 149–154, 1994.

[11] T. E. Weaver and R. R. Grunstein, "Adherence to continuous positive airway pressure therapy: the challenge to effective treatment," *Proceedings of the American Thoracic Society*, vol. 5, no. 2, pp. 173–178, 2008.

[12] A. M. Sawyer, N. S. Gooneratne, C. L. Marcus, D. Ofer, K. C. Richards, and T. E. Weaver, "A systematic review of CPAP adherence across age groups: clinical and empiric insights for developing CPAP adherence interventions," *Sleep Medicine Reviews*, vol. 15, no. 6, pp. 343–356, 2011.

[13] R. Budhiraja, S. Parthasarathy, C. L. Drake et al., "Early CPAP use identifies subsequent adherence to CPAP therapy," *Sleep*, vol. 30, no. 3, pp. 320–324, 2007.

[14] M. E. Billings, D. Auckley, R. Benca et al., "Race and residential socioeconomics as predictors of CPAP adherence," *Sleep*, vol. 34, no. 12, pp. 1653–1658, 2011.

[15] M. K. Means, C. S. Ulmer, and J. D. Edinger, "Ethnic differences in continuous positive airway pressure (CPAP) adherence in veterans with and without psychiatric disorders," *Behavioral Sleep Medicine*, vol. 8, no. 4, pp. 260–273, 2010.

[16] A. B. Platt, S. H. Field, D. A. Asch et al., "Neighborhood of residence is associated with daily adherence to CPAP therapy," *Sleep*, vol. 32, no. 6, pp. 799–806, 2009.

[17] T. Simon-Tuval, H. Reuveni, S. Greenberg-Dotan, A. Oksenberg, A. Tal, and A. Tarasiuk, "Low socioeconomic status is a risk factor for CPAP acceptance among adult OSAS patients requiring treatment," *Sleep*, vol. 32, no. 4, pp. 545–552, 2009.

[18] M. J. Joo and J. J. Herdegen, "Sleep apnea in an urban public hospital: assessment of severity and treatment adherence," *Journal of Clinical Sleep Medicine*, vol. 3, no. 3, pp. 285–288, 2007.

[19] B. S. Gerber, Y. I. Cho, A. M. Arozullah, and S.-Y. D. Lee, "Racial differences in medication adherence: a cross-sectional study of medicare enrollees," *American Journal Geriatric Pharmacotherapy*, vol. 8, no. 2, pp. 136–145, 2010.

[20] M. T. Roth, D. A. Esserman, J. L. Ivey, and M. Weinberger, "Racial disparities in the quality of medication use in older adults: baseline findings from a longitudinal study," *Journal of General Internal Medicine*, vol. 25, no. 3, pp. 228–234, 2010.

[21] L. E. Egede, M. Gebregziabher, K. J. Hunt et al., "Regional, geographic, and racial/ethnic variation in glycemic control in a national sample of veterans with diabetes," *Diabetes Care*, vol. 34, no. 4, pp. 938–943, 2011.

[22] C. M. Trinacty, A. S. Adams, S. B. Soumarai et al., "Racial differences in long-term adherence to oral antidiabetic drug therapy: a longitudinal cohort study," *BMC Health Services Research*, vol. 9, article 24, 2009.

[23] H. B. Bosworth, B. Powers, J. M. Grubber et al., "Racial differences in blood pressure control: potential explanatory factors," *Journal of General Internal Medicine*, vol. 23, no. 5, pp. 692–698, 2008.

[24] C. Iber, S. Ancoli-Israel, A. Chesson, and S. F. Quan, "The AASM manual for the scoring of sleep and associated events: rules, terminology and technical specifications," American Academy of Sleep Medicine, Westchester, Ill, USA, 2007.

[25] C. A. Kushida, A. Chediak, R. B. Berry et al., "Clinical guidelines for the manual titration of positive airway pressure in patients with obstructive sleep apnea," *Journal of Clinical Sleep Medicine*, vol. 4, pp. 157–171, 2008.

[26] R. D. Wells, K. E. Freedland, R. M. Carney, S. P. Duntley, and E. J. Stepanski, "Adherence, reports of benefits, and depression among patients treated with continuous positive airway pressure," *Psychosomatic Medicine*, vol. 69, no. 5, pp. 449–454, 2007.

[27] S. M. Scharf, L. Seiden, J. DeMore, and O. Carter-Pokras, "Racial differences in clinical presentation of patients with sleep-disordered breathing," *Sleep and Breathing*, vol. 8, no. 4, pp. 173–183, 2004.

[28] H. M. Engleman, N. Asgari-Jirhandeh, A. L. McLeod, C. F. Ramsay, I. J. Deary, and N. J. Douglas, "Self-reported use of CPAP and benefits of CPAP therapy: a patient survey," *Chest*, vol. 109, no. 6, pp. 1470–1476, 1996.

26

Prevalence of Sleep Disorders and Their Impacts on Occupational Performance: A Comparison between Shift Workers and Nonshift Workers

Zohreh Yazdi,[1] Khosro Sadeghniiat-Haghighi,[2] Ziba Loukzadeh,[3] Khadijeh Elmizadeh,[4] and Mahnaz Abbasi[1]

[1] *Metabolic Disease Research Center, Qazvin University of Medical Sciences, Qazvin 34139-8-3731, Iran*
[2] *Occupational Sleep Research Center, Tehran University of Medical Sciences, Tehran 5583-1-4155, Iran*
[3] *Department of Occupational Medicine, Industrial Diseases Research Center, Shahid Sadoughi University of Medical Sciences, Yazd 89151-7-3143, Iran*
[4] *Social Determinants of Health Research Center, Qazvin University of Medical Sciences, Qazvin, Qazvin 34139-8-3731, Iran*

Correspondence should be addressed to Ziba Loukzadeh; loukzadehziba@yahoo.com

Academic Editor: Liborio Parrino

The consequences of sleep deprivation and sleepiness have been noted as the most important health problem in our modern society among shift workers. The objective of this study was to investigate the prevalence of sleep disorders and their possible effects on work performance in two groups of Iranian shift workers and nonshift workers. This study was designed as a cross-sectional study. The data were collected by PSQI, Berlin questionnaire, Epworth Sleepiness Scale, Insomnia Severity Index, and RLS Questionnaire. Occupational impact of different sleep disorders was detected by Occupational Impact of Sleep Disorder questionnaire. These questionnaires were filled in by 210 shift workers and 204 nonshift workers. There was no significant difference in the age, BMI, marital status, and years of employment in the two groups. Shift workers scored significantly higher in the OISD. The prevalence of insomnia, poor sleep quality, and daytime sleepiness was significantly higher in shift workers. Correlations between OISD scores and insomnia, sleep quality, and daytime sleepiness were significant. We concluded that sleep disorders should receive more attention as a robust indicator of work limitation.

1. Introduction

The consequences of sleep deprivation and sleepiness have been noted as the most important health problem in our modern society among shift workers. These consequences include increase in mortality, morbidity, accidents and errors, absenteeism in workplace, decrease in productivity, and deterioration of personal and professional relationships [1–3].

The prevalence of sleep disorders is common in shift workers but is often underdiagnosed [4]. The association between sleep disorders and shift work is bidirectional. Shift work induces some sleep complaints such as insomnia, poor sleep quality, and daytime sleepiness. On the other hand, underlying sleep disorders decrease workers' capabilities to adapt with shift working and increase accidents at work [5, 6].

Insomnia is the most prevalent sleep disorder among the adults. The estimated prevalence of difficulty in initiating and maintaining sleep is about 30% [7]. In spite of this reality, relationship between insomnia and work performance has received little attention in researches [8].

It is estimated that 4% of males and 2% of females suffer from obstructive sleep apnea (OSA) and the majority of patients are thought to be undiagnosed. Certainly, investigators have shown that OSA is associated with large increase in healthcare costs in working age adults [9, 10]. However, few studies have specifically surveyed the impact of undiagnosed

TABLE 1: Baseline characteristics in two groups of shift workers and nonshift workers.

Characteristics	Shift workers N = 210	Nonshift workers N = 204	P value
Age	33.7 ± 5.9	35.1 ± 10.9	0.1
BMI	22.8 ± 3.1	23.5 ± 4.4	0.08
Marital status (married)	173 (%)	159 (%)	0.31
Educational status	9.3 ± 3.6	12.9 ± 5.1	0.04
Years of employment	12.1 ± 8.5	13.7 ± 10.3	0.086
OISD	27.2 ± 9.8	16.1 ± 10.3	0.001

OSA and resultant sleepiness on work disabilities such as work absences and decreased productivity [11]. A recent study has reported that the combination of OSA and resultant excessive daytime sleepiness contributes to work disability in patients who underwent overnight polysomnography [12].

There are few studies regarding work disabilities due to other sleep disorders such as restless legs syndrome, periodic limb movement syndrome, and parasomnia. But theoretically, all of these sleep disorders are generally associated with either sleep fragmentation or decreased sleep quality [13].

Sleep quality is an important clinical construct for being healthy people. Poor sleep quality can be an important symptom of many sleep disorders and other medical diseases and might even have a direct effect on increased mortality [14].

Despite the high prevalence of sleep disorders, there are few studies on their effects on work limitations. Verster et al. assessed the validity of the Occupational Impact of Sleep Questionnaire in Dutch language. According to their results Dutch version OISD was a suitable instrument to estimate the occupational impact of sleep disorders. Also, they showed that poor sleepers had higher scores of OISD compared to good sleepers [8].

The aim of this study was to evaluate the prevalence of sleep disorders and their possible effects on work performance in two groups of Iranian shift workers and nonshift workers.

2. Materials and Methodology

A self-administered questionnaire was submitted to all workers employed in textile factory. A total of 225 shift workers and 245 nonshift workers participated in this study. All the participants were informed about the objectives of the study and the methods used during the survey. Each participant received the questionnaire and completed it during the work hours.

The Persian version of the questionnaires was used to detect the sleep disorders in workers. Insomnia Severity Index, Berlin questionnaire, Epworth Sleepiness Scale, and Pittsburg Sleep Quality Index were used to screen insomnia, obstructive sleep apnea, daytime sleepiness, and sleep quality, respectively [15–17]. Berlin questionnaire consists of three categories. The first, second, and third categories have

questions about snoring, daytime somnolence, and existence of high blood pressure, respectively. The patient is considered high risk for OSA if two or more categories are positive [18].

We used the four minimal IRLSSG clinical criteria for screening of RLS in participants. All cases who responded positively to the first three questions of questionnaire were considered to have RLS [19].

We used the Occupational Impact of Sleep Disorder (OISD) questionnaire to detect the occupational impact of sleep disorders. This questionnaire included 23 items, and each item was organized into four levels as follows: "Never," "Rarely," "Sometimes," and "Often," with a numeric value of 0, 1, 2, and 3, respectively, and a total score from 0 to 96 [8]. At first, we translated the OISD questionnaire by bilingual expert panel of sleep physicians and occupational medicine specialist. In the translation process, we choose an easily understandable style and a wording with the same meanings of original questionnaire. Then we back-translated into English by another two translators, who did not participate in any of the previous steps. At last, individuals who were fluent in English compared original OISD with the final back-translated form. The OISD internal consistency in our study was high with a Cronbach's alpha of 0.83.

SPSS for windows version 13 was used for statistical analysis. Summary statistics for descriptive data were obtained for means and standard deviations. We used Cronbach's alpha to test internal consistency reliabilities and Pearson correlation coefficients to compute correlations among the measures. Student's t-tests and chi-square analyses were performed to look for group differences. For all data, a P value of <0.05 was considered statistically significant.

3. Results

A total of 470 questionnaires were completed including 210 shift workers and 204 nonshift workers. Incompletely filled questionnaires were excluded from the study. All participants were male, and the mean age was 34.8 ranging from 22 to 45. Table 1 shows sociodemographic data of participants. There were no significant differences in the age, BMI, marital status, and years of employment.

Shift workers reported lower education compared with nonshift workers and scored significantly higher in the OISD, indicating they tolerated more occupational impacts of sleep disorders than nonshift workers (27.2 versus 16.1; $P = 0.001$).

The prevalence of insomnia, poor sleep quality, and daytime sleepiness was significantly higher in shift workers than nonshift workers (Table 2).

Table 3 shows that the correlations between OISD scores and insomnia, sleep quality, and daytime sleepiness are high and significant. Correlations are stronger in the shift workers group. There is not any correlation between OISD scores and RLS and sleep apnea in both groups.

4. Discussion

This study evaluated the impacts of sleep disorders on occupational performance in an industrial setting. The major

TABLE 2: Prevalence of different types of sleep disorders in two groups of shift workers and nonshift workers.

		Shift workers	Nonshift workers	P value
Insomnia	Yes	26 (12.4%)	14 (6.8%)	P = 0.02
	No	184 (87.6%)	190 (93.1%)	
Sleep quality	Poor sleep quality	43 (20.4%)	21 (10.3%)	P = 0.004
	Better sleep quality	167 (79.5%)	183 (89.7%)	
ESS	With ESS	21 (10%)	13 (6.4%)	P = 0.041
	Without ESS	189 (90%)	191 (93.6%)	
RLS	Yes	22 (10.5%)	14 (6.8%)	P > 0.05
	No	188 (89.5%)	190 (93.1%)	
Sleep apnea	Yes	15 (7.1%)	17 (8.3%)	P > 0.05
	No	195 (92.8%)	187 (91.6%)	

TABLE 3: Correlations between different types of sleep disorders with OISD in two groups of shift workers and nonshift workers.

	Insomnia	Sleep quality	ESS	RLS	Sleep apnea
OISD in shift workers	0.52*	0.48*	0.39**	0.14	0.04
OISD in nonshift workers	0.37*	0.36*	0.21*	0.06	0.11

*$P < 0.05$; **$P < 0.01$.

finding of this study was a significant increase in sleep disorders among the shift workers than in nonshift workers. In addition, occupational impacts of these sleep disorders were more profound in this group. Despite the high prevalence of different sleep disorders in the general population, there is a lack of studies on the harmful effects of these disorders on job performance [8]. Overall, the result of our study is consistent with limited studies performed in this field. In a study about OSA that was conducted in patients admitted to a sleep clinic, it was found that patients with excessive daytime sleepiness (assessed by the Epworth Sleepiness Scale) were more likely to suffer from work limitation in time management, work efficiency, and mental interpersonal relationship. They did not find such correlation in OSA patients without daytime sleepiness [12].

In another study it was found that excessive daytime sleepiness is related to increased rate of stress and interpersonal tensions at work [11]. In addition, several studies have reported improvement in work performance after treatment of OSA patients with excessive daytime sleepiness [10, 20].

In our study, the prevalence of EDS was higher in shift workers than in nonshift workers and in both groups it was accompanied by higher OISD scores. Also, our study showed that there was no difference between the prevalence of OSA in shift workers and nonshift workers on the basis of the Berlin questionnaire. They also found no relation between OSA and the scores that resulted from OISD questionnaire. The absence of this relation can be attributed to the small number of cases detected to have OSA using the Berlin questionnaire.

In many studies, the prevalence of insomnia has been evaluated in general population and shift workers and the results of these studies show that insomnia is more prevalent in shift workers in contrast to general population [4, 14, 21]. In this regard the result of our study is consistent with other

studies. As the results of our study show, among the sleep disorders, insomnia and low sleep quality had the highest correlation with the incidence of negative occupational impacts. As impaired daily functioning is one of the diagnostic items for detecting sleep disorders, the above correlation is completely logical. In another study using sleep50 questionnaire for evaluation of sleep disorders, researchers showed powerful association between insomnia negative occupational impacts [8].

Other studies have also shown the same results. Previous studies have revealed that it is twice more probable for workers with insomnia to lose their work. They have lower self-confidence and occupational satisfaction and lower efficacy in work. In addition, patients with insomnia disorder are 3 times more prone to dangerous road accidents. The studies have also shown that these workers have 1.4 times more absence from work than the workers without insomnia [22–26]. It seems that, with the use of the OISD questionnaire, it is possible to prevent these complications at the first stages. On the other hand, it is obvious that absence from work is the end point of the problems in waking up on time to work and on time arrival and the ability to work the whole work time. Thus, assessment of the above problems in questionnaire is very important and necessary for occupational investigations.

Another considerable result of the present study is more prevalence of poor sleep quality in the shift workers in contrast to nonshift workers. In both groups, poor sleep quality culminated in negative impacts on work performance. Of course this impact was stronger in shift workers than the others. In one study performed in Denmark there was a meaningful association between the OISD questionnaire and the quality of sleep [8].

It is necessary to say that the relation between the quality of sleep and occupational performance is two-sided. On one hand, low quality of sleep can result in poor work performance and work accidents. On the other hand, problems occurring while working can culminate in sleep disorders [25]. Knudsen et al. in their study showed that the workers who had work accidents resulting in work absence in the recent past year were more prone to insomnia disorder and poor sleep quality [26].

Different factors can affect sleep quality including personal characteristics sleep biology, circadian rhythm, and shifting work [27]. Our study revealed that poor quality of sleep can be seen in both shift workers and nonshift workers with a meaningful higher prevalence in the former. Different studies have reported higher incidence of tension, depression, and tiredness in shift workers. They are not spiteful when awaking and are more tired along the day. This is due to discrepancy between circadian rhythm and sleeping and awaking time in these populations [28, 29].

In the present study, we found no statistical difference in the prevalence of RLS among the shift workers and nonshift workers. Also, there was no statistical correlation between the scores from OISD questionnaire and the presence of RLS. In this regard, our results are different from the results of another study that evaluated the prevalence of RSL in shift and nonshift workers [30]. The present discrepancy can be due to small number of cases complaining about RSL in our study.

In the study, we showed the scores from OISD questionnaire to be significantly higher in shift workers than in nonshift workers. In some studies that used other questionnaires to assess the work ability index, they showed that this index was different among shift and nonshift workers both in males and females [31]. In different studies, different questionnaires have been designed to evaluate the occupational impact and work limitations due to sleep disorders in various populations. In most of these studies the effects of OSA on work limitation have been evaluated [11, 12, 32].

We used the related standard questionnaire to diagnose each sleep disorder and this is a positive point of our study. As a point of weakness, we evaluated various sleep disorders only subjectively and we did not use objective tests such as polysomnography. The other limiting factor of the paper is the fact that all the participants in the study are male, so we cannot extrapolate the results to the female shift workers.

It is suggested that in future studies the result of questionnaires be evaluated in different groups of sleep disorder proved on the basis of subjective methods. It is also suggested to investigate the effect of treatment on the scores of patients. However, in further studies on OISD the effect of different variables including age, sex, and various personality characteristics such as preferred sleep time can be evaluated. Furthermore, for the validity assessment of the questionnaire, the association between the questionnaire results and the incidence of work errors and accidents can be investigated.

Referring to our study results, OISD questionnaire is a suitable tool for assessment of the effect of sleep disorders on work ability. We propose that the efficacy of this questionnaire be evaluated in different groups of workers like HCWs, professional drivers, pilots, workers who spent long hours in front of a computer screen, and overall workers with heavy work load.

Abbreviations

PSQI: Pittsburg Sleep Quality Index
ESS: Epworth Sleepiness Scale
ISS: Insomnia Severity Index
OISD: Occupational Impact of Sleep Disorder questionnaire.

Conflict of Interests

The authors declare that there is no conflict of interests regarding the publication of this paper.

References

[1] S. D. Kyle, K. Morgan, and C. A. Espie, "Insomnia and health-related quality of life," *Sleep Medicine Reviews*, vol. 14, no. 1, pp. 69–82, 2010.

[2] C. A. Brown, R. Berry, and A. Schmidt, "Sleep and military members: emerging issues and nonpharmacological intervention," *Sleep Disorders*, vol. 2013, Article ID 160374, 6 pages, 2013.

[3] A. Metlaine, D. Leger, and D. Choudat, "Socioeconomic impact of insomnia in working populations," *Industrial Health*, vol. 43, no. 1, pp. 11–19, 2005.

[4] A. Fido and A. Ghali, "Detrimental effects of variable work shifts on quality of sleep, general health and work performance," *Medical Principles and Practice*, vol. 17, no. 6, pp. 453–457, 2008.

[5] T. Åkerstedt, "Shift work and disturbed sleep/wakefulness," *Occupational Medicine*, vol. 53, no. 2, pp. 89–94, 2003.

[6] T. Åkerstedt, P. Fredlund, M. Gillberg, and B. Jansson, "A prospective study of fatal occupational accidents—relationship to sleeping difficulties and occupational factors," *Journal of Sleep Research*, vol. 11, no. 1, pp. 69–71, 2002.

[7] M. LeBlanc, S. Beaulieu-Bonneau, C. Mérette, J. Savard, H. Ivers, and C. M. Morin, "Psychological and health-related quality of life factors associated with insomnia in a population-based sample," *Journal of Psychosomatic Research*, vol. 63, no. 2, pp. 157–166, 2007.

[8] J. C. Verster, B. David, K. Morgan, and B. Olivier, "Validation of the Dutch occupational impact of sleep questionnaire (OISQ)," *Industrial Health*, vol. 46, no. 6, pp. 601–606, 2008.

[9] P. Jennum and J. Kjellberg, "Health, social and economical consequences of sleep-disordered breathing: a controlled national study," *Thorax*, vol. 66, no. 7, pp. 560–566, 2011.

[10] T. Young, J. Skatrud, and P. E. Peppard, "Risk factors for obstructive sleep apnea in adults," *The Journal of the American Medical Association*, vol. 291, no. 16, pp. 2013–2016, 2004.

[11] S. Garbarino, F. De Carli, L. Nobili et al., "Sleepiness and sleep disorders in shift workers: a study on a group of Italian police officers," *Sleep*, vol. 25, no. 6, pp. 648–653, 2002.

[12] T. A. Omachi, D. M. Claman, P. D. Blanc, and M. D. Eisner, "Obstructive sleep apnea: a risk factor for work disability," *Sleep*, vol. 32, no. 6, pp. 791–798, 2009.

[13] N. J. Wesensten, T. J. Balkin, and G. Belenky, "Does sleep fragmentation impact recuperation? A review and reanalysis," *Journal of Sleep Research*, vol. 8, no. 4, pp. 237–245, 1999.

[14] M. A. J. Kompier, T. W. Taris, and M. V. Veldhoven, "Tossing and turning-insomnia in relation to occupational stress, rumination, fatigue and well-being," *Scandinavian Journal of Work, Environment & Health*, vol. 38, no. 3, pp. 238–246, 2012.

[15] K. Sadeghniiat-Haghighi, O. Aminian, G. Pouryaghoub, and Z. Yazdi, "Efficacy and hypnotic effects of melatonin in shift-work nurses: double-blind, placebo-controlled crossover trial," *Journal of Circadian Rhythms*, vol. 6, article 10, 2008.

[16] J. Farrahi, N. Nakhaee, V. Sheibani, B. Garrusi, and A. Amirkafi, "Psychometric properties of the persian version of the Pittsburgh sleep quality index addendum for PTSD (PSQI-A)," *Sleep and Breathing*, vol. 13, no. 3, pp. 259–262, 2009.

[17] K. Sadeghniiat Haghighi, A. Montazeri, A. Khajeh Mehrizi et al., "The Epworth Sleepiness Scale: translation and validation study of the Iranian version," *Sleep Breath*, vol. 17, no. 1, pp. 419–426, 2013.

[18] N. C. Netzer, R. A. Stoohs, C. M. Netzer, K. Clark, and K. P. Strohl, "Using the Berlin Questionnaire to identify patients at risk for the sleep apnea syndrome," *Annals of Internal Medicine*, vol. 131, no. 7, pp. 485–491, 1999.

[19] A. S. Walters, C. LeBrocq, A. Dhar et al., "Validation of the International Restless Legs Syndrome Study Group rating scale for restless legs syndrome," *Sleep Medicine*, vol. 4, no. 2, pp. 121–132, 2003.

[20] H. M. Engleman, S. E. Martin, I. J. Deary, and N. J. Douglas, "Effect of continuous positive airway pressure treatment on daytime function in sleep apnoea/hypopnoea syndrome," *The Lancet*, vol. 343, no. 8897, pp. 572–575, 1994.

[21] U. M. Edéll-Gustafsson, "Sleep quality and responses to insufficient sleep in women on different work shifts," *Journal of Clinical Nursing*, vol. 11, no. 2, pp. 280–288, 2002.

[22] T. Åkerstedt and K. P. Wright Jr., "Sleep loss and fatigue in shift work and shift work disorders," *Sleep Medicine Clinics*, vol. 4, no. 2, pp. 257–271, 2009.

[23] D. Léger and V. Bayon, "Societal costs of insomnia," *Sleep Medicine Reviews*, vol. 14, no. 6, pp. 379–389, 2010.

[24] M. Daley, C. M. Morin, M. LeBlanc, J.-P. Grégoire, and J. Savard, "The economic burden of insomnia: direct and indirect costs for individuals with insomnia syndrome, insomnia symptoms, and good sleepers," *Sleep*, vol. 32, no. 1, pp. 55–64, 2009.

[25] E. R. Kucharczyk, K. Morgan, and A. P. Hall, "The occupational impact of sleep quality and insomnia symptoms," *Sleep Medicine Reviews*, vol. 16, no. 16, pp. 547–559, 2012.

[26] H. K. Knudsen, L. J. Ducharme, and P. M. Roman, "Job stress and poor sleep quality: data from an American sample of full-time workers," *Social Science and Medicine*, vol. 64, no. 10, pp. 1997–2007, 2007.

[27] M. Härmä, L. Tenkanen, T. Sjöblom, T. Alikoski, and P. Heinsalmi, "Combined effects of shift work and life-style on the prevalence of insomnia, sleep deprivation and daytime sleepiness," *Scandinavian Journal of Work, Environment and Health*, vol. 24, no. 4, pp. 300–307, 1998.

[28] S. J. Linton and I.-L. Bryngelsson, "Insomnia and its relationship to work and health in a working-age population," *Journal of Occupational Rehabilitation*, vol. 10, no. 2, pp. 169–183, 2000.

[29] C. L. Drake, T. Roehrs, G. Richardson, J. K. Walsh, and T. Roth, "Shift work sleep disorder: prevalence and consequences beyond that of symptomatic day workers," *Sleep*, vol. 27, no. 8, pp. 1453–1462, 2004.

[30] A. Sharifian, M. Firoozeh, G. Pouryaghoub et al., "Restless Legs Syndrome in shift workers: a cross sectional study on male assembly workers," *Journal of Circadian Rhythms*, vol. 7, article 12, 2009.

[31] G. Costa, "Some considerations about aging, shift work and work ability," *International Congress Series*, vol. 1280, pp. 67–72, 2005.

[32] A. T. Mulgrew, C. F. Ryan, J. A. Fleetham et al., "The impact of obstructive sleep apnea and daytime sleepiness on work limitation," *Sleep Medicine*, vol. 9, no. 1, pp. 42–53, 2007.

27

Rising Prevalence and Neighborhood, Social, and Behavioral Determinants of Sleep Problems in US Children and Adolescents, 2003–2012

Gopal K. Singh and Mary Kay Kenney

US Department of Health and Human Services, Health Resources and Services Administration, Maternal and Child Health Bureau, 5600 Fishers Lane, Room 18-41, Rockville, MD 20857, USA

Correspondence should be addressed to Gopal K. Singh; gsingh@hrsa.gov

Academic Editor: Giora Pillar

We examined trends and neighborhood and sociobehavioral determinants of sleep problems in US children aged 6–17 between 2003 and 2012. The 2003, 2007, and 2011-2012 rounds of the National Survey of Children's Health were used to estimate trends and differentials in sleep problems using logistic regression. Prevalence of sleep problems increased significantly over time. The proportion of children with <7 days/week of adequate sleep increased from 31.2% in 2003 to 41.9% in 2011-2012, whereas the prevalence of adequate sleep <5 days/week rose from 12.6% in 2003 to 13.6% in 2011-2012. Prevalence of sleep problems varied in relation to neighborhood socioeconomic and built-environmental characteristics (e.g., safety concerns, poor housing, garbage/litter, vandalism, sidewalks, and parks/playgrounds). Approximately 10% of children in neighborhoods with the most-favorable social environment had serious sleep problems, compared with 16.2% of children in neighborhoods with the least-favorable social environment. Children in neighborhoods with the fewest health-promoting amenities or the greatest social disadvantage had 37%–43% higher adjusted odds of serious sleep problems than children in the most-favorable neighborhoods. Higher levels of screen time, physical inactivity, and secondhand smoke exposure were associated with 20%–47% higher adjusted odds of sleep problems. Neighborhood conditions and behavioral factors are important determinants of sleep problems in children.

1. Introduction

Sleep problems in children have significant impacts on their health and well-being [1–4]. Inadequate sleep in children has been shown to be associated with poor academic performance, behavioral problems, poor mental and physical health, obesity and weight gain, alcohol use, accidents, and injuries [1–15]. Research also suggests that these adverse health effects vary in relation to the amount or duration of sleep problems [2–6, 12–15]. The US data show that, compared to children and adolescents who do not experience any sleep problems during the week, those who experience inadequate sleep during the entire week have 3-4 times higher risks of serious behavioral problems, 4-5 times higher risks of depression and anxiety, 2.5 times higher risk of ADD/ADHD, 3.2 times higher risk of migraine headaches, 1.5 times higher risk of being in fair/poor overall health, 1.6 times higher risk

of repeating a grade or having a problem at school, and 2.8 times higher risk of missing >2 weeks of school during a year [16–18].

Past research has examined the impact of a number of sociodemographic and behavioral factors on childhood sleep problems [1, 2, 4, 19–23]. These factors include child's age, gender, race/ethnicity, household socioeconomic status (SES), and such behavioral risk factors as physical activity, television viewing, and recreational computer use [1, 2, 4, 19–23]. Although the effects of neighborhood factors have been examined for a number of child health and behavioral outcomes such as physical inactivity, obesity, school performance, perceived health status, mental health, behavioral problems, and youth violence [16, 24–31] few studies have addressed the relationship between neighborhood environments and children's sleep problems [1, 2, 32]. To our knowledge, the impact of neighborhood social conditions and built environments on sleep problems in the US has not been fully explored using a nationally representative sample of school-aged children.

Analyzing the health effects of neighborhood environment is important because neighborhood conditions reflect the broader social and community contexts within which variations in individual health and social behaviors occur [16, 24–27, 33]. Many aspects of neighborhood environment that are thought to influence child health and behavioral outcomes, such as socioeconomic deprivation, poor housing, crime, and lack of social amenities, are potentially modifiable through social policies [16, 24, 25, 34]. Additionally, neighborhood conditions have been linked to a variety of health and behavioral outcomes among both children and adults, including obesity and physical activity, infant mortality, low birthweight, smoking, self-rated health, mental health, injury, and mortality [16, 24–26, 33]. As such, improvements in neighborhood environment have the potential to positively impact a wide range of childhood health inequalities, including those in sleep problems [16, 26]. Emphasis on the neighborhood environment and broader social structure is also consistent with the *Healthy People 2020* objectives [35].

Besides neighborhood factors, examining the sleep effects of household SES, race/ethnicity, and behavioral characteristics is important as well because they identify additional opportunities to reduce health disparities among children through targeted interventions. Moreover, health-related behaviors, which are amenable to change through public policy and social interventions, are one possible mechanism through which neighborhood, ethnic, and social factors might influence sleep patterns in children.

The National Survey of Children's Health (NSCH) allows us to explore the association between neighborhood conditions, household SES, behavioral risk factors, and childhood sleep problems in the US. In this study, we (1) examine trends in prevalence of sleep problems by child's age, gender, and race/ethnicity, (2) estimate prevalence of sleep problems by a variety of neighborhood, household, and child-level characteristics, (3) assess whether neighborhoods effects on sleep problems persist after adjusting for household SES and sociodemographic characteristics, (4) examine the potential intervening mechanisms, particularly behavioral factors of physical activity, recreational screen time, and exposure to secondhand smoke (SHS), through which neighborhood conditions may influence sleep patterns, and (5) examine whether the sleep effects of neighborhood environment and behavioral factors vary by child's age and gender.

2. Methods

Trends in prevalence of sleep problems by age, gender, and race/ethnicity were analyzed using the 2003, 2007, and 2011-2012 NSCH [18, 36–41]. However, data for the detailed analyses of neighborhood, socioeconomic, and behavioral determinants came from the 2007 NSCH because it had the most complete information on covariates, including composite neighborhood indices [18, 36, 37, 40]. All three rounds of the survey were conducted by the National Center for Health Statistics (NCHS), with funding and direction

from the Maternal and Child Health Bureau [36–39]. The purpose of the NSCH was to provide national and state-specific prevalence estimates for a variety of children's health and well-being indicators [36–39]. The surveys included an extensive array of questions about children's health and the family, including parental health, stress and coping behaviors, family activities, and parental concerns about their children [18, 36–41]. Interviews were conducted with parents, and special emphasis was placed on factors related to children's well-being.

All three rounds of the NSCH were cross-sectional telephone surveys. The 2003 survey was conducted between January 2003 and July 2004; the 2007 survey was conducted between April 2007 and July 2008; and the 2011-2012 survey was conducted between February 2011 and June 2012 [18, 36–41]. The sample size was 102,353 children <18 years of age for the 2003 survey, 91,642 for the 2007 survey, and 95,677 for the 2011-2012 survey. In each survey, the average sample size was about 1,800-2,000 children per state [18, 36–41]. In all three rounds of the survey, a random-digit-dial sample of households with children <18 years of age was selected from each of the 50 states and the District of Columbia. One child was selected from all children in each identified household to be the subject of the survey [18, 36–41]. Interviews were conducted in English, Spanish, and four Asian languages. The respondent was the parent or guardian who knew most about the child's health status and health care. All survey data were based on parental reports. The interview completion rate for the NSCH, measuring the percentage of completed interviews among known households with children, was 68.8% in 2003, 66.0% in 2007, and 54.1% for the landline sample and 41.2% for the cell-phone sample in 2011-2012 [37–39]. The overall response rate at the national level was 55.3% in 2003 and 46.7% in 2007 [37, 38].The overall response rate for the 2011-2012 survey is not yet available. Substantive and methodological details of the 2003, 2007, and 2011-2012 surveys are described elsewhere [36–41]. The NCHS Research Ethics Review Board approved all data collection procedures for each round of the survey.

The sample size for the detailed covariate analysis, based on the 2007 NSCH, was 63,352 children and adolescents aged 6–17. The dependent variable, sleep problems, was based on the question "During the past week, on how many nights did the child get enough sleep for a child his/her age?" From this question, we derived two measures of inadequate sleep: children who experienced <7 days/week of adequate sleep (or at least 1 day/week of inadequate sleep) and those who experienced <5 days/week of adequate sleep (or at least 3 days/week of inadequate sleep) [16, 17, 42]. The latter measure, representing more serious sleep problems, tends to capture the amount of sleep problems and may be clinically more relevant as it leads to stronger physical and mental health effects [16, 17, 42].

Neighborhood social conditions and built environments were the primary covariates of interest. Neighborhood social conditions included dichotomous measures of perceived neighborhood safety, presence of garbage/litter in the neighborhood, poor/dilapidated housing, and vandalism such as broken windows or graffiti [26]. We used a previously

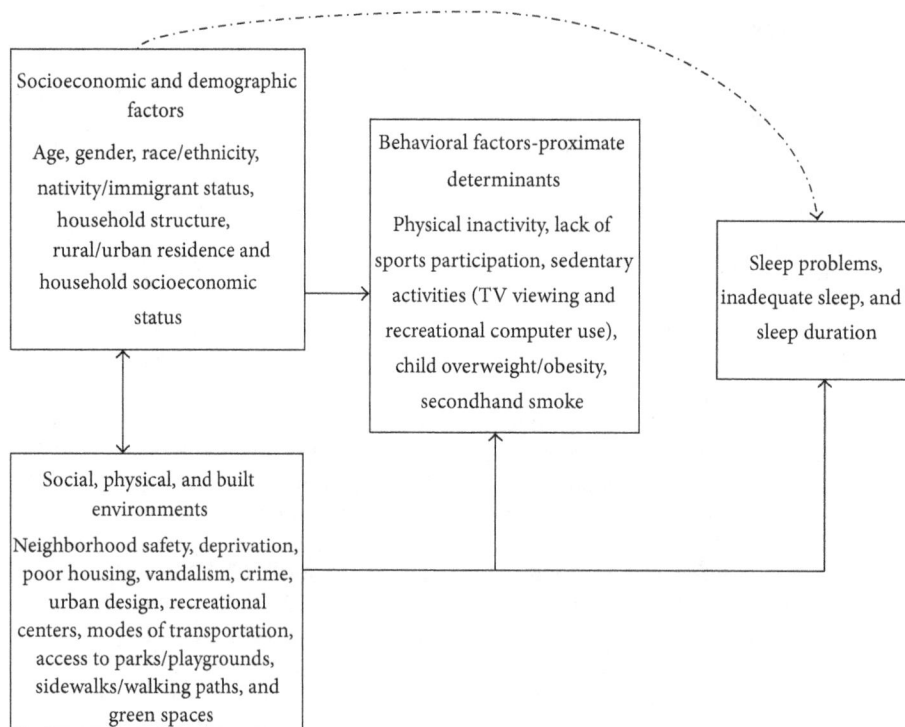

FIGURE 1: A simple model of neighborhood and sociobehavioral determinants of sleep problems in children and adolescents.

developed factor-based index of neighborhood social conditions that combined the above four neighborhood social indicators with respective factor loadings or weights of 0.52, 0.69, 0.71, and 0.72 [26]. Higher scores on the neighborhood social conditions index (alpha = 0.57) represent more favorable socioeconomic conditions. The built environment index, developed previously, consisted of 4 variables: neighborhood access to sidewalks/walking paths; parks/playgrounds; recreation or community centers; and library/bookmobile, with respective factor loadings of 0.69, 0.75, 0.66, and 0.67 [26]. Higher scores on the built environment index (alpha = 0.64) represent higher levels of health-promoting neighborhood amenities. Both indices were standardized to have a mean score of 100 and standard deviation of 20. Note that the two neighborhood indices were orthogonal or independent of each other [26]. Two indicators of household SES were used: parental education and household income/poverty levels.

We used social determinants of health framework to model links between neighborhood conditions, household socioeconomic characteristics, health-related behaviors, and childhood sleep problems (Figure 1) [16, 25, 26, 28, 43, 44]. Within this framework, neighborhood and household socioeconomic characteristics are considered underlying determinants, [16, 25, 26, 28, 43, 44] which may influence sleep patterns by creating conditions (e.g., noise, violence, and anxiety) that lead to sleep disturbance in children. They are also hypothesized to affect sleep problems indirectly through their effects on intervening psychosocial and behavioral mechanisms such as familial stress and behavioral risk factors such as physical activity, television viewing, alcohol, tobacco and substance use, and SHS exposure [16, 26, 28].

A bidirectional relationship between household SES and neighborhood conditions is postulated as neighborhood social and built environment conditions can influence household or individual education and income attainment, employment status, and housing tenure. On the other hand, age and racial/ethnic composition, household socioeconomic conditions, and place of residence can contribute significantly to the makeup of the neighborhoods, community economic development, and the kinds of social and physical amenities that might be available to neighborhood or community residents [16, 26, 28, 43, 44].

Using this framework and past research as a guide, we considered twelve covariates of childhood sleep problems, in addition to the neighborhood conditions. These included child's age, gender, race/ethnicity, nativity/immigrant status, household composition, metropolitan/non-metropolitan residence, household/parental education (<12, 12, 13–15, ≥16 years), household poverty status measured as a ratio of family income to the poverty threshold (<100%, 100–199%, 200–399%, ≥400%), television viewing, recreational computer use, physical activity levels, and SHS exposure [1, 2, 4, 16, 19–23, 26, 28]. SHS exposure was determined by whether anyone smoked inside child's home. All other covariates were measured as shown in Tables 1–4.

Income was imputed for 9% of the observations by using a multiple imputation technique [37]. For all other covariates, there were few or no missing cases, which were excluded from the multivariate analyses.

The χ^2 statistic was used to test the overall association between covariates and sleep problems. The t-statistic was used to test the difference in prevalence between any two

TABLE 1: Trends in weighted prevalence (%) of sleep problems among US children aged 6–17, 2003–2012: the National Survey of Children's Health.

| | <5 days/week of adequate sleep | | | | | | <7 days/week of adequate sleep | | | | | | % change in prevalence during 2003–2012 | |
| | 2011–2012 | | 2007 | | 2003 | | 2011–2012 | | 2007 | | 2003 | | <5 d/w of adequate sleep | <7 d/w of adequate sleep |
	%	SE	%	SE	%	SE	%	SE	%	SE	%	SE		
Total population	13.63	0.30	13.33	0.32	12.58	0.23	41.85	0.44	35.69	0.47	31.24	0.31	8.35[a]	33.96[a]
Child's age (years)														
6–8	7.82	0.48	6.68	0.43	7.49	0.42	34.43	0.85	26.06	0.89	22.81	0.59	4.41	50.94[a]
9–11	10.39	0.55	9.03	0.64	7.91	0.37	40.64	0.89	29.13	0.92	26.13	0.60	31.35[a]	55.53[a]
12–14	13.94	0.62	14.53	0.68	12.38	0.43	42.07	0.88	40.08	0.94	33.12	0.61	12.60[a]	27.02[a]
15–17	22.10	0.70	22.71	0.76	22.69	0.55	49.97	0.88	46.83	0.95	42.82	0.64	-2.60	16.70[a]
Child's sex														
Male	13.23	0.42	12.75	0.44	12.48	0.31	41.07	0.61	35.45	0.65	31.00	0.43	6.01	32.48[a]
Female	14.05	0.42	13.94	0.48	12.68	0.33	42.66	0.63	35.94	0.68	31.49	0.45	10.80[a]	35.47[a]
Race/ethnicity														
Hispanic	11.63	0.80	10.82	0.92	13.88	0.74	36.34	1.23	28.54	1.39	25.23	0.91	-16.21[a]	44.03[a]
Non-Hispanic white	14.11	0.35	13.80	0.39	12.27	0.24	45.18	0.50	39.40	0.55	33.87	0.35	15.00[a]	33.39[a]
Non-Hispanic black	14.80	0.83	15.31	0.85	13.58	0.71	40.82	1.20	32.75	1.11	29.10	0.91	8.98	40.27[a]
Non-Hispanic mixed race	15.63	1.34	12.70	1.27	13.20	1.44	43.26	1.82	38.66	2.46	31.03	1.78	18.41[a]	39.41[a]
Other[b]	12.78	1.21	12.36	1.39	9.39	1.07	35.69	1.72	28.71	1.91	24.91	1.60	36.10[a]	43.28[a]

[a]The t-test for change in prevalence between 2003 and 2012 was statistically significant at P < 0.05. [b]Includes Asians and Pacific Islanders and American Indians/Alaska Natives.

TABLE 2: Descriptive statistics of the sample for children aged 6–17 years, according to neighborhood, sociodemographic, and behavioral characteristics: the 2007 National Survey of Children's Health ($N = 63,352$).

Sociodemographic and behavioral characteristics	Unweighted number in sample	Weighted percent in sample
Index of neighborhood socioeconomic conditions		
20.78–67.09 (least favorable)	4,618	8.88
67.10–88.32	4,187	7.31
88.33–104.99	10,635	17.62
105.00–111.40 (most favorable)	42,981	66.19
Neighborhood safety		
Safe	56,356	86.57
Unsafe	6,328	13.43
Presence of garbage/litter in neighborhood		
Yes	9,427	16.04
No	53,348	83.96
Poorly kept or dilapidated/rundown housing in neighborhood		
Yes	8,717	14.21
No	53,981	85.79
Vandalism such as broken windows or graffiti in neighborhood		
Yes	6,007	11.17
No	56,757	88.83
Index of neighborhood built environment		
46.40–67.04 (low amenities)	5,121	8.53
67.05–81.39	8,227	12.02
81.40–104.99	20,306	32.40
105.00–116.40 (high amenities)	28,193	47.05
Neighborhood access to sidewalks or walking paths		
Yes	43,947	72.19
No	18,840	27.81
Neighborhood access to parks or playgrounds		
Yes	49,025	79.33
No	13,768	20.67
Neighborhood access to a recreation or community center		
Yes	39,915	64.95
No	22,132	35.05
Neighborhood access to a library or bookmobile		
Yes	54,594	86.33
No	8,122	13.67
Child's age (years)		
6–8	13,512	24.55
9–11	14,083	24.23
12–14	16,338	26.00
15–17	19,419	25.22
Child's sex		
Male	32,981	51.15
Female	30,371	48.85

TABLE 2: Continued.

Sociodemographic and behavioral characteristics	Unweighted number in sample	Weighted percent in sample
Race/ethnicity		
Non-Hispanic white	43,444	56.53
Non-Hispanic black	6,363	14.81
Hispanic	7,245	18.85
American Indian/Alaska native	818	0.83
Asian	1,452	3.33
Hawaiian/Pacific Islander	309	0.34
Non-Hispanic mixed race	2,753	3.74
Other	968	1.56
Child's nativity/immigrant status		
Born to immigrant parents	7,964	19.02
Born to US-born parents	55,388	80.98
Household composition		
Two-parent biological	41,673	62.49
Two-parent stepfamily	5,984	10.12
Single mother	10,744	19.76
Other family type	4,951	7.63
Place of residence		
Metropolitan	43,859	83.69
Non-metropolitan	19,493	16.31
Household poverty status (ratio of family income to poverty threshold)		
Below 100%	6,886	17.08
100%–199%	10,500	20.51
200%–399%	21,624	32.17
At or above 400%	24,343	30.24
Highest household or parental education level (years)		
<12	3,666	8.47
12	10,263	23.53
13–15	17,813	26.87
16+	30,193	41.13
Television watching (number of hours per day)		
<1	13,282	20.66
1	19,176	29.07
2	18,252	28.41
>2	12,151	21.87
Recreational computer use (number of hours per day)		
<1	30,663	51.30
1-2	24,036	38.23
>2	6,352	10.47
Physical activity (number of days per week)		
0	5,649	10.21
1-2	7,571	12.36
3-4	15,529	23.95
5+	34,096	53.48
Secondhand smoke exposure		
Yes	5,293	8.93
No	57,620	91.07

TABLE 3: Weighted prevalence of sleep problems among US children aged 6–17 by neighborhood, sociodemographic, and behavioral characteristics: the 2007 National Survey of Children's Health (N = 63,352).

Sociobehavioral characteristic	Less than 5 days/week of adequate sleep			Less than 7 days/week of adequate sleep		
	%	SE	P value	%	SE	P value
Index of neighborhood socioeconomic conditions			<0.001			0.282
20.78–67.09 (least favorable)	16.20	1.16		38.20	1.70	
67.10–88.32	15.46	1.37		37.80	1.96	
88.33–104.99	15.77	0.85		35.44	1.08	
105.00–111.40 (most favorable)	12.10	0.38		35.32	0.57	
Neighborhood safety			<0.001			0.588
Safe	12.87	0.34		35.89	0.50	
Unsafe	16.62	1.01		35.10	1.36	
Presence of garbage/litter in neighborhood			<0.001			<0.001
Yes	16.41	0.88		39.33	1.17	
No	12.77	0.35		35.07	0.51	
Poorly kept or dilapidated/rundown housing in neighborhood			0.005			0.083
Yes	15.68	0.91		37.76	1.27	
No	12.95	0.35		35.41	0.51	
Vandalism such as broken windows or graffiti in neighborhood			0.030			0.192
Yes	15.58	1.10		37.68	1.58	
No	13.08	0.34		35.52	0.49	
Index of neighborhood built environment			0.049			0.575
46.40–67.04 (low amenities)	15.68	1.32		35.66	1.78	
67.05–81.39	14.68	0.88		37.32	1.21	
81.40–104.99	13.53	0.56		36.03	0.81	
105.00–116.40 (high amenities)	12.61	0.48		35.38	0.7	
Neighborhood access to sidewalks or walking paths			0.500			0.985
Yes	13.22	0.40		35.76	0.58	
No	13.68	0.56		35.78	0.79	
Neighborhood access to parks or playgrounds			0.009			0.025
Yes	12.90	0.35		35.18	0.52	
No	15.22	0.81		37.85	1.06	
Neighborhood access to a recreation or community center			0.120			0.557
Yes	13.02	0.40		36.03	0.58	
No	14.10	0.57		35.45	0.80	
Neighborhood access to a library or bookmobile			0.031			0.743
Yes	13.06	0.34		35.90	0.50	
No	15.39	1.03		35.41	1.39	
Child's age (years)			<0.001			<0.001
6–8	6.68	0.43		26.06	0.89	
9–11	9.03	0.64		29.13	0.92	
12–14	14.53	0.68		40.08	0.94	
15–17	22.71	0.76		46.83	0.95	

TABLE 3: Continued.

Sociobehavioral characteristic	Less than 5 days/week of adequate sleep			Less than 7 days/week of adequate sleep		
	%	SE	P value	%	SE	P value
Child's sex			0.067			0.595
Male	12.75	0.44		35.45	0.65	
Female	13.94	0.48		35.94	0.68	
Race/ethnicity			0.040			<0.001
Non-Hispanic white	13.80	0.39		39.40	0.55	
Non-Hispanic black	15.31	0.85		32.75	1.11	
Hispanic	10.82	0.92		28.54	1.39	
American Indian/Alaska native	13.12	2.55		32.09	3.41	
Asian	12.04	2.13		26.96	2.94	
Hawaiian/Pacific Islander	13.90	3.92		36.17	7.86	
Non-Hispanic mixed race	12.70	1.27		38.66	2.46	
Other	12.32	2.40		29.01	3.02	
Child's nativity/immigrant status			<0.001			<0.001
Born to immigrant parents	10.33	0.79		27.08	1.2	
Born to US-born parents	14.04	0.35		37.71	0.49	
Household composition			<0.001			0.585
Two-parent biological	12.15	0.37		35.38	0.58	
Two-parent stepfamily	13.77	0.98		35.55	1.57	
Single mother	17.33	0.89		36.99	1.05	
Other family type	12.12	1.25		35.03	1.84	
Place of residence			0.102			0.064
Metropolitan	13.50	0.37		35.39	0.53	
Non-metropolitan	12.46	0.52		37.24	0.84	
Household poverty status (ratio of family income to poverty threshold)			0.494			<0.001
Below 100%	13.43	0.85		30.32	1.14	
100%–199%	12.94	0.76		32.29	1.06	
200%–399%	12.88	0.59		37.09	0.86	
At or above 400%	14.03	0.55		39.55	0.81	
Highest household or parental education level (years)			0.964			<0.001
<12	13.09	1.26		30.57	1.82	
12	13.73	0.77		34.29	1.07	
13–15	13.40	0.60		34.94	0.88	
16+	13.31	0.47		38.52	0.69	
Television watching (number of hours per day)			<0.001			0.996
<1	12.45	0.65		36.02	1.04	
1	12.64	0.61		35.82	0.87	
2	12.62	0.63		35.76	0.87	
>2	16.12	0.73		35.67	1.01	
Recreational computer use (number of hours per day)			<0.001			<0.001
<1	9.93	0.38		32.33	0.63	
1-2	15.89	0.60		39.03	0.79	
>2	20.93	1.17		43.05	1.59	

TABLE 3: Continued.

Sociobehavioral characteristic	Less than 5 days/week of adequate sleep			Less than 7 days/week of adequate sleep		
	%	SE	P value	%	SE	P value
Physical activity (number of days per week)			<0.001			<0.001
0	18.77	1.14		37.83	1.55	
1-2	18.13	1.17		40.65	1.42	
3-4	12.76	0.57		36.24	0.90	
5+	11.27	0.41		33.79	0.64	
Secondhand smoke exposure			<0.001			0.042
Yes	17.88	1.07		38.76	1.43	
No	12.90	0.34		35.43	0.50	

P values associated with chi-square tests for independence between each covariate and sleep problems.
Both neighborhood indices have a mean score of 100 and a standard deviation of 20.

groups or time points. Logistic regression was used to examine the association between neighborhood and behavioral characteristics and sleep problems, after adjusting for the above covariates. To account for the complex sample design of the NSCH, SUDAAN software was used to conduct all statistical analyses [45].

3. Results

3.1. Trends in the Prevalence of Sleep Problems, 2003–2012. The prevalence of sleep problems increased significantly between 2003 and 2012 (Table 1). The proportion of children with <7 days/week of adequate sleep increased from 31.2% in 2003 to 35.7% in 2007 and 41.9% in 2011-2012, whereas the prevalence of adequate sleep <5 days/week rose from 12.6% in 2003 to 13.6% in 2011-2012. The number of children aged 6–17 with at least 1 day/week of sleep problems rose from an estimated 15.1 million in 2003 to 20.5 million in 2011-2012. The increase in prevalence of sleep problems was more pronounced among children aged 6–11 and females. During 2003–2012, while children in all racial/ethnic groups experienced a marked increase in sleep problems at least 1 day/week, the prevalence of serious (≥3 days/week) sleep problems increased significantly only among white, mixed-race, and "other" children (Table 1).

3.2. Neighborhood and Sociobehavioral Disparities in Sleep Problems, 2007. Descriptive characteristics of the 2007 sample are shown in Table 2. Approximately 9% of the child population lived in neighborhoods with the most-unfavorable social or built environments. Non-Hispanic white children were the largest racial/ethnic group (56.5%), followed by Hispanics (18.9%), blacks (14.8%), and Asians (3.3%). Approximately 17% of children lived below the poverty line, and 8.5% of children had parents who had less than a high school education. Approximately 22% of children watched television >2 hours/day, while 10.2% of children were physically inactive and 8.9% were exposed to secondhand smoke. Table 3 shows observed prevalence of childhood sleep problems in 2007 according to various neighborhood, sociodemographic, and behavioral characteristics. The prevalence of sleep problems varied significantly in relation to

neighborhood socioeconomic and built-environmental characteristics. Approximately 10% of children in neighborhoods with the most-favorable social environment had serious sleep problems, compared with 16.2% of children in neighborhoods with the least-favorable social environment. Children living in unfavorable neighborhoods that were characterized by safety concerns, garbage/litter in streets/sidewalks, poor/dilapidated housing, or vandalism had 19%–29% higher prevalence of serious sleep problems than those in more favorable neighborhoods (Table 3).

Approximately 15.7% of children in neighborhoods with the fewest health-promoting amenities had serious sleep problems, compared with 12.6% of children in neighborhoods with the most health-promoting amenities (Table 3). Specifically, children living in neighborhoods with no access to parks and playgrounds had 8% and 18% higher risks of ≥1 day/week and ≥3 days/week of sleep problems, respectively, than those with access to these amenities.

The prevalence of sleep problems was positively associated with child's age. Approximately 47% of children aged 15–17 experienced at least 1 day/week of sleep problems, compared to 26.1% of children aged 6–8. The prevalence of more serious sleep problems was 3.4 times greater among older adolescents compared to younger children. Hispanic and Asian children had fewer sleep problems than white and black children, whereas children of immigrant parents had fewer sleep problems than those with US-born parents (Table 3). Higher parental education and income were associated with a higher prevalence of at least 1 day/week of sleep problems.

In terms of behavioral effects, higher levels of physical inactivity, recreational computer use, and SHS exposure were significantly associated with both ≥1 day/week and ≥3 days/week of sleep problems. Higher levels of television viewing were associated with only more serious sleep problems (Table 3).

Since the adjusted effects of neighborhood factors, household SES, and demographic factors were generally similar in both the sociodemographic and full sociobehavioral models, we only interpret the results from the full multivariate models in Table 4. Higher risks of sleep problems associated with unfavorable neighborhood social conditions persisted even after the adjustment of sociodemographic and behavioral

TABLE 4: Logistic regression models showing covariate-adjusted odds of sleep problems among US children aged 6–17 by neighborhood, sociodemographic, and behavioral characteristics: the 2007 National Survey of Children's Health.

Neighborhood conditions and Socio-behavioral characteristics	Less than 5 days/week of adequate sleep				Less than 7 days/week of adequate sleep			
	Sociodemographic model		Full socio-behavioral model		Sociodemographic model		Full socio-behavioral model	
	Adj OR	95% CI	Adj OR	95% CI	Adj OR	95% CI	Adj OR	95% CI
Index of neighborhood socioeconomic conditions								
20.78–67.09 (least favorable)	1.48	1.21 1.80	1.43	1.18 1.75	1.37	1.16 1.60	1.35	1.15 1.59
67.10–88.32	1.38	1.10 1.73	1.38	1.11 1.72	1.22	1.03 1.45	1.22	1.03 1.45
88.33–104.99	1.45	1.25 1.69	1.42	1.22 1.65	1.12	1.00 1.26	1.11	1.00 1.25
105.00–111.40 (most favorable)	1.00	Reference	1.00	Reference	1.00	Reference	1.00	Reference
Neighborhood safety								
Safe	1.00	Reference	1.00	Reference	1.00	Reference	1.00	Reference
Unsafe	1.44	1.21 1.72	1.40	1.17 1.66	1.21	1.05 1.39	1.19	1.04 1.37
Presence of garbage/litter in neighborhood								
Yes	1.33	1.14 1.54	1.29	1.12 1.50	1.32	1.18 1.47	1.30	1.16 1.46
No	1.00	Reference	1.00	Reference	1.00	Reference	1.00	Reference
Poorly kept or dilapidated/rundown housing in neighborhood								
Yes	1.28	1.09 1.50	1.26	1.09 1.48	1.20	1.07 1.35	1.19	1.06 1.34
No	1.00	Reference	1.00	Reference	1.00	Reference	1.00	Reference
Vandalism such as broken windows or graffiti in neighborhood								
Yes	1.24	1.03 1.50	1.24	1.03 1.49	1.20	1.04 1.39	1.20	1.04 1.39
No	1.00	Reference	1.00	Reference	1.00	Reference	1.00	Reference
Index of neighborhood built environment								
46.40–67.04 (low amenities)	1.39	1.11 1.74	1.37	1.10 1.70	1.06	0.89 1.26	1.05	0.89 1.25
67.05–81.39	1.20	1.01 1.43	1.21	1.02 1.44	1.05	0.92 1.19	1.05	0.93 1.19
81.40–104.99	1.14	1.00 1.30	1.14	1.00 1.29	1.05	0.96 1.15	1.05	0.96 1.15
105.00–116.40 (high amenities)	1.00	Reference	1.00	Reference	1.00	Reference	1.00	Reference
Neighborhood access to sidewalks or walking paths								
Yes	1.00	Reference	1.00	Reference	1.00	Reference	1.00	Reference
No	1.10	0.97 1.24	1.10	0.97 1.24	0.98	0.90 1.07	0.98	0.90 1.07
Neighborhood access to parks or playgrounds								
Yes	1.00	Reference	1.00	Reference	1.00	Reference	1.00	Reference
No	1.21	1.05 1.40	1.20	1.04 1.38	1.07	0.96 1.18	1.06	0.96 1.18
Neighborhood access to a recreation or community center								
Yes	1.00	Reference	1.00	Reference	1.00	Reference	1.00	Reference
No	1.13	1.01 1.27	1.11	0.99 1.25	1.00	0.92 1.09	1.00	0.91 1.09
Neighborhood access to a library or bookmobile								
Yes	1.00	Reference	1.00	Reference	1.00	Reference	1.00	Reference
No	1.24	1.05 1.47	1.24	1.05 1.47	1.05	0.92 1.20	1.05	0.92 1.20

TABLE 4: Continued.

Neighborhood conditions and Socio-behavioral characteristics	Less than 5 days/week of adequate sleep				Less than 7 days/week of adequate sleep			
	Sociodemographic model		Full socio-behavioral model		Sociodemographic model		Full socio-behavioral model	
	Adj OR	95% CI	Adj OR	95% CI	Adj OR	95% CI	Adj OR	95% CI
Child's age (years)								
6–8	1.00	Reference	1.00	Reference	1.00	Reference	1.00	Reference
9–11	1.38	1.12 1.71	1.33	1.08 1.64	1.20	1.05 1.36	1.18	1.04 1.34
12–14	2.40	2.02 2.85	2.13	1.79 2.54	1.95	1.73 2.20	1.86	1.64 2.10
15–17	4.06	3.45 4.78	3.37	2.83 4.01	2.54	2.25 2.86	2.35	2.06 2.67
Child's sex								
Male	1.00	Reference	1.00	Reference	1.00	Reference	1.00	Reference
Female	1.11	0.99 1.24	1.08	0.96 1.21	1.02	0.94 1.11	1.00	0.92 1.09
Race/ethnicity								
Non-Hispanic white	1.17	0.92 1.49	1.18	0.92 1.51	1.28	1.08 1.51	1.29	1.09 1.53
Non-Hispanic black	1.16	0.90 1.50	1.11	0.86 1.45	0.98	0.81 1.18	0.98	0.81 1.18
Hispanic	1.00	Reference	1.00	Reference	1.00	Reference	1.00	Reference
American Indian/Alaska native	1.06	0.65 1.75	1.08	0.67 1.76	0.97	0.68 1.38	0.98	0.69 1.40
Asian	1.21	0.78 1.87	1.17	0.76 1.82	0.94	0.67 1.31	0.92	0.65 1.29
Hawaiian/Pacific Islander	1.16	0.58 2.31	1.21	0.62 2.38	1.20	0.59 2.46	1.22	0.60 2.51
Non-Hispanic mixed race	1.06	0.77 1.46	1.07	0.78 1.48	1.35	1.04 1.74	1.38	1.06 1.78
Other	0.63	0.34 1.20	0.61	0.32 1.19	0.59	0.36 0.96	0.59	0.36 0.97
Child's nativity/immigrant status								
Born to immigrant parents	0.80	0.65 0.98	0.78	0.63 0.96	0.72	0.62 0.84	0.71	0.61 0.83
Born to US-born parents	1.00	Reference	1.00	Reference	1.00	Reference	1.00	Reference
Household composition								
Two-parent biological	1.00	Reference	1.00	Reference	1.00	Reference	1.00	Reference
Two-parent stepfamily	1.01	0.83 1.22	0.98	0.81 1.19	0.96	0.82 1.12	0.95	0.81 1.11
Single mother	1.39	1.16 1.65	1.35	1.13 1.60	1.12	1.00 1.27	1.11	0.99 1.26
Other family type	0.92	0.69 1.23	0.89	0.66 1.20	1.01	0.84 1.22	1.01	0.83 1.22
Place of residence								
Metropolitan	1.15	1.01 1.29	1.13	1.00 1.28	0.98	0.89 1.07	0.97	0.88 1.06
Non-metropolitan	1.00	Reference	1.00	Reference	1.00	Reference	1.00	Reference
Household poverty status (ratio of family income to poverty threshold)								
Below 100%	0.93	0.74 1.16	0.88	0.70 1.10	0.78	0.66 0.93	0.77	0.65 0.91
100%–199%	0.86	0.71 1.04	0.83	0.69 1.00	0.79	0.69 0.91	0.79	0.69 0.90
200%–399%	0.89	0.77 1.03	0.87	0.75 1.01	0.93	0.84 1.03	0.92	0.83 1.02
At or above 400%	1.00	Reference	1.00	Reference	1.00	Reference	1.00	Reference
Highest household or parental education level (years)								
<12	0.95	0.72 1.25	0.86	0.65 1.13	0.90	0.72 1.12	0.87	0.70 1.08
12	0.91	0.77 1.08	0.85	0.71 1.01	0.87	0.77 0.98	0.86	0.76 0.97
13–15	0.93	0.80 1.08	0.89	0.77 1.03	0.86	0.78 0.96	0.86	0.77 0.96
16+	1.00	Reference	1.00	Reference	1.00	Reference	1.00	Reference

TABLE 4: Continued.

Neighborhood conditions and Socio-behavioral characteristics	Less than 5 days/week of adequate sleep				Less than 7 days/week of adequate sleep			
	Sociodemographic model		Full socio-behavioral model		Sociodemographic model		Full socio-behavioral model	
	Adj OR	95% CI	Adj OR	95% CI	Adj OR	95% CI	Adj OR	95% CI
Television watching (number of hours per day)								
<1			1.00	Reference			1.00	Reference
1			0.97	0.82 1.14			0.95	0.84 1.08
2			0.94	0.79 1.11			0.95	0.85 1.08
>2			1.07	0.89 1.28			0.91	0.79 1.05
Recreational computer use (number of hours per day)								
<1			1.00	Reference			1.00	Reference
1-2			1.22	1.07 1.40			1.08	0.98 1.18
>2			1.41	1.17 1.69			1.20	1.02 1.41
Physical activity (number of days per week)								
0			1.47	1.22 1.77			1.21	1.04 1.41
1-2			1.45	1.21 1.75			1.30	1.13 1.49
3-4			1.07	0.93 1.22			1.08	0.98 1.19
5+			1.00	Reference			1.00	Reference
Secondhand smoke exposure								
Yes			1.23	1.04 1.46			1.07	0.94 1.23
No			1.00	Reference			1.00	Reference

Sociodemographic logistic models included child's age, sex, race/ethnicity, nativity, household composition, metropolitan/nonmetropolitan residence, household poverty and education levels, and neighborhood social conditions or built environments. The full logistic model included neighborhood conditions and sociodemographic and behavioral covariates.

characteristics. Children in neighborhoods with the most unfavorable social conditions had 35% and 43% higher adjusted odds of ≥1 day/week and ≥3 days/week of sleep problems, respectively, than their counterparts from the most-favorable neighborhood social environment. Each of the specific neighborhood social conditions was significantly related to both sleep measures. Children in neighborhoods with safety concerns, garbage/litter, poor/dilapidated housing, and vandalism had 40%, 29%, 26%, and 24% higher adjusted odds of serious sleep problems than children in neighborhoods without these unfavorable conditions, respectively (Table 4).

The built environment index was only significantly related to more serious sleep problems. Children in neighborhoods with the fewest health-promoting amenities had 37% higher adjusted odds of serious sleep problems than children in neighborhoods with the most amenities. Not having an access to parks/playgrounds or a library/bookmobile was associated with 20%–24% higher adjusted odds of serious sleep problems. While there were no significant gender differentials in sleep problems, older adolescents aged 15–17 had, respectively, 2.4 and 3.4 times higher odds of ≥1 day/week and ≥3 day/week of sleep problems than children aged 6–8. No significant racial/ethnic differentials were found for serious sleep problems; however, non-Hispanic white and mixed-race children had 29% and 38% higher adjusted odds of experiencing at least 1 day/week of sleep problems than Hispanic children. Nativity remained a stronger risk factor, with children born to immigrant parents having 22%–29% lower odds of sleep problems than children of US-born parents. Children in single-mother households had 35% higher adjusted odds of serious sleep problems than those in two-parent households. Although household education or income was not significantly related to serious sleep problems, children from higher-SES households were significantly more likely to experience at least 1 day/week of sleep problems than children from lower-SES households (Table 4).

Neighborhood environments and household SES partly accounted for the effects of behavioral factors on sleep problems. Children with no physical activity had 21% and 47% higher adjusted odds of ≥1 day/week and ≥3 day/week of sleep problems, respectively, than children who exercised at least 5 days/week. Children with >2 hours/day of recreational computer use had 20% and 41% higher adjusted odds of ≥1 day/week and ≥3 day/week of sleep problems, respectively, than children with <1 hour/day of computer use. Children exposed to SHS had 23% higher adjusted odds of serious sleep problems than those without exposure (Table 4).

We also examined interaction models of neighborhood, household SES, and behavioral factors by child's age (6–11, 12–17) and gender. However, none of the interactions were statistically significant, and the effects of the covariates on sleep problems were similar for males and females and for younger and older children and adolescents (data not shown).

4. Discussion

Sleep problems are increasingly being recognized as an important public health problem in the United States [3]. Our study showed a marked and consistent increase in the prevalence of childhood sleep problems between 2003 and 2012. Currently, half of all adolescents aged 15–17 and more than one-third of young children aged 6–8, and approximately 21 million school-aged children and adolescents in the US are reported to have at least 1 day/week of sleep problems. What might account for this substantial increase in prevalence? It is conceivable that changes in the social, built, or obesogenic environments, demographic composition of the population, and physical inactivity levels or other sedentary activities may have contributed to the rise in sleep problems among US children—but a more formal analysis of the 2003, 2007, and 2011-2012 National Surveys of Children's Health is needed to shed more light on the rising trend.

To our knowledge, our study is the first to examine variations in sleep problems according to a variety of neighborhood and behavioral factors using a large, nationally representative sample of school-aged children and adolescents. In addition to neighborhood influences, assessing effects of screen time, physical inactivity, and SHS exposure on sleep problems in children represented an important aspect of our study. Increased risks of sleep problems associated with excess television viewing, recreational screen time, physical inactivity, and SHS exposure were independent of neighborhood conditions and household SES, and are consistent with those reported previously in the US and international studies [1, 4, 19, 20, 22, 23].

Neighborhood effects reported here are consistent with limited research that shows higher risks of sleep problems in children associated with unsafe school or neighborhood environment and greater area-based neighborhood distress or socioeconomic disadvantage [1, 2, 32]. In our study, the association between neighborhood factors and sleep problems was not explained or mediated by household SES and behavioral characteristics. Thus, most of the neighborhood effects reported here appear to be either direct or operate through psychosocial or behavioral mechanisms (such as parental stress, family conflict, family cohesiveness, social support, alcohol and substance use) that we did not consider in our analysis.

While neighborhood effects on childhood obesity, physical activity, and mental health have been shown to vary according to child's age and gender, [16, 24, 26, 28] we did not find similar patterns for sleep problems. Thus, when it comes to sleep problems, boys and girls as well as younger and older children appear to be equally vulnerable to unfavorable neighborhood environments.

Higher prevalence of sleep problems in children from higher-SES households is consistent with the patterns observed previously for children and adults in the US and elsewhere [1, 2, 19, 46]. However, some studies have shown an inverse association between SES and sleep problems [4, 20, 47]. The inconsistent SES patterns in sleep behavior across studies may partly be due to differences in sleep measures and data sources [1].

A major strength of our study includes estimating the effects of a variety of neighborhood conditions and composite indices of neighborhood environment on children's sleep problems. Another important contribution of this study is the concurrent evaluation of the impact of both neighborhood factors and health behaviors on sleep problems. Although many features of the neighborhood environment may directly lead to sleep problems (such as noise, violence, and safety fears), we have identified possible casual pathways such as excessive television viewing, physical inactivity, recreational screen time, and SHS exposure which are potentially modifiable through public health policies. Examining specific features of the neighborhood environment brings us closer to intervention (e.g., better amenities, built environments, neighborhood revitalization, crime reduction, affordable housing, community safety, and safe streets) that could lead to better sleep health. The other strengths of our study include the large sample size, the generalizability of our findings, and examination of whether sleep effects of neighborhood conditions, household SES, and behavioral factors vary by age and gender.

This study has limitations. Children's behavioral measures, including sleep behavior, in the NSCH were based on parental reports and may not accurately reflect the true prevalence, particularly among older adolescents. However, prevalence of inadequate sleep reported here is consistent with that reported in other epidemiologic studies [1, 48, 49]. Moreover, previous research has indicated self- or parental reports to be reliable and valid reports of children's sleep patterns and disturbances and has shown satisfactory agreement between objective measures such as actigraphy and parent-report or survey-based measures [50–54]. Second, although neighborhood characteristics considered in our study are important measures of the social environment, they are perceived or parent-reported measures. While subjective ratings of the neighborhood environment may result in underestimation of the neighborhood effects on sleep health, both subjective and objective measures of the neighborhood environment are needed [26, 33]. Third, same-source bias is a possible limitation since neighborhood conditions and sleep problems were reported by the same respondents [16, 55]. The effects of neighborhood conditions on sleep problems could have been underestimated if disadvantaged individuals provided a more positive assessment of neighborhood environment [16, 33, 55]. Individuals in disadvantaged neighborhoods may be more optimistic about their neighborhood situation and, consequently, may downgrade the severity of problems facing their neighborhood surroundings, a phenomenon called "psychological adjustment" [16, 33, 55]. Fourth, our sleep measures were based on parental response to a single question regarding adequacy of child's sleep. No information in the survey was available about sleep quality, sleep duration, and types of sleep problems such as obstructive sleep apnea, difficulty falling or staying asleep through the night, and daytime sleepiness. Fifth, because of the cross-sectional nature of the NSCH, causal inferences about the relationships between neighborhood environment, household SES, behavioral factors, and childhood sleep problems cannot be drawn [16, 17, 26]. Sixth, as with most sample surveys, the potential for nonresponse bias exists for the NSCH, implying that the sample interviewed differed from the targeted child population in a systematic fashion [37]. Since response rates in the NSCH tend to be lower in urban areas and low-income and ethnic-minority populations, differential nonresponse bias might affect (most likely underestimate) the impact of neighborhood disadvantage, individual SES, and race/ethnicity on sleep problems [37]. However, the nonresponse adjustment to the sampling weights in the NSCH might have reduced the potential magnitude of these biases [37]. Lastly, the increased use of cell/mobile phone use in recent years, especially among young, minority, renters, and low-income adults, may be an additional source of noncoverage bias for landline only surveys such as the 2007 NSCH [56, 57].

In conclusion, the evidence presented here suggests that favorable neighborhood conditions and positive health behaviors are significantly associated with reduced risk of sleep problems in children, which, in turn, may support reductions in overall child health inequalities given the wide-ranging health effects of poor sleep. While behavioral changes such as increased physical activity, reduced television viewing and computer use, and reduced exposure to secondhand smoke can be beneficial in promoting children's sleep health, social policy measures aimed at improving the broader social and physical environments can be vital to improving overall child health in general and their sleep health in particular. Continued surveillance and monitoring of the prevalence of childhood sleep problems as well as its determinants are essential in order to better understand the role of broader societal factors and health behaviors and to design effective public health interventions, including public awareness and educational campaigns [46].

Human Subjects Review

No IRB approval was required for this study, which is based on the secondary analysis of a public-use federal database.

Conflict of Interests

The authors declare no conflict of interests.

Disclaimer

The views expressed are the authors' and not necessarily those of the Health Resources and Services Administration or the US Department of Health and Human Services.

References

[1] A. Smaldone, J. C. Honig, and M. W. Byrne, "Sleepless in America: inadequate sleep and relationships to health and well-being of our nation's children," *Pediatrics*, vol. 119, supplement 1, pp. S29–S37, 2007.

[2] M. Moore, H. L. Kirchner, D. Drotar, N. Johnson, C. Rosen, and S. Redline, "Correlates of adolescent sleep time and variability in sleep time: the role of individual and health related characteristics," *Sleep Medicine*, vol. 12, no. 3, pp. 239–245, 2011.

[3] H. R. Colten and B. M. Altevogt, *Sleep Disorders and Sleep Deprivation: An Unmet Public Health Problem*, Institute of Medicine, National Academies Press, Washington, DC, USA, 2006.

[4] A. M. Moran and D. E. Everhart, "Adolescent sleep: review of characteristics, consequences, and intervention," *Journal of Sleep Disorders: Treatment & Care*, vol. 1, no. 2, pp. 1–8, 2012.

[5] E. J. Paavonen, K. Räikkönen, J. Lahti et al., "Short sleep duration and behavioral symptoms of attention-deficit/hyperactivity disorder in healthy 7- to 8-year-old children," *Pediatrics*, vol. 123, no. 5, pp. e857–e864, 2009.

[6] A. R. Wolfson and M. A. Carskadon, "Understanding adolescents' sleep patterns and school performance: a critical appraisal," *Sleep Medicine Reviews*, vol. 7, no. 6, pp. 491–506, 2003.

[7] H. Taras and W. Potts-Datema, "Sleep and student performance at school," *Journal of School Health*, vol. 75, no. 7, pp. 248–254, 2005.

[8] S. Ravid, I. Afek, S. Suraiya, E. Shahar, and G. Pillar, "Sleep disturbances are associated with reduced school achievements in first-grade pupils," *Developmental Neuropsychology*, vol. 34, no. 5, pp. 574–587, 2009.

[9] J. A. Owens, "Sleep disorders and attention-deficit/hyperactivity disorder," *Current Psychiatry Reports*, vol. 10, no. 5, pp. 439–444, 2008.

[10] B. H. Hansen, B. Skirbekk, B. Oerbeck, T. Wentzel-Larsen, and H. Kristensen, "Associations between sleep problems and attentional and behavioral functioning in children with anxiety disorders and ADHD," *Behavioral Sleep Medicine*, 2013.

[11] R. Gruber, S. Michaelson, L. Bergmame et al., "Short sleep duration is associated with teacher-reported inattention and cognitive problems in healthy school-aged children," *Nature and Science of Sleep*, vol. 4, pp. 33–40, 2012.

[12] J. A. Mitchell, D. Rodriguez, K. H. Schmitz, and J. Audrain-McGovern, "Sleep duration and adolescent obesity," *Pediatrics*, vol. 131, no. 5, pp. 1–7, 2013.

[13] J. Liu, J. Hay, D. Joshi, B. E. Faught, T. Wade, and J. Cairney, "Sleep difficulties and obesity among preadolescents," *Canadian Journal of Public Health*, vol. 102, no. 2, pp. 139–143, 2011.

[14] G. E. Silva, J. L. Goodwin, S. Parthasarathy et al., "Longitudinal association between short sleep, body weight, and emotional and learning problems in Hispanic and Caucasian children," *Sleep*, vol. 34, no. 9, pp. 1197–1205, 2011.

[15] L. S. Nielsen, K. V. Danielsen, and T. I. A. Sørensen, "Short sleep duration as a possible cause of obesity: critical analysis of the epidemiological evidence," *Obesity Reviews*, vol. 12, no. 2, pp. 78–92, 2011.

[16] G. K. Singh and R. M. Ghandour, "Impact of neighborhood social conditions and household socioeconomic status on behavioral problems among US children," *Maternal and Child Health Journal*, vol. 16, supplement 1, pp. S158–S169, 2012.

[17] G. K. Singh and S. M. Yu, "The impact of ethnic-immigrant status and obesity-related risk factors on behavioral problems among US children and adolescents," *Scientifica*, vol. 2012, Article ID 648152, 14 pages, 2012.

[18] National Center for Health Statistics, *The National Survey of Children's Health (NSCH), 2007: The Public Use Data File and Documentation*, US Department of Health and Human Services, Hyattsville, Md, USA, 2009.

[19] A. R. Arman, P. Ay, N. P. Fis et al., "Association of sleep duration with socio-economic status and behavioural problems among schoolchildren," *Acta Paediatrica*, vol. 100, no. 3, pp. 420–424, 2011.

[20] K. Yolton, Y. Xu, J. Khoury et al., "Associations between secondhand smoke exposure and sleep patterns in children," *Pediatrics*, vol. 125, no. 2, pp. e261–e268, 2010.

[21] J. C. Spilsbury, A. Storfer-Isser, D. Drotar et al., "Sleep behavior in an urban US sample of school-aged children," *Archives of Pediatrics and Adolescent Medicine*, vol. 158, no. 10, pp. 988–994, 2004.

[22] J. G. Johnson, P. Cohen, S. Kasen, M. B. First, and J. S. Brook, "Association between television viewing and sleep problems during adolescence and early adulthood," *Archives of Pediatrics and Adolescent Medicine*, vol. 158, no. 6, pp. 562–568, 2004.

[23] H. M. Al-Hazzaa, A. O. Musaiger, N. A. Abahussain, H. I. Al-Sobayel, and D. M. Qahwaji, "Lifestyle correlates of self-reported sleep duration among Saudi adolescents: a multicentre school-based cross-sectional study," *Child: Care, Health and Development*, 2013.

[24] A. R. Pebley and N. Sastry, "Neighborhoods, poverty, and children's well-being," in *Social Inequality*, K. M. Neckerman, Ed., pp. 119–144, Russell Sage Foundation, New York, NY, USA, 2004.

[25] A. V. Diez Roux and C. Mair, "Neighborhoods and health," *Annals of the New York Academy of Sciences*, vol. 1186, pp. 125–145, 2010.

[26] G. K. Singh, M. Siahpush, and M. D. Kogan, "Neighborhood socioeconomic conditions, built environments, and childhood obesity," *Health Affairs*, vol. 29, no. 3, pp. 503–512, 2010.

[27] M. A. Papas, A. J. Alberg, R. Ewing, K. J. Helzlsouer, T. L. Gary, and A. C. Klassen, "The built environment and obesity," *Epidemiologic Reviews*, vol. 29, no. 1, pp. 129–143, 2007.

[28] G. K. Singh, M. D. Kogan, P. C. Van Dyck, and M. Siahpush, "Racial/ethnic, socioeconomic, and behavioral determinants of childhood and adolescent obesity in the United States: analyzing independent and joint associations," *Annals of Epidemiology*, vol. 18, no. 9, pp. 682–695, 2008.

[29] Y. Xue, T. Leventhal, J. Brooks-Gunn, and F. J. Earls, "Neighborhood residence and mental health problems of 5- to 11-year-olds," *Archives of General Psychiatry*, vol. 62, no. 5, pp. 554–563, 2005.

[30] T. Leventhal and J. Brooks-Gunn, "The neighborhoods they live in: the effects of neighborhood residence on child and adolescent outcomes," *Psychological Bulletin*, vol. 126, no. 2, pp. 309–337, 2000.

[31] G. W. Evans, "The built environment and mental health," *Journal of Urban Health*, vol. 80, no. 4, pp. 536–555, 2003.

[32] J. C. Spilsbury, A. Storfer-Isser, H. L. Kirchner et al., "Neighborhood disadvantage as a risk factor for pediatric obstructive sleep apnea," *Journal of Pediatrics*, vol. 149, no. 3, pp. 342–347, 2006.

[33] I. Kawachi and L. F. Berkman, "Introduction," in *Neighborhoods and Health*, I. Kawachi and L. F. Berkman, Eds., pp. 1–19, Oxford University Press, New York, NY, USA, 2003.

[34] J. Heymann and A. Fischer, "Neighborhoods, health research, and its relevance to public policy," in *Neighborhoods and Health*, I. Kawachi and L. F. Berkman, Eds., pp. 335–347, Oxford University Press, New York, NY, USA, 2003.

[35] US Department of Health and Human Services, Healthy People 2020, 2013, http://www.healthypeople.gov/2020/default.aspx .

[36] Health Resources and Services Administration, Maternal and Child Health Bureau, *The National Survey of Children's Health 2007: The Health and Well-Being of Children, A Portrait of States and the Nation*, US Department of Health and Human Services, Rockville, Md, USA, 2009.

[37] S. J. Blumberg, E. B. Foster, A. M. Frasier et al., "Design and operation of the National Survey of Children's Health, 2007," *Vital and Health Statistics*, vol. 1, no. 55, pp. 1–149, 2012.

[38] S. J. Blumberg, L. Olson, M. R. Frankel, L. Osborn, K. P. Srinath, and P. Giambo, "Design and operation of the National Survey of Children's Health, 2003," *Vital and Health Statistics*, vol. 1, no. 43, pp. 1–124, 2005.

[39] National Center for Health Statistics, *The National Survey of Children's Health (NSCH), 2011-2012: The Public Use Data File and Documentation*, US Department of Health and Human Services, Hyattsville, Md, USA, 2013, http://www.cdc.gov/nchs/slaits/nsch.htm.

[40] National Center for Health Statistics, *Health, United States, 2011 with Special Feature on Socioeconomic Status and Health*, US Department of Health and Human Services, Hyattsville, Md, USA, 2012.

[41] National Center for Health Statistics, *The National Survey of Children's Health (NSCH), 2003: The Public Use Data File*, US Department of Health and Human Services, Hyattsville, Md, USA, 2005, http://www.cdc.gov/nchs/slaits/nsch.htm.

[42] G. K. Singh, S. M. Yu, and M. D. Kogan, "Health, chronic conditions, and behavioral risk disparities amongUS immigrant children and adolescents," *Public Health Reports*. In press.

[43] R. Wilkinson and M. Marmot, *Social Determinants of Health: The Solid Facts*, World Health Organization, Regional Office for Europe, Copenhagen, Denmark, 2nd edition, 2003.

[44] N. Adler, J. Stewart, S. Cohen et al., *Reaching for a Healthier Life: Facts on Socioeconomic Status and Health in the US*, The John D. and Catherine T. Macarthur Foundation Research Network on Socioeconomic Status and Health, San Francisco, Calif, USA, 2009.

[45] SUDAAN, *Software for the Statistical Analysis of Correlated Data, Release 10.0.1*, Research Triangle Institute, Research Triangle Park, NC, USA, 2009.

[46] Centers for Disease Control and Prevention, "Unhealthy sleep-related behaviors-12 states, 2009," *Morbidity and Mortality Weekly Report*, vol. 60, no. 8, pp. 233–238, 2011.

[47] M. A. Stein, J. Mendelsohn, W. H. Obermeyer, J. Amromin, and R. Benca, "Sleep and behavior problems in school-aged children," *Pediatrics*, vol. 107, no. 4, article E60, 2001.

[48] National Sleep Foundation, "Children and sleep: sleep in America poll," 2004, http://www.sleepfoundation.org/sites/default/files/FINAL%20SOF%202004.pdf.

[49] National Sleep Foundation, "Teens and sleep: sleep in America poll," 2006, http://www.sleepfoundation.org/sites/default/files/2006_summary_of_findings.pdf.

[50] A. R. Wolfson, M. A. Carskadon, C. Acebo et al., "Evidence for the validity of a sleep habits survey for adolescents," *Sleep*, vol. 26, no. 2, pp. 213–216, 2003.

[51] L. J. Meltzer, K. T. Avis, S. Biggs et al., "The children's report of sleep patterns (CRSP): a self-report measure of sleep for school-aged children," *Journal of Clinical Sleep Medicine*, vol. 9, no. 3, pp. 235–245, 2013.

[52] C. A. Kushida, A. Chang, C. Gadkary, C. Guilleminault, O. Carrillo, and W. C. Dement, "Comparison of actigraphic, polysomnographic, and subjective assessment of sleep parameters in sleep-disordered patients," *Sleep Medicine*, vol. 2, no. 5, pp. 389–396, 2001.

[53] H. Werner, L. Molinari, C. Guyer, and O. G. Jenni, "Agreement rates between actigraphy, diary, and questionnaire for children's sleep patterns," *Archives of Pediatrics and Adolescent Medicine*, vol. 162, no. 4, pp. 350–358, 2008.

[54] S. W. Lockley, D. J. Skene, and J. Arendt, "Comparison between subjective and actigraphic measurement of sleep and sleep rhythms," *Journal of Sleep Research*, vol. 8, no. 3, pp. 175–183, 1999.

[55] S. Macintyre and A. Ellaway, "Neighborhoods and health: an overview," in *Neighborhoods and Health*, I. Kawachi and L. F. Berkman, Eds., pp. 20–42, Oxford University Press, New York, NY, USA, 2003.

[56] S. J. Blumberg and J. V. Luke, "Reevaluating the need for concern regarding noncoverage bias in landline surveys," *American Journal of Public Health*, vol. 99, no. 10, pp. 1806–1810, 2009.

[57] S. J. Blumberg and J. V. Luke, *Wireless Substitution: Early Release of Estimates from the National Health Interview Survey, January-June 2008*, National Center for Health Statistics, 2008, http://www.cdc.gov/nchs/data/nhis/earlyrelease/wireless200-812.pdf.

28

The Negative Effect of Carpal Tunnel Syndrome on Sleep Quality

Ashish Patel,[1,2] **Maya Deza Culbertson,**[1] **Archit Patel,**[1] **Jenifer Hashem,**[1] **Jinny Jacob,**[1] **David Edelstein,**[1] **and Jack Choueka**[1]

[1] *Maimonides Medical Center, Department of Orthopaedic Surgery, 927 49th Street, Brooklyn, NY 11219, USA*
[2] *SUNY Downstate Medical Center, 450 Clarkson Avenue, Brooklyn, NY 11203, USA*

Correspondence should be addressed to Jenifer Hashem; jhashem@maimonidesmed.org

Academic Editor: Marco Zucconi

Objective. Sleep disturbances are common in patients with carpal tunnel syndrome (CTS). This study investigates the impact of CTS on sleep quality and clarifies the magnitude of this relationship. *Methods.* This is a prospective investigation of patients with CTS. Patients responded to the Levine-Katz Carpal Tunnel and the Pittsburgh Sleep Quality Index (PSQI) questionnaires to assess symptom severity and quality, respectively. Descriptive and bivariate analyses summarized the findings and assessed the correlations between CTS severity and sleep quality parameters. *Results.* 66 patients (53F, 13M) were enrolled. Patients reported a sleep latency of 30.0 (±22.5) minutes, with a total sleep time of 5.5 (±1.8) hours nightly. Global PSQI score was 9.0 (±3.8); 80% of patients demonstrated a significant reduction in sleep quality (global PSQI score > 5). Increased CTS symptom and functional severity both resulted in a significant reduction in quality and time asleep. Both significantly correlated with subjective sleep latency, sleep disturbance, use of sleep promoting medications, daytime dysfunction, and overall global PSQI score. *Conclusions.* The findings confirm the correlation of sleep disturbances to CTS, that is, significant reduction of sleep duration and a correlation to sleep quality. Patients sleep 2.5 hours less than recommended and are at risk for comorbid conditions.

1. Introduction

The critical relationship between sleep, health, and overall well-being is gaining greater attention. The National Sleep Foundation recommends 7 to 9 sleep hours per night for adequate rest and repair [1].Unfortunately, sleep curtailment has become increasingly prevalent in modern day society due to higher demands, longer working hours, and the introduction of radio, television,and the internet [1]. Recent investigations have demonstrated the negative impact of declining sleep quality on the human body. It is thought that reductions in sleep quality results in longer exposure to elevated sympathetic nervous system activity and to waking physical and psychological stressors [2]. Consequently, there is growing evidence that significant correlations exist between poor sleep quality and the development of comorbid conditions including obesity, hypertension, diabetes mellitus, pain, and even death [2–9].

Patients with carpal tunnel syndrome (CTS) consistently report nighttime symptoms including multiple awakenings due to hand pain and numbness. It is thought that wrist malposition during sleep acutely exacerbates CTS symptoms by increasing the pressure within the carpal canal [10]. For the majority of patients, night symptoms and subsequent daytime dysfunction are the impetus to seek medical intervention. While numerous reports have quantified the impact of CTS on functional limitations [10–14], the critical relationship between CTS and sleep quality is rather limited. The authors are aware of just a single report studying the effects of CTS on sleep. Using a self-reported survey in 34 CTS patients, Lehtinen et al. [15] found that CTS results in frequent nighttime awakenings, an increase in fragmented sleep, and an increase in daytime sleepiness and dysfunction versus a control database of 1600 Finns.The magnitude and correlation of the relationship between CTS symptom severity and sleep quality was not studied. Understanding this relationship will provide improved patient education regarding sleep-related symptoms and a platform for future investigations studying outcomes of CTS treatment modalities on sleep restoration.

The objective of this study was to investigate the impact of CTS on sleep quality. Specifically, this study aims to answer the following questions: (1) to what magnitude does CTS adversely affect sleep quality and duration; (2) what areas of sleep quality are affected by CTS; and finally (3) is there a relationship between CTS functional severity and the impact on sleep quality parameters as assessed by validated outcome measures.

2. Methods

2.1. Study Sample. This study is a prospective clinical investigation of consecutive patients presenting to an outpatient orthopaedic hand surgeon's clinic with symptoms consistent with carpal tunnel syndrome (CTS). Each patient was evaluated by the senior author (Jack Choueka) and enrolled into the study if they met inclusion/exclusion criteria including age over 18, history, physical examination (i.e., sensory neuropathy or pain in the hand within the median nerve distribution, thenar muscle weakness/atrophy, and positive Tinel's and Phalen's test), and EMG data consistent with CTS. Subjects were excluded if they reported the following: previous hand trauma, previous hand surgery, inflammatory arthritis, or sleep pathology (i.e., sleep apnea, restless leg syndrome, etc.). The study was approved by our institutional review board prior to patient enrollment.

2.2. Data Collection. Once enrolled into this study, patients were asked to provide responses to a questionnaire packet, which included basic demographic information, a visual analog scale (VAS) for sleep quality and hand pain, the Levine-Katz carpal tunnel questionnaire [16] (Boston carpal tunnel questionnaire), and the Pittsburgh Sleep Quality Index (PSQI) [17].

2.2.1. Demographic Information. Demographic information collected as part of routine evaluation included age, gender, symptomatic hand, and duration of symptoms.

2.2.2. Visual Analog Scale. The Visual Analog Scale (VAS) consisted of 2 separate lines: the VAS-Pain scale and VAS-Sleep scale. Patients were asked to mark the severity of hand pain with an "X" on a 100-point scale (10 cm line): "0" indicating no pain and "100" indicating the worst pain imaginable. Patients were also asked to mark their sleep quality with an "X" on a 100-point scale (10 cm line): "0" indicating poor sleep and "100" indicating excellent sleep. The measurement in millimeters was used as the VAS score.

2.2.3. Levine-Katz Carpal Tunnel Questionnaire [16]. The Levine-Katz (Boston) carpal tunnel questionnaire is a frequently used patient-reported questionnaire to assess patients with carpal tunnel syndrome. There are 19 questions with 2 outcome scores: the symptom severity score (SSS) and the function status scale (FSS). The symptoms severity score includes multiple questions regarding pain and numbness/tingling and includes questions regarding sleep impact. The FSS assesses the patient's ability to perform activities of daily living. Each response is scored from 1 point (mildest) to 5 points (most severe) and averaged to obtain the SSS and FSS (scored 1–5). The Levine-Katz questionnaire has been proven to be reproducible, internally consistent, and responsive to clinical change.

2.2.4. Pittsburgh Sleep Quality Index [17]. The Pittsburgh Sleep Quality Index (PSQI) is a patient-reported questionnaire which assesses sleep quality over a 1-month time interval. There are 19 questions which generate seven "component" scores (scored 0–3, 0 = no pathology, 3 = greatest pathology): C1—subjective sleep quality, C2—sleep latency, C3—sleep duration, C4—habitual sleep efficiency, C5—sleep disturbances, C6—use of sleeping medication, and C7—daytime dysfunction. The sum of the component scores yields the "global PSQI Score" (0–21). The PSQI has been shown to be internally homogenous, consistent, and clinically responsive to changes in sleep 17.

2.3. Statistical Analysis. Descriptive statistics including medians, standard deviations, and minimum/maximum range were used to summarize questionnaire responses where appropriate. Bivariate analysis was used to investigate associations between sleep parameters (PSQI) and CTS parameters SSS and FSS (Levine-Katz). To address known differences in sleep quality measures based on gender and age, data were also stratified by gender and age group. Three age groups were defined: "young adults" (age 25–45), "adults" (45–65), and "elderly" (65 years or older). Analyses were carried out on all subjects and then repeated on gender- and age-stratified groups. Differences between groups were examined by ANOVA. Analysis was conducted using SPSS software (Chicago, ILL) with a level of significance set at $P < 0.05$.

3. Results

3.1. Patient Sample. 66 patients were enrolled into this study. There were 53 females and 13 males, with a median age of 55.4 ± 15.4 years (range = 24.9–85.7 years). 15 patients were classified as "young adults," 27 as "adults," and 19 as "elderly." Age data were missing for five subjects. Approximately 33% of patients had symptoms in their right hand, 33% in their left hand, and 33% in both hands. Patients reported CTS symptoms for a median duration of 12 ± 11.1 months (range = 1–48 months). There were no significant differences in symptom duration between gender or age strata.

3.2. CTS Parameters. The severity of CTS was assessed using the VAS-Pain scale and the symptom severity score (SSS) and functional status score (FSS) of the Boston carpal tunnel questionnaire. The median VAS-Pain score was 67 ± 27 mm (range = 3–100 mm). The median (standard deviation) SSS was 3.0 ± 0.8 (range = 1.5–4.5). The median FSS was 2.4 ± 0.9 (range = 1.0–4.3). Figure 1 illustrates the distribution of patients in each CTS disability group. VAS-Pain and SSS scores showed no significant differences between genders or age groups. Females exhibited significantly higher FSS scores

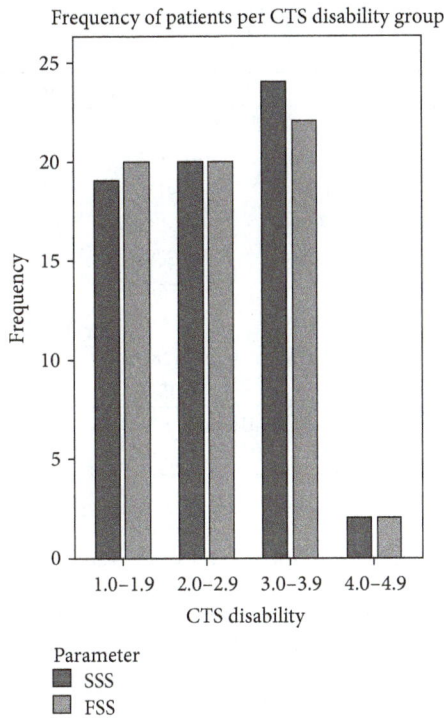

FIGURE 1: Frequency of patients versus increasing CTS disability (SSS and FSS) assessed using the Levine-Katz questionnaire.

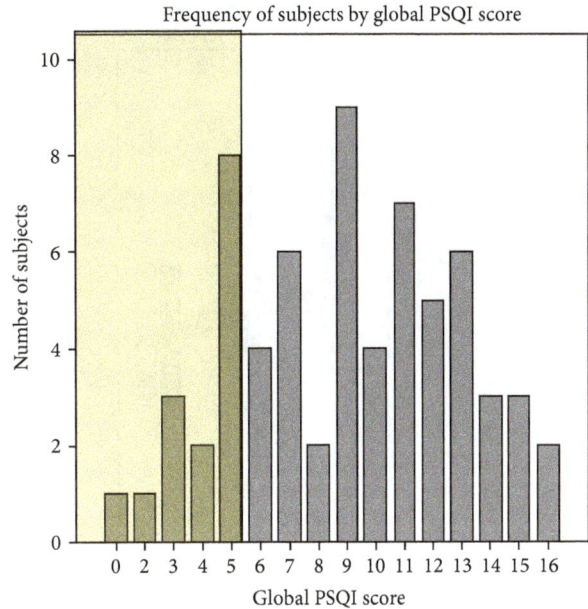

FIGURE 2: Global PSQI score over the entire study group. The shaded area is considered normal sleep.

than males (2.8 ± 0.91 for females versus 2.0 ± 0.69 for males). There was no difference in FSS between age strata.

3.3. Sleep Data.

Sleep quality was assessed using the VAS-Sleep scale and the PSQI questionnaire. The median (standard deviation) VAS-Sleep score was 40.5 (±28.7) mm (range = 0–100 mm). Patients reported a median (standard deviation) sleep latency of 30.0 (±22.5) minutes (range = 0–120 min) with a median (standard deviation) total sleep time of 5.5 (±1.8) hours (range = 1–10 hours). There were no significant differences between genders or age groups for VAS-Sleep scores, sleep latencies, or total sleep times.

The median (standard deviation) global PSQI score was 9.0 (±3.8) (range = 0–16). PSQI did not change significantly between genders or age groups. Global PSQI scores of greater than 5 are reported to indicate poor sleep quality [17]. 78% of patients had global PSQI scores greater than 5. Figure 2 illustrates the distribution of PSQI score over the entire study group. Component score analysis is illustrated in Figure 3.

3.4. CTS and Sleep Correlations.

No correlations were evident between age, gender, or duration of symptoms and sleep parameters. Significant correlations were observed between VAS-Pain and SSS/FSS ($r = 0.78$, $P < 0.000$ and $r = 0.57$, $P < 0.000$ resp.,) and between VAS-Sleep and the PSQI ($r = -47$, $P < 0.000$). Significant correlations were evident between CTS parameters (SSS/FSS), the global PSQI score, and 5 of the 7 PSQI subcomponent sleep parameters. Increasing CTS severity (SSS and/or FSS) resulted in a significant reduction in total hours asleep ($r = -0.288$, $P = 0.023$; Figure 4)

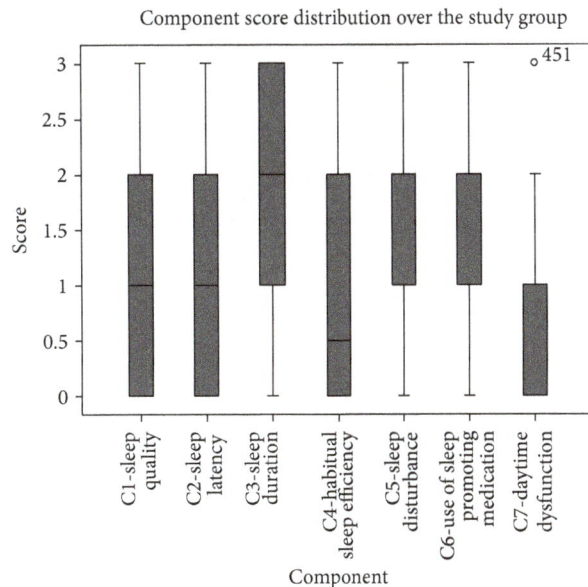

FIGURE 3: Individual sleep component analysis. Patients demonstrated sleep dysfunction in all 7 subcategories. Sleep duration, sleep disturbance, and use of sleep promoting medications were the parameters greatest effected. Bars indicate 95% min and max values.

and sleep quality ($r = -0.328$, $P = 0.008$). Increasing CTS severity (SSS/FSS) also resulted in a significant increase in sleep latency ($r = 0.339$, $P = 0.006$), sleep disturbance ($r = 0.402$, $P = 0.001$), use of sleep promoting medications ($r = 0.529$, $P < 0.000$), daytime dysfunction ($r = 0.289$, $P = 0.019$), and overall global PSQI score ($r = 0.506$, $P < 0.000$; Figure 5). CTS parameters were grouped according to the symptom severity score (SSS) and functional severity score

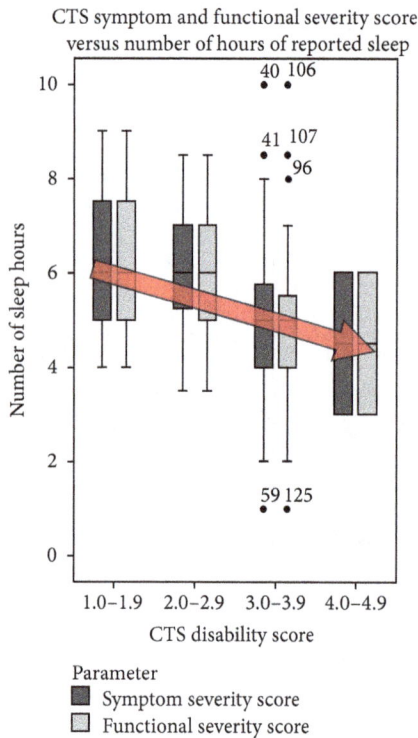

FIGURE 4: CTS disability score (SSS and FSS) versus total number of hours asleep. A significant negative correlation was demonstrated between increasing CTS and total sleep hours ($r = -0.288$, $P < 0.023$). Bars indicate 95% min and max values.

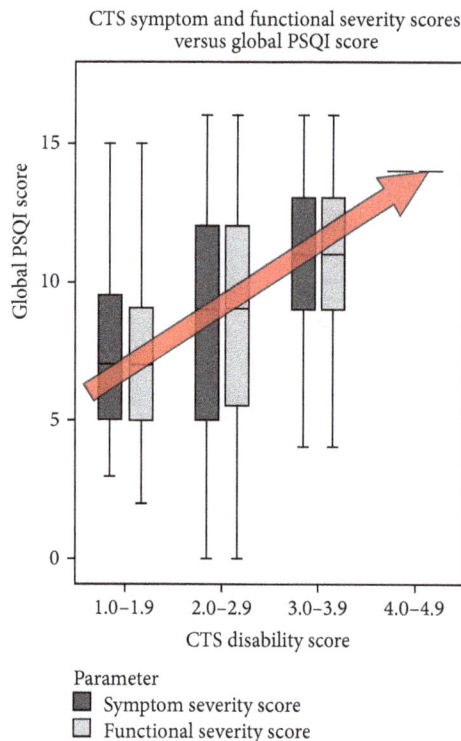

FIGURE 5: CTS disability score (SSS and FSS) versus global PSQI. A significant correlation was demonstrated between increasing CTS and increasing global PSQI score ($r = 0.506$, $P < 0.000$). Bars indicate 95% min and max values.

TABLE 1: Significant correlations of CTS and sleep parameters by gender.

Variable	By	Correlation	n	P value
Gender: Female				
VAS-Sleep	VAS-Pain	−0.3220	47	0.0273
PSQI	VAS-Pain	0.4157	47	0.0037
SSS	VAS-Sleep	−0.4358	48	0.0020
SSS	Latency	0.3391	51	0.0149
SSS	PSQI	0.5644	52	<0.0001
FSS	VAS-Sleep	−0.3498	47	0.0159
FSS	Hours of sleep	−0.2896	49	0.0435
FSS	PSQI	0.4596	51	0.0007
Gender: male				
FSS	PSQI	0.5905	13	0.0336

TABLE 2: Significant correlations of CTS and sleep parameters by age strata.

Variable	By	Correlation	n	P value
Young adults (25–45 years)				
PSQI	VAS-Pain	0.5735	14	0.0320
SSS	PSQI	0.7151	15	0.0027
FSS	VAS-Sleep	−0.6312	14	0.0155
FSS	Latency	0.7417	15	0.0016
FSS	PSQI	0.669	15	0.0064
Adults (45–65 years)				
SSS	VAS-Sleep	−0.4229	26	0.0314
Elderly (>65 years)				
No significant differences between CTS and sleep parameters				

(FSS) into discrete groups (0.0–0.9, 1.0–1.9, 2.0–2.9, 3.0–3.9, and 4.0–5.0).

When subjects were examined by gender, several significant correlations were found between CTS and sleep parameters, particularly in females. Among female subjects, significant correlations were observed between VAS-Pain and VAS-Sleep as well as VAS-Pain and PSQI scores. SSS scores in females also correlated significantly with VAS-Pain, sleep latency, and PSQI. FSS scores in females correlated to VAS-Sleep scores, hours of sleep, and PSQI. Among males, the only significant correlation found was between FSS and PSQI (Table 1).

When correlations were examined in the context of age strata, several correlations were found, primarily in young adults. In subjects young adults between the ages of 25 and 45, significant correlations with the PSQI were observed in VAS-Pain as well as SSS. Likewise, FSS functional scores were correlated with VAS-Sleep scores, sleep latency, and the PSQI. Among adults aged 45–65, the only significant correlation observed was between SSS and VAS-Sleep scores. No significant correlations were observed between CTS and sleep parameters in elderly subjects aged 65 or above (Table 2).

4. Discussion

The effect of chronic pain syndromes (i.e., lower back pain) on sleep quality/duration is well known and has been extensively studied [18–21]. Yet CTS, the most common neurocompressive disorder, which is intimately tied to sleep symptoms, has received little attention despite the frequency of this complaint. Sleep symptoms are routinely solicited and expressed during patient presentation, although it is rarely quantified or objectively used as a parameter for treatment. The majority of attention is being directed toward the patient's pain and functional symptoms. Awareness into the deleterious effects of CTS on sleep quality can help educate patients regarding the natural course of their disease. It can also provide the physician with objective data concerning the severity of the patient's condition and potentially offer criteria for treatment.

Within our cohort, ~80% of patients demonstrated clinically significant sleep disturbances (global PSQI scores > 5); a comparable group of asymptomatic subjects examined by Buysse et al., during the original characterization of the PSQI, yielded a median global score of 2.67 ($\pm$1.70) versus the median 9.0 ($\pm$3.8) observed in our cohort [17]. Furthermore, our data yielded a reported median of 5.5 hours of sleep per night, 2.5 hours less than that recommended by the National Sleep Foundation (mean 8 hours/night), and 1.2 hours less than the approximate 6.7 hours reported by control subjects in the Buysse study [1, 17]. A nightly sleep debt of this magnitude places patients at a significantly increased risk for developing or exacerbating comorbid conditions and compromising overall health and well-being.

The deleterious effects of sleep deprivation on various medical conditions have been investigated. Knutson and Turek [22] demonstrated a direct relationship between the PSQI, perceived sleep debt, and HbA1c levels; from this, the authors purport that optimizing sleep duration/quality may improve glucose regulation in type II diabetics. Gangwisch et al. demonstrated significantly increased rates of developing hypertension in subjects that slept <5 hours/night. Additionally, the 10–20% reduction in blood pressure during sleep over 24-hour periods is only partially attained by these subjects [2]. Similar findings have been confirmed by other investigators, including Sampaio et al, who found that reduced sleep quality in elderly patients correlated with higher body mass indices and increased risks of depression; this and similar studies add to the body of evidence indicating that that sleep deprivation results in significant harm to one's health [3, 4, 23–25].

Previous work on sleep disturbances in patients contending with chronic pain reinforces the notion that pain disorders result in significant sleep disruptions that can cause subsequent health problems. A study by Covarrubias-Gomez and Mendoza-Reyes on the effects of chronic, nonmalignant pain on sleep found that 89% of subjects (276/311) exhibited poor sleep quality, defined as PSQI scores of 5 or above [26]. Similarly, Shyen et al. reported increased delays in sleep onset, sleep anxiety, and sleep disordered breathing as well as night awakening episodes and parasomnias in children with idiopathic juvenile arthritis [27]. In addition to the effects of pain on sleep, recent work suggests a mechanism for the exacerbation of pain response following sleep disruption. A 2013 functional imaging study employing positron emission and magnetic resonance imaging to elucidate the relationship between pain response and mu opioid receptor (MOR) activity found a positive correlation between sleep disruption and MOR-ligand binding potential [28]. This preliminary study suggests a potential feedback loop that can further intensify both chronic pain and sleep disturbances.

During this investigation, the PSQI and the symptom severity score and functional status score from the Levine-Katz carpal tunnel questionnaire revealed important relationships between sleep and CTS. The symptom severity score, as expected, was directly correlated with the PSQI due to its inherent inclusion of sleep impact questions. More interestingly, the increasing FSS (which does not have the same direct correlation to sleep impact) demonstrated that patients experienced a linear decrease in sleep quality (global PSQI score). More specific results showed that increasing severity of CTS (SSS and FSS) was found to increase the time required to fall asleep and decreased total sleep time (PSQI questions 1 and 4). As CTS pathology worsened, so did night pain. Careful examination of questionnaire responses revealed a significant relationship between CTS severity and the frequency of night time awakenings: specifically from pain attacks (PSQI questions 6 and 13). Patients more frequently turned to sleep promoting medications (question 15) to reduce their nightly sleep debt. Additionally, escalating sleep deprivation was found to lead to increasing daytime dysfunction, possibly compromising work and social activities. This cascade of events equates to increasing morbidity to the patient and is often the impetus for seeking medical intervention.

Several limitations exist in this investigation. Firstly, although comorbid sleep pathology was queried during patient enrollment, extensive screening, that is, sleep polysomnography testing, was not implemented prior to data collection. Patients with undiagnosed sleep disturbances may have been recruited into this investigation. Secondly, additional objective measures of CTS severity (i.e., grip strength) were not collected routinely for this study. These objective data would have complemented subjective patient reported questionnaire responses. Finally, quantitative nerve conduction data was not collected to study the correlation between symptom severity, nerve injury, and sleep quality. However, Chang et al. [29] in their study from 2008 have indicated that there is no definitive correlation between the Levine Katz questionnaire (SSS/FSS) and nerve injury as assessed by electrophysiologic data. In addition, this study has raised the interesting question of a cyclic style "cause and effect" of sleep deprivation and functionality in activities of daily life where pain and dysfunction as assessed by the FSS were directly correlated to decreased sleep quality. It is likely that the decreased sleep quality further reduced the FSS score since the activities of daily living were directly affected by sleep deprivation.

CTS is the most common neurocompressive disorder in human population with approximately 250,000–300,000 carpal tunnel releases preformed in the United States each year [30]. Sleep symptoms are frequently reported in patients with CTS, although they are generally given limited attention. This study has established the preliminary relationships between subjective CTS severity (using patient-reported questionnaires) and the subsequent effect on subjective sleep quality (using patient-reported questionnaires). This study sheds some light on a critical relationship that is poorly understood and hopes to raise awareness of the negative impacts of carpal tunnel syndrome on a variety of sleep parameters. Future research in this field will attempt to investigate the impact of operative and nonoperative treatment on the resolution of CTS symptoms and the subsequent effect on sleep quality.

Disclosure

Level of evidence is prognostic, Level II.

Conflict of Interests

The authors declare that there is no conflict of interests regarding the publication of this paper.

Acknowledgment

Funding was obtained from Maimonides Medical Center Research Foundation grant.

References

[1] NSF, "Sleep in America," Poll. Washington, National Sleep Foundation, Washington, DC, USA, 2002, http://www.sleep-foundation.org/.

[2] J. E. Gangwisch, S. B. Heymsfield, B. Boden-Albala et al., "Short sleep duration as a risk factor for hypertension: analyses of the first National Health and Nutrition Examination Survey," Hypertension, vol. 47, no. 5, pp. 833–839, 2006.

[3] F. P. Cappuccio, L. D'Elia, P. Strazzullo, and M. A. Miller, "Sleep duration and all-cause mortality: a systematic review and meta-analysis of prospective studies," Sleep, vol. 33, no. 5, pp. 585–592, 2010.

[4] F. P. Cappuccio, L. D'Elia, P. Strazzullo, and M. A. Miller, "Quantity and quality of sleep and incidence of type 2 diabetes: a systematic review and meta-analysis," Diabetes Care, vol. 33, no. 2, pp. 414–420, 2010.

[5] J. E. Gangwisch, D. Malaspina, B. Boden-Albala, and S. B. Heymsfield, "Inadequate sleep as a risk factor for obesity: analyses of the NHANES I," Sleep, vol. 28, no. 10, pp. 1289–1296, 2005.

[6] K. L. Knutson, P. J. Rathouz, L. L. Yan, K. Liu, and D. S. Lauderdale, "Stability of the Pittsburgh sleep quality index and the epworth sleepiness questionnaires over 1 year in early middle-aqed adults: the CARDIA study," Sleep, vol. 29, no. 11, pp. 1503–1506, 2006.

[7] K. L. Knutson, A. M. Ryden, B. A. Mander, and E. Van Cauter, "Role of sleep duration and quality in the risk and severity of type 2 diabetes mellitus," Archives of Internal Medicine, vol. 166, no. 16, pp. 1768–1774, 2006.

[8] M. Trento, F. Broglio, F. Riganti et al., "Sleep abnormalities in type 2 diabetes may be associated with glycemic control," Acta Diabetologica, vol. 45, no. 4, pp. 225–229, 2008.

[9] R. Wolk and V. K. Somers, "Sleep and the metabolic syndrome," Experimental Physiology, vol. 92, no. 1, pp. 67–78, 2007.

[10] S. J. McCabe, A. L. Uebele, V. Pihur, R. S. Rosales, and I. Atroshi, "Epidemiologic associations of carpal tunnel syndrome and sleep position: is there a case for causation?" Hand, vol. 2, no. 3, pp. 127–134, 2007.

[11] J. N. Katz, E. Losina, B. C. Amick 3rd, A. H. Fossel, L. Bessette, and R. B. Keller, "Predictors of outcomes of carpal tunnel release," Arthritis and Rheumatism, vol. 44, no. 5, pp. 1184–1193, 2001.

[12] M. E. Leit, R. W. Weiser, and M. M. Tomaino, "Patient-reported outcome after carpal tunnel release for advanced disease: a prospective and longitudinal assessment in patients older than age 70," Journal of Hand Surgery, vol. 29, no. 3, pp. 379–383, 2004.

[13] M. Okada, O. Tsubata, S. Yasumoto, N. Toda, and T. Matsumoto, "Clinical study of surgical treatment of carpal tunnel syndrome: open versus endoscopic technique," Journal of Orthopaedic Surgery, vol. 8, no. 2, pp. 19–25, 2000.

[14] A. J. Rege and J. L. Sher, "Can the outcome of carpal tunnel release be predicted?" Journal of Hand Surgery, vol. 26, no. 2, pp. 148–150, 2001.

[15] I. Lehtinen, T. Kirjavainen, M. Hurme, H. Lauerma, K. Martikainen, and E. Rauhala, "Sleep-related disorders in carpal tunnel syndrome," Acta Neurologica Scandinavica, vol. 93, no. 5, pp. 360–365, 1996.

[16] D. W. Levine, B. P. Simmons, M. J. Koris et al., "A self-administered questionnaire for the assessment of severity of symptoms and functional status in carpal tunnel syndrome," Journal of Bone and Joint Surgery A, vol. 75, no. 11, pp. 1585–1592, 1993.

[17] D. J. Buysse, C. F. Reynolds III, T. H. Monk, S. R. Berman, and D. J. Kupfer, "The Pittsburgh sleep quality index: a new instrument for psychiatric practice and research," Psychiatry Research, vol. 28, no. 2, pp. 193–213, 1989.

[18] O. Gureje, G. E. Simon, and M. Von Korff, "A cross-national study of the course of persistent pain in primary care," Pain, vol. 92, no. 1-2, pp. 195–200, 2001.

[19] F. J. Keefe, M. E. Rumble, C. D. Scipio, L. A. Giordano, and L. M. Perri, "Psychological aspects of persistent pain: current state of the science," Journal of Pain, vol. 5, no. 4, pp. 195–211, 2004.

[20] G. J. Macfarlane, J. McBeth, and A. J. Silman, "Widespread body pain and mortality: prospective population based study," British Medical Journal, vol. 323, no. 7314, pp. 662–664, 2001.

[21] R. Marin, T. Cyhan, and W. Miklos, "Sleep disturbance in patients with chronic low back pain," American Journal of Physical Medicine and Rehabilitation, vol. 85, no. 5, pp. 430–435, 2006.

[22] K. L. Knutson and F. W. Turek, "The U-shaped association between sleep and health: the 2 peaks do not mean the same thing," Sleep, vol. 29, no. 7, pp. 878–879, 2006.

[23] S. Ikehara, H. Iso, C. Date et al., "Association of sleep duration with mortality from cardiovascular disease and other causes for japanese men and women: the JACC study," Sleep, vol. 32, no. 3, pp. 295–301, 2009.

[24] K. L. Knutson, K. Spiegel, P. Penev, and E. Van Cauter, "The metabolic consequences of sleep deprivation," Sleep Medicine Reviews, vol. 11, no. 3, pp. 163–178, 2007.

[25] R. A. C. Sampaio, P. Y. S. Sampaio, M. Yamada, T. Tsuboyama, and H. Arai, "Self-reported quality of sleep is associated with bodily pain, vitality and cognitive impairment in Japanese older adults," Geriatrics & Gerontology International, 2013.

[26] A. Covarrubias-Gomez and J. J. Mendoza-Reyes, "Evaluation of sleep quality in subjects with chronic nononcologic pain," *Journal of Pain and Palliative Care Pharmacotherapy*, vol. 27, no. 3, pp. 220–224, 2013.

[27] S. Shyen, B. Amine, S. Rostom, D. Badri et al., "Sleep and its relationship to pain, dysfunction, and disease activity in juvenile idiopathic arthritis," *Clinical Rheumatology*, 2013.

[28] C. M. Campbell, S. C. Bounds, H. Kuwabara et al., "Individual variation in sleep quality and duration is related to cerebral mu opioid receptor binding potential during tonic laboratory pain in healthy subjects," *Pain Medicine*, vol. 14, no. 12, pp. 1882–1892, 2013.

[29] C.-W. Chang, Y.-C. Wang, and K.-F. Chang, "A practical electrophysiological guide for non-surgical and treatment of carpal tunnel syndrome," *Journal of Hand Surgery E*, vol. 33, no. 1, pp. 32–37, 2008.

[30] R. B. Keller, A. M. Largay, D. N. Soule, and J. N. Katz, "Maine carpal tunnel study: small area variations," *Journal of Hand Surgery*, vol. 23, no. 4, pp. 692–696, 1998.

29

Daytime Sleepiness: Associations with Alcohol Use and Sleep Duration in Americans

Subhajit Chakravorty,[1,2] **Nicholas Jackson,**[3] **Ninad Chaudhary,**[2,4] **Philip J. Kozak,**[5] **Michael L. Perlis,**[2] **Holly R. Shue,**[6] **and Michael A. Grandner**[2]

[1] *MIRECC VISN-4, Philadelphia Veterans Affairs Medical Center, University & Woodland Avenues, Philadelphia, PA 19104, USA*
[2] *Perelman School of Medicine, University of Pennsylvania, Philadelphia, PA 19104, USA*
[3] *University of Southern California, Los Angeles, CA 90033, USA*
[4] *West Chester University of Pennsylvania, West Chester, PA 19383, USA*
[5] *School of Veterinary Medicine, University of Pennsylvania, Philadelphia, PA 19104, USA*
[6] *Children's Hospital of Philadelphia, Philadelphia, PA 19104, USA*

Correspondence should be addressed to Subhajit Chakravorty; subhajit.chakravorty@uphs.upenn.edu

Academic Editor: Michel M. Billiard

The aim of the current analysis was to investigate the relationship of daytime sleepiness with alcohol consumption and sleep duration using a population sample of adult Americans. Data was analyzed from adult respondents of the National Health and Nutritional Examination Survey (NHANES) 2007-2008 (N = 2919) using self-reported variables for sleepiness, sleep duration, and alcohol consumption (quantity and frequency of alcohol use). A heavy drinking episode was defined as the consumption of ≥5 standard alcoholic beverages in a day. Logistic regression models adjusted for sociodemographic variables and insomnia covariates were used to evaluate the relationship between daytime sleepiness and an interaction of alcohol consumption variables with sleep duration. The results showed that daytime sleepiness was reported by 15.07% of the subjects. In univariate analyses adjusted for covariates, an increased probability of daytime sleepiness was predicted by decreased log drinks per day [OR = 0.74 (95% CI, 0.58–0.95)], a decreased log drinking frequency [0.90 (95% CI, 0.83–0.98)], and lower sleep duration [OR = 0.75 (95% CI, 0.67–0.84)]. An interaction between decreased sleep duration and an increased log heavy drinking frequency predicted increased daytime sleepiness (P = 0.004). Thus, the effect of sleep duration should be considered when evaluating the relationship between daytime sleepiness and heavy drinking.

1. Introduction

Daytime sleepiness is highly prevalent. 19.5% of Americans suffer from moderate sleepiness and 11% suffer from severe sleepiness [1]. These prevalence rates are of concern given that daytime sleepiness affects nearly every aspect of human functioning and is a substantial risk factor for accidents and injuries [2]. The combination of daytime sleepiness and at-risk vocations vulnerable to such negative effects magnifies the risk for adverse outcomes of accidents, for example, sleepiness in truck drivers, airline pilots, medical personnel, mass transit operators, and so forth [3]. The perils associated

with these conditions underscore the need to identify factors that may serve to aggravate sleepiness, or may serve as vulnerability for sleepiness. One such condition may be the use of or the abuse of alcohol.

To date, some studies have been undertaken to evaluate the relationship between daytime sleepiness and alcohol consumption. The outcomes from these studies were inconsistent. Acute drinking episodes were found to be associated with complaints of sleepiness (as a component of hangover symptoms) [4] and an acute impairment in objective measures of flying the following day (after an acute drinking episode) [5]. In contrast, increased alcohol consumption

(>7 drinks per week) has been shown to be associated with a decreased likelihood of excessive daytime sleepiness in the elderly [6]. These studies differed in several ways, including the following: the duration of alcohol use (i.e., acute versus chronic use), the age of the cohort studied, and the sleep duration immediately prior to the study (or the typical total sleep duration).

The last of these issues is the role of sleep duration, which is particularly important as an increased consumption of alcohol has been independently associated with short sleep duration in some prior epidemiological studies [7–9]. Sleep duration has been investigated as a moderator in this relationship between alcohol consumption and sleepiness in a few laboratory-based studies. Some of these studies involved paradigms with partial sleep restriction and some with sleep extension (longer than typical ad lib sleep). In the *partial sleep deprivation studies*, Rupp and colleagues found that nocturnal alcohol consumption prior to bedtime and in conjunction with a partial sleep restriction increased the sleepiness at night (as compared to those who did not consume alcohol) [10]. Roehrs and colleagues found that despite an increase in the sleep latency on the Multiple Sleep Latency Test (MSLT) with partial sleep deprivation and moderate nocturnal alcohol consumption, no interaction between alcohol consumption and sleep deprivation was seen [11]. Similarly, a study by Horne and colleagues failed to show a difference in daytime sleepiness in the sleep-deprived conditions, with or without afternoon alcohol consumption, by using a different paradigm [12]. In the *sleep extension studies*, Lumley and colleagues found no differences in objective sleepiness on MSLT in subjects with an 11-hour total time in bed and morning alcohol consumption (as compared to normal sleep or partial sleep deprivation conditions) [13]. In another study, Roehrs and colleagues found that sleep extension with a 10-hour time in bed and morning alcohol consumption showed a decreased objectively measured sleepiness with a MSLT test [14].

As can be seen from the above summary, the data to date are mixed. If trends are evident it appears that heavy alcohol consumption is associated with shorter sleep durations, and objective daytime sleepiness may be associated with acute alcohol use/alcohol abuse in association with sleep deprivation. These findings must be considered tentative, as there are only a few studies with mixed results, and the alcohol measures are not well operationalized. With respect to the alcohol measures, the variables used rarely allow for a comprehensive assessment that takes into account dose (amount of alcohol per occasion), use frequency (number of occasions using alcohol per day or week), and use in the hazardous range (the presence of heavy drinking, and the frequency of heavy drinking as defined as the use of ≥5 drinks per session) [15, 16].

Accordingly, using a nationally representative sample, we explored the interactions between self-reported alcohol consumption and sleep duration variables and their association to daytime sleepiness while controlling for covariates and symptoms related to several intrinsic sleep disorders.

2. Methods

2.1. Design and Setting. This investigation utilized the 2007-2008 National Health and Nutrition Examination Survey (NHANES). This annual survey, conducted by the Centers for Disease Control and Prevention, assesses the demographic, health, and nutritional characteristics in the US population through in-person interviews, physical examinations, and laboratory tests. The unweighted response rate for the overall sample was 78.4%. In order to compensate for underrepresentation, African Americans, Hispanics, and adults over 60 were over-sampled [17].

2.2. Sample Size. Out of the initial participants ($N = 10,149$), we excluded children and adolescents <18 years of age ($N = 3921$), those with a lifetime history of drug use ($N = 1896$), those without response to outcome variables ($N = 21$), and those missing data on predictor variables ($N = 1079$), and covariates ($N = 313$). The final sample consisted of 2919 subjects. Drug use history was assessed for any lifetime use of marijuana, cocaine, methamphetamine, or illicit opiates individually; the response was coded dichotomously as "yes"/ "no."

2.3. Measures

2.3.1. Sleep. (a) Daytime sleepiness (DS) was assessed with the question, "In the past month, how often did you feel excessively or overly sleepy during the day?" (b) Sleep Duration (SD) was investigated with the question, "How much sleep do you usually get at night on weekdays or workdays?" This question was similar to that used in prior studies [18, 19]. (c) Insomnia symptoms: (i) difficulty falling asleep (DFA) was assessed using the question "In the past month, how often did you have trouble falling asleep?" (ii) difficulty maintaining sleep (AWAK) was assessed with the question "In the past month, how often did you wake up during the night and had trouble getting back to sleep?" (iii) Nonrestorative sleep (NRS) was evaluated with the question,"In the past month, how often did you feel unrested during the day, no matter how many hours of sleep you have had?" The responses to the DS, SL, AWAK, and SQ variables were presented with the following severity options: "0" (never), "1" (rarely: 1 time/ month), "2" (sometimes: 2–4 times/month), "3" (often: 5–15 times/month), and "4" (almost always: 16–30 times/month). The response to the SD variable was recorded as a number, rounded to the nearest decimal point and was assessed as a continuous variable.

2.3.2. Alcohol-Related Variables. The quantity of alcohol in a drink was evaluated in terms of a standard alcoholic drink [20]. The alcohol consumption variables used in this investigation were in line with those used in prior studies, and included the following [16, 21]: (a) drinks/day: this variable was assessed with "In the past 12 months, on those days that you drank alcoholic beverages, on an average, how many drinks did you have?" (b) drinking frequency was investigated using the question "In the past 12 months, how often did you drink any type of alcoholic beverage?" (c) heavy drinking status was assessed using the question

"In the past 12 months, on how many days did you have 5 or more drinks of any alcoholic beverage?" (d) heavy drinking frequency was evaluated using the question, "In the past 12 months, on how many days did you have 5 or more drinks of any alcoholic beverage?" Drinks/day, drinking frequency and binge-drinking frequency were recorded continuously as number of days. Heavy drinking status was recorded dichotomously, as "present" or "absent."

2.3.3. Covariates. The variables included in these analyses included, age, gender, race/ethnicity (White, Black/African American, Hispanic, and other), marital status, education, income, body mass index (BMI; objectively measured), depression (over past two weeks), anxiety (days anxious in past month), access to health insurance, physical health, mental health, exercise, and smoking (smoking days in past month). All the above-mentioned questions were assessed as part of the NHANES interview with the responses being self-reported by the subjects.

2.4. Statistical Analysis. Two-year full sample weights were used to adjust for unequal probability of being selected among noncoverage or nonresponse population, as recommended [17]. Daytime sleepiness was assessed with the question, "In the past month, how often did you feel excessively or overly sleepy during the day?" Daytime sleepiness was assessed as a dichotomous variable ("presence" or "absence" of daytime sleepiness) based on the distribution of the response. The sleep duration was assessed as a continuous variable. Alcohol consumption was assessed using four variables, including, drinks/day, drinking frequency, heavy drinking status, and heavy drinking frequency. Heavy drinking status was assessed as a dichotomous variable ("presence" or "absence" of heavy drinking). The remaining 3 alcohol variables were assessed as continuous variables, drinks/day, drinking frequency, and heavy drinking frequency. Log_n transformation was conducted for the variables including, drinks/day, drinking frequency, and heavy drinking frequency because of the skewness in the data, prior to the bivariate and multivariable analyses. Some of the covariates were dichotomized because of the skewed distribution and included insomnia variables (reporting a complaint ≥5 times a month/<5 times a month), depression, and anxiety symptoms (symptoms <15 days/≥15 days over last month). The relationships between daytime sleepiness (dependent variable) and alcohol consumption variables were assessed using multinomial logistic regression analyses. This relationship was assessed using three different models to adjust for covariates. Model 1 assessed the crude relationship between daytime sleepiness and the alcohol consumption variables or sleep duration. Model 2 assessed the relationship in model 1, adjusted for the covariates mentioned above. Model 3 assessed for this relationship in Model 2, further adjusted for insomnia symptoms. Interactive models evaluated for the presence of 2-way interactions, of whether the effects of one alcohol consumption variable depended on levels of a second category, that is, the sleep duration in predicting daytime sleepiness. Analyses were conducted using Stata version 12 (StataCorp LP, Stata Statistical Software: Release 12. College Station, TX).

3. Results

3.1. Subjects. The average subject in this study which was middle-aged female, college graduate, who identified herself as of Caucasian race, non-Hispanic in ethnicity, married, was overweight and had health insurance, Table 1.

3.2. Sleep-Related Characteristics. Daytime sleepiness was reported by 15.07% of the subjects. The mean (SD) sleep duration was 6.91 (SD = 1.36) hours. Amongst them, 56.72% had sleep duration within the normal range (7-8 hours a night), 36.12% had short sleep duration (≤6 hours a night), and 7.16% had long sleep duration (≥8 hours a night), with nonrestorative sleep being the commonest insomnia symptom (22.32%), Table 1.

3.3. Alcohol Consumption. The average subject reported an alcohol consumption in the moderate range with a mean (SD) alcohol consumption of 1.25 (SD = 2.28) drinks per day within the last 12 months. Amongst those drinking alcohol in the past 12 months, 9.77% of the respondents reported heavy drinking (≥5 drinks a day), and with a heavy drinking frequency of 4.23 (SD = 27.18) days of over the last 12 months, Table 1.

3.4. The Relationship of Daytime Sleepiness with Alcohol Consumption and Sleep Duration

3.4.1. Alcohol Consumption. Subjects with daytime sleepiness reported lower alcohol consumption as compared to those without daytime sleepiness (0.99 ± 1.65 drinks and 1.29 ± 2.38 drinks resp., $P = 0.002$). In analyses adjusted for sociodemographic variables and insomnia covariates, a decreased risk of daytime sleepiness was predicted by log drinks per day, that is, each percent increase in the number of alcoholic drinks per day [OR = 0.74 (95% CI, 0.58–0.95), $P = 0.019$]. A similar relationship of a decreased risk of daytime sleepiness was seen with increased log drinking frequency, that is, each percent increase in the frequency of drinking and with nonsignificant trends for log binge-drinking frequency predicting a lower risk of daytime sleepiness, Table 2.

3.4.2. Sleep Duration. Those with daytime sleepiness reported a lower sleep duration as compared to those without daytime sleepiness (6.38 ± 1.63 hours and 7.00 ± 1.28 hours, resp., $P < 0.0001$). In analyses adjusted for sociodemographic variables and insomnia covariates, a decreased probability of daytime sleepiness was predicted by higher sleep duration [OR = 0.75 (95% CI, 0.67–0.84), $P < 0.001$], Table 2.

3.5. Interactions between Alcohol Consumption and Sleep Duration on Daytime Sleepiness. In models adjusted for covariates, an interaction between a decreased sleep duration and an increased log frequency of binge-drinking predicted increased daytime sleepiness ($P = 0.004$), such that with each percent increase in the binge-drinking frequency and

TABLE 1: Baseline demographics.

Variable	Categories	Mean/%	S.D.
Age (years)		53.1	17.4
Gender	Female	57.84%	
Race	White	68.05%	
	Black	10.20%	
	Other	21.76%	
Ethnicity	Hispanic	14.71%	
BMI (Kg/m^2)		29.1	6.6
Mental health	Days with poor mental health (past month)	3.21	7.30
Anxiety	≥15 days (past month)	12.61%	
Depression	≥15 days (past month)	6.01%	
Exercise (in minutes)	Moderate/vigorous exercise	124	187
Education	College graduate	26.51%	
	Less than high school	21.30%	
	High school graduate	25.88%	
	Some college education	26.31%	
Income (per year)	>75,000	29.79%	
	<20,000	17.24%	
	20,000–25,000	7.65%	
	25,000–35,000	12.45%	
	35,000–45,000	10.40%	
	45,000–55,000	8.78%	
	55,000–65,000	7.03%	
	65,000–75,000	6.66%	
General heath	Excellent	16.77%	
	Very good	29.57%	
	Good	34.31%	
	Poor	15.80%	
	Very poor	3.55%	
Marital status	Married	63.04%	
	Widowed	9.43%	
	Divorced/separated	11.11%	
	Never married	12.29%	
	Living with partner	4.13%	
Insurance status	Insured	85.35%	
Caffeine use	Present	91.06%	
Smoker	Yes	11.03%	
Daytime sleepiness	Present	15.07%	
Sleep duration	Sleep duration (hrs)	6.91	1.36
Insomnia symptoms	Difficulty falling asleep (DFA, ≥5 nights/month)	16.05%	
	Difficulty maintaining sleep (AWAK, ≥5 nights/month)	18.15%	
	Nonrestorative sleep (NRS, ≥5 nights/month)	22.32%	
Alcohol quantity	Drinks/day (past 12 months)	1.25	2.28
Drinking frequency	Drinking days (past 12 months)	40.9	85.8
Heavy drinking status	Present (past 12 months)	9.77%	
Heavy drinking frequency	Heavy drinking days (past 12 months)	4.23	27.18

S.D.: standard deviation.

TABLE 2: Associations of daytime sleepiness with alcohol variables and sleep duration.

Predictor	Subgroup	Model 1		Model 2		Model 3	
		OR (95% CI)	P	OR (95% CI)	P	OR (95% CI)	P
Alcohol	Log drinks/day	0.72 (0.58–0.90)	0.0046	0.78 (0.60–1.01)	0.0557	0.74 (0.58–0.95)	0.0197
	Log drinking frequency	0.87 (0.81–0.93)	0.0001	0.91 (0.84–0.99)	0.0297	0.90 (0.83–0.98)	0.0129
	Heavy drinking status	0.68 (0.43–1.07)	0.0971	0.76 (0.48–1.21)	0.2471	0.71 (0.45–1.11)	0.1311
	Log heavy drinking frequency	0.87 (0.74–1.02)	0.0805	0.89 (0.75–1.06)	0.1891	0.88 (0.75–1.04)	0.1366
Sleep duration	Hours	0.71 (0.64–0.80)	<0.0001	0.75 (0.67–0.84)	<0.0001	0.75 (0.67–0.84)	<0.0001

OR: odds ratio, CI: confidence interval, P: P value, and mo: months.
Model 1: unadjusted model.
Model 2: adjusted for age, BMI, gender, race, marital status, education, income, depression, insurance, health status, anxiety, mental health, and exercise.
Model 3: model 2 + insomnia status.

TABLE 3: Daytime sleepiness and its association with an interaction of alcohol consumption variables on sleep duration.

Moderating variable	Model 1 (P)	Model 2 (P)	Model 3 (P)
Log drinks/day	0.131	0.627	0.626
Log drinking frequency	0.323	0.628	0.602
Heavy drinking status	0.059	0.286	0.289
Log heavy drinking frequency	**0.005**	**0.003**	**0.004**

P: P value.
Model 1: unadjusted model.
Model 2: adjusted for age, BMI, gender, race, marital status, education, income, depression, insurance, health status, anxiety, mental health, and exercise.
Model 3: model 2 + insomnia status.

a decrease in the sleep duration in hours, there was an increased probability of reporting daytime sleepiness; see Table 3, and Figure 1. No significant interactions between other alcohol consumption variables and sleep duration predicted daytime sleepiness.

4. Discussion

The association between subjective sleepiness as it relates to alcohol consumption and sleep duration from a population perspective is currently unknown. In this study, we explored this relationship using data from the 2007-2008 NHANES survey using self-reported measures. In univariate analyses, the presence of daytime sleepiness was inversely associated with the drinks per day, drinking frequency, and sleep duration. In the final model adjusted for covariates, an interaction between heavy drinking frequency and sleep duration predicted daytime sleepiness, such that an increased probability of daytime sleepiness was reported with each percent increase in the frequency of heavy drinking and a decrease in the sleep duration (in hours).

Short sleep duration has been linked with heavy alcohol consumption on one hand [7–9] and with daytime drowsiness on the other hand [22, 23]. Heavy alcohol consumption has been linked with next day symptoms of tiredness [24], and with an impaired performance [5]. It is therefore possible that sleepiness is reliably produced with a higher intensity and periodicity of alcohol consumption along with insufficient habitual sleep duration. The sleep duration may be decreased by the heavy alcohol consumption itself, or from insufficiency based on the need or opportunity of functioning in a 24-hour society, and/or the presence of intrinsic sleep disorders like insomnia or obstructive sleep apnea syndrome. In light

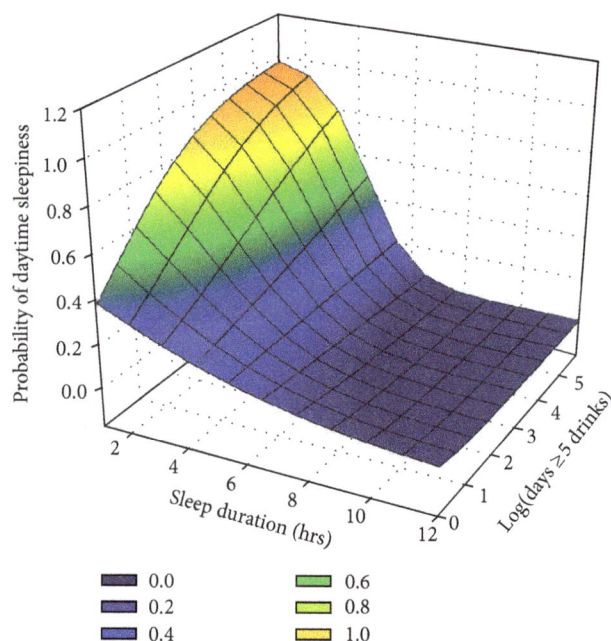

FIGURE 1: Surface model of the interaction between heavy drinking frequency and sleep duration on daytime sleepiness.

of the above it is easier to comprehend our findings of an interaction between heavy drinking and a decreased sleep duration predicting sleepiness.

Evaluating this relationship from another perspective, it is possible that after the alcohol is metabolized in the latter half of the night, the sleep is shallow and fragmented sleep as shown previously [24, 25]. This shallow and/or fragmented sleep may lead the subject to a state of subacute sleep deprivation with continued heavy drinking over time, leading to complaints of daytime sleepiness [4]. Our results differ from those of Pack and colleagues [6] as their study did not account for the sleep duration or for any heavy drinking and showed results similar to our bivariate analysis. In addition, our study adjusted for the effect of gender as a covariate, as well as body mass index and insomnia symptoms in the analyses.

Some of the limitations associated with this study include the following: the cross-sectional nature of the study precludes determination of the cause and effect between the variables; the dichotomous nature of sleepiness complaint prevents us from differentiating relationships associated with varying intensities of the daytime sleepiness; the lack of additional data on the drinking pattern across genders (in a calendar format) over the past year (in days, months, or years) or the pattern of drinking on weekdays versus weekends; and the lack of data on the circadian pattern of sleep and sleepiness as well as caffeine and alcohol consumption. Despite its weaknesses, this is one of the first studies at the population level that shows the presence of a complex relationship between alcohol consumption and sleep duration, on daytime sleepiness.

In conclusion, an inverse relationship of the probability of daytime sleepiness with the intensity and the frequency of alcohol consumption was seen in adult respondents from a nationally representative US sample. Once the duration of sleep was factored in, an interaction between the frequency of heavy drinking and sleep duration predicted an increased probability of daytime sleepiness. These results extend the findings from prior laboratory-based studies to a population sample. Future studies will need to further clarify this complex relationship further using more detailed information on alcohol use, sleepiness in the context of circadian phase and the ascending versus the descending limbs of alcohol concentrations as seen in a prior laboratory study [26], and the association with hangover symptoms. In addition, studies are also warranted to tease apart the role of gender differences in this relationship considering the gender related differences in sleepiness and alcohol consumption.

Conflict of Interests

None of the authors (Subhajit Chakravorty, Nicholas Jackson, Michael A. Grandner, Ninad Chaudhary, Philip J. Kozak, Holly R. Shue, and Michael L. Perlis) have reported any actual or any potential conflict of interests with the subject matter of the paper.

Authors' Contribution

Subhajit Chakravorty conceptualized, analyzed, and drafted the paper. Nicholas Jackson worked in data analyses and collaborated with the drafting of this paper. Ninad Chaudhary collaborated with the drafting of this paper. Philip J. Kozak collaborated with the drafting of this paper. Michael L. Perlis collaborated in conceptualization and drafting this paper. Holly R. Shue collaborated with the drafting of this paper.

Michael A. Grandner collaborated in conceptualizing the study, analyzing the data, and drafting of this paper.

Acknowledgments

The content of this publication does not represent the views of the Department of Veterans Affairs, the United States Government, or any of the collaborating institutions.

References

[1] M. M. Ohayon, "Determining the level of sleepiness in the American population and its correlates," *Journal of Psychiatric Research*, vol. 46, no. 4, pp. 422–427, 2012.

[2] T. B. Young, "Epidemiology of daytime sleepiness: definitions, symptomatology, and prevalence," *Journal of Clinical Psychiatry*, vol. 65, no. 16, pp. 12–16, 2004.

[3] J. S. Durmer and D. F. Dinges, "Neurocognitive consequences of sleep deprivation," *Seminars in Neurology*, vol. 25, no. 1, pp. 117–129, 2005.

[4] R. Penning, A. McKinney, and J. C. Verster, "Alcohol hangover symptoms and their contribution to the overall hangover severity," *Alcohol and Alcoholism*, vol. 47, no. 3, pp. 248–252, 2012.

[5] J. A. Yesavage and V. O. Leirer, "Hangover effects on aircraft pilots 14 hours after alcohol ingestion: a preliminary report," *The American Journal of Psychiatry*, vol. 143, no. 12, pp. 1546–1550, 1986.

[6] A. I. Pack, D. F. Dinges, P. R. Gehrman, B. Staley, F. M. Pack, and G. Maislin, "Risk factors for excessive sleepiness in older adults," *Annals of Neurology*, vol. 59, no. 6, pp. 893–904, 2006.

[7] M. A. Schuckit and L. I. Bernstein, "Sleep time and drinking history: a hypothesis," *The American Journal of Psychiatry*, vol. 138, no. 4, pp. 528–530, 1981.

[8] C. D. Palmer, G. A. Harrison, and R. W. Hiorns, "Association between smoking and drinking and sleep duration," *Annals of Human Biology*, vol. 7, no. 2, pp. 103–107, 1980.

[9] J. P. Chaput, J. McNeil, J. P. Despres, C. Bouchard, and A. Tremblay, "Short sleep duration is associated with greater alcohol consumption in adults," *Appetite*, vol. 59, no. 3, pp. 650–655, 2012.

[10] T. L. Rupp, C. Acebo, E. van Reen, and M. A. Carskadon, "Effects of a moderate evening alcohol dose. I: sleepiness," *Alcoholism*, vol. 31, no. 8, pp. 1358–1364, 2007.

[11] T. Roehrs, J. Yoon, and T. Roth, "Nocturnal and next-day effects of ethanol and basal level of sleepiness," *Human Psychopharmacology*, vol. 6, no. 4, pp. 307–311, 1991.

[12] J. A. Horne, L. A. Reyner, and P. R. Barrett, "Driving impairment due to sleepiness is exacerbated by low alcohol intake," *Occupational and Environmental Medicine*, vol. 60, no. 9, pp. 689–692, 2003.

[13] M. Lumley, T. Roehrs, D. Asker, F. Zorick, and T. Roth, "Ethanol and caffeine effects on daytime sleepiness/alertness," *Sleep*, vol. 10, no. 4, pp. 306–312, 1987.

[14] T. Roehrs, A. Zwyghuizen-Doorenbos, V. Timms, F. Zorick, and T. Roth, "Sleep extension, enhanced alertness and the sedating effects of ethanol," *Pharmacology Biochemistry and Behavior*, vol. 34, no. 2, pp. 321–324, 1989.

[15] D. A. Dawson, "Defining risk drinking," *Alcohol Research and Health*, vol. 34, no. 2, pp. 144–156, 2011.

[16] J. Tsai, E. S. Ford, C. Li, and G. Zhao, "Past and current alcohol consumption patterns and elevations in serum hepatic enzymes among US adults," *Addictive Behaviors*, vol. 37, no. 1, pp. 78–84, 2012.

[17] C. D. C. Centers for Disease Control Prevention, *National Health and Nutrition Examination Survey Data (NHANES), 2007-2008*, Hyattsville, Md, USA, 2010.

[18] P. M. Krueger and E. M. Friedman, "Sleep duration in the united states: a cross-sectional population-based study," *American Journal of Epidemiology*, vol. 169, no. 9, pp. 1052–1063, 2009.

[19] M. A. Grandner, N. Jackson, J. R. Gerstner, and K. L. Knutson, "Dietary nutrients associated with short and long sleep duration. Data from a nationally representative sample," *Appetite*, vol. 64, pp. 71–80, 2013.

[20] N.I.A.A.A, "Rethinking drinking: what is at-risk or heavy drinking," http://rethinkingdrinking.niaaa.nih.gov/whatcountsdrink/whatsastandarddrink.asp.

[21] S. Liangpunsakul, "Relationship between alcohol intake and dietary pattern: findings from NHENES III," *World Journal of Gastroenterology*, vol. 16, no. 32, pp. 4055–4060, 2010.

[22] H. P. A. van Dongen, G. Maislin, J. M. Mullington, and D. F. Dinges, "The cumulative cost of additional wakefulness: dose-response effects on neurobehavioral functions and sleep physiology from chronic sleep restriction and total sleep deprivation," *Sleep*, vol. 26, no. 2, pp. 117–126, 2003.

[23] M. A. Grandner and D. F. Kripke, "Self-reported sleep complaints with long and short sleep: a nationally representative sample," *Psychosomatic Medicine*, vol. 66, no. 2, pp. 239–241, 2004.

[24] B. Feige, H. Gann, R. Brueck et al., "Effects of alcohol on polysomnographically recorded sleep in healthy subjects," *Alcoholism*, vol. 30, no. 9, pp. 1527–1537, 2006.

[25] J. T. Arnedt, D. J. Rohsenow, A. B. Almeida et al., "Sleep following alcohol intoxication in healthy, young adults: effects of sex and family history of alcoholism," *Alcoholism*, vol. 35, no. 5, pp. 870–878, 2011.

[26] E. van Reen, T. L. Rupp, C. Acebo, R. Seifer, and M. A. Carskadon, "Biphasic effects of alcohol as a function of circadian phase," *Sleep*, vol. 36, no. 1, pp. 137–145, 2013.

30

Screening for Sleep Apnoea in Mild Cognitive Impairment: The Utility of the Multivariable Apnoea Prediction Index

Georgina Wilson,[1] Zoe Terpening,[1] Keith Wong,[2] Ron Grunstein,[2] Louisa Norrie,[1] Simon J. G. Lewis,[1] and Sharon L. Naismith[1]

[1] *Healthy Brain Ageing Clinic, Brain & Mind Research Institute, University of Sydney, 94 Mallett Street, Camperdown, NSW 2050, Australia*
[2] *Woolcock Institute of Medical Research, University of Sydney, Glebe, NSW 2050, Australia*

Correspondence should be addressed to Sharon L. Naismith; sharon.naismith@sydney.edu.au

Academic Editor: Marco Zucconi

Purpose. Mild cognitive impairment (MCI) is considered an "at risk" state for dementia and efforts are needed to target modifiable risk factors, of which Obstructive sleep apnoea (OSA) is one. This study aims to evaluate the predictive utility of the multivariate apnoea prediction index (MAPI), a patient self-report survey, to assess OSA in MCI. *Methods.* Thirty-seven participants with MCI and 37 age-matched controls completed the MAPI and underwent polysomnography (PSG). Correlations were used to compare the MAPI and PSG measures including oxygen desaturation index and apnoea-hypopnoea index (AHI). Receiver-operating characteristics (ROC) curve analyses were performed using various cut-off scores for apnoea severity. *Results.* In controls, there was a significant moderate correlation between higher MAPI scores and more severe apnoea (AHI: $r = 0.47$, $P = 0.017$). However, this relationship was not significant in the MCI sample. ROC curve analysis indicated much lower area under the curve (AUC) in the MCI sample compared to the controls across all AHI severity cut-off scores. *Conclusions.* In older people, the MAPI moderately correlates with AHI severity but only in those who are cognitively intact. Development of further screening tools is required in order to accurately screen for OSA in MCI.

1. Introduction

Mild cognitive impairment (MCI) is a syndrome defining a transitional stage between normal ageing and dementia. Clinically, it is defined as cognitive decline greater than expected for an individual's age and education, but with preservation of daily functioning [1]. Since there is a conversion rate to dementia of around 50% in five years, MCI is often considered an "at risk" state. Importantly, in this critical period, there is opportunity to implement secondary prevention strategies targeting modifiable risk factors. Research to date has identified that a range of cardiovascular, psychological, and lifestyle factors are associated with an increased conversion to dementia. However, there has been a paucity of research addressing sleep. This is despite the fact that sleep disturbance is a common symptom of dementia [2], associated with decreased cognitive and daily functioning, reduced quality of life, and increased carer burden [3].

Sleep disturbance in older people is multifaceted and includes age-related changes to sleep macro- and microarchitecture, medical comorbidity, mood disturbance, and alterations in circadian rhythm [3, 4]. In addition, the prevalence of nocturnal respiratory disturbance increases with age, and, in particular, obstructive sleep apnoea (OSA) affects 70% of men and 56% of women over the age of 65 years [5], a figure which is markedly increased from that observed in the general adult population, where the prevalence is only around 2–7% [6]. OSA is characterised by repetitive partial or complete collapse of the pharyngeal airway during sleep and can affect brain functioning in many ways including intermittent hypoxemia, sleep fragmentation, and consequent hypersomnolence. The prevalence of OSA in older adults with a neurodegenerative disorder is less well understood. Studies have shown that up to 40% of institutionalised Alzheimer's disease (AD) patients suffer from OSA [7] and that untreated OSA can exacerbate the primary cognitive and functional deficits associated with this disorder. In MCI, there are few detailed studies, but some data suggests that OSA may be linked to impaired language function [8].

Although research investigating links between OSA and dementia are in their infancy, there is mounting evidence linking OSA to cognitive decline in younger cohorts with poorer performance in the domains of processing speed, attention, learning/memory, and executive functioning [9, 10]. Moreover, longitudinal studies have further confirmed that OSA is a predictor of cognitive decline [11]. Pathophysiologically, there appear to be at least two primary contributors to cognitive decline, namely, hypoxic brain changes due to oxygen desaturation (associated with repetitive apnoeas or hypopnoeas) and/or sleep fragmentation due to frequent arousals or awakenings. It has been postulated that hypoxemia and sleep fragmentation contribute differentially to neuropsychological dysfunction in OSA, with the former being specifically linked to executive deficits and the latter being linked to changes in processing speed [9, 12]. Disruption to sleep microarchitecture from sleep fragmentation may also impede sleep-related memory consolidation [13].

Treatment for OSA, such as continuous airway pressure (CPAP), has been shown to decrease sleep disturbance in patients with AD and OSA [14] and, although the cognitive benefits of CPAP are not yet clear, some studies have shown positive improvement in neuropsychological functioning [7, 15]. Overall, there is evidence suggesting that, even in established dementia, there may be merit in addressing this problem and this may be even greater if intervention targeted critical "at risk" periods such as MCI. In order to effectively detect OSA at the population level, it is necessary to have effective screening tools. Currently, overnight polysomnography (PSG) represents the gold standard for evaluating respiratory disturbance providing detailed data on airflow, oxygen saturation, and sleep cycle. It is, therefore, an accurate diagnostic tool for OSA. The apnoea-hypopnoea index (AHI: number of apnoeas/hypopnoeas per hour of sleep) is commonly used as an indicator of OSA severity. However, there are many barriers to the assessment of patients in overnight sleep laboratory facilities. The process is costly and requires qualified staff to run and interpret complex data, which is often time consuming and associated with long waiting lists [6]. Older people may also be reluctant to leave their homes and often an adaptation night is required in order to capture the usual sleep pattern [16]. Therefore, there has been a drive to develop validated screening instruments for OSA that are easily administered and cost-effective.

One of the common screening tools that has been developed for use in OSA generally is the multivariable apnoea prediction (MAP) survey which predicts apnoea risk as a score between 0 (low risk) and 1 (high risk) termed the multivariate apnoea prediction index (MAPI) [17]. The predictive ability of the MAPI was determined by receiver operating characteristics (ROC) curve analysis offering good sensitivity and specificity for the detection of respiratory

disturbance [17] in younger cohorts, where the optimum MAPI value was determined to be 0.50. The MAPI has been validated for use in sleep and nonsleep disorder clinical samples and primary care settings, in order to discriminate between people likely and unlikely to have OSA [18–20]. Also, in one elderly sample with excessive daytime sleepiness, the MAPI demonstrated a predictive utility that was comparable to that obtained in sleep disorder clinic samples. In addition, it was also identified that, compared to BMI alone (which by itself is a very strong predictor of OSA in adult samples), the symptom questions on the survey were necessary to obtain adequate predictive value in the older population with excessive daytime sleepiness [19].

To our knowledge, no study has previously examined the utility of the MAP questionnaire in those patients with MCI who are "at risk" of dementia. We proposed that, if the MAPI was found to be a reliable method for screening OSA in this cohort, it may be an effective method of screening older people for OSA and may negate the need for formal overnight PSG studies. Therefore, the main objective of this study was to determine the predictive utility of the MAPI for determining AHI in older people and specifically in patients with MCI.

2. Method

2.1. Patients. Thirty-seven older adults over 50 years of age meeting Petersen's criteria for MCI [21] (mean age = 65.5 years, SD = 9.0) were recruited from the Healthy Brain Ageing Clinic at the Brain and Mind Research Institute, University of Sydney, Australia. In accordance with these criteria, patients were classified as having MCI if they performed at 1.5 standard deviations below their predictive level of intelligence on at least one neuropsychological test. Thirty-seven age-matched controls were recruited from the community via local community advertisement (mean age = 63.5 years, SD = 8.7). Exclusion criteria included history of stroke, head injury with a loss of consciousness for more than 30 minutes; neurological disease (e.g., Parkinson's disease, epilepsy); psychotic illness; medical conditions known to affect cognition (e.g., cancer); mini-mental state examination (MMSE) score <24; diagnosis of dementia; illicit substance use; shift workers, transmeridian travel within 60 days before overnight laboratory assessment; and use of medication known to affect sleep and/or melatonin secretion including beta-blockers, lithium or benzodiazepines or sedative hypnotics. Prior to overnight PSG assessment, patients were also required to abstain from alcohol and caffeinated drinks for 48 and 24 hours respectively.

2.2. Clinical Assessment. All controls and patients received comprehensive clinical assessments by an old age psychiatrist who interviewed patients regarding medical history including current medications, heart disease, hypertension, and diabetes. Physical measurements including height, weight, and BMI were also taken. The cumulative illness rating scale (CIRS) [22] total score (the sum of all the scores of all categories) was used to evaluate overall medical burden. Global cognitive functioning was measured by the mini-mental state examination (MMSE) [23]. As described elsewhere [24], all participants were further assessed by a clinical neuropsychologist, who confirmed MCI diagnosis and that the patient did not meet criteria for dementia. Individuals were also diagnosed with multi- or single domain MCI (depending on if there were deficits in more than one cognitive domain) and amnestic (only memory impairment) or nonamnestic MCI [25]. This study was approved by the University of Sydney Institutional Ethics committee and all participants gave written informed consent.

2.3. Measures

2.3.1. Polysomnography.
All participants underwent standard nocturnal PSG which included electroencephalography (EEG), electrooculography (EOG), electromyography (EMG), and pulse oximetry. A subset of participants (MCI = 24; controls = 25) also had nasal airflow (using a nasal pressure transducer or thermistor) and respiratory effort (using thoracic and abdominal bands) measured which enabled AHI to be calculated. Sleep architecture stages were scored by an experienced sleep technician using standardised criteria [26] modified for older subjects [27]. The main outcome variables used in this study included AHI (obtained for a subset of participants), oxygen desaturation index (ODI), and average oxygen desaturation (obtained for all participants). Apnoea was defined as complete cessation of airflow on the nasal pressure transducer or thermistor for at least 10 seconds. Hypopnoea was defined as a reduction of nasal airflow >50% with either a 3% desaturation or an arousal [28]. AHI was calculated as the total number of apnoeas and hypopnoeas divided by the total sleep time, giving the number of apnoeas/hypopnoeas per hour of sleep. ODI was calculated as the number of oxygen desaturations >3% per hour of sleep.

2.3.2. Self-Report

(a) Multivariable Apnoea Prediction Survey [17]. All participants completed the MAP survey, which predicts apnoea risk using demographic data and self-reported apnoea symptoms. Three frequency questions as well as gender, age, height, and weight (to calculate BMI) are used to produce a MAPI between 0 (low risk) and 1 (high risk). The three questions determine the frequency that the patient has experienced loud snoring, snoring or gasping, cessation of breathing, or struggle for breath in the last month. Together, the questions produce a score referred to as Index 1.

(b) The Pittsburgh Sleep Quality Index (PSQI) [29]. This was used to determine an overall subjective measure of sleep quality over the previous month. The questionnaire consists of 17 items with most questions rated on a 4-point Likert scale. The PSQI provides a global score based on the components of quality, latency, duration, efficiency, disturbance, use of sleeping medication, and daytime dysfunction.

2.4. Statistical Analyses.
Statistical analysis was conducted using the statistical package for social sciences (SPSS) version 20. Independent samples t-tests were used for normally distributed variables to compare the descriptive statistics for

controls versus MCI patients. To investigate the association between BMI and OSA in our whole sample, independent t-tests were used with AHI $\geq$ 5. Chi-square tests were used for categorical variables, except where Fisher's exact test was used to analyse medical conditions including heart disease, hypertension, and diabetes. Pearson correlations were employed to examine the associations between normally distributed variables and all other correlations used Spearman rank. All analyses were two-tailed with an alpha level of 0.05.

To determine the predictive utility of the MAPI in our sample of older adults, receiver-operating characteristics (ROC) curve analysis was performed using the program *MedCalc* version 12.2.1.0. ROC curves were generated using cutoff scores of AHI $\geq$ 5, AHI $\geq$ 15 and AHI $\geq$ 30. These particular cut-offs were chosen on the basis of the values typically used to classify severity of OSA in older adults [28]. The sensitivity (true positive rate) is plotted in function of 1-specificity (false positive rate). The Youden index, defined as "sensitivity + specificity − 1," was used to determine the optimal MAPI cut-off points in each analysis, where equal weight was given to the sensitivity and specificity of the test.

3. Results

Descriptive data for the sample including clinical and sleep variables is presented in Table 1. Of the 37 MCI patients, 27 were of the nonamnestic type and 10 had amnestic MCI. Twenty-eight MCI patients had multiple cognitive domains affected and nine had only a single domain. No significant differences in terms of age, BMI, height, or weight were identified between the controls and those with MCI. As expected, the MMSE scores were significantly lower in the MCI sample ($P < 0.01$). Those with MCI had a significantly higher medical burden as evidenced by the CIRS total score ($P = 0.012$). No significant differences were found between the MCI and control groups in terms of diagnosis of hypertension ($P = 0.33$), diabetes ($P = 0.26$), or heart disease ($P = 0.67$). For the whole sample, no significant differences were found regarding BMI and OSA (AHI $\geq$ 5: t-value (df) = −0.483 (47), $P = 0.63$).

Of the control sample with AHI data, 68.0% had an AHI $\geq$ 5; 28.0% AHI $\geq$ 15, and 8.0% AHI $\geq$ 30. Within the MCI sample with AHI data, 70.8% had an AHI $\geq$ 5; 41.7% AHI $\geq$ 15; and 16.7% AHI $\geq$ 30. Table 1 shows that the two groups did not differ significantly in terms of self-reported sleep quality (PSQI) or PSG-derived apnoea measures. There was a trend for a greater proportion of controls (54.2%) to have central sleep apnoea (CSA) compared to those with MCI (26.1%) (χ^2 (1) = 3.45, $P = 0.05$).

As expected, AHI correlated significantly with ODI and average oxygen desaturations in both the MCI ($r = 0.59$, $P = 0.002$ and $r = 0.78$, $P < 0.001$, resp.) and control ($r = 0.78$, $P < 0.001$ and $r = 0.72$, $P < 0.001$, resp.) group (not shown in the table).

Correlation of MAPI with Apnoea Measures. Table 2 shows that, in the control group, a modest but significant correlation was observed between higher MAPI scores and more severe apnoea (AHI) ($P = 0.017$) as well as more frequent oxygen

TABLE 1: A comparison of clinical, self-report, and polysomnographic data between MCI and control subjects.

	Control Mean ± SD	MCI Mean ± SD	t value (df)/z	P value
Clinical				
Age (years)	63.5 ± 8.7	65.5 ± 9.0	−0.98 (71)	0.333
Body mass index	27.1 ± 4.0	27.6 ± 5.5	−0.43 (72)	0.669
Weight (kg)	75.9 ± 14	78.0 ± 16	−0.60 (72)	0.552
Height (cm)	167 ± 10	168 ± 11	−0.43 (72)	0.668
CIRS, total score	3.0 ± 2.3	5.9 ± 6.4	−2.57 (67)	**0.012***
MMSE score	29.2 ± 1.1	28.1 ± 1.5	3.75 (72)	**<0.001****
Self-report				
MAPI	0.3 ± 0.2	0.4 ± 0.2	−1.30 (72)	0.199
PSQI, global score	5.4 ± 4.0	7.0 ± 3.4	−1.83 (69)	0.072
PSQI, sleep efficiency (%)	77.6 ± 10	75.5 ± 14	0.63 (68)	0.533
Overnight polysomnography				
Apnoea-hypopnoea index	11.9 ± 10	16.4 ± 16	−1.20 (47)	0.236
Total sleep time (minutes)	377 ± 73	385 ± 100	−0.41 (72)	0.682
Sleep efficiency (%)	77.6 ± 10	75.6 ± 14	0.73 (72)	0.468
WASO (mins)	96.9 ± 53	97.9 ± 56	−0.08 (72)	0.938
Lowest oxygen desaturation (%)	87.6 ± 5.0	87.9 ± 8.4	−0.19 (72)	0.854
Average oxygen desaturation (%)	4.1 ± 1.4	6.5 ± 13	−1.10 (72)	0.273
Oxygen desaturation index	23.9 ± 21.6	39.3 ± 65.4	−1.21	0.228
Non-REM sleep AHI	9.5 ± 9.9	14.2 ± 15	−1.31 (47)	0.198
REM sleep AHI	18.6 ± 15	19.8 ± 16	−0.11 (47)	0.916

*$P < 0.05$, **$P < 0.01$.

MCI: mild cognitive impairment; CIRS: cumulative illness rating scale; MMSE: mini-mental state examination; MAPI: multivariable aponea prediction index; PSQI: pittsburgh sleep quality index; AHI: apnoea-hypopnoea index; WASO: wake after sleep onset; REM: rapid eye movement.

desaturations (ODI) ($P = 0.010$). However, the correlation in the MCI sample was nonsignificant. There was also a significant difference between the correlation coefficients for MAPI and AHI between the MCI and control sample (Fishers r to z transformation, $z = 2.15$, $P = 0.032$), although this was not found between the MAPI and ODI correlation coefficients.

Interestingly, MAPI and age were inversely correlated in the MCI sample only (Table 2). As this finding is unusual, the relationship between age and BMI (a major predictor in the MAPI) was investigated in the MCI sample. These variables were also found to be inversely correlated, but this relation was not statistically significant ($r = -0.11$, $P = 0.525$).

ROC Curve Analysis. Table 3 displays the ROC curve data for the whole sample, MCI, and control participants and Table 4 shows the area under the curve (AUC) data. Table 3 indicates the specificity and sensitivity for the optimal cut-off MAPI scores to various AHI scores as determined by ROC curve analysis. When detecting any degree of OSA (i.e., AHI ≥ 5) in the whole sample, the optimum cut-off score for older adults on the MAPI was 0.29 with a sensitivity of 67.65% and specificity of 60.00%. Rather surprisingly, when detecting severe OSA (i.e., AHI ≥ 30), the optimal cut-off score was paradoxically lower, at 0.15, which afforded improved sensitivity (100.00%) but at a trade-off for specificity (18.60%). However, in our sample, only few participants were diagnosed with severe OSA (MCI: 4; controls: 2). To

TABLE 2: Correlation coefficients between the MAPI and clinical and polysomnographic data for controls ($n = 37$) and patients with mild cognitive impairment (MCI) ($n = 37$).

	MAPI Controls	MAPI MCI
Age	**0.458****	−0.165
Body mass index	**0.491****	**0.499****
MMSE score	−0.086	−0.084
CIRS, total score	0.325	0.287
Apnoea-hypopnoea index (nonparametric test)	**0.474*** ($n = 25$)	−0.141 ($n = 24$)
Average oxygen desaturation (non-parametric test)	0.279	−0.144
Oxygen desaturation index (non-parametric test)	**0.418****	−0.077
Lowest oxygen desaturations	−0.308	−0.180

*$P < 0.05$, **$P < 0.01$.

MAPI: multivariable apnoea prediction index; CIRS: cumulative illness rating scale; MMSE: mini-mental state examination.

detect mild OSA (AHI ≥ 15), the MAPI cut-off score (0.21) is also lower than AHI ≥ 5 with an improved sensitivity of 88.24% but lower specificity of 31.25%.

In control participants, the AUC was greater at every cut-off score of AHI as compared to the corresponding findings in the MCI sample (Table 3). The optimum cut-off score for

TABLE 3: ROC curve analysis demonstrating optimal MAPI scores according to various apnoea-hypopnoea index (AHI) scores for the whole sample, MCI, and control sample.

	Whole sample (n = 49)			MCI sample (n = 24)			Control sample (n = 25)		
	AHI ≥ 5	AHI ≥ 15	AHI ≥ 30	AHI ≥ 5	AHI ≥ 15	AHI ≥ 30	AHI ≥ 5	AHI ≥ 15	AHI ≥ 30
AUC	0.567	0.580	0.502	0.576	0.504	0.650	0.699	0.671	0.761
Sensitivity	67.65*	88.24*	100.00*	88.24*	20.00*	75.00*	82.35*	100.00*	100.00*
Specificity	60.00*	31.25*	18.60*	42.86*	64.29*	70.00*	75.00*	38.89*	52.17*
MAPI cutoff	(0.29)	(0.21)	(0.15)	(0.65)	(0.56)	(0.27)	(0.27)	(0.22)	(0.33)

ROC: receiver operating characteristic; MAPI: multivariable aponea prediction index; AHI: apnoea-hypopnoea index; AUC: area under the curve. *Criterion corresponding with the highest Youden index.

TABLE 4: ROC curve analysis demonstrating the area under the curve (AUC) values according to various apnoea-hypopnoea index (AHI) scores for the whole sample (n = 48), control (n = 25), and MCI (n = 24) samples.

AHI	Sample	AUC (95% CI)
AHI ≥ 5	Whole	0.567 (0.323, 0.837)
	Control	0.699 (0.349, 0.968)
	MCI	0.576 (0.099, 0.816)
AHI ≥ 15	Whole	0.580 (0.161, 0.500)
	Control	0.671 (0.173, 0.643)
	MCI	0.504 (0.351, 0.872)
AHI ≥ 30	Whole	0.502 (0.084, 0.334)
	Control	0.761 (0.306, 0.732)
	MCI	0.650 (0.457, 0.881)

ROC: receiver operating characteristic; AHI: apnoea-hypopnoea index; AUC: area under the curve; MCI: mild cognitive impairment.

suspicion of OSA (AHI ≥ 5) in the MCI sample was much higher (MAPI of 0.65) compared to controls (MAPI of 0.27) with decreased specificity. In the MCI group, when detecting severe OSA (AHI ≥ 30), the cut-off score was lower (0.27) than was found in controls (0.33). For detecting mild OSA (AHI ≥ 15), the MAPI cut-off score in the MCI sample (0.56) was higher compared to the control (0.22) and whole sample (0.22).

The AUCs for MAPI, Index 1, and BMI were also compared simultaneously between MCI and controls (data not shown). In the MCI sample, there was a reduced ability of Index 1 to discriminate between an AHI ≤ 5 and AHI ≥ 5 (AUC = 0.353). There was also a significant positive correlation found between Index 1 and overall MAPI score in the MCI group ($r = 0.353$, $P = 0.048$), a relationship that was not observed in controls.

4. Discussion

This is the first study to investigate the utility of the MAP survey in patients with MCI and in comparison to healthy older controls. The results show that, in this sample of patients, the use of the MAPI to predict sleep apnoea offers significantly reduced utility as compared to studies in other age groups and clinical samples.

An analysis of this entire sample of older people found that, to detect severe sleep apnoea (AHI ≥ 30), the MAPI cut-off score was determined to be lower than all other severities of OSA, a finding which is in contrast to that expected. However, it is noted that only small numbers of participants had an AHI above this cutoff, thus preventing valid conclusions to be drawn regarding the utility of the tool for severe OSA.

Importantly, however, analysis of subsamples of MCI patients and controls showed that there was a significant difference in correlations between AHI and MAPI amongst controls versus MCI, suggesting that the relationship between MAPI and AHI differs according to the presence of cognitive impairment. Specifically, ROC curve analysis also showed that the MAPI is less valid in the MCI sample compared to healthy controls, with consistently lower AUC irrespective of the cutoff used in the MCI group. While it is not possible from this study alone to definitively ascertain why the MAPI is unsuitable for those with MCI, we suspect it is due to MCI patients having poor recall of sleep-wake disturbances and/or failing to report their symptoms due to their cognitive impairments. This was supported by our AUC data, which found a reduced ability of Index 1 of the MAPI to detect the presence of OSA (as measured by AHI) in the MCI group, which was not evident in controls. Another possible explanation could be that the factors that load heavily on the MAPI may not have great utility within an MCI or an older adult population. Although no significant difference emerged in common conditions associated with OSA (hypertension, heart disease, or diabetes) between the MCI and control groups, the CIRS indicated that the MCI group did have higher medical burden. Also, BMI is a factor which loads heavily on the MAPI; however, within the whole sample, there was no significant difference found between BMI and people with or without OSA (defined as AHI ≥ 5 or AHI ≥ 10). Therefore, rather than factors traditionally used to derive OSA risk such as BMI, other factors may be pertinent to the development of sleep apnoea in this age group, such as upper airway collapsibility from changes in structures surrounding the pharynx or age-related differences in respiratory control. It was also interesting to find that MAPI and age were inversely correlated in the MCI sample, as were age and BMI. Increasing BMI and age are important risk factors for OSA in the normal population; therefore, this unusual finding in our MCI sample could provide some explanation for the nonsignificant results in this subset of participants. PSG-confirmed AHI would not consider age or BMI whereas the MAPI is heavily weighted on these risk factors. Therefore, AHI may be more reliable in this group.

The MAP survey has been specifically derived to detect OSA raising the possibility that our MCI sample may actually be suffering from other sleep disorders such as CSA. Whilst having an elevated AHI on PSG, this disturbance would not be registered by the MAP survey. The pathophysiology underlying CSA is related to a failure in signalling from the brain to the muscles of ventilation resulting in cessation of breathing [30]. Unlike OSA, CSA does not trigger increased respiratory effort to breathe, and therefore loud snoring (a key component of the MAPI) is not a common symptom. However, CSA is not more prevalent in our MCI sample suggesting this is not a factor affecting the results found.

Evidently, our findings suggest that PSG remains the most reliable method for evaluating OSA in patients with MCI. Other self-report questionnaires such as the Epworth sleepiness scale have also been shown to only correlate poorly with AHI [31] suggesting that symptomatology is not always concordant with apnoea severity. However, future studies could be focused on alternative methods of PSG, such as home monitoring devices, which might prove both efficacious and well tolerated in MCI cohorts [32, 33]. In conclusion, although the MAP survey is an inexpensive and easy-to-administer screening instrument, its poor specificity reduces its clinical utility for patients with MCI.

Conflict of Interests

The authors declare that there is no conflict of interests regarding the publication of this paper.

Acknowledgments

The authors would like to thank the patients and controls who kindly participated in this study. They gratefully acknowledge the contributions of old age psychiatrist Dr. Matt Paradise, neuropsychologists Dr. Keri Diamond and Dr. Loren Mowszowski, and Chronobiologist A/Professor Naomi Rogers. They would also like to thank all BMRI sleep lab technicians as well as Tony Ip and Stergos Pates and for their assistance with PSG acquisition and scoring, respectively. A/Professor Simon J. G. Lewis is supported by an NHMRC Practitioner Fellowship. Professor Ron Grunstein is supported by an NHMRC Practitioner Fellowship. A/Professor Sharon L. Naismith is supported by an NHMRC Career Development Award.

References

[1] S. Gauthier, B. Reisberg, M. Zaudig et al., "Mild cognitive impairment," *The Lancet*, vol. 367, no. 9518, pp. 1262–1270, 2006.

[2] J.-M. Yu, I.-J. Tseng, R.-Y. Yuan, J.-J. Sheu, H.-C. Liu, and C.-J. Hu, "Low sleep efficiency in patients with cognitive impairment," *Acta Neurologica Taiwanica*, vol. 18, no. 2, pp. 91–97, 2009.

[3] S. L. Naismith, S. J. Lewis, and N. L. Rogers, "Sleep-wake changes and cognition in neurodegenerative disease," *Progress in Brain Research*, vol. 190, pp. 21–52, 2011.

[4] N. Wolkove, O. Elkholy, M. Baltzan, and M. Palayew, "Sleep and aging: 1. Sleep disorders commonly found in older people,"

Canadian Medical Association Journal, vol. 176, no. 9, pp. 1299–1304, 2007.

[5] S. Ancoli-Israel, D. F. Kripke, M. R. Klauber, W. J. Mason, R. Fell, and O. Kaplan, "Sleep-disordered breathing in community-dwelling elderly," *Sleep*, vol. 14, no. 6, pp. 486–495, 1991.

[6] N. M. Punjabi, "The epidemiology of adult obstructive sleep apnea," *Proceedings of the American Thoracic Society*, vol. 5, no. 2, pp. 136–143, 2008.

[7] J. R. Cooke, L. Ayalon, B. W. Palmer et al., "Sustained use of CPAP slows deterioration of cognition, sleep, and mood in patients with Alzheimer's disease and obstructive sleep apnea: a preliminary study," *Journal of Clinical Sleep Medicine*, vol. 5, no. 4, pp. 305–309, 2009.

[8] S. J. Kim, J. H. Lee, D. Y. Lee, J. H. Jhoo, and J. I. Woo, "Neurocognitive dysfunction associated with sleep quality and sleep apnea in patients with mild cognitive impairment," *American Journal of Geriatric Psychiatry*, vol. 19, no. 4, pp. 374–381, 2011.

[9] S. Naismith, V. Winter, H. Gotsopoulos, I. Hickie, and P. Cistulli, "Neurobehavioral functioning in obstructive sleep apnea: differential effects of sleep quality, hypoxemia and subjective sleepiness," *Journal of Clinical and Experimental Neuropsychology*, vol. 26, no. 1, pp. 43–54, 2004.

[10] N. Canessa and L. Ferini-Strambi, "Sleep-disordered breathing and cognitive decline in older adults," *The Journal of the American Medical Association*, vol. 306, no. 6, pp. 654–655, 2011.

[11] K. Yaffe, A. M. Laffan, S. L. Harrison et al., "Sleep-disordered breathing, hypoxia, and risk of mild cognitive impairment and dementia in older women," *The Journal of the American Medical Association*, vol. 306, no. 6, pp. 613–619, 2011.

[12] K. Jones and Y. Harrison, "Frontal lobe function, sleep loss and fragmented sleep," *Sleep Medicine Reviews*, vol. 5, no. 6, pp. 463–475, 2001.

[13] J. G. McCoy and R. E. Strecker, "The cognitive cost of sleep lost," *Neurobiology of Learning and Memory*, vol. 96, no. 4, pp. 564–582, 2011.

[14] J. R. Cooke, S. Ancoli-Israel, L. Liu et al., "Continuous positive airway pressure deepens sleep in patients with Alzheimer's disease and obstructive sleep apnea," *Sleep Medicine*, vol. 10, no. 10, pp. 1101–1106, 2009.

[15] C. A. Kushida, D. A. Nichols, T. H. Holmes et al., "Effects of continuous positive airway pressure on neurocognitive function in obstructive apnea patients: the Apnea Positive Pressure Long-term Efficacy Study (APPLES)," *Sleep*, vol. 35, no. 12, pp. 1593–1602, 2012.

[16] A. Wauquier, B. Van Sweden, G. A. Kerkhof, and H. A. C. Kamphuisen, "Ambulatory first night sleep effect recording in the elderly," *Behavioural Brain Research*, vol. 42, no. 1, pp. 7–11, 1991.

[17] G. Maislin, A. I. Pack, N. B. Kribbs et al., "A survey screen for prediction of apnea," *Sleep*, vol. 18, no. 3, pp. 158–166, 1995.

[18] K. K. H. Wong, M. P. Jones, G. Marks, N. Zwar, and R. R. Grunstein, "Development of a diagnostic model for sleep apnea in primary care," Poster session presented at: World Sleep, 2011.

[19] G. Maislin, I. Gurubhagavatula, R. Hachadoorian et al., "Operating characteristics of the multivariable apnea prediction index in non-clinic populations," *Sleep*, vol. 26, 2003, abstract A247.

[20] I. Gurubhagavatula, G. Maislin, and A. I. Pack, "An algorithm to stratify sleep apnea risk in a sleep disorders clinic population," *American Journal of Respiratory and Critical Care Medicine*, vol. 164, no. 10 I, pp. 1904–1909, 2001.

[21] R. C. Petersen and J. C. Morris, "Mild cognitive impairment as a clinical entity and treatment target," *Archives of Neurology*, vol. 62, no. 7, pp. 1160–1163, 2005.

[22] B. S. Linn, M. W. Linn, and L. Gurel, "Cumulative illness rating scale," *Journal of the American Geriatrics Society*, vol. 16, no. 5, pp. 622–626, 1968.

[23] M. F. Folstein, S. E. Folstein, and P. R. McHugh, "'Mini mental state'. A practical method for grading the cognitive state of patients for the clinician," *Journal of Psychiatric Research*, vol. 12, no. 3, pp. 189–198, 1975.

[24] S. L. Naismith, N. L. Rogers, I. B. Hickie, J. MacKenzie, L. M. Norrie, and S. J. G. Lewis, "Sleep well, think well: sleep-wake disturbance in mild cognitive impairment," *Journal of Geriatric Psychiatry and Neurology*, vol. 23, no. 2, pp. 123–130, 2010.

[25] B. Winblad, K. Palmer, M. Kivipelto et al., "Mild cognitive impairment—beyond controversies, towards a consensus: report of the International Working Group on Mild Cognitive Impairment," *Journal of Internal Medicine*, vol. 256, no. 3, pp. 240–246, 2004.

[26] K. Rechtschaffen, *A Manual of Standardized Terminology, Techniques and Scoring System for Sleep Stages of Human Subjects*, vol. 204, National Institutes of Health, U. S. National Institute of Neurological Diseases and Blindness, Neurological Information Network, Bethesda, Md, USA, 1968, Edited by: A. Rechtschaffen and A. Kales, http://catalogue.nla.gov.au/Record/823711.

[27] W. B. Webb and L. M. Dreblow, "A modified method for scoring slow wave sleep of older subjects," *Sleep*, vol. 5, no. 2, pp. 195–199, 1982.

[28] W. W. Flemons, D. Buysse, S. Redline et al., "Sleep-related breathing disorders in adults: recommendations for syndrome definition and measurement techniques in clinical research. The Report of American Academy of Sleep Medicine Task Force," *Sleep*, vol. 22, no. 5, pp. 667–689, 1999.

[29] D. J. Buysse, C. F. Reynolds III, T. H. Monk, S. R. Berman, and D. J. Kupfer, "The Pittsburgh Sleep Quality Index: a new instrument for psychiatric practice and research," *Psychiatry Research*, vol. 28, no. 2, pp. 193–213, 1989.

[30] D. J. Eckert, A. S. Jordan, P. Merchia, and A. Malhotra, "Central sleep apnea: pathophysiology and treatment," *Chest*, vol. 131, no. 2, pp. 595–607, 2007.

[31] E. M. Weaver, V. Kapur, and B. Yueh, "Polysomnography vs self-reported measures in patients with sleep apnea," *Archives of Otolaryngology—Head and Neck Surgery*, vol. 130, no. 4, pp. 453–458, 2004.

[32] L. M. Rofail, K. K. H. Wong, G. Unger, G. B. Marks, and R. R. Grunstein, "The utility of single-channel nasal airflow pressure transducer in the diagnosis of OSA at home," *Sleep*, vol. 33, no. 8, pp. 1097–1105, 2010.

[33] L. M. Rofail, K. K. H. Wong, G. Unger, G. B. Marks, and R. R. Grunstein, "Comparison between a single-channel nasal airflow device and oximetry for the diagnosis of obstructive sleep apnea," *Sleep*, vol. 33, no. 8, pp. 1106–1114, 2010.

31

The Relationship between Nocturnal Hypoxemia and Left Ventricular Ejection Fraction in Congestive Heart Failure Patients

Mohammad Mirzaaghazadeh,[1] **Mehrzad Bahtouee,**[2] **Fariba Mehdiniya,**[1] **Nasrollah Maleki,**[1] **and Zahra Tavosi**[2]

[1] *Department of Internal Medicine, Imam Khomeini Hospital, Ardabil University of Medical Sciences, Ardabil 6368134497, Iran*
[2] *Department of Internal Medicine, Shohadaye Khalije Fars Hospital, Bushehr University of Medical Sciences, Bushehr, Iran*

Correspondence should be addressed to Nasrollah Maleki; malekinasrollah@yahoo.com

Academic Editor: Michel M. Billiard

Congestive heart failure (CHF) is a major cause of mortality and morbidity. Among patients with heart failure, sleep disordered breathing (SDB) is a common problem. Current evidence suggests that SDB, particularly central SDB, is more prevalent in patients with CHF than in the general population, but it is underdiagnosed as SDB symptoms that are less prevalent in CHF. The main aims of this study were to determine the relationship between nocturnal hypoxemia and left ventricular ejection fraction in patients with chronic heart failure. By means of echocardiography, 108 patients with left ventricular ejection fraction ≤45% were divided into mild, moderate, and severe CHF. Hypoxemia was recorded overnight in the hospital and was measured by portable pulse oximetry. In the 108 patients with CHF, 44 (40.7%) were severe, 17 (15.7%) moderate, and 47 (43.6%) mild CHF. 95 (88%) of patients with CHF had abnormal patterns of nocturnal hypoxemia suggestive of Cheyne-Stokes respiration. Ejection fraction correlated negatively with dip frequency. There was no correlation between nocturnal hypoxemia with BMI and snoring. This study confirms strong associations between sleep apnea and heart disease in patients with CHF. Overnight oximetry is a useful screening test for Cheyne-Stokes respiration in patients with known heart failure.

1. Introduction

Sleep related breathing disorders (SRBD) refer to an abnormal respiratory pattern (e.g., apneas, hypopneas, or respiratory effort related arousals) or an abnormal reduction in gas exchange (e.g., hypoventilation) during sleep. They tend to repetitively alter sleep duration and architecture, resulting in daytime symptoms, signs, or organ system dysfunction. Sleep related breathing disorders are best characterized by polysomnography that has captured one or more periods of rapid eye movement (REM) sleep, as severe perturbations can be common during REM sleep [1, 2]. Sleep apnea is hypothesized to increase the risk of developing cardiovascular disease (CVD) and hypertension. Initial support for this hypothesis came from several population studies of snoring and CVD outcomes, suggesting that those who snore are more likely to develop hypertension, myocardial infarction, and stroke [3–5]. Two types of sleep disordered breathing are common among patients with heart failure: obstructive sleep apnea (OSA) and Cheyne-Stokes breathing (CSB).

1.1. Prevalence. While OSA is more common than CSB in the general population, CSB may be more common than OSA in patients with heart failure [6, 7]. Single-center observational studies estimate that the prevalence of SRBD may be as high as 50 percent among all patients with heart failure and as high as 70 percent among patients with heart failure who are referred to a sleep laboratory [6–9]. The prevalence may be even higher among patients with acute decompensated heart failure, as suggested by a study that detected an apnea hypopnea index ≥10 events per hour of sleep in 22 out of 29 such patients (76 percent) [10].

1.2. Risk Factors. Risk factors for SRBD in patients with heart failure vary according to the type of SRBD. With respect to CSB, risk factors include male gender, advanced age, atrial fibrillation, and hypocapnia (i.e., transcutaneous carbon dioxide ≤38 mmHg) [9]. With respect to OSA, risk factors include advanced age and an increasing body mass index (BMI).

1.3. Pathogenesis. The pathogenesis of OSA involves abnormalities in pharyngeal anatomy, pharyngeal function, and ventilatory control. In patients with heart failure, edema of the upper airway is an additional factor that may contribute to pharyngeal airway narrowing [11]. The pathogenesis of CSB is uncertain, but the favored hypothesis is based on the observation that patients who have heart failure and CSB tend to have lower arterial carbon dioxide tensions ($PaCO_2$) than patients who have heart failure without CSB [12, 13]. The net effect is oscillation of ventilation between apnea and hyperpnea. Elimination of the hypocapnia with inhaled CO_2, continuous positive airway pressure (CPAP), or oxygen can markedly attenuate CSB [14–17]. Both OSA and CSB can impair systolic and diastolic cardiac function by a variety of mechanisms. First, intermittent hypoxemia and arousals induce adrenergic surges that may lead to heart disease progression. Second, the extremely negative intrapleural pressures increase ventricular transmural wall stress and afterload [18].

1.4. Clinical Manifestations. A sleep history should be sought from both the patient and the spouse because, in many cases, it is only the spouse who is aware of the abnormal ventilatory pattern. SRBD can be asymptomatic or symptomatic in patients who have heart failure [19]. When OSA is the predominant type of SRBD, poor sleep quality and snoring are common. As a result, sleep disruption and easy fatigability often exist and may be out of proportion to the severity of the heart failure. However, sleepiness is relatively uncommon in patients with heart failure for reasons that remain unclear [20]. When CSB is the predominant type of SRBD, symptoms due to CSB may be indistinguishable from those due to the heart failure [6]. Symptoms of poor sleep quality (e.g., excessive daytime sleepiness) are subtle and generally unreliable. Occasionally, patients with CSB report paroxysmal nocturnal dyspnea (due to the hyperpnea that follows an apnea) [21]. SRBD may contribute to nocturnal angina in patients with heart failure, presumably due to hypoxemia and catecholamine surges [21]. In addition, recurrent arrhythmias may occur, such as atrial fibrillation or ventricular tachycardia [9, 22]. These arrhythmias often occur in the absence of any symptoms or signs of SRBD. Thus, a high index of suspicion should be maintained and evaluation for SRBD should be considered in heart failure patients with recurrent arrhythmias.

1.5. Diagnosis. The diagnostic evaluation of suspected SRBD is the same for patients with or without heart failure. An in-laboratory overnight polysomnogram is the gold standard diagnostic test. In-home portable monitoring is also available.

The 2005 American College of Cardiology/American Heart Association (ACC/AHA) guidelines on the diagnosis and treatment of chronic heart failure indicate that screening for SRBD is reasonable in selected patients (e.g., those with risk factors) [23].

1.6. Prognosis. Heart failure accompanied by SRBD is associated with a worse prognosis than heart failure in the absence of SRBD [24]. With respect to OSA, a prospective cohort study followed up 164 patients who had heart failure and a left ventricular ejection fraction of 45 percent or less [25]. At a mean of three years, patients who had OSA (defined as an AHI of at least 15 events per hour) had a higher cardiac mortality than patients who did not have OSA (8.7 versus 4.2 deaths per 100 patient-years). With respect to CSB, a prospective cohort study followed up 62 patients with NYHA class II to III heart failure [26]. At a mean of 28 months, cardiac mortality was associated with an AHI greater than 30 events per hour. The AHI was a better predictor of cardiac mortality than demographic variables, Holter monitoring, exercise studies, echocardiography, or autonomic testing. CSB was found to predict mortality in numerous other studies of patients with heart failure [7, 27–30].

1.7. Treatment. With respect to the impact of heart failure therapy on SRBD, case series and observational studies suggest that the following interventions are associated with improved SRBD: medical management (e.g., ACE inhibitors, beta blockers, and diuretics) [11, 25, 31, 32], cardiac transplantation [33–35], cardiac resynchronization (i.e., biventricular pacing) [36–38], and left ventricular assist device (LVAD) implantation [39]. For patients who have heart failure complicated by OSA or CSB, positive airway pressure may improve cardiac function, blood pressure, exercise capacity, and quality of life [15, 28, 40–46]. The possible role of theophylline in patients with heart failure complicated by SRBD was evaluated in a doubleblind crossover trial of 15 such patients who received either theophylline or placebo twice daily for five days [47].

2. Materials and Methods

The current cross-sectional study is a descriptive, analytical one that was conducted on 108 patients referred to the Imam Hospital from November 2010 to March 2011, who had been hospitalized due to CHF. CHF diagnosis was performed based on history, clinical examination, and echocardiography. Given the prevalence of heart failure as 14% in Iran and considering that, in accordance with previous studies, approximately 51% of these patients suffer from sleep disorders resulting from changes in arterial oxygen pressure, the sample size for this study was estimated as 108 patients. Inclusion criteria for this study included patients with systolic CHF (congestive heart failure) (EF less than or equal to 45%) and people with chronic obstructive pulmonary diseases (COPD) and patients with unstable CHF were excluded.

TABLE 1: Distribution of patients according to age and body mass index.

Variable	Number	Minimum	Maximum	Mean	SD
Age	108	35	86	65.42	11.40
BMI (Kg/m^2)	108	20	38	26.93	3.74

Information on age, sex, BMI, and sleep patterns of patients was obtained. Spirometric examinations were performed on patients with CHF, and patients with COPD diagnosis based on medical history, physical examination, and spirometry were excluded. Then, eligible patients underwent pulse oximetry from the night until the next morning using DC-68B (Shenzhen Creative Industry wrist oximeter).

In this study, the statistical software SPSS V16 was used for data analysis. The tests including chi-square, t-test, Pearson correlation coefficient, and ANOVA were used for obtained data analysis. The significance level was determined as less than or equal to 0.05.

3. Results

In this study, 108 patients with stable chronic heart failure were studied; 52 patients (48.1%) were males and 56 patients (51.9%) were females. The patients' age range was 35–86 years with a mean of 65.42 ± 11 years, and the patients, BMI was between 20 and 38 with a mean of 26.93 ± 3.74. 73 patients (67.6%) had a BMI greater than or equal to 25 and 35 patients (32.4%) had a BMI less than 25 (Table 1). Patients were studied regarding sleep disorders. 62 patients (57.4%) were snoring at night, and only 18 patients (16.7%) complained of daytime sleepiness. The patients were classified regarding ejection fraction into three groups, including mild failure (ejection fraction between 40 and 45 percent), moderate failure (ejection fraction between 35 and 40 percent), and severe failure (less than or equal to 34 percent of ejection fraction). The results showed that 47 patients (43.6%) had mild heart failure; 17 patients (15.7%) had moderate heart failure; and 44 patients (40.7%) were with severe heart failure.

The patients were also examined regarding the percentage of their nocturnal sleep duration suffered from hypoxia. The results showed that 42.6% of patients experienced hypoxia in 10% of their total nocturnal recording time; 9.1% of patients had suffered from hypoxia in 40–70% of their total nocturnal recording time; 5.4% of patients had hypoxia in more than 75% of their total nocturnal recording time; and in 12% of patients, hypoxia was not observed in total nocturnal recording time. During evaluating the patients about daily hypoxia (during waking hours), the results showed that only 6.5% of the patients experience arterial oxygen desaturation at the time of awakening.

Patients with different levels of ejection fraction and with different levels of arterial oxygen desaturation were compared (Table 2). The results showed that patients with mild heart failure in the majority of arterial blood oxygen saturation levels had the least hypoxia time; however, the analysis of variance showed no significant difference between the three groups of patients. Thus, Pearson correlation test was

also performed to investigate the relationship between levels of arterial oxygen desaturation and ejection fraction. The results showed that, at levels of arterial oxygen desaturation between 80–84%, 75–79%, and 65–69%, there is a significant correlation between the two variables of arterial oxygen saturation percentage and ejection fraction, so that with decrease in ejection fraction, the arterial oxygen desaturation in patients increases.

The arterial oxygen desaturation was also calculated according to patients' gender. The results showed that arterial oxygen desaturation rate in women is higher than in men; however, performing t-test showed no statistically significant differences between the two groups (P = 0.43). The correlation test was also performed between arterial oxygen desaturation and the age of patients; however, no significant correlation was found between these two variables (P = 0.07).

Arterial oxygen desaturation in patients with complaints of sleep disorders and without sleep disorders was examined. The results showed that the decline in arterial oxygen saturation is higher in patients with nocturnal snoring than patients without snoring at night; however, performing independent t-test showed no significant differences between the two groups (P = 0.90). The mean arterial oxygen desaturation rate was also compared in two groups of patients with BMI greater than or equal to 25 and less than 25. The results showed that patients with a BMI greater than or equal to 25 have a greater mean arterial oxygen desaturation rate than patients with lower BMI; however, the independent t-test showed no significant differences between the two groups (P = 0.72).

4. Discussion

Heart failure (HF) is a major cause of mortality and morbidity [48] and is associated with progressively severe symptoms, chronic disability, and impaired quality of life [6]. Sleep-disordered breathing (SDB) is known to occur frequently in patients with stable but severe HF [6, 19, 48] and may be a predictor of poor prognosis [29]. Sleep related breathing disorders (SRBD) appear to be common even among patients whose heart failure is optimally managed. SDB is present in approximately three-fourths of patients with symptomatic or decompensated systolic heart failure [45, 46]. The prevalence is very high even in those with stable chronic heart failure [6, 47, 48]. Cross-sectional analyses from Sleep Heart Health Study data revealed an adjusted odds ratio of 2.2 for self-reported heart failure amongst subjects with OSA.

In this study, 88% of patients with heart failure experienced SRBD during their total nocturnal recording time. In a study by Javaheri et al. in 1998, 51% of male patients with stable heart failure had SRBD, 40% of which was central sleep apnea type (CSA) and 11% was obstructive sleep apnea type (OSA) [6]. In another study in China by Wang et al. conducted on 195 patients with heart failure, the SRBD was seen in 80% of patients, 53% of OSA type and 27% of CSA type [49]. In a study by Rao et al. performed in 2006 in the United Kingdom, the SRBD prevalence was reported on average as 24% [50]. In a study by Lanfranchi et al., the SRBD was found

TABLE 2: Correlation between the two variables of arterial oxygen saturation percentage and ejection fraction in study patients.

Arterial oxygen saturation percentage	Mild CHF (mean ± SD)	Moderate CHF (mean ± SD)	Severe CHF (mean ± SD)	P value
60–65%	0.17 ± 0.41	0.11 ± 0.25	0.34 ± 0.65	0.16
65–70%	0.22 ± 0.58	0.11 ± 0.20	0.32 ± 0.47	0.31
70–75%	0.68 ± 1.75	1.73 ± 6.51	0.81 ± 1.13	0.42
75–80%	1.84 ± 6.09	3.85 ± 11.26	2.57 ± 3.69	0.57
80–85%	3.90 ± 8.11	7.23 ± 12.17	5.84 ± 8.75	0.36
85–89%	12.77 ± 15.52	14.02 ± 16.67	16.04 ± 18.40	0.65

in 55% of patients with asymptomatic heart failure with LVEF less than 40% [19, 26]; but in a study by Tremel et al., 82% of patients with heart failure had SRBD [51]. A prospective cohort study followed up 108 patients who visited a heart failure clinic with stable heart failure, which was defined as clinical stability without hospitalizations or medication changes within the past 30 days [52]. SRBD was detected in 61 percent of patients and was independently associated with the presence of atrial fibrillation and a worse New York Heart Association (NYHA) functional class.

In the present study, no significant relationship was found between age and arterial oxygen desaturation. In a study by Staniforth et al. in 1998 performed on 104 patients, no significant relationship was found between age and arterial oxygen saturation. In this study, the nocturnal pulse oximetry was identified as a useful screening test for Cheyne-Stokes respiration in patients with heart failure [53]. However, in a study by Sin et al. to evaluate risk factors of CSA and OSA performed on 450 patients with heart failure, the patients with CSA were older than patients with OSA [9]. In a study by Liu et al. in 2006 on 56 elderly patients with CHF, 67.9% of patients had SRBD and the OSA prevalence was higher in older patients [54]. Male gender may be a risk factor for CSA because, in general, men have a less stable sleep architecture than women, with a greater number of sleep-wake transitions and shorter slow-wave sleep, which may predispose to respiratory control system instability and central apneas [55].

In our study, patients with a BMI greater than 25 had a mean arterial oxygen desaturation higher than patients with a lower BMI; however, no statistically significant difference was found between the two groups. Considering that polysomnography was not available in our study and evaluation of arterial oxygen desaturation was performed by using a portable pulse oximetry, there was no possibility to differentiate patients with OSA from CSA. However, since the prevalence of CSA in patients with cardiac failure is more than OSA, we expect that most of our patients have CSA, and the lack of significant correlation between BMI and arterial oxygen desaturation can be explained in this regard. In Javaheri et al.'s study, high BMI was more common only in patients with OSA [6]. In Sin et al.'s study, high BMI was significantly correlated with OSA. In this study, high BMI association with OSA, which was more in men, was due to android pattern of obesity in them [9].

In the present study, snoring at night (nocturnal snoring) was seen in 57.4% of patients. In heart failure patients who had nocturnal snoring, the mean arterial oxygen desaturation was more than in patients without this clinical symptom; but there was no statistically significant difference between the two groups. In Javaheri et al.'s study, 78% of patients with OSA had nocturnal snoring, and only 28% of patients with CSA had nightly snoring [6].

In our study, daytime sleepiness was seen in only 16.7% of the patients. In Wang et al.'s study, patients with heart failure who had SRBD were not mentioning daytime sleepiness [49]. The first goal in the treatment of SDB in CHF is to optimize CHF treatment. Conservative measures for OSA such as weight reduction, avoidance of supine position during sleep, and avoiding alcohol and sedative medications before sleep are also useful. Nocturnal CPAP therapy may be useful in treating SDB in CHF [56].

In the present study, there was a significant correlation between the severity of arterial oxygen desaturation rate and ejection fraction. In similar studies by Staniforth et al. [53], Javaheri et al. [6], and Shahar et al. [57], a significant correlation between decreased ejection fraction and arterial oxygen desaturation was seen.

5. Conclusion

Several studies in recent years have demonstrated the close relationship between sleep related breathing disorders (SRBD) and systolic heart failure. In the present study, 88% of patients with heart failure experienced SRBD during their total nocturnal recording time. Unfortunately, in clinical treatment of systolic heart failure, SRBD is hardly considered.

Conflict of Interests

The authors declare that there is no conflict of interests regarding the publication of this paper.

References

[1] C. Iber, S. Ancoli-Israel, A. L. Chesson et al., *The AASM Manual for the Scoring of Sleep and Associated Events*, American Academy of Sleep Medicine, West Chester, Ill, USA, 2007.

[2] G. M. Loughlin, R. T. Brouillette, L. J. Brooke et al., "Standards and indications for cardiopulmonary sleep studies in children,"

American Journal of Respiratory and Critical Care Medicine, vol. 153, no. 2, pp. 866–878, 1996.

[3] R. D'Alessandro, C. Magelli, G. Gamberini et al., "Snoring every night as a risk factor for myocardial infarction: a case-control study," *British Medical Journal*, vol. 300, no. 6739, pp. 1557–1558, 1990.

[4] M. Koskenvuo, J. Kaprio, and T. Telakivi, "Snoring as a risk factor for ischaemic heart disease and stroke in men," *British Medical Journal*, vol. 294, no. 6563, pp. 16–19, 1987.

[5] P. G. Norton and E. V. Dunn, "Snoring as a risk factor for disease: an epidemiological survey," *British Medical Journal*, vol. 291, no. 6496, pp. 630–632, 1985.

[6] S. Javaheri, T. J. Parker, J. D. Liming et al., "Sleep apnea in 81 ambulatory male patients with stable heart failure: types and their prevalences, consequences, and presentations," *Circulation*, vol. 97, no. 21, pp. 2154–2159, 1998.

[7] U. Corrà, M. Pistono, A. Mezzani et al., "Sleep and exertional periodic breathing in chronic heart failure: prognostic importance and interdependence," *Circulation*, vol. 113, no. 1, pp. 44–50, 2006.

[8] S. Javaheri, T. J. Parker, L. Wexler et al., "Occult sleep-disordered breathing in stable congestive heart failure," *Annals of Internal Medicine*, vol. 122, no. 7, pp. 487–492, 1995.

[9] D. D. Sin, F. Fitzgerald, J. D. Parker, G. Newton, J. S. Floras, and T. D. Bradley, "Risk factors for central and obstructive sleep apnea in 450 men and women with congestive heart failure," *American Journal of Respiratory and Critical Care Medicine*, vol. 160, no. 4, pp. 1101–1106, 1999.

[10] M. Padeletti, P. Green, A. M. Mooney, R. C. Basner, and D. M. Mancini, "Sleep disordered breathing in patients with acutely decompensated heart failure," *Sleep Medicine*, vol. 10, no. 3, pp. 353–360, 2009.

[11] C. B. Bucca, L. Brussino, A. Battisti et al., "Diuretics in obstructive sleep apnea with diastolic heart failure," *Chest*, vol. 132, no. 2, pp. 440–446, 2007.

[12] M. Naughton, D. Benard, A. Tam, R. Rutherford, and T. D. Bradley, "Role of hyperventilation in the pathogenesis of central sleep apneas in patients with congestive heart failure," *American Review of Respiratory Disease*, vol. 148, no. 2, pp. 330–338, 1993.

[13] P. Hanly, N. Zuberi, and R. Gray, "Pathogenesis of Cheyne-Stokes respiration in patients with congestive heart failure: relationship to arterial PCO2," *Chest*, vol. 104, no. 4, pp. 1079–1084, 1993.

[14] R. D. Steens, T. W. Millar, S. Xiaoling et al., "Effect of inhaled 3% CO2 on Cheyne-Stokes respiration in congestive heart failure," *Sleep*, vol. 17, no. 1, pp. 61–68, 1994.

[15] M. T. Naughton, D. C. Benard, P. P. Liu, R. Rutherford, F. Rankin, and T. D. Bradley, "Effects of nasal CPAP on sympathetic activity in patients with heart failure and central sleep apnea," *American Journal of Respiratory and Critical Care Medicine*, vol. 152, no. 2, pp. 473–479, 1995.

[16] M. T. Naughton, D. C. Benard, R. Rutherford, and T. D. Bradley, "Effect of continuous positive airway pressure on central sleep apnea and nocturnal PCO2 in heart failure," *American Journal of Respiratory and Critical Care Medicine*, vol. 150, no. 6 I, pp. 1598–1604, 1994.

[17] P. J. Hanley, T. W. Millar, D. G. Steljes, R. Baert, M. A. Frais, and M. H. Kryger, "The effect of oxygen on respiration and sleep in patients with congestive heart failure," *Annals of Internal Medicine*, vol. 111, no. 10, pp. 777–782, 1989.

[18] A. Malhotra, V. V. Muse, and E. J. Mark, "Case 12-2003: an 82-year-old man with dyspnea and pulmonary abnormalities," *New England Journal of Medicine*, vol. 348, no. 16, pp. 1574–1585, 2003.

[19] P. A. Lanfranchi, V. K. Somers, A. Braghiroli, U. Corra, E. Eleuteri, and P. Giannuzzi, "Central sleep apnea in left ventricular dysfunction: prevalence and implications for arrhythmic risk," *Circulation*, vol. 107, no. 5, pp. 727–732, 2003.

[20] M. Arzt, T. Young, L. Finn et al., "Sleepiness and sleep in patients with both systolic heart failure and obstructive sleep apnea," *Archives of Internal Medicine*, vol. 166, no. 16, pp. 1716–1722, 2006.

[21] K. A. Franklin, J. B. Nilsson, C. Sahlin, and U. Näslund, "Sleep apnoea and nocturnal angina," *The Lancet*, vol. 345, no. 8957, pp. 1085–1087, 1995.

[22] S. Javaheri, "Effects of continuous positive airway pressure on sleep apnea and ventricular irritability in patients with heart failure," *Circulation*, vol. 101, no. 4, pp. 392–397, 2000.

[23] S. A. Hunt, W. T. Abraham, M. H. Chin et al., "ACC/AHA 2005 Guideline Update for the Diagnosis and Management of Chronic Heart Failure in the Adult: a report of the American College of Cardiology/American Heart Association Task Force on Practice Guidelines (Writing Committee to Update the 2001 Guidelines for the Evaluation and Management of Heart Failure): developed in collaboration with the American College of Chest Physicians and the International Society for Heart and Lung Transplantation: endorsed by the Heart Rhythm Society," *Circulation*, vol. 112, article e154, 2005.

[24] H. Wang, J. D. Parker, G. E. Newton et al., "Influence of obstructive sleep apnea on mortality in patients with heart failure," *Journal of the American College of Cardiology*, vol. 49, no. 15, pp. 1625–1631, 2007.

[25] D. S. Dark, S. K. Pingleton, G. R. Kerby et al., "Breathing pattern abnormalities and arterial oxygen desaturation during sleep in the congestive heart failure syndrome. Improvement following medical therapy," *Chest*, vol. 91, no. 6, pp. 833–836, 1987.

[26] P. A. Lanfranchi, A. Braghiroli, E. Bosimini et al., "Prognostic value of Nocturnal Cheyne-Stokes respiration in chronic heart failure," *Circulation*, vol. 99, no. 11, pp. 1435–1440, 1999.

[27] L. J. Findley, C. W. Zwillich, and S. Ancoli-Israel, "Cheyne-Stokes breathing during sleep in patients with left ventricular heart failure," *Southern Medical Journal*, vol. 78, no. 1, pp. 11–15, 1985.

[28] D. D. Sin, A. G. Logan, F. S. Fitzgerald, P. P. Liu, and T. D. Bradley, "Effects of continuous positive airway pressure on cardiovascular outcomes in heart failure patients with and without Cheyne-Stokes respiration," *Circulation*, vol. 102, no. 1, pp. 61–66, 2000.

[29] P. J. Hanly and N. S. Zuberi-Khokhar, "Increased mortality associated with Cheyne-Stokes respiration in patients with congestive heart failure," *American Journal of Respiratory and Critical Care Medicine*, vol. 153, no. 1, pp. 272–276, 1996.

[30] T. Brack, I. Thüer, C. F. Clarenbach et al., "Daytime Cheyne-Stokes respiration in ambulatory patients with severe congestive heart failure is associated with increased mortality," *Chest*, vol. 132, no. 5, pp. 1463–1471, 2007.

[31] P. Solin, P. Bergin, M. Richardson, D. M. Kaye, E. H. Walters, and M. T. Naughton, "Influence of pulmonary capillary wedge pressure on central apnea in heart failure," *Circulation*, vol. 99, no. 12, pp. 1574–1579, 1999.

[32] J. T. Walsh, R. Andrews, R. Starling, A. J. Cowley, I. D. A. Johnston, and W. J. Kinnear, "Effects of captopril and oxygen

on sleep apnoea in patients with mild to moderate congestive cardiac failure," *British Heart Journal*, vol. 73, no. 3, pp. 237–241, 1995.

[33] D. K. Murdock, C. E. Lawless, and H. S. Loeb, "The effect of heart transplantation on Cheyne-Stokes respiration associated with congestive heart failure," *Journal of Heart Transplantation*, vol. 5, no. 2, pp. 336–337, 1986.

[34] H. M. Braver, W. C. Brandes, M. A. Kubiet, M. C. Limacher, R. M. Mills Jr., and A. J. Block, "Effect of cardiac transplantation on Cheyne-Stokes respiration occurring during sleep," *American Journal of Cardiology*, vol. 76, no. 8, pp. 632–634, 1995.

[35] D. R. Mansfield, P. Solin, T. Roebuck, P. Bergin, D. M. Kaye, and M. T. Naughton, "The effect of successful heart transplant treatment of heart failure on central sleep apnea," *Chest*, vol. 124, no. 5, pp. 1675–1681, 2003.

[36] M. L. Stanchina, K. Ellison, A. Malhotra et al., "The impact of cardiac resynchronization therapy on obstructive sleep apnea in heart failure patients: a pilot study," *Chest*, vol. 132, no. 2, pp. 433–439, 2007.

[37] A.-M. Sinha, E. C. Skobel, O.-A. Breithardt et al., "Cardiac resynchronization therapy improves central sleep apnea and Cheyne-Stokes respiration in patients with chronic heart failure," *Journal of the American College of Cardiology*, vol. 44, no. 1, pp. 68–71, 2004.

[38] A. Sharafkhaneh, H. Sharafkhaneh, A. Bredikus, C. Guilleminault, B. Bozkurt, and M. Hirshkowitz, "Effect of atrial overdrive pacing on obstructive sleep apnea in patients with systolic heart failure," *Sleep Medicine*, vol. 8, no. 1, pp. 31–36, 2007.

[39] M. Padeletti, A. Henriquez, D. M. Mancini, and R. C. Basner, "Persistence of Cheyne-Stokes breathing after left ventricular assist device implantation in patients with acutely decompensated end-stage heart failure," *Journal of Heart and Lung Transplantation*, vol. 26, no. 7, pp. 742–744, 2007.

[40] T. D. Bradley, A. G. Logan, R. J. Kimoff et al., "Continuous positive airway pressure for central sleep apnea and heart failure," *New England Journal of Medicine*, vol. 353, no. 19, pp. 2025–2033, 2005.

[41] D. R. Mansfield, N. C. Gollogly, D. M. Kaye, M. Richardson, P. Bergin, and M. T. Naughton, "Controlled trial of continuous positive airway pressure in obstructive sleep apnea and heart failure," *American Journal of Respiratory and Critical Care Medicine*, vol. 169, no. 3, pp. 361–366, 2004.

[42] Y. Kaneko, J. S. Floras, K. Usui et al., "Cardiovascular effects of continuous positive airway pressure in patients with heart failure and obstructive sleep apnea," *New England Journal of Medicine*, vol. 348, no. 13, pp. 1233–1241, 2003.

[43] L. A. Smith, M. Vennelle, R. S. Gardner et al., "Auto-titrating continuous positive airway pressure therapy in patients with chronic heart failure and obstructive sleep apnoea: a randomized placebo-controlled trial," *European Heart Journal*, vol. 28, no. 10, pp. 1221–1227, 2007.

[44] R. N. Khayat, W. T. Abraham, B. Patt, M. Roy, K. Hua, and D. Jarjoura, "Cardiac effects of continuous and bilevel positive airway pressure for patients with heart failure and obstructive sleep apnea: a pilot study," *Chest*, vol. 134, no. 6, pp. 1162–1168, 2008.

[45] T. Köhnlein, T. Welte, L. B. Tan, and M. W. Elliott, "Assisted ventilation for heart failure patients with Cheyne-Stokes respiration," *European Respiratory Journal*, vol. 20, no. 4, pp. 934–941, 2002.

[46] M. Arzt, J. S. Floras, A. G. Logan et al., "Suppression of central sleep apnea by continuous positive airway pressure and transplant-free survival in heart failure: a post hoc analysis of the Canadian Continuous Positive Airway Pressure for Patients with Central Sleep Apnea and Heart Failure Trial (CANPAP)," *Circulation*, vol. 115, no. 25, pp. 3173–3180, 2007.

[47] S. Javaheri, T. J. Parker, L. Wexler, J. D. Liming, P. Lindower, and G. A. Roselle, "Effect of theophylline on sleep-disordered breathing in heart failure," *New England Journal of Medicine*, vol. 335, no. 8, pp. 562–567, 1996.

[48] R. Schulz, A. Blau, J. Börgel et al., "Sleep apnoea in heart failure," *European Respiratory Journal*, vol. 29, no. 6, pp. 1201–1205, 2007.

[49] H.-Q. Wang, G. Chen, J. Li et al., "Subjective sleepiness in heart failure patients with sleep-related breathing disorder," *Chinese Medical Journal*, vol. 122, no. 12, pp. 1375–1379, 2009.

[50] A. Rao, P. Georgiadou, D. P. Francis et al., "Sleep-disordered breathing in a general heart failure population: relationships to neurohumoral activation and subjective symptoms," *Journal of Sleep Research*, vol. 15, no. 1, pp. 81–88, 2006.

[51] F. Tremel, J.-L. Pépin, D. Veale et al., "High prevalence and persistence of sleep apnoea in patients referred for acute left ventricular failure and medically treated over 2 months," *European Heart Journal*, vol. 20, no. 16, pp. 1201–1209, 1999.

[52] M. Macdonald, J. Fang, S. D. Pittman, D. P. White, and A. Malhotra, "The current prevalence of sleep disordered breathing in congestive heart failure patients treated with beta-blockers," *Journal of Clinical Sleep Medicine*, vol. 4, no. 1, pp. 38–42, 2008.

[53] A. D. Staniforth, W. J. M. Kinnear, R. Starling, and A. J. Cowley, "Nocturnal desaturation in patients with stable heart failure," *Heart*, vol. 79, no. 4, pp. 394–399, 1998.

[54] H.-X. Liu, P. Huang, Y.-C. Chen et al., "Relationship between chronic congestive heart failure and sleep-disordered breathing in elderly patients," *Journal of Southern Medical University*, vol. 26, no. 6, pp. 847–848, 2006.

[55] K. I. Hume, F. Van, and A. Watson, "A field study of age and gender differences in habitual adult sleep," *Journal of Sleep Research*, vol. 7, no. 2, pp. 85–94, 1998.

[56] S. Javaheri, E. B. Caref, E. Chen, K. B. Tong, and W. T. Abraham, "Sleep apnea testing and outcomes in a large cohort of medicare beneficiaries with newly diagnosed heart failure," *American Journal of Respiratory and Critical Care Medicine*, vol. 183, no. 4, pp. 539–546, 2011.

[57] E. Shahar, C. W. Whitney, S. Redline et al., "Sleep-disordered breathing and cardiovascular disease: cross-sectional results of the sleep heart health study," *American Journal of Respiratory and Critical Care Medicine*, vol. 163, no. 1, pp. 19–25, 2001.

32

Clinically Diagnosed Insomnia and Risk of All-Cause and Diagnosis-Specific Disability Pension: A Nationwide Cohort Study

Catarina Jansson,[1] **Kristina Alexanderson,**[1] **Göran Kecklund,**[2] **and Torbjörn Åkerstedt**[1,2]

[1] *Division of Insurance Medicine, Department of Clinical Neuroscience, Karolinska Institutet, Berzelius väg 3, 6th Floor, 171 77 Stockholm, Sweden*
[2] *Stress Research Institute, Stockholm University, 106 91 Stockholm, Sweden*

Correspondence should be addressed to Catarina Jansson; catarina.jansson@ki.se

Academic Editor: Michael J. Thorpy

Background. Insomnia and disability pension are major health problems, but few population-based studies have examined the association between insomnia and risk of disability pension. *Methods.* We conducted a prospective nationwide cohort study based on Swedish population-based registers including all 5,028,922 individuals living in Sweden on December 31, 2004/2005, aged 17–64 years, and not on disability or old age pension. Those having at least one admission/specialist visit with a diagnosis of disorders of initiating and maintaining sleep (insomnias) (ICD-10: G47.0) during 2000/2001–2005 were compared to those with no such inpatient/outpatient care. All-cause and diagnosis-specific incident disability pension were followed from 2006 to 2010. Incidence rate ratios (IRRs) and 95% confidence intervals (CIs) were estimated by Cox regression. *Results.* In models adjusted for prior sickness absence, sociodemographic factors, and inpatient/specialized outpatient care, associations between insomnia and increased risks of all-cause disability pension (IRR 1.35, 95% CI 1.09–1.67) and disability pension due to mental diagnoses (IRR 1.86, 95% CI 1.38–2.50) were observed. After further adjustment for insomnia medications these associations disappeared. No associations between insomnia and risk of disability pension due to cancer, circulatory, or musculoskeletal diagnoses were observed. *Conclusion.* Insomnia seems to be positively associated with all-cause disability pension and disability pension due to mental diagnoses.

1. Introduction

Insomnia is defined as complaint of or difficulty initiating or maintaining sleep or experiencing nonrestorative sleep that impairs daily social, occupational, or other functioning [1, 2]. Insomnia is a large and increasing health problem worldwide [3–5], associated with substantial costs for individuals, employers, and society [3]. The prevalence of insomnia in the adult population ranges from 4 to 50%, while fewer, that is, about 6–15%, are diagnosed with insomnia [1, 2, 4, 6]. The etiology of sleep disorders such as insomnia is multifactorial [7] and studies have shown that such disorders are associated with older age, female sex, low socioeconomic status (SES), and work-related stress [2, 3, 7, 8]. Moreover,

insomnia has been suggested to adversely influence quality of life [1], work capacity [9], and endocrinology, immunology, and metabolism [10]. Thus, insomnia is associated with a wide range of health problems and diseases such as hypertension, inflammation, obesity, cardiovascular disease, cognitive and intellectual impairment, and mental disorders, predominantly depression and anxiety [1, 4, 11].

Disability pension is another major health problem, entailing severe social, economic, and health-related consequences for individuals and a considerable economic burden for society [12–14]. About 8% of the Swedish population aged 16–64 years were on disability pension in March 2010 of which disability pensions due to musculoskeletal and mental diagnoses were the most common [14]. Known risk factors for all-cause disability pension include high age, female sex, low SES, being unmarried, living in smaller places, adverse psychosocial and physical working conditions, poor self-rated health, chronic disease, obesity, smoking, and factors measured in late adolescence [14–17]. Moreover, disability pension is generally preceded by sickness absence [12], but the majority of those who are sickness absent are not granted disability pensions.

Despite adverse economic and health-related consequences of both insomnia and disability pension, few studies have focused on the influence of insomnia on early exit from the labor market [6, 9]. However, an association between insomnia and disability pension might be expected [9], potentially mediated by reduced work capacity, poor self-rated health [18], or other diseases [4]. Some prior cohort studies have examined sleep problems/insomnia and risk of disability pension [1, 6, 19, 20]. Existing evidence is, however, inconclusive [6] due to different definitions of outcomes, data sources, social security settings, and response rates [21]. Moreover, most previous studies are based on smaller and/or selected, that is, not population-based, samples, including only self-reported, not clinically diagnosed, sleep problems or insomnia [1, 6, 19, 20, 22, 23]. Thus, the aim of the present study was to—for the first time—examine insomnia diagnosed in inpatient and specialized outpatient care and risk of incident disability pension using a nationwide population-based prospective cohort study including data regarding several potential confounders.

2. Methods

2.1. Study Design. This prospective cohort study consists of all 5,620,619 individuals who were registered as living in Sweden on December 31, 2004, and December 31, 2005, respectively, and on December 31, 2005, were 17–64 years old. By using the Personal Identity Number (a unique ten-digit number assigned to all Swedish residents) data from the following nationwide, population-based registers were linked: (1) *Longitudinal Integration Database for Health Insurance and Labor Market Studies* (LISA), held by Statistics Sweden, including data for cohort definition, potential confounders (i.e., sociodemographic factors), old age pension, and follow-up regarding migration; (2) *Micro Data for Analysis of the Social Insurance database* (MiDAS), held by the Swedish Social Insurance Agency, including outcome data regarding all-cause and diagnosis-specific disability pension and data regarding old age pension; (3) the *National Patient Register* (PAR); (4) the *Swedish Prescribed Drug Register*; and (5) the *Causes of Death Register*, all held by the National Board of Health and Welfare, including exposure data (i.e., insomnia), potential confounders (i.e., inpatient/specialized outpatient care and medications), and mortality data, respectively. The study was approved by the Regional Ethical Review Board in Stockholm, Sweden.

2.2. Insomnia. Exposure data was based on inpatient and specialized outpatient care (PAR data) where inpatient/outpatient diagnoses are classified according to *The International Statistical Classification of Diseases and Related Health* *Problems, Tenth Revision* (ICD-10). Insomnia was defined as having at least one admission/hospitalization or at least one specialist visit with a diagnosis of disorders of initiating and maintaining sleep (insomnias) (ICD-10, chapter VI: G47.0). Inpatient care was based on admissions during 2000–2005 and specialized outpatient care on visits during 2001–2005 (i.e., nationwide outpatient care data, not including primary care, available since 2001). We constructed five different exposure variables regarding insomnia in- and outpatient care with main and/or secondary diagnoses, studied separately and combined, dichotomized a priori into (i) no insomnia (G47.0) in-/outpatient care during 2000–2005/2001–2005 (unexposed/reference group) and (ii) at least one admission/specialist visit with insomnia (G47.0) during 2000–2005/2001–2005.

2.3. Incident Disability Pension. The Swedish social insurance system includes sickness benefits covering up to 80% of lost income when work capacity is reduced due to disease or injury among all adult residents with income from work or unemployment benefits. Disability pension may be granted when a disease or injury has led to permanent work incapacity, covering up to 64% of lost income. Old age pension is mostly granted at 65 years but may be granted earlier. To identify all incident disability pensions we used MiDAS, comprising all disability pensions granted among Swedish residents since 1993. Disability pensions were defined as incident disability pensions received during follow-up, 2006–2010. Disability pension diagnoses are classified according to ICD-10. We analyzed all-cause disability pension and diagnosis-specific disability pension due to common diagnostic groups regarding disability pension and/or common chronic diseases. Thus, the following main diagnoses were studied: (i) malignant and benign tumors (ICD-10, chapter II: C00-C97, D00-D48), (ii) mental and behavioral disorders (ICD-10, chapter V: F00-F99), (iii) diseases of the circulatory system (ICD-10, chapter IX: I00-I99), and (iv) diseases of the musculoskeletal system and connective tissue (ICD-10, chapter XIII: M00-M99).

2.4. Exclusions of Cohort Members. The cohort included 5,620,619 individuals. After excluding 30 individuals who were erroneously registered as alive in 2005, 28,131 individuals with early old age pension starting before or at January 1, 2005, and 563,536 individuals with ongoing or newly granted disability pension in 2005, respectively, 5,028,922 individuals were included in the statistical analyses.

2.5. Statistical Analyses. The cohort members were followed from January 1, 2006 to December 31, 2010, December 31 of the year the participant turned 65, date of emigration, date of death, or date of an incident disability pension, whichever came first. Incidence rate ratios (IRRs) and 95% confidence intervals (CIs) were estimated by Cox proportional hazards models [24], using time since entry into the cohort as underlying time scale and the PHREG procedure in SAS, release 9.2 (SAS Institute Inc. Cary, NC). Data were analyzed in crude and multivariable models. The following potential confounders, that is, known risk factors for insomnia and all-cause disability pension, respectively, were successively adjusted for: *prior sickness absence*, that is, sickness benefits (in three predefined categories: (i) no sickness benefits, (ii) 1–179 sick-leave days, and (iii) 180+ sick-leave days); *age* (in 10-year intervals, reference group "17–24 years"); *sex* (reference group "men"); *education* (in three categories, reference group "high educational level that is more than 12 years"); *region of residence* (in three categories, reference group "larger cities"); *summarized number of hospitalization days*, that is, inpatient data, and *summarized number of specialist visits*, that is, outpatient data (i.e., two variables in three categories: (i) 0 hospitalization days/visits (reference group), (ii) ≤median hospitalization days/visits, and (iv) >median hospitalization days/visits); and finally *medical treatment for diseases of the nervous system, that is, psycholeptics/insomnia medications*, that is, prescribed, dispensed, and purchased drugs classified according to the following Anatomical Therapeutic Chemical (ATC) codes: antipsychotics (N05A), anxiolytics (N05B), and hypnotics and sedatives (N05C) (dichotomized as (i) no purchased antipsychotics, anxiolytics, or hypnotics and sedatives and (ii) at least one purchase of prescribed antipsychotics, anxiolytics, or hypnotics and sedatives). Prior sickness absence was based on sickness benefits during 2003–2005, sociodemographic factors on registration on December 31, 2005, inpatient care on admissions during 2000–2005, specialized outpatient care on visits during 2001–2005, and insomnia medications on purchases during July–December 2005 (i.e., nationwide data available since July 2005). Summarized number of hospitalization days/visits was based on main ICD-10 diagnoses only and in- and outpatient diagnoses regarding normal delivery, singleton (ICD-10, 080); chapter XVI (perinatal conditions) and chapter XXI (factors of significance for health and for contacts with health care, except for e-codes) were not included. Stratified analyses by sex (as female sex is a risk factor for both insomnia and disability pension) and insomnia medications were also performed. Observations with missing data on any of the covariates included in the models were excluded from the analyses. The number of missing data was, however, few (Tables 1 and 2).

3. Results

3.1. Characteristics of Study Participants. The 5,028,922 study participants together contributed with almost 24 million person-years at risk of incident disability pension during follow-up, 2006–2010 (Table 2). Insomnia inpatient/specialized outpatient care, that is, the exposure, was rare, including in total only 632 exposed individuals (0.01%). The distributions across the adjusted factors for insomnia inpatient/outpatient care combined, including both secondary + main diagnoses (ICD-10 G47.0), are shown in Table 1. The all-cause disability pension incident rate (IR) was high within all categories of the factors adjusted for and highest in the age category 55–64 years (IR 13.96), among women (IR 7.22), among persons with low educational level (IR 9.32), among those living in smaller cities/rural areas (IR

7.05), among those with long-term prior sickness absence (IR 82.30), among those with hospitalization days (IR 19.20) and specialists visits (IR 13.86) above the median, respectively, and among those having at least one purchase of antipsychotics, anxiolytics, hypnotics, or sedatives (IR 36.10) (Table 1). The most common incident disability pension diagnoses during follow-up were mental and musculoskeletal diagnoses (data not shown).

3.2. All-Cause Disability Pension. In total, we observed 142,192 incident disability pensions during follow-up, 2006–2010, more among women (82,311, 58%) compared to men (59,881, 42%) (Table 1). Three- to sixfold increased risks of all-cause disability pension were observed among persons having insomnia inpatient or outpatient specialized care regarding all five exposure variables in the crude models (IRR 5.08, 95% CI 4.11–6.28 (insomnia in-/outpatient care combined, main/secondary G47.0 diagnosis)) (Table 2). There were no major differences regarding having insomnia as a main or secondary diagnosis. After successive adjustment for prior sickness absence, sociodemographic factors, and summarized inpatient/specialized outpatient care, the positive associations regarding insomnia inpatient care, secondary diagnosis and insomnia outpatient care, main diagnosis, were no longer significant, while insomnia inpatient care, main diagnosis, insomnia outpatient care, secondary diagnosis, and combined insomnia in-/outpatient care remained, although attenuated (IRR 1.35, 95% CI 1.09–1.67 (insomnia in-/outpatient care, main/secondary G47.0 diagnosis)). After further adjustment for insomnia medications, the positive associations regarding these exposures also became nonsignificant (Table 2). We also adjusted for hypnotics and sedatives separately (i.e., ATC code N05C; hypnotics and sedatives combined), but the influence on the associations was similar as when adjusting for antipsychotics, anxiolytics, hypnotics, and sedatives combined (data not shown). Both hypnotics and hypnotics and sedatives combined were strongly associated with increased risks of all-cause disability pension in the fully adjusted model (hypnotics: IRR 1.97, 95% CI 1.94–2.00, hypnotics and sedatives combined: IRR 2.19, 95% CI 2.16–2.22).

In the stratified analyses, a similarly increased risk of all-cause disability pension was observed among men having insomnia in-/outpatient care in the model adjusted for prior sickness absence, sociodemographic factors, and inpatient/specialized outpatient care (IRR 1.56, 95% CI 1.14–2.13), but this association became nonsignificant after additional adjustment for insomnia medications. Among women, a positive association between insomnia and risk of all-cause disability pension was observed in the model adjusted for prior sickness absence and sociodemographic factors (IRR 1.37, 95% CI 1.02–1.82) that became nonsignificant after further adjustment for in-/outpatient care and insomnia medications. Among the majority having no purchase of prescribed insomnia medications in 2005, there was a positive association between insomnia and risk of all-cause disability pension (IRR 1.51, 95% CI 1.08–2.13), while among the 225,076 individuals having at least one purchase of insomnia

TABLE 1: Number of participants, person-years, all incident disability pensions (DPs), and incidence rates (IRs) by the adjusted factors.

	No. of exposed (%) (insomnia)[b]	No. of participants (%)[a]	Person-years	No. of incident DPs	IR[c]
Age groups (year); Dec. 31, 2005					
17–24	53 (>0)	846,146 (17)	4,133,741	15,026	3.64
25–34	97 (>0)	1,100,539 (22)	5,359,645	12,757	2.38
35–44	138 (>0)	1,182,671 (23)	5,760,797	26,222	4.55
45–54	196 (>0)	1,012,125 (20)	4,889,723	37,901	7.75
55–64	148 (>0)	887,441 (18)	3,601,907	50,286	13.96
Sex; Dec. 31, 2005					
Male	321 (>0)	2,611,409 (52)	12,352,585	59,881	4.85
Female	311 (>0)	2,417,513 (48)	11,393,229	82,311	7.22
Education; Dec. 31, 2005[d]					
High educational level (more than 12 years)	226 (>0)	1,681,493 (33)	4,236,610	29,918	3.73
Medium educational level (10–12 years)	295 (>0)	2,379,667 (47)	11,313,525	68,007	6.01
Low educational level (0–9 years)	110 (>0)	919,722 (18)	8,010,680	39,464	9.32
Missing		48,040 (1)			
Region of residence; Dec. 31, 2005[e]					
Larger cities	257 (>0)	1,896,500 (38)	8,968,370	44,142	4.92
Medium sized cities	215 (>0)	1,806,371 (36)	8,537,511	54,047	6.33
Smaller cities/rural areas	160 (>0)	1,326,051 (26)	6,239,934	44,003	7.05
Prior sickness absence; 2003–2005					
No sickness benefits	319 (>0)	3,949,089 (79)	18,891,108	39,962	2.12
1–179 reimbursed sick-leave days	137 (>0)	833,572 (17)	3,943,005	27,193	6.90
180+ reimbursed sick-leave days	176 (>0)	246,261 (5)	911,700	75,037	82.30
Inpatient care; admission: 2000–2005					
0 hospitalization days	239 (>0)	3,897,245 (78)	18,549,913	75,199	4.05
≤median summarized hospitalization days	160 (>0)	613,853 (12)	2,886,232	22,649	7.85
>median summarized hospitalization days	233 (>0)	517,824 (10)	2,309,668	44,344	19.20
Outpatient care; 2001–2005					
0 specialist visits	15 (>0)	1,823,960 (36)	8,718,627	18,216	2.09
≤median summarized specialist visits	186 (>0)	1,836,577 (37)	8,759,807	37,182	4.24
>median summarized specialist visits	431 (>0)	1,368,385 (27)	6,267,380	86,794	13.86
Antipsychotics, anxiolytics, hypnotics, and sedatives combined[f]; July–Dec. 2005					
No prescribed medications	380 (>0)	4,801,705 (95)	22,792,763	107,788	4.73
At least one purchase of prescribed medications	252 (>0)	227,217 (5)	953,051	34,404	36.10
Total (missing excluded)	567	5,028,922 *(4,980,882)*			

[a]Observations with missing data on any characteristic included in the study were excluded from the estimation of person-years, number of incident DPs and IRs.

[b]Insomnia in-/outpatient care (ICD-10: G47.0, main/secondary diagnosis).

[c]IRs per 100,000 person-years for all-cause DP; follow-up, 2006–2010.

[d]Statistics Sweden derives the attained "highest education" based on information regarding education according to the Swedish Standard Classification of Education. We classified SES based on education into three commonly used categories.

[e]"Region of residence" is based on "H-regions," that is, homogenous regions regarding the population base, a categorization by Statistics Sweden based on municipalities according to the local and regional population bases following the scale urban-rural. We categorized these regions into three categories.

[f]The Swedish Prescribed Drug Register contains data on drugs (ATC codes) but lacks information on indication of treatment, which prohibits identification of specific disease groups and it is not possible to link drugs bought over-the-counter to individual persons.

medication, no association between insomnia and risk of all-cause disability pension was observed (Table 3).

3.3. Disability Pension due to Mental Diagnoses. In total, 55,811 incident disability pensions due to mental diagnoses were observed during follow-up, although only 43 among the exposed. A positive association between insomnia and risk of disability pension due to mental diagnoses was observed after adjustment for prior sickness absence, sociodemographic factors, and in-/outpatient care (IRR 1.86, 95% CI 1.38–2.50 (insomnia in-/outpatient care combined, main/secondary G47.0 diagnosis)), but after further adjustment for insomnia medications this association became nonsignificant (data not shown).

TABLE 2: Total cohort. Insomnia and risk of all-cause incident disability pension (DP), Swedish nationwide cohort study; follow-up, 2006–2010[a].

In-/outpatient care with diagnoses of disorders of initiating and maintaining sleep (ICD-10: G 47.0)	No. of participants (%)	Person-years	No. of DPs	Crude IRR (95% CI)	Adjusted IRR (95% CI)[b]	Adjusted IRR (95% CI)[c]	Adjusted IRR (95% CI)[d]	Adjusted IRR (95% CI)[e]
Insomnia inpatient care (G47.0 main diagnosis)								
0 admissions/hospitalization due to insomnia, 2000–2005 (unexposed)	4,980,748 (100.00)	23,560,231	137,370	1.00 (reference)	1.00 (reference)	1.00 (reference)	1.00 (reference)	1.00 (reference)
At least one admission due to insomnia, 2000–2005	134 (0.00)	584	19	5.29 (3.38–8.30)	1.34 (0.86–2.10)	1.30 (0.83–2.04)	1.20 (1.18–1.21)	0.79 (0.50–1.23)
Insomnia inpatient care (G47.0 secondary diagnosis)								
0 admissions/hospitalization due to insomnia, 2000–2005 (unexposed)	4,980,799 (100.00)	23,560,431	137,382	1.00 (reference)	1.00 (reference)	1.00 (reference)	1.00 (reference)	1.00 (reference)
At least one admission due to insomnia, 2000–2005	83 (0.00)	384	7	3.10 (1.49–6.45)	0.94 (0.45–1.97)	1.18 (0.56–2.47)	0.98 (0.47–2.05)	0.70 (0.33–1.47)
Insomnia outpatient care (G47.0 main diagnosis)								
0 specialist visits due to insomnia, 2001–2005 (unexposed)	4,980,552 (99.99)	23,559,370	137,348	1.00 (reference)	1.00 (reference)	1.00 (reference)	1.00 (reference)	1.00 (reference)
At least one specialist visit due to insomnia, 2001–2005	330 (0.01)	1,445	41	4.70 (3.47–6.37)	1.30 (0.96–1.76)	1.33 (0.98–1.80)	1.17 (0.86–1.58)	0.83 (0.61–1.12)
Insomnia outpatient care (G47.0 secondary diagnosis)								
0 specialist visits due to insomnia, 2001–2005 (unexposed)	4,980,743 (100.00)	23,560,223	137,367	1.00 (reference)	1.00 (reference)	1.00 (reference)	1.00 (reference)	1.00 (reference)
At least one specialist visit due to insomnia, 2001–2005	139 (0.00)	591	22	6.14 (4.05–9.31)	1.89 (1.24–2.87)	2.22 (1.46–3.36)	1.97 (1.30–2.99)	1.50 (0.99–2.27)
Insomnia in-/outpatient care (G47.0 main/secondary diagnosis)								
0 admissions/visits due to insomnia, 2000/2001–2005 (unexposed)	4,980,251 (99.99)	23,558,071	137,304	1.00 (reference)	1.00 (reference)	1.00 (reference)	1.00 (reference)	1.00 (reference)
At least one admission/visit due to insomnia, 2000/2001–2005	631 (0.01)	2,744	85	5.08 (4.11–6.28)	1.47 (1.19–1.82)	1.52 (1.23–1.88)	1.35 (1.09–1.67)	0.96 (0.78–1.19)
Total	4,980,882	23,560,815	137,389					

[a]The numbers of participants, person-years, and incident DPs are from the adjusted models where missing observations were excluded. In the crude models the number of missing observations = 0. The small number of missing observations for education, family situation, and country of birth is shown in Table 1.
[b]IRRs adjusted for prior sickness absence.
[c]IRRs adjusted for prior sickness absence, age, sex, education, and region of residence.
[d]IRRs adjusted for prior sickness absence, age, sex, education, region of residence, inpatient care, and specialized outpatient care.
[e]IRRs adjusted for prior sickness absence, age, sex, education, region of residence, inpatient care, specialized outpatient care, and medications (i.e., antipsychotics, anxiolytics, hypnotics, and sedatives).

TABLE 3: Stratified analyses. Insomnia and risk of all-cause incident disability pension (DP), Swedish nationwide cohort study; follow-up, 2006–2010.

In-/outpatient care with diagnoses of initiating and maintaining sleep (ICD-10: G 47.0)	No. of participants (%)	Person-years	No. of DPs	Crude IRR (95% CI)	Adjusted IRR (95% CI)[a]	Adjusted IRR (95% CI)[b]	Adjusted IRR (95% CI)[c]	Adjusted IRR (95% CI)[d]
Subcohort: men								
Insomnia in-/outpatient care (G47.0 main/secondary diagnosis)								
0 admissions/visits due to insomnia, 2000/2001–2005 (unexposed)	2,585,422 (99.99)	12,254,479	57,137	1.00 (reference)	1.00 (reference)	1.00 (reference)	1.00 (reference)	1.00 (reference)
At least one admission/visit due to insomnia, 2000/2001–2005	320 (0.01)	1,428	39	5.59 (4.09–7.64)	1.52 (1.11–2.08)	1.77 (1.29–2.42)	1.56 (1.14–2.13)	1.08 (0.79–1.47)
Subcohort: women								
Insomnia in-/outpatient care (G47.0 main/secondary diagnosis)								
0 admissions/visits due to insomnia, 2000/2001–2005 (unexposed)	2,394,829 (99.99)	11,303,591	80,167	1.00 (reference)	1.00 (reference)	1.00 (reference)	1.00 (reference)	1.00 (reference)
At least one admission/visit due to insomnia, 2000/2001–2005	311 (0.01)	1,316	46	4.76 (3.57–6.35)	1.44 (1.08–1.92)	1.37 (1.02–1.82)	1.21 (0.91–1.62)	0.89 (0.67–1.19)
Subcohort: no insomnia medications								
Insomnia in-/outpatient care (G47.0 main/secondary diagnosis)								
0 admissions/visits due to insomnia, 2000/2001–2005 (unexposed)	4,755,427 (99.99)	22,613,214	103,607	1.00 (reference)	1.00 (reference)	1.00 (reference)	1.00 (reference)	
At least one admission/visit due to insomnia, 2000/2001–2005	379 (0.01)	1,723	33	4.10 (2.92–5.74)	1.61 (1.15–2.27)	1.65 (1.17–2.32)	1.51 (1.08–2.13)	
Subcohort: insomnia medications[e]								
Insomnia in-/outpatient care (G47.0 main/secondary diagnosis)								
0 admissions/visits due to insomnia, 2000/2001–2005 (unexposed)	224,824 (99.99)	944,857	33,697	1.00 (reference)	1.00 (reference)	1.00 (reference)	1.00 (reference)	
At least one admission/visit due to insomnia, 2000/2001–2005	252 (0.01)	1,022	52	1.40 (1.07–1.84)	0.88 (0.67–1.16)	0.91 (0.70–1.20)	0.84 (0.64–1.10)	

[a]IRRs adjusted for prior sickness absence.
[b]IRRs adjusted for prior sickness absence, age, sex (i.e., only in subcohorts for insomnia medications), education, and region of residence.
[c]IRRs adjusted for prior sickness absence, age, sex (i.e., only in subcohorts for insomnia medications), education, region of residence, inpatient care, and specialized outpatient care.
[d]IRRs adjusted for prior sickness absence, age, sex, education, region of residence, inpatient care, specialized outpatient care, and medications (i.e., antipsychotics, anxiolytics, hypnotics, and sedatives).
[e]At least one purchase of antipsychotics, anxiolytics, hypnotics, and sedatives; July–December 2005.

3.4. Disability Pension due to Musculoskeletal Diagnoses. In total, 39,941 incident disability pensions due to musculoskeletal diagnoses were observed, although only 12 among the exposed. A positive association between insomnia and risk of disability pension due to musculoskeletal diagnoses was observed in the crude model (IRR 6.14, 95% 4.05–9.31 (insomnia in-/outpatient care combined, main/secondary G47.0 diagnosis)), but after adjustment no association was observed (data not shown).

3.5. Disability Pension due to Cancer and Circulatory Diagnoses. In total, 4,630 disability pensions due to cancer diagnoses and 9,876 disability pensions due to circulatory diagnoses were observed. No associations between insomnia and risk of disability pension due to these diagnoses were observed (data not shown).

4. Discussion

To our knowledge, this is the first nationwide cohort study of insomnia and risk of disability pension. We observed associations between insomnia and increased risks of all-cause disability pension and disability pension due to mental diagnoses even after adjustment for prior sickness absence, sociodemographic factors, and summarized inpatient/specialized outpatient care in the total cohort and among men analyzed separately. The strongest association was observed regarding disability pension due to mental diagnoses. After adjustment for insomnia medications these associations became nonsignificant. No associations between insomnia and risk of disability pension due to cancer, circulatory, or musculoskeletal diagnoses were observed.

Hitherto, to our knowledge, there are only four previous cohort studies, performed in Norway and Finland and based on smaller or not population-based samples, of insomnia and risk of disability pension [1, 6, 19, 20, 22, 23]. In these studies, positive associations of similar strengths as in the present study between self-reported insomnia/sleep problems and risk of all-cause disability pension and disability pension due to mental diagnoses were observed, although none of these studies adjusted for prior sickness absence or insomnia medications. In contrast to our findings, positive associations between sleep problems and disability pension due to nervous, circulatory, and musculoskeletal diagnoses and injuries were observed in some prior studies [6, 19, 23], which might be due to clinically diagnosed insomnia being rare in our study or our more comprehensive adjustment for potential confounders. That the positive associations became nonsignificant after adjustment for insomnia medications may be due to insomnia being secondary to, for example, depression or other disorders. Another potential explanation is limited power as there were few individuals with a clinical diagnosis of insomnia and/or that those with self-reported insomnia symptoms may have been included in the reference group. Although a low prevalence of insomnia inpatient/specialized outpatient care was expected, the observed figures are extremely low and may suggest presence of underdiagnosis. Thus, for insomnia outpatient care,

secondary diagnosis, the point estimate was increased also after adjustment for insomnia medications. In addition, the adjustment for insomnia medications might partly adjust for those treated for insomnia or a mental disorder in primary care as well as inpatient/specialized outpatient care. Hypnotic drugs are among the most widely used treatments in adult medicine, although the indication may not be sleep-related since physicians often use another diagnosis if they believe that insomnia is secondary to other conditions [25] and a cross-sectional association between self-reported sleep disorders and register-based hypnotics (ATC code N05C) has been observed [26]. In the present study, insomnia medications were strongly associated with an increased risk of disability pension. Thus, potential overadjustment due to collinearity between clinically diagnosed insomnia and insomnia medications may have been introduced in our study by the adjustment for hypnotics. In addition, the present study is the first to adjust for prior sickness absence.

In contrast, even after adjustment for inpatient and specialized outpatient care (including, e.g., ICD-10, chapter V; mental and behavioral disorders), we observed a strong positive association between insomnia and risk of disability pension due to mental diagnoses. One potential explanation is that mental disorders might be in the causal pathway/mediators between insomnia and disability pension or that insomnia is an early symptom of a mental disorder which may be the underlying cause of both insomnia and disability pension [10, 26].

Among men, we found a positive association between insomnia and risk of all-cause disability pension after adjustment for prior sickness absence, sociodemographic factors, and in-/outpatient care, potentially explained by some risk factors for disability pension being more common among men with insomnia. That no association between insomnia and risk of disability pension was found among those with at least one purchase of insomnia medications might be due to limited power as the point estimates were increased or that disability pension was more common in the reference group.

An important strength of this study is the population-based nationwide prospective study design, including the whole Swedish population aged 17–64 years, entailing high statistical power and avoiding selection bias. The availability of objectively measured register data regarding clinically diagnosed insomnia, incident disability pension, and covariates with no or very few missing and the possibility to adjust for several potential confounders are other major strengths. The need to adjust for physical and mental disorders when studying consequences of poor sleep has been stressed [20]. The follow-up and detection of incident disability pensions are complete due to the high quality and nationwide coverage of the Swedish population-based registers used [27–29]. Limitations include potential underestimation of the exposure as insomnia inpatient and specialized outpatient care is rare in Sweden because insomnia symptoms often are untreated or treated in primary care. Studies have shown that mild and even severe insomniacs do not always seek help for treatment [2, 3]. This may have resulted in limited statistical power to ascertain weak associations or attenuated the associations observed. Moreover, many individuals with self-reported insomnia symptoms were probably included in our reference, that is, "unexposed," group, although our exposure definition may have identified patients with the most severe insomnia as insomnia diagnoses are adequately and thoughtfully made by the treating physician. Another potential limitation is that data regarding potential confounders such as adverse life style factors and work-related stress were not included in the nationwide registers, although some of these factors are associated with low SES and should partly be adjusted for by our adjustment for SES based on education.

Early exit from work is a serious challenge for workplaces, employees, and social security and it has been stressed that sleep problems warrant attention in occupational health to prevent reduced work capacity, disability pension, and morbidity [6, 30]. If insomnia symptoms are detected early it may help prevent early exit from work and provide tools for supporting employees continuing their work careers until normal retirement age [6].

5. Conclusions

This population-based nationwide cohort study demonstrates increased risks of all-cause disability pension and disability pension due to mental diagnoses among individuals with clinically diagnosed insomnia after adjustment for prior sickness absence, several sociodemographic factors, and inpatient/specialized outpatient care, although these associations disappeared after adjustment for insomnia medications. Thus, early detection of insomnia symptoms may prevent disability pension.

Conflict of Interests

The authors declare that they have no conflict of interests.

Acknowledgment

This study was funded by the Swedish Council for Working Life and Social Research (Grant no. 2009-1758 (Stockholm Stress Center) and Grant no. 2007-1762). The funder had no role in the study design, data collection, statistical analyses, interpretation of data, writing of the paper, or the decision to submit the paper for publication.

References

[1] B. Sivertsen, S. Overland, D. Neckelmann et al., "The long-term effect of insomnia on work disability: the HUNT-2 historical cohort study," *American Journal of Epidemiology*, vol. 163, no. 11, pp. 1018–1024, 2006.

[2] A. G. Wade, "The societal costs of insomnia," *Neuropsychiatric Disease and Treatment*, vol. 7, no. 1, pp. 1–18, 2011.

[3] D. Léger and V. Bayon, "Societal costs of insomnia," *Sleep Medicine Reviews*, vol. 14, no. 6, pp. 379–389, 2010.

[4] J. E. Ferrie, M. Kumari, P. Salo, A. Singh-Manoux, and M. Kivimäki, "Sleep epidemiology-A rapidly growing field," *International Journal of Epidemiology*, vol. 40, no. 6, Article ID dyr203, pp. 1431–1437, 2011.

[5] S. Stranges, W. Tigbe, F. X. Gómez-Olivé, M. Thorogood, and N. B. Kandala, "Sleep problems: an emerging global epidemic? Findings from the INDEPTH WHO-SAGE study among more than 40,000 older adults from 8 countries across Africa and Asia," *Sleep*, vol. 35, no. 8, pp. 1173–1181, 2012.

[6] T. Lallukka, P. Haaramo, E. Lahelma, and O. Rahkonen, "Sleep problems and disability retirement: a register-based follow-up study," *American Journal of Epidemiology*, vol. 173, no. 8, pp. 871–881, 2011.

[7] P. C. Zee and F. W. Turek, "Sleep and health: everywhere and in both directions," *Archives of Internal Medicine*, vol. 166, no. 16, pp. 1686–1688, 2006.

[8] T. Åkerstedt, "Psychosocial stress and impaired sleep," *Scandinavian Journal of Work, Environment and Health*, vol. 32, no. 6, pp. 493–501, 2006.

[9] E. R. Kucharczyk, K. Morgan, and A. P. Hall, "The occupational impact of sleep quality and insomnia symptoms," *Sleep Medicine Reviews*, vol. 16, no. 6, pp. 547–559, 2012.

[10] H. Westerlund, K. Alexanderson, T. Åkerstedt, L. M. Hanson, T. Theorell, and M. Kivimäki, "Work-related sleep disturbances and sickness absence in the Swedish working population, 1993–1999," *Sleep*, vol. 31, no. 8, pp. 1169–1177, 2008.

[11] T. Akerstedt, G. Kecklund, L. Alfredsson, and J. Selen, "Predicting long-term sickness absence from sleep and fatigue," *Journal of Sleep Research*, vol. 16, no. 4, pp. 341–345, 2007.

[12] K. Alexanderson, M. Kivimäki, J. E. Ferrie et al., "Diagnosis-specific sick leave as a long-term predictor of disability pension: a 13-year follow-up of the GAZEL cohort study," *Journal of Epidemiology and Community Health*, vol. 66, no. 2, pp. 155–159, 2012.

[13] J. Narusyte, A. Ropponen, K. Silventoinen et al., "Genetic liability to disability pension in women and men: a prospective population-based twin study," *PLoS ONE*, vol. 6, no. 8, Article ID e23143, 2011.

[14] E. Johansson, O. Leijon, D. Falkstedt, A. Farah, and T. Hemmingsson, "Educational differences in disability pension among Swedish middle-aged men: role of factors in late adolescence and work characteristics in adulthood," *Journal of Epidemiology and Community Health*, vol. 66, no. 10, pp. 901–907, 2012.

[15] S. Reinholdt, M. Upmark, and K. Alexanderson, "Health-selection mechanisms in the pathway towards a disability pension," *Work*, vol. 37, no. 1, pp. 41–51, 2010.

[16] A. Ropponen, J. Narusyte, K. Alexanderson, and P. Svedberg, "Stability and change in health behaviours as predictors for disability pension: a prospective cohort study of Swedish twins," *BMC Public Health*, vol. 11, p. 678, 2011.

[17] A. Samuelsson, K. Alexanderson, A. Ropponen, P. Lichtenstein, and P. Svedberg, "Incidence of disability pension and associations with socio-demographic factors in a Swedish twin cohort," *Social Psychiatry and Psychiatric Epidemiology*, vol. 47, no. 12, pp. 1999–2009, 2012.

[18] A. Steptoe, V. Peacey, and J. Wardle, "Sleep duration and health in young adults," *Archives of Internal Medicine*, vol. 166, no. 16, pp. 1689–1692, 2006.

[19] P. Salo, T. Oksanen, B. Sivertsen et al., "Sleep disturbances as a predictor of cause-specific work disability and delayed return to work," *Sleep*, vol. 33, no. 10, pp. 1323–1331, 2010.

[20] B. Sivertsen, S. Øverland, S. Pallesen et al., "Insomnia and long sleep duration are risk factors for later work disability. the Hordaland Health Study," *Journal of Sleep Research*, vol. 18, no. 1, pp. 122–128, 2009.

[21] U. Bültmann, M. B. Nielsen, I. E. Madsen, H. Burr, and R. Rugulies, "Sleep disturbances and fatigue: independent predictors of sickness absence? A prospective study among 6538 employees," *European Journal of Public Health*, vol. 23, no. 1, pp. 123–128, 2012.

[22] S. Overland, N. Glozier, B. Sivertsen et al., "A comparison of insomnia and depression as predictors of disability pension: the HUNT study," *Sleep*, vol. 31, no. 6, pp. 875–880, 2008.

[23] P. Haaramo, O. Rahkonen, E. Lahelma, and T. Lallukka, "The joint association of sleep duration and insomnia symptoms with disability retirement—a longitudinal, register-linked study," *Scandinavian Journal of Work, Environment & Health*, vol. 38, no. 5, pp. 427–435, 2012.

[24] N. E. Breslow and N. E. Day, "Statistical methods in cancer research. Volume II—the design and analysis of cohort studies," *IARC Scientific Publications*, no. 82, pp. 1–406, 1987.

[25] D. F. Kripke, R. D. Langer, and L. E. Kline, "Hypnotics' association with mortality or cancer: a matched cohort study," *BMJ Open*, vol. 2, no. 1, Article ID e000850, 2012.

[26] P. Salo, J. Vahtera, M. Hall et al., "Using repeated measures of sleep disturbances to predict future diagnosis-specific work disability: a cohort study," *Sleep*, vol. 35, no. 4, pp. 559–569, 2012.

[27] Causes of Death 2009, "The National Board of Health and Welfare," 2011.

[28] J. F. Ludvigsson, E. Andersson, A. Ekbom et al., "External review and validation of the Swedish national inpatient register," *BMC Public Health*, vol. 11, p. 450, 2011.

[29] B. Wettermark, N. Hammar, C. M. Fored et al., "The new Swedish Prescribed Drug Register Opportunities for pharmacoepidemiological research and experience from the first six months," *Pharmacoepidemiology and Drug Safety*, vol. 16, no. 7, pp. 726–735, 2007.

[30] B. Floderus, S. Göransson, K. Alexanderson, and G. Aronsson, "Self-estimated life situation in patients on long-term sick leave," *Journal of Rehabilitation Medicine*, vol. 37, no. 5, pp. 291–299, 2005.

Permissions

All chapters in this book were first published in SD, by Hindawi Publishing Corporation; hereby published with permission under the Creative Commons Attribution License or equivalent. Every chapter published in this book has been scrutinized by our experts. Their significance has been extensively debated. The topics covered herein carry significant findings which will fuel the growth of the discipline. They may even be implemented as practical applications or may be referred to as a beginning point for another development.

The contributors of this book come from diverse backgrounds, making this book a truly international effort. This book will bring forth new frontiers with its revolutionizing research information and detailed analysis of the nascent developments around the world.

We would like to thank all the contributing authors for lending their expertise to make the book truly unique. They have played a crucial role in the development of this book. Without their invaluable contributions this book wouldn't have been possible. They have made vital efforts to compile up to date information on the varied aspects of this subject to make this book a valuable addition to the collection of many professionals and students.

This book was conceptualized with the vision of imparting up-to-date information and advanced data in this field. To ensure the same, a matchless editorial board was set up. Every individual on the board went through rigorous rounds of assessment to prove their worth. After which they invested a large part of their time researching and compiling the most relevant data for our readers.

The editorial board has been involved in producing this book since its inception. They have spent rigorous hours researching and exploring the diverse topics which have resulted in the successful publishing of this book. They have passed on their knowledge of decades through this book. To expedite this challenging task, the publisher supported the team at every step. A small team of assistant editors was also appointed to further simplify the editing procedure and attain best results for the readers.

Apart from the editorial board, the designing team has also invested a significant amount of their time in understanding the subject and creating the most relevant covers. They scrutinized every image to scout for the most suitable representation of the subject and create an appropriate cover for the book.

The publishing team has been an ardent support to the editorial, designing and production team. Their endless efforts to recruit the best for this project, has resulted in the accomplishment of this book. They are a veteran in the field of academics and their pool of knowledge is as vast as their experience in printing. Their expertise and guidance has proved useful at every step. Their uncompromising quality standards have made this book an exceptional effort. Their encouragement from time to time has been an inspiration for everyone.

The publisher and the editorial board hope that this book will prove to be a valuable piece of knowledge for researchers, students, practitioners and scholars across the globe.

List of Contributors

Constance H. Fung
Geriatric Research Education and Clinical Center (GRECC), Veterans Administration Greater Los Angeles Healthcare System, North Hills, CA 91343, USA
David Geffen School of Medicine, University of California, Los Angeles, CA 90095, USA

Stella Jouldjian
Geriatric Research Education and Clinical Center (GRECC), Veterans Administration Greater Los Angeles Healthcare System, North Hills, CA 91343, USA

Lara Kierlin
Oregon Sleep Associates, Portland, OR 97210, USA

Kazuya Fujihara, Satoru Kodama, Chika Horikawa, Sakiko Yoshizawa, Ayumi Sugawara and Reiko Hirasawa
Department of Internal Medicine, Faculty of Medicine, Tsukuba University, Japan
Department of Internal Medicine, Faculty of Medicine, Niigata University, 1-754 Asahimachi, Niigata, Niigata 951-8510, Japan

Hitoshi Shimano
Department of Internal Medicine, Faculty of Medicine, Tsukuba University, Japan

Yoko Yachi, Akiko Suzuki, Osamu Hanyu and Hirohito Sone
Department of Internal Medicine, Faculty of Medicine, Niigata University, 1-754 Asahimachi, Niigata, Niigata 951-8510, Japan

Cary A. Brown
Department of Occupational Therapy, University of Alberta, 2-64 Corbett Hall, Edmonton, AB, Canada T6G 2G4

Patricia Wielandt
Occupational Therapy, Central Queensland University, Building 6, Bruce Highway, Rockhampton, QLD 4702, Australia

Donna Wilson
Faculty of Nursing, Edmonton Clinic Health Academy, University of Alberta, 87 Avenue, Edmonton, AB, Canada T6G 1C9

Allyson Jones and Katelyn Crick
Department of Physical Therapy, University of Alberta, 3-44C Corbett Hall, Edmonton, AB, Canada T6G 2G4

Esther Yuet Ying Lau
Sleep Laboratory, Department of Psychology, 6/F Jockey Club Tower, The University of Hong Kong, Pokfulam Road, Hong Kong

Gail A. Eskes
Department of Psychiatry, Dalhousie University, Halifax, NS, Canada
Department of Psychology, Dalhousie University, Halifax, NS, Canada
Department of Medicine, Dalhousie University, Halifax, NS, Canada

Debra L. Morrison
Department of Medicine, Dalhousie University, Halifax, NS, Canada
Sleep Clinic and Laboratory, Queen Elizabeth II Health Sciences Centre, Halifax, NS, Canada

Malgorzata Rajda
Department of Psychiatry, Dalhousie University, Halifax, NS, Canada
Sleep Clinic and Laboratory, Queen Elizabeth II Health Sciences Centre, Halifax, NS, Canada

Kathleen F. Spurr
School of Health Sciences, Dalhousie University, Halifax, NS, Canada

Nicholas D. Taylor and Gary D. Fireman
Psychology Department, Suffolk University, 41 Temple Street, Boston, MA 02114, USA

Ross Levin
Independent Practice, 25 West 86th Street No. 3, New York, NY 10024, USA

Meredith Bessey and Jennifer Richards
Department of Psychology & Neuroscience, Dalhousie University, P.O. Box 15000, Halifax, NS, Canada B3H4R2

Penny Corkum
Department of Psychology & Neuroscience, Dalhousie University, P.O. Box 15000, Halifax, NS, Canada B3H4R2
IWK Health Centre, 5850 University Avenue, Halifax, NS, Canada B3K 6R8
Colchester East Hants ADHD Clinic, 600 Abenaki Road, Truro, NS, Canada B2N 5A1

Alon Reshef and Boaz Bloch
Psychiatric Department, Emek Medical Center, Afula, Israel
Technion — Israel Institute of Technology, Haifa, Israel

Limor Vadas
Psychiatric Department, Emek Medical Center, Afula, Israel
Department of Psychology and the Center for Psychobiological Research, Yezreel Academic College, Emek Yezreel 19300, Israel

Shai Ravid
Psychiatric Department, Emek Medical Center, Afula, Israel

Ilana Kremer
Technion—Israel Institute of Technology, Haifa, Israel
Mazra Mental Health Center, Akko, Israel

Iris Haimov
Department of Psychology and the Center for Psychobiological Research, Yezreel Academic College, Emek Yezreel 19300, Israel

Carl Stepnowsky
Health Services Research & Development Unit, Veterans Affairs San Diego Healthcare System, San Diego, CA 92161, USA
Department of Medicine, University of California, San Diego, CA 92037, USA

Tania Zamora
Health Services Research & Development Unit, Veterans Affairs San Diego Healthcare System, San Diego, CA 92161, USA

Robert Barker
Pulmonary Service, Veterans Affairs San Diego Healthcare System, San Diego, CA 92161, USA

Lin Liu
Department of Family and Preventive Medicine, University of California, San Diego, CA 92037, USA

Kathleen Sarmiento
Department of Medicine, University of California, San Diego, CA 92037, USA
Pulmonary Service, Veterans Affairs San Diego Healthcare System, San Diego, CA 92161, USA

N. Katz
Sleep Laboratory, Assuta Medical Services and Wolfson Hospital, 69710 Holon, Israel

Y. Adir
Pulmonary Unit, Carmel Hospital and Clalit Health Care, 34362 Haifa, Israel

T. Etzioni
Sleep Clinic, Clalit Health Care, 34362 Haifa, Israel
Sleep Laboratory, Rambam Health Care Campus, P.O. Box 9602, 31096 Haifa, Israel
Department of Pediatrics, Carmel Hospital and Faculty of Medicine, Technion-Israel Institute of Technology, 34362 Haifa, Israel

E. Kurtz
Sleep Clinic, Clalit Health Care, 34362 Haifa, Israel

G. Pillar
Sleep Laboratory, Rambam Health Care Campus, P.O. Box 9602, 31096 Haifa, Israel
Department of Pediatrics, Carmel Hospital and Faculty of Medicine, Technion-Israel Institute of Technology, 34362 Haifa, Israel

Annie Vallières
École de psychologie, Université Laval, Québec, QC, Canada G1V A06
Centre d'étude des troubles du sommeil, Centre de recherche de l'institut universitaire en santé mentale de Québec, Québec, QC, Canada G1J 2G3
Centre de recherche du centre hospitalier universitaire en santé mentale duQuébec, Québec, QC, Canada G1V 4G2

Tijana Ceklic and Célyne H. Bastie
École de psychologie, Université Laval, Québec, QC, Canada G1V A06
Centre d'étude des troubles du sommeil, Centre de recherche de l'institut universitaire en santé mentale de Québec, Québec, QC, Canada G1J 2G3

Colin A. Espie
Nuffield Department of Clinical Neurosciences, Sleep & Circadian Neuroscience Institute, University of Oxford, Oxford OX3 9DU, UK

Pei-Li Chien and Ruo-Yan Siao
Department of Preventive Medicine, Taiwan Adventist Hospital, No. 424, Section 2, Bade Road, Songshan District, Taipei 105, Taiwan

Hui-Fang Su and Pi-Ching Hsieh
Department of Health Care Management, National Taipei University of Nursing and Health Sciences, No. 89, Nei-Chiang Street, Wanhua District, Taipei 10845, Taiwan

Pei-Ying Ling
Department of Obstetrics and Gynecology, Taiwan Adventist Hospital, No. 424, Section 2, Bade Road, Songshan District, Taipei 105, Taiwan

Hei-Jen Jou
Department of Obstetrics and Gynecology, Taiwan Adventist Hospital, No. 424, Section 2, Bade Road, Songshan District, Taipei 105, Taiwan
Department of Obstetrics and Gynecology, National Taiwan University Hospital, No. 7, Zhongshan S. Road, Zhongzheng District, Taipei 100, Taiwan

M. Ataide and O. G. Lins
Pós-Graduação em Neuropsiquiatria e Ciências do Comportamento, Universidade Federal de Pernambuco, Recife, PE, Brazil

C. M. R. Franco
Hospital das Clinicas, Universidade Federal de Pernambuco, Recife, PE, Brazil

Juan Carlos Vélez, Clarita Barbosa, Asterio Andrade and Megan Frye
Centro de Rehabilitación Club de Leones Cruz del Sur, Punta Arenas, Suiza 01441, Chile

Aline Souza, Samantha Traslaviña, Adaeze Wosu, Bizu Gelaye and Michelle A. Williams
Department of Epidemiology, Multidisciplinary International Research Training Program, Harvard University School of Public Health, Boston, MA 02131, USA

Annette L. Fitzpatrick
Departments of Epidemiology and Global Health, University of Washington, Seattle, WA 98195, USA

Forugh Rafii and Fatemeh Oskouie
Center for Nursing Care Research and School of Nursing and Midwifery, Iran University of Medical Sciences, Rashid Yasemi Street, Valiasr Avenue, P.O. Box 19395-4798, Tehran 19964, Iran

Mahnaz Shoghi
School of Nursing and Midwifery, Iran University of Medical Sciences, Rashid Yasemi Street, Valiasr Avenue, P.O. Box 19395-4798, Tehran 19964, Iran

Anders Broström
Department of Nursing Science, School of Health Sciences, Jönköping University, 551 11 Jönköping, Sweden
Department of Clinical Neurophysiology, Linköping University Hospital, 581 85 Linköping, Sweden

Per Nilsen
Division of Health Care Analysis, Faculty of Health Sciences, Department of Health and Society, Linköping University, 581 83 Linköping, Sweden

Benjamin Gardner
Health Behaviour Research Centre, Department of Epidemiology and Public Health, University College London, London, WC1E 6BT, UK

Peter Johansson
Department of Cardiology, Linköping University Hospital, 581 85 Linköping, Sweden

Martin Ulander
Department of Clinical Neurophysiology, Linköping University Hospital, 581 85 Linköping, Sweden
Departement of Clinical and Experimental Medicine, Division of Clinical Neurophysiology, Faculty of Health Sciences, Linköping University, 581 83 Linköping, Sweden

Bengt Fridlund
School of Health Sciences, Jönköping University, 551 11 Jönköping, Sweden

Kristofer Årestedt
Faculty of Health and Life Sciences, Linnaeus University, 391 82 Kalmar, Sweden
Department of Medicine and Health Sciences, Linköping University, 581 83 Linköping, Sweden
Palliative Research Centre, Ersta Sköndal University College and Ersta Hospital, 100 61 Stockholm, Sweden

Jo Spong and David J. Berlowitz
Institute for Breathing and Sleep, Austin Hospital, Heidelberg, VIC 3084, Australia

Gerard A. Kennedy
Institute for Breathing and Sleep, Austin Hospital, Heidelberg, VIC 3084, Australia
School of Social Sciences & Psychology, Victoria University, St. Albans, VIC 3021, Australia

Douglas J. Brown
Victorian Spinal Cord Service, Austin Hospital, Heidelberg, VIC 3084, Australia

Stuart M. Armstrong
Brain Sciences Institute, Swinburne University, Hawthorn, VIC 3122, Australia
The Bronowski Institute of Behavioural Neuroscience, Kyneton, VIC 3444, Australia

Cary A. Brown, Robyn Berry and Ashley Schmidt
Department of Occupational Therapy, Faculty of Rehabilitation Medicine, University of Alberta, 2-64 Corbett Hall, Edmonton, AB, Canada T6G 2G4

Maria-Lucia Muntean
Paracelsus Elena Klinik, Klinik Straße 16, 34128 Kassel, Germany
Department of Neurosciences, University of Medicine and Pharmacy, Victor Babes Straße 43, 400012 Cluj-Napoca, Romania

Friederike Sixel-Döring
Paracelsus Elena Klinik, Klinik Straße 16, 34128 Kassel, Germany

Claudia Trenkwalder
Paracelsus Elena Klinik, Klinik Straße 16, 34128 Kassel, Germany
Department of Neurosurgery, University of Göttingen, Robert Koch Straße 40, 37075 Göttingen, Germany

Geovanny F. Perez, Shehlanoor Huseni and Khrisna Pancham
Division of Pulmonary and Sleep Medicine, Children's National Medical Center, Washington, DC 20010, USA

Maria J. Gutierrez
Division of Pediatric Rheumatology, Allergy & Immunology, Pennsylvania State University College of Medicine, Hershey, PA 17033, USA

Carlos E. Rodriguez-Martinez
Department of Pediatrics, School of Medicine, Universidad Nacional de Colombia, Bogota, Colombia
Department of Pediatric Pulmonology and Pediatric Critical Care Medicine, School of Medicine, Universidad El Bosque, Bogota, Colombia
Research Unit, Military Hospital of Colombia, Bogota, Colombia

Cesar L. Nino
Department of Electronics Engineering, Javeriana University, Bogota, Colombia

Gustavo Nino
Division of Pulmonary and Sleep Medicine, Children's National Medical Center, Washington, DC 20010, USA
Department of Integrative Systems Biology and Center for Genetic Medicine Research, Children's National Medical Center, George Washington University, Washington, DC 20010, USA

Mihaela Teodorescu
James B. Skatrud Pulmonary/Sleep Research Laboratory, Medical Service, William S. Middleton Memorial Veterans Hospital, Madison, WI, USA
Section of Allergy, Pulmonary and Critical Care Medicine, USA
Center for Sleep Medicine and Sleep Research/Wisconsin Sleep, University of Wisconsin School of Medicine and Public Health, Madison, WI, USA

David A. Polomis
Section of Allergy, Pulmonary and Critical Care Medicine, USA
Ronald E. Gangnon
Department of Biostatistics and Medical Informatics and Population Health Sciences, University of Wisconsin School of Medicine and Public Health, Madison, WI, USA

Jessica E. Fedie
James B. Skatrud Pulmonary/Sleep Research Laboratory, Medical Service, William S. Middleton Memorial Veterans Hospital, Madison, WI, USA
Section of Allergy, Pulmonary and Critical Care Medicine, USA

Flavia B. Consens and Ronald D. Chervin
Department of Neurology and Sleep Disorders Center, University of Michigan Health System, Ann Arbor, MI, USA

Mihai C. Teodorescu
James B. Skatrud Pulmonary/Sleep Research Laboratory, Medical Service, William S. Middleton Memorial Veterans Hospital, Madison, WI, USA
Center for Sleep Medicine and Sleep Research/Wisconsin Sleep, University of Wisconsin School of Medicine and Public Health, Madison, WI, USA
Section of Geriatrics and Gerontology, University of Wisconsin School of Medicine and Public Health, Madison, WI, USA

Mehdi Zobeiri
Department of Internal Medicine, School of Medicine, Imam Reza Hospital, Kermanshah University of Medical Sciences, Kermanshah, Iran

Azita Shokoohi
Kermanshah University of Medical Sciences, Kermanshah, Iran

Lena Mallon and Jan-Erik Broman
Department of Neuroscience, Psychiatry, Uppsala University, SE-75185 Uppsala, Sweden

Torbjörn Åkerstedt
Stress Research Institute, Stockholm University, SE-10691 Stockholm, Sweden

Jerker Hetta
Department of Clinical Neuroscience, Psychiatry, Karolinska Institutet, SE-14186 Stockholm, Sweden

Amanda Hellström
School of Health Science, Blekinge Institute of Technology, 371 79 Karlskrona, Sweden
Department of Health Sciences, Lund University, 221 00 Lund, Sweden

Patrik Hellström
School of Health Science, Blekinge Institute of Technology, 371 79 Karlskrona, Sweden

Ania Willman
School of Health Science, Blekinge Institute of Technology, 371 79 Karlskrona, Sweden
Department of Care Science, Malmö University, 205 06 Malmö, Sweden

Cecilia Fagerström
School of Health Science, Blekinge Institute of Technology, 371 79 Karlskrona, Sweden
Blekinge Centre of Competence, 371 81 Karlskrona, Sweden

Joseph V. Pergolizzi Jr.
Department of Medicine, School of Medicine, Johns Hopkins University, Baltimore, MD 21205, USA
Department of Anesthesiology, Georgetown University School of Medicine, Washington, DC 20057, USA
Department of Pharmacology, School of Medicine in Philadelphia, Temple University, PA 19140, USA

Robert Taylor Jr.
NEMA Research, Inc., Naples, FL 34108, USA

Robert B. Raffa
School of Pharmacy, Temple University, Philadelphia, PA 19140, USA

Srinivas Nalamachu
Kansas University Medical Center, Kansas City, KS 66160, USA
International Clinical Research, Leawood, KS 66211, USA

Maninder Chopra
Kirax Pharmaceuticals, Bonita Springs, FL 34134, USA

Montserrat Diaz-Abad
Division of Pulmonary and Critical Care Medicine, Sleep Disorders Center, University of Maryland School of Medicine, 685West Baltimore Street, MSTF 800, Baltimore, MD 21201-1192, USA

Wissam Chatila, Irene Swift, Gilbert E. D'Alonzo and Samuel L. Krachman
Division of Pulmonary, Critical Care, and Sleep Medicine, Temple University School of Medicine, 3401 North Broad Street, Philadelphia, PA 19140, USA

Matthew R. Lammi
Section of Pulmonary and Critical Care Medicine, Louisiana State University Health Sciences Center, 433 Bolivar Street New Orleans, LA 70112, USA

Zohreh Yazdi and Mahnaz Abbasi
Metabolic Disease Research Center, Qazvin University of Medical Sciences, Qazvin 34139-8-3731, Iran

Khosro Sadeghniiat-Haghighi
Occupational Sleep Research Center, Tehran University of Medical Sciences, Tehran 5583-1-4155, Iran

Ziba Loukzadeh
Department of Occupational Medicine, Industrial Diseases Research Center, Shahid Sadoughi University of Medical Sciences, Yazd 89151-7-3143, Iran

Khadijeh Elmizadeh
Social Determinants of Health Research Center, Qazvin University of Medical Sciences, Qazvin, Qazvin 34139-8-3731, Iran

Gopal K. Singh and Mary Kay Kenney
US Department of Health and Human Services, Health Resources and Services Administration, Maternal and Child Health Bureau, 5600 Fishers Lane, Room 18-41, Rockville, MD 20857, USA

Ashish Patel
Maimonides Medical Center, Department of Orthopaedic Surgery, 927 49th Street, Brooklyn, NY 11219, USA
SUNY Downstate Medical Center, 450 Clarkson Avenue, Brooklyn, NY 11203, USA

Maya Deza Culbertson, Archit Patel, Jenifer Hashem, Jinny Jacob, David Edelstein and Jack Choueka
Maimonides Medical Center, Department of Orthopaedic Surgery, 927 49th Street, Brooklyn, NY 11219, USA

Subhajit Chakravorty
MIRECC VISN-4, Philadelphia Veterans Affairs Medical Center, University &Woodland Avenues, Philadelphia, PA 19104, USA
Perelman School of Medicine, University of Pennsylvania, Philadelphia, PA 19104, USA

Nicholas Jackson
University of Southern California, Los Angeles, CA 90033, USA

Ninad Chaudhary
Perelman School of Medicine, University of Pennsylvania, Philadelphia, PA 19104, USA
West Chester University of Pennsylvania, West Chester, PA 19383, USA

Philip J. Kozak
School of Veterinary Medicine, University of Pennsylvania, Philadelphia, PA 19104, USA

Michael L. Perlis and Michael A. Grandner
Perelman School of Medicine, University of Pennsylvania, Philadelphia, PA 19104, USA

Holly R. Shue
Children's Hospital of Philadelphia, Philadelphia, PA 19104, USA

Georgina Wilson, Zoe Terpening, Louisa Norrie, Simon J. G. Lewis and Sharon L. Naismith
Healthy Brain Ageing Clinic, Brain & Mind Research Institute, University of Sydney, 94 Mallett Street, Camperdown, NSW 2050, Australia

Keith Wong and Ron Grunstein
Woolcock Institute of Medical Research, University of Sydney, Glebe, NSW2050, Australia

Mohammad Mirzaaghazadeh, Fariba Mehdiniya and NasrollahMaleki
Department of Internal Medicine, Imam Khomeini Hospital, Ardabil University of Medical Sciences, Ardabil 6368134497, Iran

Mehrzad Bahtouee and Zahra Tavosi
Department of Internal Medicine, Shohadaye Khalije Fars Hospital, Bushehr University of Medical Sciences, Bushehr, Iran

Catarina Jansson and Kristina Alexanderson
Division of Insurance Medicine, Department of Clinical Neuroscience, Karolinska Institutet, Berzelius väg 3, 6th Floor, 171 77 Stockholm, Sweden

Göran Kecklund
Stress Research Institute, Stockholm University, 106 91 Stockholm, Sweden

Torbjörn Åkerstedt
Division of Insurance Medicine, Department of Clinical Neuroscience, Karolinska Institutet, Berzelius väg 3, 6th Floor, 171 77 Stockholm, Sweden
Stress Research Institute, Stockholm University, 106 91 Stockholm, Sweden